CLINICAL MANAGEMENT OF THE AIRWAY

James T. Roberts, M.D., M.A.

Assistant Professor of Anesthesiology
Harvard Medical School
Associate Anesthetist
Department of Anesthesia
Massachusetts General Hospital
Boston, Massachusetts

W.B. SAUNDERS COMPANY
A Division of Harcourt Brace & Company
Philadelphia   London   Toronto   Montreal   Sydney   Tokyo

W.B. SAUNDERS COMPANY
A Division of
Harcourt Brace & Company

The Curtis Center
Independence Square West
Philadelphia, Pennsylvania 19106

Library of Congress Cataloging-in-Publication Data

Clinical management of the airway /
[edited by] James T. Roberts.—1st ed.

p. cm.

ISBN 0–7216–3670–5

1. Lungs—Diseases, Obstructive.   I. Roberts, James T. (James
   Thomas). [DNLM: 1. Airway Obstruction—therapy.
   2. Airway Obstruction—diagnosis.   3. Intubation.
   WF 145 C6414 1994]

RC776.O3C53 1994

616.2–dc20

DNLM/DLC   93-12115

Clinical Management of the Airway   ISBN 0–7216–3670–5

Printed in the United States of America.

Last digit is the print number: 9   8   7   6   5   4   3   2   1

To my wife, Charlene,
whose persistent good nature in the face of 4:30 alarm clocks
never ceases to amaze me.
God bless you.

Contributors

Amr E. Abouleish, M.D.
Assistant Professor and Director, Pediatric Anesthesia, Department of Anesthesiology, University of Texas Medical Branch, Galveston, Texas

Paul H. Alfille, M.D.
Instructor, Harvard Medical School; Assistant in Anesthesia and Director, Thoracic Anesthesia, Department of Anesthesia, Massachusetts General Hospital, Boston, Massachusetts

Mark S. Allen, M.D.
Consultant in the Section of General Thoracic Surgery, Mayo Clinic; Assistant Professor of Surgery, Mayo Medical School, Rochester, Minnesota

Pamela Angle, M.D.
Resident in Anesthesia, Department of Anesthesia, Massachusetts General Hospital, Boston, Massachusetts

Louis P. Bucky, M.D.
Resident in Plastic and Reconstructive Surgery, Department of Surgery, Massachusetts General Hospital, Harvard Medical School, Boston, Massachusetts

William H. Campbell, M.D., M.B.A., F.R.C.P.(C.)
Clinical Fellow in Anesthesia, Harvard Medical School; Chief Resident, Department of Anesthesia, Massachusetts General Hospital, Boston, Massachusetts

George G. Collee, M.B.Ch.B., F.F.A.R.C.S.(Eng)
Consultant Anesthetist, The Royal Free Hospital, London, United Kingdom

Charles J. Coté, M.D.
Professor of Anesthesia, Northwestern University Medical School; Vice Chairman, Department of Anesthesia, Children's Memorial Hospital, Chicago, Illinois

Anne-Marie Cros, M.D.
Department of Anesthesiology, Centre Hospitalier Universitaire, Hôpital Pellegrin, Bordeaux, France

David J. Cullen, M.D., M.S.
Professor of Anesthesia, Harvard Medical School; Anesthetist, Department of Anesthesia, Massachusetts General Hospital, Boston, Massachusetts

Frederick J. Curlin IV, M.D.
Resident in Anesthesia, Massachusetts General Hospital, Boston, Massachusetts

Carl G. W. Dahlberg, M.D.
Associate Medical Director for Intensive Care Medicine, St. Luke's Episcopal Hospital; Clinical Assistant Professor, Baylor College of Medicine, Houston, Texas

Harold J. DeMonaco, M.S.
Director, Pharmacy Department, Massachusetts General Hospital, Boston, Massachusetts

William T. Denman, M.B.Ch.B., F.R.C.Anaes.
Instructor in Anesthesia, Harvard Medical School; Assistant in Anesthesia, Massachusetts General Hospital, Boston, Massachusetts

Stephen F. Dierdorf, M.D.
Professor of Anesthesia, Indiana University School of Medicine; Director, Anesthesia Section, Richard L. Roudebush Veterans Affairs Medical Center; Staff Anesthesiologist, Riley Children's Hospital, Indianapolis, Indiana

Roland D. Eavey, M.D., F.A.A.P., F.A.C.S.
Assistant Professor, Department of Otology and Laryngology, Harvard Medical School; Director, ENT Pediatric Services, Massachusetts Eye and Ear Infirmary, Boston, Massachusetts

Abdel R. El-Ganzouri, M.D.
Associate Professor of Anesthesiology, Rush-Presbyterian–St. Luke's Medical Center, Chicago, Illinois

Steven Elia, M.D., F.R.C.P.C.
Staff Physician, Internal Medicine, Toronto East General Hospital, University of Toronto, and North York Branson Hospital, Toronto, Ontario, Canada

Jeffrey J. Fredberg, M.D.
Professor of Bioengineering and Physiology, Harvard School of Public Health, Boston, Massachusetts

Max L. Goodman, M.D.
Associate Professor of Pathology, Harvard Medical School; Director, ENT Pathology, Massachusetts Eye and Ear Infirmary; Associate Pathologist, Massachusetts General Hospital, Boston, Massachusetts

Takahisa Goto, M.D.
Clinical Fellow in Anesthesia, Department of Anesthesia, Harvard Medical School; Fellow in Critical Care, Department of Anesthesia, Massachusetts General Hospital, Boston, Massachusetts

Alexander W. Gotta, M.D.
Professor of Clinical Anesthesiology, State University of New York Health Science Center at Brooklyn; Chief of Anesthesiology, King's County Hospital Center, Brooklyn, New York

Nishan G. Goudsouzian, M.D., M.S.
Associate Professor of Anesthesia, Harvard Medical School; Anesthetist, Massachusetts General Hospital, Boston, Massachusetts

Reginald E. Greene, M.D.
Associate Radiologist in Chief, Massachusetts General Hospital; Professor of Radiology, Harvard Medical School, Boston, Massachusetts; Chairman of Radiology at Health Care (Scotland)

Hermes C. Grillo, M.D.
Professor of Surgery, Harvard Medical School; Chief of General Thoracic Surgery, Massachusetts General Hospital, Boston, Massachusetts

Charles A. Hales, M.D.
Associate Professor of Medicine, Harvard Medical School; Associate Professor, Harvard/MIT Division of Health Sciences and Technology; Physician, and Associate Director, Pulmonary/Critical Care Unit, Massachusetts General Hospital, Boston, Massachusetts

Don G. Han, M.D.
Assistant Professor of Anesthesiology, Mount Sinai School of Medicine, New York, New York

Victor Hoffstein, Ph.D., M.D., F.R.C.P.(C.)
Professor of Medicine, University of Toronto; Head, Respiratory Division, St. Michael's Hospital, Toronto, Ontario, Canada

William E. Hurford, M.D.
Assistant Professor of Anesthesia, Harvard Medical School; Associate Anesthetist, Massachusetts General Hospital, Boston, Massachusetts

Calvin Johnson, M.D.
Assistant Professor, Anesthesia, Wayne State University; Chief of Anesthesia, Hutzel Hospital, Detroit, Michigan

Michael P. Joseph, M.D.
Assistant Professor of Laryngology and Otology, Harvard Medical School; Associate in Otolaryngology, Massachusetts Eye and Ear Infirmary, Boston, Massachusetts

Praveen Khilnani, M.D.
Director, Pediatric Intensive Care Unit, Henrico Doctors' Hospital and Johnston Willis Hospital, Richmond, Virginia

Michael C. Lawlor, D.O., M.S.
Assistant Professor, Anesthesiology, Wayne State University; Staff Anesthesiologist, Hutzel Hospital, Detroit, Michigan

Lawrence Mason, M.D.
Assistant Professor, Anesthesia, Wayne State University; Staff Anesthesiologist, Hutzel Hospital, Detroit, Michigan

Douglas J. Mathisen, M.D.
Associate Professor of Surgery, Harvard Medical School; Associate Visiting Surgeon, Massachusetts General Hospital, Boston, Massachusetts

Charles J. McCabe, M.D.
Assistant Professor of Surgery, Harvard Medical School; Associate Chief, Emergency Services, Massachusetts General Hospital, Boston, Massachusetts

Ashby C. Moncure, M.D.
Associate Clinical Professor of Surgery, Harvard Medical School; Visiting Surgeon, Massachusetts General Hospital, Boston, Massachusetts

William Panza, M.D.
Instructor in Anesthesia, Tufts University School of Medicine; Assistant Anesthetist, New England Medical Center, Boston, Massachusetts

Andrew Patterson, M.D.
Resident in Anesthesiology, Department of Anesthesia, Massachusetts General Hospital, Boston, Massachusetts

Ben Z. Pilch, M.D.
Assistant Professor of Pathology, Harvard Medical School; Associate Pathologist, Massachusetts General Hospital, and Assistant Pathologist in Otolaryngology, Massachusetts Eye and Ear Infirmary, Boston, Massachusetts

Richard Pino, M.D., Ph.D.
Resident in Anesthesia, Department of Anesthesia, Massachusetts General Hospital, Boston, Massachusetts

Allan P. Reed, M.D.
Associate Professor of Anesthesiology, Mount Sinai School of Medicine, New York, New York

James T. Roberts, M.D., M.A.
Assistant Professor of Anesthesiology, Harvard Medical School; Associate Anesthetist, Department of Anesthesia, Massachusetts General Hospital, Boston, Massachusetts

Norbert Rolf, M.D.
Research Fellow, Department of Anesthesia, Massachusetts General Hospital, Boston, Massachusetts; Resident in Anesthesiology, Universitaetskliniken Muenster, Klinik f. Anaesthesiologie und Operative Intensivmedizin, Muenster, Germany

Reid Rubsamen, M.D.
Clinical Instructor in Anesthesia, Stanford University School of Medicine; Clinical Faculty, Stanford Hospital, San Francisco, California

Daniel C. Shannon, M.D.
Professor of Pediatrics, Harvard Medical School; Professor of Health Sciences, Harvard/MIT School of Health Science and Technology; Chief, Pediatric Pulmonary Unit, Massachusetts General Hospital, Boston, Massachusetts

Kenneth E. Shepherd, M.D.
Staff Anesthesiologist, Department of Anesthesia, Massachusetts General Hospital, Boston, Massachusetts

George D. Shorten, M.B., F.F.A.R.C.S.(I.), F.C.Anaes.
Instructor in Anesthesia, Harvard Med-

ical School; Fellow in Cardiac Anesthesia, Beth Israel Hospital, Boston, Massachusetts

Depak Soni, M.D.
Senior Fellow, Pulmonary and Critical Care Unit, Massachusetts General Hospital, Harvard Medical School, Boston, Massachusetts; Attending Physician, Pulmonary and Critical Care Sections, Department of Medicine, The Fairfax Hospital, Falls Church, Virginia

Denise J. Strieder, M.D.
Associate Professor of Pediatrics, Harvard Medical School; Pediatrician, Massachusetts General Hospital, Boston, Massachusetts

Colleen A. Sullivan, M.B.Ch.B.
Clinical Professor of Anesthesiology, State University of New York, Health Science Center at Brooklyn; Clinical Director, Department of Anesthesiology, University Hospital of Brooklyn, Brooklyn, New York

I. David Todres, M.D.
Associate Professor in Anesthesia (Pediatrics), Harvard Medical School; Anesthetist, Pediatrician, and Director, Neonatal and Pediatric Intensive Care Units, Massachusetts General Hospital, Boston, Massachusetts

José G. Venegas, Ph.D.
Assistant Professor, Department of Anesthesia/Bioengineering, Harvard

Medical School; Assistant Biomedical Engineer, Massachusetts General Hospital, Boston, Massachusetts

John C. Wain, M.D.
Assistant Professor, Harvard Medical School; Assistant Surgeon, Massachusetts General Hospital, Boston, Massachusetts

Alfred L. Weber, M.D.
Professor of Radiology, Harvard Medical School; Chief of Radiology, Massachusetts Eye and Ear Infirmary; Radiologist, Massachusetts General Hospital, Boston, Massachusetts

Mark A. Weiner, D.O.
Anesthesiologist, Premier Anesthesia of Toledo, and Department of Anesthesia, Parkview Hospital, Toledo, Ohio

Jeffrey White, M.D.
Reading Anesthesia Group, Reading, California

Donna J. Wilson, R.N., M.S.N., R.R.T.
Pulmonary Clinical Nurse Specialist, Memorial Sloan-Kettering Cancer Center, New York, New York

George R. Wodicka, Ph.D.
Assistant Professor of Electrical Engineering, Purdue University, West Lafayette, Indiana

Preface

Clinical Management of the Airway is designed to help the clinician maximize successful management of airway problems. The first section (Chapters 1 and 2) provides a foundation of airway anatomy and pathology; the second section (Chapters 3 to 8) presents basic laboratory, surgical, bedside, and bronchoscopic techniques for assessing the adequacy of the airway, as well as the latest methods of airway sound analysis; the third section (Chapters 9 to 25) emphasizes methods and problems of securing the airway, including time-honored approaches, as well as the latest flexible fiberoptic methods, the laryngeal mask airway, and a chapter on the failed intubation in the patient with a compromised airway; the fourth section (Chapters 26 to 42) covers management of specific airway problems, including chapters on the burned airway, infections of the airway, tracheal stenosis, major and minor hemoptysis, high-frequency ventilation. lasers and the airway, maxillofacial trauma, and drug interactions and the airway.

Contributions to this text were made by emergency room specialists, surgeons, anesthesiologists, internists, radiologists, pathologists, and basic scientists, each examining the airway from a different perspective. This diversity should provide greater insight into airway problems and strengthen the clinician's understanding of airway function.

JAMES T. ROBERTS, M.D., M.A.

I thank my secretary, Ms. Mary Farr, for her devoted efforts on my behalf.

Contents

SECURING THE AIRWAY

MANAGING SPECIFIC AIRWAY PROBLEMS

INTRODUCTION

CHAPTER 1

Functional Anatomy of the Airway

James T. Roberts, M.D., M.A.,
and Richard Pino, M.D., Ph.D.

The anatomy of the airway may be viewed from many different vantage points, depending on the interests and objectives of the physician. The surgeon who is performing a tracheostomy needs different information than that required by the anesthesiologist who is attempting a difficult awake intubation. This chapter has been designed as a general review of airway anatomy, including cartilaginous and bony supports, blood supply, innervation, and functional implications. It can serve as a primer for the house officer who is attempting initial airway management, as well as for the more experienced clinician who desires a review of the functional anatomy of the airway.

NASAL PASSAGES

The nasal passages are the most fixed structures of the respiratory tract (Figs. 1–1 to 1–3). Each passage has an anterior opening (naris), four sides, and a posterior opening (choana). The anterior, movable, portion of the nose has a framework of five distinct cartilage plates. One of these, the septal cartilage, comprises at least half of the medial wall (septum) of the nose. Nine bones make up the borders of the nasal canal. The palatine bone is a component of each wall. The maxilla is part of three walls, the roof being the excep-

tion. With the palatine bone, the maxilla forms the floor. The nasal and frontal bones are found only in the roof (with the ethmoid, sphenoid, vomer, and palatine bones), and the inferior turbinate and lacrimal bones are located only as part of the lateral wall with the ethmoid, sphenoid, and palatine bones. The superior and middle turbinates are part of the ethmoid bone. Infants are obligate nose breathers and consequently have a higher ratio of anatomic dead space to tidal volume than do adults. Patent nasal passages are critical, as exemplified by the newborn with choanal atresia, whose respirations must be emergently supported.

The mucosa that covers these bony and cartilaginous supports is the functional component of the nasal passages, as well as of the paranasal sinuses. It is composed of an epithelium, subepithelial connective tissue, glands, nerves, and blood vessels.[1] The squamous epithelium of the nares is a sturdy, stratified layer with hairs, ie, vibrissae, which prevent coarse particulates from further passage into the nasal canals. The inner lining of the nasal canal and paranasal sinuses is covered by a respiratory epithelium. Most of the cells are pseudostratified ciliated columnar. As the name implies, the cells are columnar, in a single layer, and *look* stratified only because their nuclei are at different levels. Goblet cells that secrete mu-

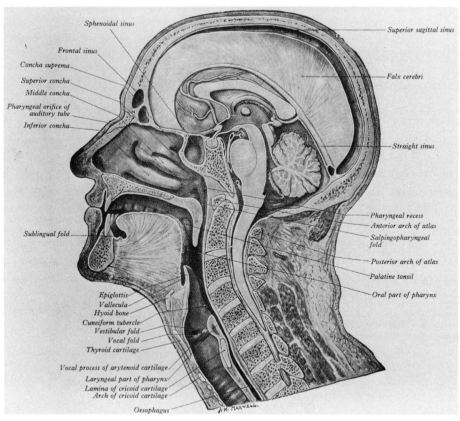

Figure 1–1. A sagittal section through the nose, mouth, pharynx, and larynx. (From Williams PL, Warwick R. Gray's Anatomy, 36th ed. London: Churchill Livingstone, 1980; with permission.)

cus, brush cells that produce a more serous secretion, precursor basal cells, and cells of the enteroendocrine system that produce locally acting peptides (also called APUD cells, an abbreviation for amine precursor uptake and decarboxylation) are integral components of the epithelium. Tubuloalveolar glands in the submucosa, similar to seromucous salivary glands, open onto the epithelial surface. The seromucous layer on the surface of the epithelium helps to trap inhaled particles that are not stopped by the vibrissae. The action of the underlying cilia is to propel this layer toward the nasopharynx, where it is either expectorated or swallowed. The collagen-rich subepithelial tissue bears abundant macrophages that ingest foreign material, which breach in the epithelium. A comparison of the dimensions of the rather large nasal passages as seen in a skeleton versus the smaller size seen in life readily demonstrates the thickness of the mucosa.

In addition to the respiratory epithelium, the bipolar sensory cells, branches of cranial nerve (CN) I, and their supportive elements are located in the roof as they penetrate the cribriform plate of the ethmoid bone. The sensory innervation of the nasal mucosa is largely via the pterygopalatine branches of the maxillary division of the trigeminal nerve (CN V). Trigeminal nerve pain, as anyone with a toothache knows, is often excruciating. Therefore, topical anesthesia of the nasal mucosa must be complete prior to a nasotracheal intubation.

The vascular supply to the nasal passages is predominantly derived from the third part of the maxillary artery, a branch of the external carotid artery. The anterior part of the nasal canal is supplied by branches of the anterior ethmoid artery, a branch of the ophthalmic artery. This anastomoses anteriorly with branches of the facial artery. The latter location is a common site of nose bleeds. The sphenopalatine artery supplies most of the lateral wall and septum. A branch descends anteriorly along the nasal septum to anastomose with a branch of the greater palatine artery. Epistaxis involving the branches of the sphenopalatine artery can be brisk and should

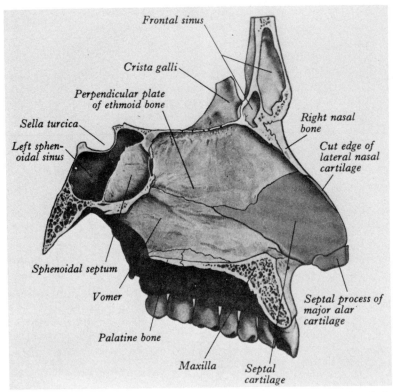

Figure 1–2. The nasal septum. (From Williams PL, Warwick R. Gray's Anatomy, 36th ed. London: Churchill Livingstone, 1980; with permission.)

not be taken lightly. Veins accompany these arteries and drain into the pterygoid plexus, cavernous sinus, and superior sagittal sinus.

There is a rich anastomosis of arteries and veins in the nasal mucosa. Arterial arcades generously supply capillaries under the epithelium.[2] These rich plexuses serve to warm inspired air before it moves to more distal portions of the respiratory tract. Over the middle and inferior turbinates, the nasal mucosa is thickened to form "swell bodies" that are similar to erectile tissue. Via constrictive adrenergic nerve fibers from the superior cervical ganglion and cholinergic vasodilatory nerve fibers from the pterygopalatine ganglion, there is a cyclic engorgement of the swell bodies of each nasal passage. This helps the epithelium recover from the desiccating effects of the entering dry air.

The structure–function aspects of the nasal mucosa have implications for the intubated patient. With inflammation, the increased vascular permeability of the nasal mucosa might effect a total occlusion of the nasal passage. Prior to intubation attempts, alpha agonists, such as phenylephrine and oxymetazoline, will shrink the mucosa and decrease the risk of

bleeding. Tracheal intubation, whether nasal or oral, bypasses the warming and particulate trapping functions of the mucosa. Finally, a prolonged nasotracheal intubation may be associated with inflammation of the nasal mucosa and blockage of paranasal sinus drainage; this may lead to sinusitis with retrograde spread of the infection via the venous drainage into the dural venous sinuses.

ORAL CAVITY

The oral cavity has four sides and is contiguous posteriorly with the oropharynx. The roof is the hard palate (palatine and maxillary bones), which is actually the underside of the floor of the nasal cavity, and the soft palate (Figs. 1–1, 1–4, and 1–5). The soft palate is a mucosa-covered skeletal muscle that assists in closing off of the nasal cavity during swallowing and helps to maintain a patent pharynx during breathing. The palatoglossus (CN X) and palatopharyngeus (CN X) muscles tense the soft palate along with the musculus uvulae (CN X) and tensor veli palatini (CN V) (Fig. 1–6). The palatoglossus also helps to pull the

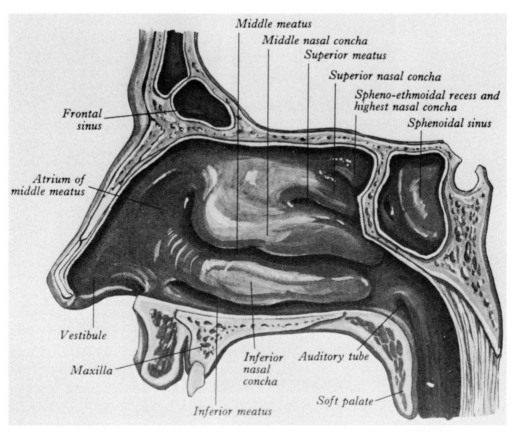

Figure 1–3. The lateral aspect of the nasal cavity and nasopharynx. (From Williams PL, Warwick R. Gray's Anatomy, 36th ed. London: Churchill Livingstone, 1980; with permission.)

tongue superiorly while also lifting the larynx during swallowing. These two muscles, with their overlying mucosa, make up the faucial pillars. These faucial pillars are the border between the oral cavity and the oropharynx. The levator veli palatini (CN X) raises the soft palate.

The mandible forms the structural framework for the floor of the mouth. The temporomandibular joint (TMJ) is the most critical joint involved in the process of endotracheal intubation. It is the only diarthrotic (movable) joint in the head. Most diarthrotic joints are made up of hyaline cartilage, which covers the articular surface of bones, and a single joint space, which contains synovial fluid produced by a synovial membrane. In contrast, the coronoid process of the mandible and the articular tubercle of the temporal bone are lined by fibrocartilage. Furthermore, the TMJ has two synovial compartments, which are separated by a fibrocartilage articular disc. This arrangement allows for depression (opening), elevation (closing), protrusion, retraction, and side-

to-side movements. The lateral pterygoid muscles protrude the jaw, whereas retraction is done by part of the temporalis muscles. In addition to the medial pterygoids and masseters, the temporalis muscles close the jaw. The strength of these muscles should not be underestimated and often poses formidable problems with intubation attempts. The approach to intubation of a patient with trismus secondary to pain (eg, a patient with a tonsillar abscess) is different from that of a patient with trismus secondary to radiation fibrosis. If the mouth cannot be opened because of pain, the administration of anesthetics and muscle relaxants often enables passive mouth opening and direct laryngoscopy. In contrast, the fibrotic jaw is relatively fixed and is not relaxed by anesthetic agents. Usually, an awake fiberoptic (nasal or oral) or blind nasal intubation is required. Dislocation of the jaw may occur spontaneously, as with a yawn, or after wide mouth opening before direct laryngoscopy. Because of the mobility at the TMJ, the mandible is displaced anteriorly into the infratemporal

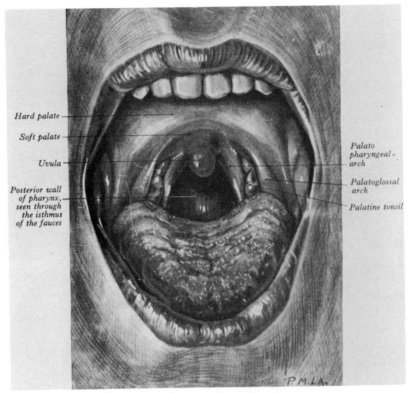

Hard palate
Soft palate
Uvula
Posterior wall
of pharynx,
seen through
the isthmus
of the fauces

Palato
pharyngeal-
arch
Palatoglossal
arch
Palatine tonsil

Figure 1–4. The oral cavity. (From Williams PL, Warwick R. Gray's Anatomy, 36th ed. London: Churchill Livingstone, 1980; with permission.)

fossa and is pulled upward. Reduction is done by depressing the jaw to overcome the traction of the muscles, followed by posterior movement into place.

The tongue forms the bulk of the floor of the mouth and is relatively larger in children. It includes the genioglossus (from the mandible), the hyoglossus (from the hyoid bone), and the styloglossus (from the styloid process of the temporal bone); these are all innervated by CN XII. The genioglossus is the protruder of the tongue and helps to maintain a patent airway. Cyclic genioglossus activity in coordination with excursions of the diaphragm during breathing has been observed.[3] The sensory innervation of the tongue is via the trigeminal nerve (CN V, mandibular division) for general sensation, the facial nerve (CN VII) for taste to the anterior two thirds, and the glossopharyngeal nerve (CN IX) for the remainder of general sensation and taste. The glossopharyngeal nerve is found just underneath the palatoglossal arch (anterior faucial pillar) adjacent to the tongue and can be blocked here with local anesthetics (see Fig. 1–6). The subject of taste does have relevance to airway management if one remembers that lidocaine spray,

used topically to anesthetize oral structures, is bitter and often offensive to patients. The size of the tongue relative to the size of the oral cavity, as predicted by the Mallampati test,[4] indicates the relative ease of visualization of the glottis during laryngoscopy.

Although the buccal mucosa is the lateral wall of the oral cavity in edentulous individuals, the teeth are the functional lateral walls in most patients and are often barriers to laryngoscopy. The space between the teeth and the buccal mucosa is called the vestibule. Protuberant maxillary incisors may make viewing of the larynx by direct larygoscopy difficult because they impose a limitation on the manipulation of the laryngoscope blade. Removable prosthodontic appliances should be removed prior to intubation attempts, because they can be displaced posteriorly and cause airway obstruction. Missing, chipped, and loose teeth should be noted. As discussed previously, the muscles of mastication are very powerful and can easily compress an endotracheal tube, thereby preventing ventilation. Equally disturbing is the closure of teeth on hard plastic Yankauer suction catheters. For these reasons, it is useful to place an oropharyngeal airway

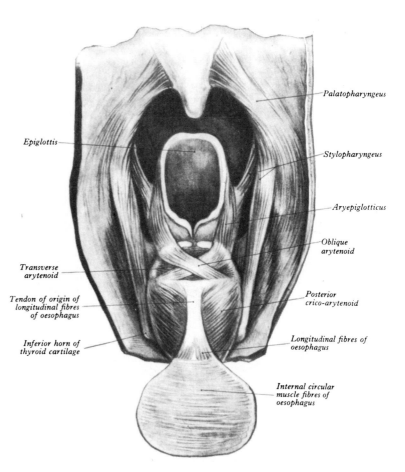

Palatopharyngeus

Epiglottis

Stylopharyngeus

Aryepiglotticus

Oblique arytenoid

Transverse arytenoid

Posterior crico-arytenoid

Tendon of origin of longitudinal fibres of oesophagus

Inferior horn of thyroid cartilage

Longitudinal fibres of oesophagus

Internal circular muscle fibres of oesophagus

Figure 1–5. The posterior aspect of the larynx and pharynx. (From Williams PL, Warwick R. Gray's Anatomy, 36th ed. London: Churchill Livingstone, 1980; with permission.)

to limit mouth closure; soft-suction catheters are also useful. If capped teeth are present, one may use a bite block fashioned from cotton gauze.

The teeth form a natural oral airway. They allow the correct anatomic approximation of the maxilla and mandible. If the tone of the tongue muscles is intact, the teeth create a space between the tongue and palate. By protruding the mandible (subluxation), the base of the tongue is moved further anteriorly, thereby facilitating ventilation. In edentulous patients, including children, cephalad pressure on the mandible easily compresses the tongue against the palate and posteriorly into the oropharynx, creating an obstruction. The absence of teeth makes fitting a mask difficult, especially if the alveolar ridge has receded. In these patients, an oropharyngeal airway facilitates ventilation by creating a space between the tongue and the hard palate, and also by preventing posterior displacement of the tongue into the pharynx.

At the entrance to the oropharynx is a sentinel of lymphoid tissue known as Waldey-

er's ring. This consists of the lingual tonsil at the base of the tongue and bilateral palatine tonsils (see Fig. 1–4) between each palatoglossal and palatopharyngeal arch. Completing the ring are the nasopharyngeal and tubal tonsils, discussed below. Inflammation of these lymphoid tissues may obstruct breathing efforts in awake patients and may make direct laryngoscopy difficult via size or associated masseter muscle trismus. Relaxation of the palatoglossus and palatopharyngeus muscles in the supine, sedated patient may further hinder efforts at ventilation. Occasionally, one sees severe postoperative bleeding in tonsils as a result of the rich blood supply from the ascending pharyngeal branch of the external carotid artery, as well as branches from the maxillary and facial arteries.

The sublingual, submandibular, and parotid salivary glands usually pose a problem to endotracheal intubation secondary to their secretion of saliva. One obvious exception is their enlargement secondary to malignancy or inflammation, which may distort the airway structures.

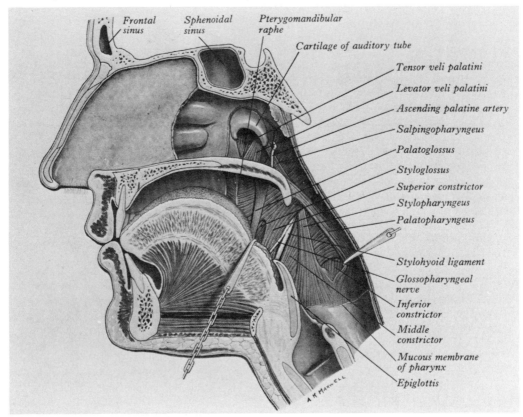

Figure 1–6. A sagittal section of the head showing the oral cavity and pharynx. (From Williams PL, Warwick R. Gray's Anatomy, 36th ed. London: Churchill Livingstone, 1980; with permission.)

THE PHARYNX

The pharynx is a muscular tube, covered by a mucosa and submucosa, which has lateral and posterior walls (see Figs. 1–1, 1–5, and 1–6). Anteriorly, the nasal cavities and mouth open into the nasopharynx and oropharynx, respectively. The pharynx extends from the base of the skull to the esophagus and epiglottis. Three circumferential muscles, the superior, middle, and inferior constrictors, are innervated by the vagus nerve (Fig. 1–7). The superior constrictor arises from the mandible and the pterygoid and pterygomandibular raphe and inserts into a median raphe. This median raphe is attached superiorly to the occipital bone. The middle constrictor is between the hyoid bone, stylohyoid ligament, and median raphe. The inferior constrictor connects the median raphe with the thyroid and cricoid cartilages of the larynx and is discussed below. Superficial to the constrictors are the stylopharyngeus (CN IX), palatopharyngeus (CN X), and salpingopharyngeus (CN X) muscles. The salpingopharyngeus muscle often is not present or is very small. The function of the constrictors is to propel food toward the esophagus, whereas the remaining muscles assist in raising the larynx during swallowing.

The nasopharynx begins at the choanae at the level of the first cervical vertebra. The inferior opening of the auditory (eustachian) tube is located just posterior to the inferior turbinate. This largely cartilaginous tube is a conduit for equalizing the pressure between the middle ear and the environment. The tensor veli palatini, levator veli palatini, and stylopharyngeus help to open the auditory tube at the nasopharynx. The tubal tonsils are present in this region.

On the posterior wall of the nasopharynx is an accumulation of lymphoid tissue, the nasopharyngeal tonsils (adenoids). Although these regress with age, they may hinder breathing through the nose when enlarged. A soft-suction catheter passed through the nose and into the nasopharynx of a child may dislodge a nasopharyngeal tonsil and lead to a more distal airway obstruction.

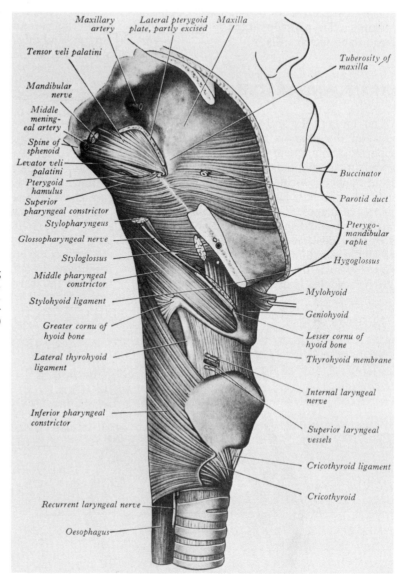

Figure 1–7. Muscles supporting the pharynx. (From Williams PL, Warwick R. Gray's Anatomy, 36th ed. London: Churchill Livingstone, 1980; with permission.)

The oropharynx begins past the palatopharyngeal arches, across from the bodies of the third and fourth cervical vertebrae. The oropharynx is attached anteriorly to the base of the tongue via condensations of connective tissue covered with mucosa. These are the median glossoepiglottic and two lateral glossoepiglottic folds. The valleculae are between these folds. In addition to these ligaments, the hyoepigastric ligament is between the hyoid bone and epiglottis. During intubation with a Macintosh laryngoscope blade, the tip of the blade contacts the hyoepiglottic ligament in the valleculae and helps to raise the epiglottis anteriorly.

The innervation of the musculature has been presented previously. The trigeminal nerve, via the palatine and nasopalatine branches, and the glossopharyngeal nerve are the sensory innervation of the nasopharynx. The glossopharyngeal nerve also innervates sensory receptors of the oropharynx, with the exception of the superior laryngeal nerve (internal branch), which transmits afferent impulses from the base of the tongue and the valleculae. The response to CN IX and CN X stimulation is important in laryngoscopy. Afferent fibers from these nerves form a reflex arc, with the sympathetic nerves leading to the heart and blood vessels. If this sensory input is not blocked by anesthetics or blunted by opiates, attempts at laryngoscopy often result in hypertension and tachycardia.[5]

LARYNX AND TRACHEA

The larynx[6] (Figs. 1–1, 1–8 to 1–11) sits between the pharynx and trachea. It is the uppermost component of the respiratory tract, is the organ of phonation, and protects the distal tracheobronchial tree from entry by foreign material. It includes three single and three paired cartilages. The largest is the thyroid cartilage, a shield-shaped hyaline cartilage that is opened posteriorly and forms the base on which the remaining components interplay (see Figs. 1–7 to 1–10). The laryngeal prominence (Adam's apple) is the midline anterior protuberance. At the posterior borders of the thyroid cartilage are vertical processes, called superior and inferior horns. The epiglottis is a single, tear-shaped structure made of elastic cartilage. It is the uppermost portion of the larynx and is the key structure to identify during endotracheal intubation. The epiglottis (see Figs. 1–9 and 1–10) is attached to the posterior border of the thyroid cartilage by the thyroepiglottic ligament. The epiglottis of the child is wider than long (omega shaped) and is at a 45-degree angle to the trachea.

Beneath the thyroid cartilage is the cricoid cartilage at the level of the C6 and C4 vertebrae in adults and children, respectively (see Figs. 1–7 to 1–10). It is shaped like a signet ring, with the widest portion posterior, and is the only complete cartilage ring found in the respiratory tract. In children, the cricoid cartilage is the narrowest portion of the larynx

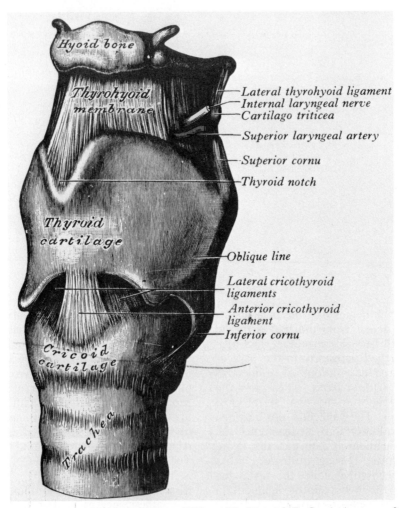

Figure 1–8. The anterior aspect of the larynx. (From Williams PL, Warwick R. Gray's Anatomy, 36th ed. London: Churchill Livingstone, 1980; with permission.)

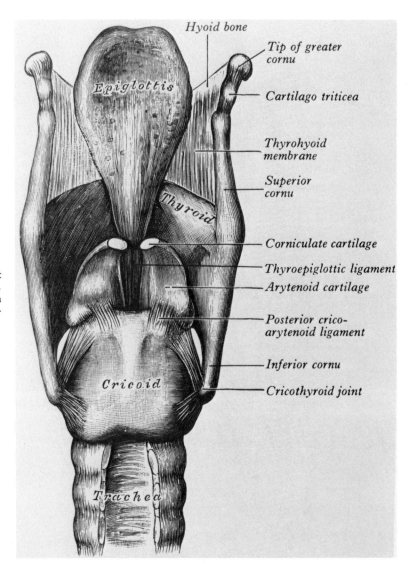

Figure 1–9. The posterior aspect of the larynx. (From Williams PL, Warwick R. Gray's Anatomy, 36th ed. London: Churchill Livingstone, 1980; with permission.)

and is the limiting factor in selecting an appropriate endotracheal tube. Furthermore, because it is a complete ring and small in a child, any edema of the mucosa will severely compromise the airway. The cricoid articulates with the inferior horn of the thyroid cartilage by a freely movable joint. The paired arytenoid cartilages articulate at the posterosuperior aspect of the cricoid cartilage (see Fig. 1–9). Each arytenoid has an anterior process, the vocal process, to which the vocal ligament is attached. A lateral process is the insertion site of several muscles. Atop each arytenoid is a triangular corniculate cartilage, attached by a perichondrium. The cricoarytenoid joint allows medial and lateral sliding, rotation, and anteroposterior tilting. The cricothyroid membrane (conus elasticus) is a tough, elastic connective tissue sheet that spans anteriorly from the medial process of the arytenoids to the thyroid cartilage and inferiorly to the cricoid cartilage. It is through this cricothyroid membrane that translaryngeal nerve blocks, emergent oxygenation via jet ventilation through intravenous catheters, and cricothyroidotomies are performed.[7] The condensation of fibers in the anterior midline is the cricothyroid ligament. The paired superior border between each arytenoid and the thyroid cartilage is thickened and called the vocal ligament. The cricoid cartilage is attached to the first tracheal ring.

Eight pairs of intrinsic muscles affect movement of the laryngeal skeleton (Figs. 1–5 and 1–12). Although the initial study of these muscles and their actions may seem complex, a consideration of a few concepts may add simplification. First, all muscles are named by

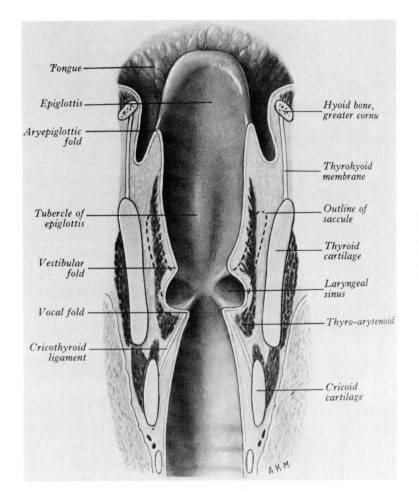

Figure 1–10. A coronal section through the larynx and trachea. (From Williams PL, Warwick R. Gray's Anatomy, 36th ed. London: Churchill Livingstone, 1980; with permission.)

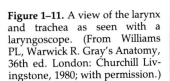

Figure 1–11. A view of the larynx and trachea as seen with a laryngoscope. (From Williams PL, Warwick R. Gray's Anatomy, 36th ed. London: Churchill Livingstone, 1980; with permission.)

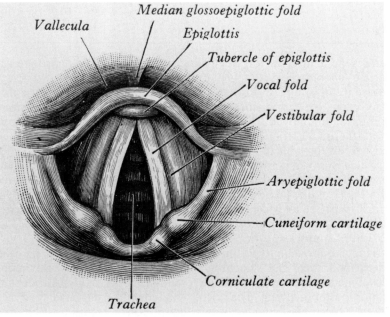

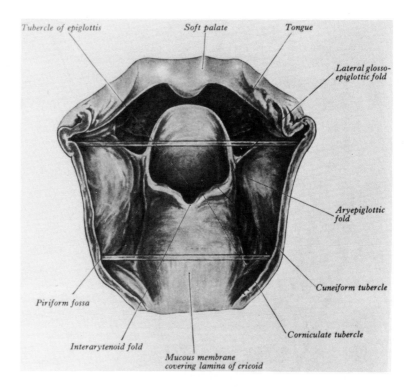

Figure 1–12. The laryngeal inlet. (From Williams PL, Warwick R. Gray's Anatomy, 36th ed. London: Churchill Livingstone, 1980; with permission.)

their points of attachment. Second, as with any muscle, to affect movement at a joint, the muscle must cross that joint; this is usually at the best mechanical advantage. Third, for the arytenoids, the lateral process is the site of muscle attachment. Fourth, muscles from the cricoid cartilage cause pivoting at the cricoarytenoid joint, whereas the other muscles create sliding motions. Finally, the vagus nerve supplies all of the intrinsic muscles of the larynx. The cricothyroid is via the external branch of the superior laryngeal nerve of the vagus, whereas the remainder are supplied by vagal fibers of the recurrent laryngeal nerves.

The cricothyroid spans the joint between the inferior process of the thyroid cartilage and the cricoid cartilage (Fig. 1–13). Contraction moves the thyroid anterior and inferior, thereby placing tension on the vocal ligaments. The posterior cricoarytenoids pass over the cricoarytenoid joints to attach to the lateral arytenoid processes. This pivots the lateral processes posteriorly and the anterior processes more laterally, with the result of widening the rima glottis, the space between the vocal ligaments. Conversely, the lateral cricoarytenoids pivot the arytenoid cartilages in the opposite direction, approximating the vocal cords. The transverse and oblique arytenoids move the vocal cords closer together via sliding at the joints. A sphincter function is performed

by the thyroarytenoid. The vocalis muscle is made up of fascicles of the thyroarytenoid that are located in the lateral aspects of the vocal ligaments. This muscle contracts the vocal ligament. Finally, the thyroepiglottis muscle helps to bring the epiglottis posterior and over the laryngeal opening.

Overlying the muscles and cartilages of the larynx is a mucosa. In several places, the mucosa covers ligaments and has an identifiable structure (see Figs. 1–11 and 1–12). As discussed previously, when contiguous with the tongue and epiglottis, the mucosa forms the medial and lateral glossoepiglottic folds, with the valleculae in between. The pyriform recess is created by the fold of the pharyngeal mucosa over the lateral wall of the larynx, and this recess is one place to look when foreign body aspiration is suspected. In addition, the pyriform recess is directly over the course of the superior laryngeal nerve, and cotton planchettes soaked in lidocaine may be placed in the pyriform recesses to externally block the superior laryngeal nerve. On the interior of the larynx, the aryepiglottic folds cover the aryepiglottic ligaments. The quadrangular membrane is a thin sheet of connective tissue that underlies the aryepiglottic fold. The small cuneiform cartilages are located in the aryepiglottic folds. The vestibular folds, or false vocal cords, are created by the mucosa that covers

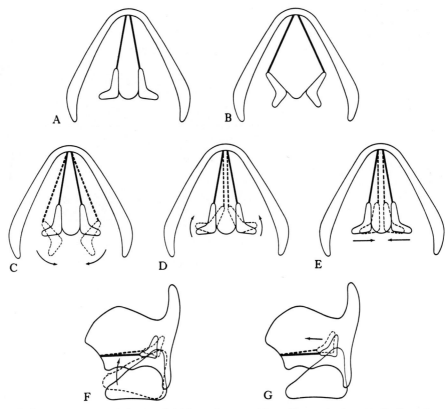

Figure 1–13. Different positions of the vocal folds and arytenoid cartilages. *A*, At rest. *B*, Forced expiration. *C*, Abduction by contraction of the posterior cricoarytenoids. *D*, Adduction by contraction of the lateral cricoarytenoids. *E*, Contraction of the transverse arytenoids. *F*, Tension by the cricothyroid. *G*, Relaxation by the thyroarytenoids. (From Williams PL, Warwick R. Gray's Anatomy, 36th ed. London: Churchill Livingstone, 1980; with permission.)

the thyroarytenoid muscles. It is the approximation of the vestibular folds by the thyroarytenoid muscle that may cause laryngospasm. The true vocal cords are the vocal folds covered by mucosa. The space between the vestibule and vocal cords is a depression known as the laryngeal ventricle.

The histologic structure of the mucosa is a reflection of its function.[1] The stratified squamous epithelium covering the epiglottis gradually is transformed into a respiratory epithelium. Laryngeal glands open onto the epithelial surface. The secretions on the surface, as in the nasal cavity and nasopharynx, entrap particulates. These particles are thrust toward the oropharynx via the cilia of the epithelium, the motion of which is called the mucociliary escalator, or by coughing. In some individuals (eg, smokers) the respiratory epithelium undergoes metaplasia into this stratified squamous type. Although the mucosa is itself protected by this transformation, the prime function of protection of the airway is lost. Stratified squamous epithelium normally cov-

ers the vocal cords. The mucosa of the lingual side of the epiglottis is not as adherent as on the laryngeal front. Because of this asymmetry, enlargement of the epiglottis, when inflamed, is usually adjacent to the tongue. The subepithelial lamina propria of the larynx is rich in mast cells, a readily available source of vasoactive substances that contribute to laryngeal edema when they are stimulated. A variety of receptors are present in the mucosa. Mechanical, chemical, and thermal agents may stimulate these receptors, initiating autonomic respiratory reflexes. Specific stimulants include the laryngoscope, endotracheal tube, secretions, aspiration of stomach contents, inhalation of volatile gases, inflation or deflation of the lungs, and burns. Salivation, coughing, gagging, vomiting, laryngospasm, and bronchospasm are among the reflexes that may be initiated.[8, 9]

The larynx is supported in place by a series of ligaments and extrinsic muscles, mostly via the horseshoe-shaped hyoid bone.[6, 7] These ligaments are the stylohyoid, thyrohyoid, and cricothyroid. The thyroepiglottic and cricothyroid muscles, discussed previously, are sometimes classified as extrinsic muscles because they do not insert on the arytenoids, although they are intralaryngeal. The inferior pharyngeal constrictor is attached to the thyroid cartilage at the oblique line, a linear protuberance that runs from the superior horn downward to the anterior thyroid border. This muscle also arises from the lateral portions of the cricoid cartilage and inserts onto a median raphe. It is innervated by the vagus nerve. The palatopharyngeus, the muscular component of the posterior faucial pillar, is inserted into the soft palate and the posterior part of the thyroid cartilage. The strap muscles of the neck, through their insertion onto the larynx (sternothyroid) or the hyoid bone (omohyoid, sternohyoid, stylohyoid), stabilize the larynx, similarly to the rigging on a ship's mast. These muscles are innervated by a loop of the first and second cervical nerves, the ansa cervicalis, also known as the descendens hypoglossi. Branches of the third and fourth cervical nerves also innervate the infrahyoid muscles. A common misconception is that the ansa cervicalis is a branch of the hypoglossal nerve. Although these fibers "ride" with this nerve, they do not originate in the hypoglossal nucleus.

The characterization of a larynx as anterior is often made by anesthesiologists. This assessment is usually made by Mallampati criteria[4] and the presence of a space of less than three fingerbreaths submandibular to the thyroid cartilage. On direct laryngoscopy, the vocal cords are not readily visible unless the larynx is moved posteriorly by pressure on the cricoid cartilage. In reality, "anterior" larynx is a misnomer. Because the mandible is smaller, the root of the tongue is more posterior and is more difficult to displace by the laryngoscope blade; this is the reason why the larynx is not readily seen.

The trachea begins at its fibrous tissue connection with the cricoid cartilage at about the seventh cervical vertebra and descends into the superior mediastinum. It includes 16 to 20 C-shaped rings of hyaline cartilage that are opened posteriorly. The opening is spanned by the trachealis muscle, which is innervated by the vagus nerve. The mucosa is of the respiratory type, the same as is found in the larynx. The vessels within the tracheal muscosa have a perfusion pressure of approximately 25 mm Hg; therefore, inflation of an endotracheal tube cuff at pressures greater than 25 mm Hg will compromise the blood flow of the mucosa.

At the fifth thoracic vertebra, the trachea divides into right and left primary (mainstem) bronchi. A midline ridge, the carina, is a landmark at the division and is looked for during endotracheal intubation by fiberoptic methods. The right mainstem bronchus is wider and at less of an angle with the trachea, as compared to the left mainstem bronchus. For this reason, insertion of an endotracheal tube too deeply will result in the intubation of the right mainstem bronchus. Similarly, aspirated foreign bodies are more likely to settle in the right lung. The length of the trachea is approximately 11 cm. Because the distance from the tip of an endotracheal tube to the top of the tube's cuff is 7 cm, there is only about 4 cm between the tip of the tube and the carina (assuming that the upper end of the cuff is flush against the vocal folds). This places the tip of the endotracheal tube in the middle one third of the trachea.

THE THYROID GLAND, BLOOD VESSELS, AND NERVES IN THE NECK

The larynx and trachea share anatomic relationships with other neck structures (Figs. 1–1, 1–7, and 1–14). Posterior and slightly to the left of the larynx and trachea is the esophagus. It arises at the inferior constrictor posterior to the glottis and descends within the neck into the thorax. The cricoid cartilage is attached posteriorly to the esophagus by a cricoesophageal ligament. The lumen of the esophagus can be occluded by compressing it between the cricoid cartilage and the sixth cervical vertebra.[10] This is often done during intubation attempts, in order to prevent reflux of gastric contents until the airway can be protected with an endotracheal tube. Commonly known as "cricoid pressure," this occlusion is called the Sellick maneuver.[10] The recurrent laryngeal nerves run between the esophagus and the trachea.

The carotid sheaths enclose the common carotid artery (medial), internal jugular vein (lateral), vagus nerve (posteromedial), and sympathetic trunks (medial). At the level of the thyroid cartilage, the common carotid artery bifurcates into its internal and external branches. Branches of the external carotid artery provide virtually all the blood to the larynx and pharynx, and to most of the nasal cavity and trachea as well.[11]

The thyroid gland is bilobed and embraces

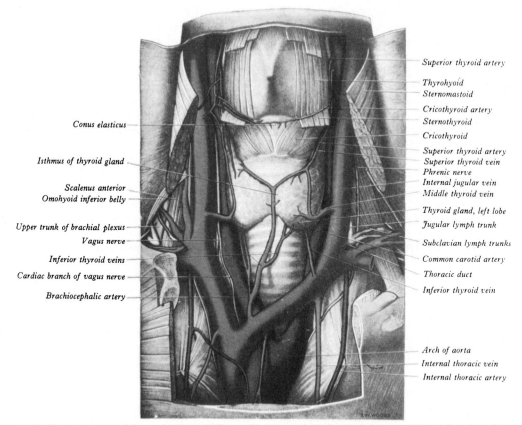

Superior thyroid artery

Thyrohyoid
Sternomastoid

Cricothyroid artery
Sternothyroid

Cricothyroid

Superior thyroid artery
Superior thyroid vein
Phrenic nerve
Internal jugular vein
Middle thyroid vein

Thyroid gland, left lobe

Jugular lymph trunk

Subclavian lymph trunks

Common carotid artery

Thoracic duct

Inferior thyroid vein

Arch of aorta
Internal thoracic vein
Internal thoracic artery

Conus elasticus

Isthmus of thyroid gland

Scalenus anterior
Omohyoid inferior belly

Upper trunk of brachial plexus
Vagus nerve

Inferior thyroid veins

Cardiac branch of vagus nerve

Brachiocephalic artery

Figure 1–14. The structures of the neck. (From Williams PL, Warwick R. Gray's Anatomy, 36th ed. London: Churchill Livingstone, 1980; with permission.)

the thyroid cartilage superiorly and extends to the fifth cervical vertebra inferiorly. It covers the carotid sheath, inferior constrictor, superior laryngeal nerve, and recurrent laryngeal nerves. In the midline, the lobes are connected by an isthmus from the second to fourth tracheal rings. The strap muscles are superficial to the thyroid gland.

The blood supply to the thyroid gland is intimately connected to that of the larynx and trachea. The superior thyroid artery from the external carotid artery arises at the upper border of the thyroid cartilage and descends to supply the upper pole of the gland and the larynx, as well as the superior laryngeal artery. The internal branch of the superior laryngeal nerve courses over the posterior aspect of the hyoid bone (where it can be anesthetized) and pierces the thyrohyoid membrane with this artery. The external branch of the superior laryngeal nerve travels over the inferior constrictor to innervate the cricothyroid muscle. The inferior poles of the thyroid gland are supplied by the inferior thyroid artery from

the thyrocervical trunk of the subclavian artery. A branch of this, the inferior laryngeal artery, accompanies the recurrent laryngeal nerve into the region just posterior to the cricothyroid articulation. The recurrent laryngeal nerves are in danger of damage during a thyroidectomy. Unilateral severance results in the unopposed action of the cricothyroid muscle and ipsilateral adduction of the cord to the midline. Bilateral damage is more life threatening, with both cords in unopposed adduction, leading to complete airway obstruction. There is a rich anastomosis of these vessels posterior to the trachea and larynx, leaving the anterior surface above the isthmus relatively vessel free. This provides the surgeon with a potential nonbloody field for a tracheostomy. The venous drainage of the larynx and thyroid tissue is via the superior and middle thyroid veins (into the internal jugular vein) and the inferior thyroid veins (into the superior vena cava). Lymphatic drainage is via pathways parallel to the arteries into pretracheal, prelaryngeal, and paratracheal lymph nodes.

The mediastinal part of the trachea is posterior to the thymus gland, superior vena cava, arch of the aorta, left brachiocephalic vein, and the brachiocephalic artery. Fistulae between the trachea and brachiocephalic artery have occurred following prolonged endotracheal intubation, usually using high-pressure, cuffed endotracheal tubes.

References

1. Sorokin SP. The respiratory system. In Weiss L (ed). Cell and Tissue Biology: A Textbook of Histology, 6th ed. Baltimore: Urban and Schwarzenberg, 1988; p. 751.
2. Dawes JDK, Prichard MML. Studies of the vascular arrangements of the nose. J Anat 87:311, 1953.
3. Onal E, Lopata M, O'Conner TD. Diaphragmatic and genioglossal electromyelogram response to CO_2 rebreathing in humans. J Appl Physiol 50:1052, 1981.
4. Mallampati SR, Gatt SP, Guigino LD, et al. A clinical sign to predict difficult tracheal intubation: A prospective study. Can Anaesth Soc J 32:429, 1985.
5. Stoelting RK. Circulatory changes during direct laryngoscopy and tracheal intubation. Anesthesiology 47:381, 1977.
6. Roberts JT. Functional anatomy of the larynx. Int Anesthesiol Clin 28:101–106, 1990.
7. Benumof J. Management of the difficult airway: With special emphasis on awake tracheal intubation. Anesthesiology 75:1087, 1991.
8. Rex M. A review of the structural and functional bases of laryngospasm and a discussion of the nerve pathways involved in the reflex and its clinical significance in man and animals. Br J Anaesth 42:891, 1970.
9. Widdecombe J. Respiratory reflexes. In Handbook of Physiology, vol. 1. Washington, D.C.: American Physiology Society, 1984; p. 585.
10. Sellick B. Cricoid pressure to control regurgitation of stomach contents during induction of anesthesia. Lancet 2:404, 1961.
11. Williams PL, Warwick R. Gray's Anatomy, 36th ed. Philadelphia: W. B. Saunders, 1980.

CHAPTER 2

Airway Pathology

Max L. Goodman, M.D., and Ben Z. Pilch, M.D.

The airway system includes the oral cavity, nasal cavities and paranasal sinuses, pharynx, larynx, and trachea. The common pathologic lesions for these regions are discussed in this chapter.

ORAL CAVITY

Lesions of the oral cavity are presented in the following groupings: anomalies, benign exophytic lesions, cysts of the jaws, odontogenic tumor (ameloblastoma), fibro-osseous lesions of the jaw, salivary gland neoplasms, leukoplakia, and malignant neoplasms.

Anomalies of the Mouth. Anomalies of the mouth of importance are the clefts of the face from non-union of the processes that form the face and jaws. *Cleft lip* (cheiloschisis) usually involves the upper lip and may be unilateral or bilateral. It arises from non-union of the globular processes with the maxillary process. Cleft lip may vary from a slight indentation to involve the alveolar process or extend into the palate. *Cleft palate* may occur without cleft lip. The cleft palate anomaly may be associated with oxycephaly, polydactylism, and syndactylism. Patients with large cleft palate defects have regurgitation of food through the nose and problems with speech development.[4, 5]

Benign Exophytic Lesions of the Oral Cavity. Those most frequently observed in decreasing frequency and anatomic locations are (1) tori involving palate and mandible; (2) irritation fibromas involving gingival mucosa,

lip, tongue, and palate; (3) hemangiomas (pyogenic granuloma) involving lip, buccal areas, and tongue; (4) papillomas involving tongue and lips; and (5) mucoceles involving lip and buccal areas.[1–3]

Tori are nodular growths of bone that involve the palate in about 66% of the cases and the mandible in 33% of the cases.[6] Torus palatinus often takes the form of an irregular bony ridge along the mid-line of the palate. Torus mandibularis often presents as a shelf or ledge of bone along the inner aspect of the mandible, extending from the molar area to the mid-line; it may be bilateral. Histologically, tori are composed of lamellar or compact bone in irregular patterns. The importance of these lesions is usually related to their interference with the use of prosthetic devices.

Irritation fibroma includes the designations fibromas, fibrous epulides, fibrous hyperplasia, and fibroepithelial polyps.[2] They are most common in the gingiva; often, they can be related to chronic irritation, caused by dentures or prosthetic devices. Usually, the lesions are solitary and enlarge slowly, but occasionally they may be multiple and the growth may be rapid. Histologically, they are characterized by dense fibrous tissue with scant vascularity, occasional chronic inflammatory cells in perivascular areas, and, not infrequently, focal calcifications and, rarely, focal ossifications. The mucosa over the lesions is usually intact, with focal hyperplastic areas. If the mucosa is ulcerated, some active inflammatory response is present, with granulation tissue in the ulcerated area. Simple excision is usually curative, but recurrences are observed if the causal factors are not altered.

Hemangiomas and pyogenic granuloma are often difficult to separate on histologic grounds and may be grouped together.[7] Both may present as papillary bluish or red masses to flattened, broad-based, slightly raised lesions involving the gingiva, tongue, or buccal areas. The gingival hyperplasia associated with pregnancy simulates pyogenic granuloma. Histologically, the lesions are characterized by capillary to cavernous vascular proliferations. Vascular thrombosis and organization may be associated with calcification and, rarely, ossification (phleboliths). After thrombosis of vascular lesions, focal areas of fibrosis and scarring are present.

Angiomatous syndromes must be considered in dealing with oral cavity hemangiomas. *Osler-Weber-Rendu syndrome* is characterized by multiple capillary telangiectases involving face and body sites, with episodes of recurrent bleeding.[8] *Sturge-Weber syndrome* is a congenital syndrome characterized by venous angiomas of the leptomeninges, ipsilateral telangiectasia of the trigeminal region, contralateral hemiplegia, choroidal angioma with late glaucoma, intracranial calcifications, mental retardation, and epileptic seizures.[9, 10] Angiomas of the mouth in this syndrome may involve the gingiva to the extent that the teeth are partially obliterated. *Maffucci's syndrome* is characterized by enchondromas of bone and multiple hemangiomas with phleboliths.[11] The hemangiomas are usually located on the skin, but the oral cavity may be involved.

Squamous papillomas are common in the oral areas, and they may be located in the mucosa of the cheek, gingiva, palate, lips, and tongue.[2, 12] They present as pedunculated or broad-based lesions, varying in size from millimeters to centimeters. Histologically, they are characterized by squamous epithelial hyperplasia with a thin, fibrovascular stalk. Trauma may result in focal ulcerations with inflammatory cell responses. The hyperplastic mucosa may exhibit focal cellular atypicalities and perinuclear vacuolization (koilocytosis) suggestive of papilloma virus infection.[13]

Mucoceles are associated with minor salivary glands or the sublingual gland. The common sites are the lips, cheeks, the tip of the tongue, and the floor of mouth.[14] Histologically, the lesion consists of cystic spaces that contain mucoid and cellular debris, and which often are lined by connective tissue or partially lined by compressed duct or squamous epithelium. The surrounding connective tissue contains vacuolated macrophages and chronic inflammatory cells. The adjacent salivary gland tissue often shows focal periductal and interstitial chronic inflammatory cell infiltrates and focal duct ectasia. In the floor of mouth, the cysts are larger and may be termed ranulas. Occasionally, a floor of mouth mucocele may dissect along the fascial planes to become a plunging ranula and present as a submental neck mass.[15] To prevent recurrences of floor of mouth mucoceles, excision of the involved sublingual gland is recommended.[16]

Dermoid cysts and *enteric cysts* may be encountered in the floor of mouth area.[17, 18] Rarely, thyroglossal duct cysts occur in the foramen cecum area.[19] Usually, the thyroglossic duct lesions present as anterior neck masses, below the hyoid bone.[20]

Odontogenic Cysts. Intraosseous cysts may be divided into (1) fissural cysts (nasopalatine, median palatal, median mandibular, globulomaxillary, nasolabial); (2) odontogenic cysts (keratocyst, dentigerous, radicular); and (3) bone cysts (aneurysmal and unicameral bone cysts). Of these groupings, only the odontogenic cysts are discussed.

The *odontogenic keratocyst* may be referred to as a primordial cyst. It is thought to represent maldevelopment of the enamel organ, with cystification replacing tooth development. The more common location is the third molar area of the mandible. The cysts range in size from millimeters to several centimeters, with complete replacement of bone possible over long periods of time.[21] Histologically, the cyst is lined by stratified, slightly keratinizing squamous epithelium, which is regular and narrow in width, with folded invagination into surrounding connective tissue. Groups of epithelial cells some distance from the main cyst may be present with focal microcystic changes (daughter cysts). A characteristic feature of keratocyst is its propensity for recurrence if it is not completely excised.[22]

Dentigerous cysts occur in relation to tooth development, with attachments to the crown of the tooth and the accumulation of fluid between the crown and follicular epithelium of enamel development (follicular cyst). Dentigerous cysts affect only the permanent teeth.[21] Usually the cysts are small, but occasionally deformity may be present. Histologically, the cysts are lined by squamous epithelium in thin layers, with occasional mucus-producing cells. Odontogenic epithelial buds may be present in the surrounding fibrous stroma. The tooth and cyst relationship is easily documented on radiographic studies, and this relationship may be destroyed at surgical excision of the tooth and cyst. Rarely, ameloblastomas may arise in the wall of a dentigerous cyst.

Radicular cysts are usually small and occur at the apical area of the tooth root secondary to an inflammatory response from dental caries. Epithelial nests normally present around the roots of teeth (cell rests of Malassez) are stimulated by the inflammatory reaction to proliferate and extend into the granulation tissue. The epithelial proliferation may develop cystification to produce a squamous, epithelium-lined cyst surrounded by granulation tissue.[21] Following tooth extractions, the radicular cyst may remain in the bone and is termed a residual cyst. Histologically, the squamous epithelial proliferations are irregular, and eosinophilic deposits (Rushton bodies) may be present in the epithelial areas. The inflammatory response may include cholesterol granulomata secondary to hemorrhage.

Odontogenic Neoplasms. These include ameloblastoma, adenomatoid odontogenic tumor, calcifying epithelial odontogenic tumor, calcifying odontogenic cyst, ameloblastic fibroma, odontoma (complex and compound), dentinoma, cementoma, and myxofibroma. Of this group, the more common ameloblastoma is discussed.

Ameloblastoma represents about 1% of all oral tumors, with a peak incidence in the fourth decade of life. The most common location is the mandible (80%), in the molar or ramus areas.[23, 24] Symptoms are few until dental problems or facial deformity develops. The tumor may produce extensive bone destruction. Bone fractures and extensions into soft tissues are late manifestations of ameloblastoma. Not infrequently, the radiographic appearance is described as unilocular or multilocular cysts. Grossly, the tumor produces fusiform enlargements of bone. Cut surface of bone shows replacement by gray-white to yellowish-brown tumor that occasionally may have cystic areas. Histologically, the tumor has large nests of epithelial cells in a thin connective tissue stroma (follicular pattern) or anastomosing cords or strands of epithelial cells in a fibrous stroma (plexiform pattern). The epithelial structures mimic the developing tooth germ, with peripheral basaloid ameloblasts and a central area simulating the stellate reticulum of normal enamel organ. The stellate areas often show microcystification and degenerated eosinophilic material. Keratinization and intercellular bridges may be observed, and, rarely, a granular cytoplasm is seen in the stellate cells. The connective tissue may have prominent vascularity. Peripheral (extraosseous) ameloblastomas may simulate basal cell carcinoma.[25, 26] Ameloblastomas have a great propensity for recurrence if they are incompletely excised.[27]

Fibro-osseous Lesions of the Jaw. These include the following designations: (1) brown tumor of hyperparathyroidism, (2) giant cell reparative granuloma, (3) fibrous dysplasia, (4) ossifying fibroma, (5) cementifying fibroma, (6) cherubism, and (7) Paget's disease of bone.

Hyperparathyroidism may result in osteitis fibrosa cystica ("brown tumor" of bone), which occasionally involves the jaws.[28] It has been suggested that this development is probably related to bone turnover due to masticatory stresses.[29, 30] Grossly, the brown tumor forms a mass that expands bone. Radiologically, the jaw shows a radiolucent area that is well defined. Histologically, the morphology is identical to reparative giant cell granuloma. Giant cells of the osteoclastic type, which have an irregular distribution, are a characteristic feature. Areas of hemorrhage with hemosiderin deposits are numerous, in a dense fibrous tissue proliferation. Occasional trabeculae of woven bone are present in the fibrous tissue.

Giant cell granuloma may present as a predominantly soft-tissue gingival lesion with focal bone involvement (giant cell epulis) or predominantly as a bone lesion (reparative granuloma).[31, 32] It usually occurs in young adults; females are affected more frequently than males. The anatomic location is most common in the mandible in tooth-bearing areas. Radiographically, the appearance is a bone radiolucency that may suggest multilocular growth. Histologically, the morphology is identical to the brown tumor of hyperparathyroidism.

Giant cell granuloma is thought possibly to result from intramedullary hemorrhage or trauma. It is important to separate these lesions from primary giant cell tumors of bone, which are considered to be neoplasms.[32–34] The giant cell granuloma is a benign condition, although occasional recurrences may develop.

Ossifying fibroma, cementifying fibroma, and fibrous dysplasia share several common histologic features, and recognition of individual entities requires clinical–pathologic–radiologic correlations to establish a diagnosis.

Fibrous dysplasia of bone may manifest as monostotic or polyostotic lesions in childhood or adolescence, and the possibility of Albright's syndrome (polyostotic bone lesions, cutaneous pigmentation, endocrine disorders, and precocious puberty) should be excluded.[35] The skeletal distribution of fibrous dysplasia is varied, but when the upper limb is involved, the skull bones may be involved.[36] It is estimated that approximately 10% of fibrous dysplasias of bone involve skull bones. The maxilla is more frequently involved in monostotic fibrous dysplasia. The symptoms are often minor, with gradual development of facial asymmetry or bone fracture from minimal trauma as the presenting complaint. Grossly, the bone appears hypertrophied, and extensive lesions produce distortion and obstruction of paranasal sinuses and nasal cavities.

Radiographically, the diffuse involvement of bone with a ground-glass translucency is characteristic.[35] Histologically, the bone is replaced by fibrous tissue with varying patterns of woven-bone trabeculae. Occasionally, the woven-bone patterns are minimal, with a predominately fibrous tissue proliferation. The fibrous dysplasia lesions tend to stabilize on completion of skeletal growth. Conservative surgical management is the treatment of choice.

Ossifying fibroma presents as a localized tumor of bone, rather than as diffuse enlargement of bone, as seen in fibrous dysplasia.[37] The mandible is involved more frequently than the maxilla, and occasionally the lesions may be multifocal.[38] Radiographically, the lesion produces a radiolucent area that is well defined, with a thin osteosclerotic rim. Occasionally, the lesions merge with the peripheral marginal bone patterns.

Histologically, the fibroblastic and woven-bone patterns are similar to fibrous dysplasia. Features that may be observed in ossifying fibroma are osteoblastic rimming of the woven-bone trabeculae and occasional osteoclasts among the bone fragments. These findings are not usually seen in fibrous dysplasia. The biologic behavior of ossifying fibroma tends to be self-limiting, but occasionally the lesion continues to increase in size, simulating a neoplasm, and it may involve large areas of bone, simulating fibrous dysplasia.

Cementifying fibroma is histologically similar to fibrous dysplasia and ossifying fibroma of the jaws. It characteristically has abundant cementum deposits in the fibrous stroma, as well as woven-bone trabeculae. Both fibrous dysplasia and ossifying fibroma of the jaws may have varying degrees of cementum-like deposits. Radiographically, the cementifying fibroma lesions tend to be multiple and usually occur at the apices of the mandibular incisor teeth.[39, 40]

Most of the lesions are picked up as incidental findings in the radiographic examination of the teeth. Therefore, it tends to be observed in adults, rather than in children. Occasionally, the cementifying fibroma produces a large lesion that has been termed "giant cementifying fibroma."[41]

Cherubism refers to hereditary fibrous dysplasia of the jaws, recognized by Jones in 1933.[42] The maxillary and mandibular enlargements produce hypertelorism, irregularly placed deciduous teeth, upper displacement of eye globes, and fullness of the cheeks and submandibular areas. The radiographic examinations usually show well-defined areas of radiolucency, occasionally with sclerotic or ground-glass appearances.[43, 44] Histologically, the bone is replaced by fibrous tissue proliferations that contain various amounts of woven bone, giant cells, and hemorrhagic areas. Surgical intervention is often required for cosmetic effects, although the lesions tend to regress after puberty.[45]

Paget's disease of bone refers to repeated episodes of osteolysis followed by excessive repair that results in increased bone mass and skeletal deformity.[46] It is seen in older adults. The skull is frequently involved in Paget's disease of bone. The maxilla is more commonly involved than the mandible. The bony enlargement may result in facial deformities, denture malfunction, difficulty in extractions of teeth, and bone fractures with minimal trauma. Radiographically, the bone involvement shows alternating areas of lucency and increased density (cotton wool effect).[47]

Histologically, the changes are osteoclastic resorption and fibrosis with increased vascularity, followed by osteoid deposits and bone deposition in irregular distribution without ensheathed lamellar haversian canal patterns. This process continues with disruption of normal bone architecture, which results in a mosaic bone pattern and loss of tensile strength. In the jaws, the increased bone metabolism stimulates hyperplastic cementum deposits along the roots of the teeth, resulting in ankylosis of the teeth.[48] The increased bone metabolism in Paget's disease of bone results in higher incidence of osteosarcoma, especially in the presence of multiple bone involvement. The increased vascularity of bone in Paget's disease may result in arterial–venous shunts with increased cardiac output and thereby contribute to cardiac failure. Calcitonin, mithramycin, and diphosphonate compounds may produce improvements in patients with Paget's disease of bone.[46]

Leukoplakia. Leukoplakia refers to white patch or plaque that persists after attempts to scrape it away. The incidence of leukoplakia in association with oral cancer varies from 10% to 60%.[49] Lesions that correlate with in situ carcinoma changes have confluent erythematous areas or speckled erythematous areas. Bouquot and Gorlin reported age-specific prevalence rates of oral leukoplakia to be 2.7 lesions per 1000 for young adults and 43.0 lesions per 1000 for adults over 70 years of age.[50] Most investigators have been unable to establish the risk of malignant transformation of oral leukoplakia. Follow-up data have suggested a range of 4% to 36%.[51] Histologically, leukoplakia represents keratosis and epithelial hyperplasia. The squamous epithelial cell atypicalities vary from minimal to marked. The marked atypicalities are thought to have the ability to progress into in situ carcinoma. Some observers have suggested intraepithelial neoplasia for the atypicalities that suggest in situ carcinoma. "Hairy" leukoplakia (oral condyloma planus) has been recognized among human immunodeficiency virus (HIV) positive individuals or acquired immunodeficiency syndrome (AIDS) patients.[52] This lesion is characterized by parakeratosis, koilocytotic changes, and surface candidiasis.[53, 54]

Malignant Neoplasms. *Squamous cell carcinoma* is the predominant malignancy of the oral cavity. The percent of oral carcinoma to all body cancers varies by country, from 1% in Norway to 47% in India. Industrial countries have a rate that varies from 3% to 7%.[3] Predisposing factors include tobacco and alcohol abuse. Grossly, squamous cell carcinomas can present as exophytic papillary growths to ulcerated, indurated tumors. Early carcinoma may present with a granular mucosal surface, indurated nodule, or superficial ulcer that bleeds on manipulation. The more common anatomic locations are the tongue, floor of mouth, and retromolar trigone areas.

The histology of squamous cell carcinoma varies from well-differentiated keratinizing neoplasms to poorly differentiated anaplastic neoplasms, with the majority of the neoplasms demonstrating intermediate or moderately differentiated patterns. The infiltrative borders are irregular, with small clusters of cells or individual cells. Squamous cell carcinoma may extensively involve the lymphatics.

The oral cavity carcinomas may produce metastases to the ipsilateral submandibular lymph nodes and jugular lymph nodes.[55] The prognosis for oral cancer is related to the stage of the tumor at time of diagnosis.[56-58]

Verrucous carcinoma is a subtype of squamous cell carcinoma characterized by a broad-based, verrucous growth that may extend for several centimeters. Histologically, the appearance is that of hyperplastic squamous epithelium without evidence of nuclear anaplasia. It is separated from verrucous hyperplasia by the presence of pushing borders and a dense inflammatory response. Verrucous carcinoma usually does not metastasize. It is important to exclude the coexistence of foci of less well-differentiated squamous carcinoma. Surgery is the treatment of choice for verrucous carcinoma, although radiation therapy may be used to control the tumor.[59-61]

Sarcomas of all types occur in the oral cavity areas, but the most frequent is the osteogenic sarcoma of bone with chondroblastic features.[62, 63] Kaposi's sarcoma may be seen in the oral cavity and mucous membrane areas, and its association with AIDS may result in a high incidence in certain patient populations.[64] Grossly, it may appear as small, hemorrhagic plaques in the mucosa. Histologically, Kaposi's sarcoma is characterized by a spindle cell and vascular proliferation with infiltrative patterns. Occasionally, it may simulate granulation tissue, and the diagnosis is difficult to establish.

Salivary Gland Neoplasms. These represent a variegated group of tumors. Anatomic distribution of salivary gland tumors is best illustrated by Willis's rule of tens: "for every 100 parotid neoplasms, there will be 10 submandibular gland neoplasms, 10 minor salivary gland neoplasms, and 1 sublingual gland neoplasm."[65] The palate is the most frequent site of salivary gland neoplasms of the oral cavity.[66]

Pleomorphic adenoma (mixed tumor) presents as a rounded, firm, nodular mass that may have been present for long periods of time. Grossly, the tumors have a sharp demarcation from adjacent tissues and tend to separate easily. It is recommended that rims of normal tissue be excised with these tumors, in order to reduce the possibility of recurrence. Histologically, the pleomorphic adenoma has epithelial and mesenchymal patterns in a wide variety of combinations. The mesenchymal components are thought to be a product of the myoepithelial cells, justifying the term pleomorphic adenoma. Approximately 5% of the pleomorphic adenomas develop malignancies.[67-69]

Adenoid cystic carcinoma may be confused with pleomorphic adenoma both clinically and histologically. Adenoid cystic carcinoma is a low-grade neoplasm that may persist for years before the aggressive growth becomes apparent.[70, 71] Clinically, it presents as a mucosal thickening and induration or as submucosal nodules. Grossly, the tumors are infiltrative rather than well demarcated. Histologically, they manifest three growth patterns: tubular, cribriform, and solid with infiltrative borders. The malignancy has a propensity to extend along nerves, blood vessels, and ducts. Bone involvement may be difficult to demonstrate by radiographic studies, because it penetrates around bone trabeculae and down haversian canals with minimal bone resorption or destruction.[72] The patient prognosis for this neoplasm probably is best related to the extent of tumor at the time of diagnosis, rather than to cell patterns.[73, 74]

Polymorphous low-grade adenocarcinoma of minor salivary glands represents a low-grade carcinoma that in part simulates pleomorphic adenoma and adenoid cystic carcinoma. The multiple epithelial patterns and myxoid-to-hyalinized stroma are like pleomorphic adenomas in nature, and the infiltrative extensions with perineural and perivascular invasions simulate adenoid cystic carcinoma. The palate is the most frequent location of this neoplasm. It has a propensity for recurrence and local extensions, but rarely metastasizes. Recurrent tumors may simulate adenoid cystic carcinoma to the extent that they are designated adenoid cystic carcinoma rather than polymorphous low-grade adenocarcinoma.[75–78]

Mucoepidermoid carcinoma of salivary glands manifests in two patterns, a low-grade neoplasm and a high-grade neoplasm. This tumor is more frequent in the major salivary glands, where it represents about 5% to 10% of salivary gland neoplasms. It is less frequent in minor salivary gland locations.[79] The low-grade mucoepidermoid carcinoma presents similarly to the pleomorphic adenoma, as a slowly enlarging painless mass; occasionally, it may simulate inflammatory lesions. The high-grade mucoepidermoid carcinoma presents with rapid growth, pain, and ulceration.[80] Grossly, the low-grade mucoepidermoid carcinoma appears encapsulated and cystic. The high-grade mucoepidermoid carcinoma is solid and infiltrative. Histologically, the low-grade tumor shows irregular fibrosis, with mucous-secreting epithelium and squamous epithelium, in ductal and cystic patterns. High-grade mucoepidermoid carcinoma has focal squamous epithelial differentiation, with nuclear anaplasia and scant evidence of mucous-secreting cells. Fibrosis is prominent, with diffuse infiltrative extensions.

The recurrence rate for low-grade tumors is about 15% over a 5-year period. The high-grade carcinomas are aggressive, with about a 25% 5-year survival rate. The patients with intermediate histologic patterns of mucoepidermoid carcinoma tend to behave similarly to those with low-grade tumors, and the histologic morphology simulates high-grade tumors.[81]

Necrotizing sialometaplasia occurs predominately in palatal areas and mimics mucoepidermoid carcinoma or squamous cell carcinoma in small biopsy specimens.[82] It is a benign ulcerative lesion that develops over a short time period.[83] Histologically, the tissues show infarct-type necrosis, with squamous metaplasia of residual salivary gland ducts and pseudoepitheliomatous hyperplasia of squamous epithelium at the ulcerated margin. This is associated with an inflammatory response of acute and chronic inflammatory cells. The cause of the lesion is unknown, but pressure on the palatal artery as it passes through the foramen is a possible explanation. In other locations, the lesion is related to tissue injuries or vascular thromboses.[84]

Sjögren's syndrome (lymphoepithelial lesion) refers to chronic inflammatory changes and hyposecretion of the lacrimal and salivary glands, resulting in keratoconjunctivitis sicca and xerostomia. Often, the patients have clinical evidence of connective tissue disease.[85] The major salivary glands and minor salivary glands may develop tumor-like masses or diffuse enlargements, and there is occasionally massive lymphadenopathy. Histologically, the lesion is characterized by a dense lymphoid infiltrate that contains germinal centers, associated with epithelial–myoepithelial proliferations of ducts. Occasionally, the epithelial–myoepithelial nests may simulate carcinoma. The dense lymphoid infiltrates may simulate lymphoma. About 6% of the patients with Sjögren's syndrome develop malignant lymphoma.[86–88] It is thought that Sjögren's syndrome probably represents an autoimmune reaction.[89]

Macroglossia may be produced by congential hyperplasia, vascular tumors (hemangioma and lymphangioma), or extensive amyloid deposits (amyloidosis). Amyloid deposits may be localized or diffuse and primary or secondary. Histologically, amyloid material is a homogeneous eosinophilic deposit of proteins that appear acellular and produce compression atrophy and replacement of normal structures. Occasionally, there are foreign-body giant cell reactions to the amyloid deposits and occasional plasma cell infiltrates. Histochemically, amyloid deposits stain with Congo red reagents, which produces an apple-green birefringence on polarization.[90, 91]

NASAL CAVITIES AND PARANASAL SINUSES

Inflammatory polyps, most of which are allergic in orgin, represent a common cause of obstruction of air flow through the nasal cavities or paranasal sinuses. In contrast to neoplastic polypoid lesions, inflammatory polyps are usually bilateral and translucent to light.[92] Histologically, they are characterized by submucosal edema with scattered eosinophils and chronic inflammatory cells. The turbinates may be involved by inflammatory polyps. Treatment involves establishing an open airway and identifying the causative agents.[93, 94]

Acute and chronic sinusitis and rhinitis are often related to allergies or obstructive masses. Any lesion that obstructs the sinus drainage predisposes to sinus infection. Recurrent episodes of sinus infection induce mucous secretions, which accumulate in an obstructed sinus to produce a mucopyocele. The mucopyocele may induce bone resorption and deformities of the involved anatomic areas. Treatment is aimed at relieving the obstruction and establishing sinus drainage. The frontal sinus areas may require obliteration with adipose tissue.[95]

Granulomatous lesions that may result in sinus and nasal deformities are syphilis,[96] sarcoidosis,[97] tuberculosis,[98] rhinoscleroma,[99] Wegener's granulomatosis,[100] relapsing polychrondritis,[101] and lethal mid-line granuloma (polymorphic reticulosis, angiocentric malignant lymphoma).[102] Fungal lesions most frequently encountered in the paranasal sinuses and nasal cavities are *aspergilloma* or fungus ball in an obstructed sinus without tissue invasion and *mucormycosis.*[103] Occasionally, *Aspergillus* fungi may invade the tissues to produce vasculitis, microabscesses, and granulomata with giant cells.[103] The fungus in mucormycosis is invasive into the tissues, with vascular thrombosis and tissue necrosis. It occurs in diabetic or immune-suppressed patients and requires emergency debridement to permit patient survival.[104]

Systemic *Wegener's granulomatosis* manifests with lesions in the upper airways, lung, and kidneys.[105] Localized lesions that precede the systemic involvement are now recognized.[106] The upper airway lesion varies from mucosal crusting to large, destructive, ulcerative involvement. Histologically, Wegener's granulomatosis is characterized by the presence of collagen degeneration; palisading histiocytes; giant cells; inflammatory cell infiltrates with eosinophils; microabscesses; and vasculitis involving arteries, veins, and capillaries.[107] Nasal bone destruction may result in a saddle-nose deformity. The antineutrophil cystoplasmic antibody elevation in the serum of patients with Wegener's granulomatosis has been helpful in establishing the diagnosis.[108] Early lesions of Wegener's granulomatosis may respond to cyclophosphamide therapy and steroids, without progression to systemic involvement.

Angiocentric malignant lymphoma, previously termed lethal mid-line granuloma, is discussed with the granulomatous lesions because the ulcerative clinical presentation is easily confused with granulomatous lesions. It is a lymphoproliferative lesion characterized by an angiocentric, angioinvasive, pleomorphic infiltrate of lymphocytes, plasma cells, eosinophils, histiocytes, and atypical lymphoid cells with immunoblastic features.[109] A T-cell phenotype has been identified in some of the lesions.[110, 111] Vascular thrombosis and necrosis produces ulceration associated with secondary infection in the surface areas. Angiocentric malignant lymphoma may have an indolent course with a good response to single-agent chemotherapy, or may progress to systemic lymphoma.[112] Radiation therapy has been effective in some patients.

Pyogenic granuloma (polypoid granulation tissue, lobular capillary hemangioma) is a polypoid vascular proliferation that may occur in several locations, but which is commonly encountered on the nasal septum.[113] Repeated trauma, as seen with "nose pickers," is the usual etiologic agent. Slight manipulation of the polypoid lesions may produce epistaxis. Simple excision is curative.

Angiofibroma (juvenile nasopharyngeal angiofibroma) is a rare tumor, and is seen predominately in juvenile males. It usually presents with nasal obstruction or episodes of epistaxis. Anatomic locations tend to be in the nasopharynx and posterolateral wall of the nasal cavity. The tumor is similar to a vascular sponge that continues to bleed from simple biopsy injuries and can bleed extensively at time of resection.[114] Histologically, it is characterized by a fibrovascular stroma that contains numerous vascular spaces, some of which are partially surrounded by smooth muscle without evidence of elastic fibers. Blood loss from surgical excisions has varied from 2 to 37 pints. Angiographic studies with embolization of the tumor vessels have reduced the blood loss to accepted levels at the time of surgical excision. Angiofibromas recur if incompletely excised.[115] Occasionally, the tumors regress after puberty. Radiation therapy has been used in some centers to control this tumor, but the possibility of a radiation-induced malignancy must be considered in this age group.[116]

Other vascular tumors that may be seen in the sinonasal areas are hemangioma, hemangiopericytoma, angiomyoma, and angiosarcoma.[113] Most of the neoplastic lesions of the nasal cavity and paranasal sinus may present as polypoid masses with varying degrees of obstruction or other related symptons.

Inverted papilloma (Schneiderian papilloma) represents a benign, neoplastic proliferation of respiratory epithelium. In contrast to the bilaterality of allergic or inflammatory polyps, these lesions tend to be unilateral.[117] The papillomas have a propensity for recurrences, and approximately 5% develop malignant alterations into squamous cell carcinoma. Anatomic locations in order of frequency are lateral nasal wall, maxillary sinus, nasal cavity and sinus areas, and nasal septum.[118] Grossly, the papillary masses are opaque to light, in contrast to the translucency of inflammatory polyps, and tend to bleed upon manipulation. Histologically, the inverted papilloma is characterized by papillary and inverting patterns of hyperplastic respiratory epithelium, with varying degrees of transitional epithelial and squamous epithelial differentiation. Mucinous microcysts in the proliferating epithelium and inflammatory cell infiltrates of the epithelium and stroma are usually present. The nasal septal lesions have fungiform papillary patterns, and the maxillary sinus tumors often exhibit an oxyphilic, cylindrical cell morphology with abundant mucous production (cylindrical cell papilloma).[119]

Some of the inverted papilloma lesions have stained with papilloma virus antibodies, suggesting the possibility of a viral cause for some of the tumors.[120] A lateral rhinotomy with removal of all visible tumor and adjacent mucosa reduces the incidence of recurrences.

Squamous cell carcinoma is the most frequent malignancy of the paranasal sinuses and nasal cavities. Approximately 80% of the lesions originate in the maxillary sinus; the remainder originate from the ethmoid and nasal cavity areas.[121] Primary malignancies of the sphenoid and frontal sinuses are rare. Carcinomas arising in the superior nasal septal areas, antroethmoid areas, and posterior nasal cavity region tend to be biologically aggressive with poorly differentiated cellular patterns. Carcinomas in other locations tend to be well to moderately differentiated.[122]

The symptomatology for sinus cancer may mimic inflammatory lesions. Tumors in oral–antral regions often present with tooth pain, loosening of teeth, or denture problems. Nasal tumors produce nasal obstruction (stuffiness), watery or bloody discharge (epistaxis), and visible tumor mass. Tumors adjacent to the orbit may result in displacement of the globe, diplopia, and occasionally a palpable mass in orbital soft tissues. Facial asymmetry and cranial nerve dysfunction may occur.[123]

The carcinomas usually spread by local extension, with metastasis developing in about 10% to 20% of the patients. The usual metastatic sites are superior jugular lymph nodes, submental lymph nodes, and retropharyngeal nodes. Effective treatment modalities include surgical excision and radiation therapy.[124]

Histologically, squamous cell carcinoma of the paranasal sinuses may have a well-differentiated, keratinizing appearance, transitional cell (nonkeratinizing) appearance, or an undifferentiated or poorly differentiated appearance. Malignancies that may be encountered in these anatomic sites include adenocarcinoma, salivary gland malignancies, malignant melanoma, olfactory neuroblastoma, malignant lymphoma, plasmacytoma, rhabdomyosarcoma, and neuroendocrine carcinoma. To establish the correct diagnosis, immunoperoxidase stains and electron microscopic studies are often required.

Malignant melanoma of the nasal cavity is rare, but important to recognize because of its poor prognosis with all treatment modalities.[125, 126]

Olfactory neuroblastoma (esthesioneuroblastoma) histologically simulates neuroblastoma and retinoblastoma of the infant, except for occurrence in an adult in the areas of the olfactory placode. It is a rare neoplasm, and the presentation is similar to other malignant nasal tumors. It is radiosensitive, but usual treatment modalities include a combination of surgery and radiation therapy.[127, 128]

Adenocarcinoma of the paranasal sinuses and nasal cavity is uncommon, and observers have noted a relation to the occupation of wood workers. Histologically, the carcinomas may be well differentiated or anaplastic, simulating intestinal carcinoma. Mucous secretions are variable. Local recurrences are frequent and metastases are rare.[129–131]

Sarcomas of all types occur in the sinus and

nasal cavity areas, but the frequency is rare; they are not discussed, except for plasmacytoma.

Plasmacytoma refers to a localized plasma cell malignancy that may be a solitary lesion of bone or an extramedullary lesion of soft tissues. Multiple myeloma (myelomatosis) represents systemic manifestation of a plasma cell malignancy with multiple sites of involvement and serum protein alterations.[132] The *extramedullary plasmacytomas* occur most frequently in the upper airway regions of the nasal cavity and nasopharynx and represent less than 1% of head and neck malignancies. They tend to be more frequent in male patients in the sixth decade or later.[133] Symptoms may vary from days to years and include pain, nasal obstruction, and epistaxis. The maxillary sinus areas are the most frequent anatomic sites. Grossly, the neoplasms are soft and gelatinous, with hemorrhagic to gray-white coloration. Histologically, the lesions are characterized by replacement of tissue structures by dense plasma cell infiltration associated with immature forms. Multinucleated pleomorphic cells and localized amyloid deposits may occur in plasmacytoma. It is important to distinguish these lesions from inflammatory processes and undifferentiated carcinoma, which represent the more frequent areas of confusion.

All patients with plasmacytoma should be thoroughly studied in order to exclude systemic manifestations of multiple myeloma. Over a 20-year period, approximately 20% to 30% of patients develop systemic multiple myeloma.[134]

Localized extramedullary plasmacytomas are usually very radiosensitive, with excellent responses. Patients should, however, be followed for recurrent tumors or systemic manifestations.

Malignant lymphoma of the paranasal sinus and nasal cavity areas are rare, and they usually manifest as large cell, diffuse-type lesions. Immunoperoxidase stains are helpful in classifying the malignant lymphomas. Recently, T-cell lymphoma of the upper air passages has been recognized, as discussed in the section on polymorphic reticulosis.[135]

NASOPHARYNX, ORAL PHARYNX, AND HYPOPHARYNX

The nasopharynx and oral pharynx contain abundant lymphoid deposits in tonsillar and adenoid areas, producing Waldeyer's ring.

Inflammatory reactions (acute and chronic tonsillitis and adenoiditis) stimulate lymphphoid tissue hyperplasia, resulting in marked enlargements of the lymphoid tissue and thereby producing varying degrees of airway obstruction. In children, the obstruction is more apparent because of the smaller airway passages.[136]

The most common problem is recurrent episodes of inflammation with persistent lymphoid hyperplasia over long periods of time. To relieve the airway obstruction, it is often necessary to resect the hyperplastic lymphoid tissue with tonsillectomies or adenoidectomies.[137]

Histologically, the tonsillar tissue shows inflammatory cell infiltrates of the cryptic epithelium and follicular lymphoid hyperplasia. The inflammatory cell infiltrates vary from polymorphonuclear leukocytes to plasma cells, eosinophils, macrophages, and lymphocytes. Fibrous bands between crypts may be seen with repeated episodes of infection and tissue destruction. The fibrous bands frequently destroy the fascial plane between tonsil and muscle, resulting in sectioning through skeletal muscle at the time of excision, which may produce excessive bleeding. The adenoid histology tends to have more prominent lymphoid hyperplasia and minimal cryptic inflammatory cell infiltrates.

The lingual tonsils are rarely excised because of the vascularity and tissue edema from trauma to the area. Steroid medications have been helpful in reducing the edema to the area if resection is necessary.

Peritonsillar abscesses (quinsy tonsillitis) are usually due to streptococcal or staphylococcal infections of the tonsil with spread to the fascial plane that covers the superior constrictor muscle, thereby resulting in tissue destruction and abscess formation. Clinically, there are episodes of sore throat with increasing pain, swelling of the soft tissues, muffled voice, and difficulty swallowing with drooling.[138] Treatment is to provide drainage and antibiotic therapy, which is followed by tonsillectomy to prevent the possibility of recurrent infection.[139]

Retropharyngeal abscesses are rare, but they are life threatening in children and occasionally in adults. Children present with difficult breathing, stridor, nasal obstruction, muffled crying, and extended head. Incision and drainage are required in order to prevent spread into other facial planes or possible rupture with asphyxiation.

Nasopharyngeal carcinoma represents a silent malignancy that produces symptoms after extensive spread of the tumor. It is an uncommon tumor in the United States, but is common in southern China and southeast Asian countries.

Etiologic considerations include genetic, environmental, and viral. Epstein-Barr virus (EBV) antibodies have been shown to be elevated in nasopharyngeal carcinoma patients, but their role as an etiologic agent has not been established.

The common sites for nasopharyngeal carcinoma are the lateral wall and roof of the nasopharynx. Clinical presentations include hearing loss, nasal obstruction, neck masses, and cranial nerve palsies. Histologically, nasopharyngeal carcinoma is composed of squamous cells with keratinized, nonkeratinized, and undifferentiated patterns. The nonkeratinizing and undifferentiated patterns are the most common and are the ones associated with elevated EBV antibody titers in the serum.

Therapy for nasopharyngeal carcinoma is radiation therapy with neck dissections for uncontrolled metastasis.[140] Tonsillar tissue may give rise to malignancies of the nasopharyngeal carcinoma type.

Malignant lymphomas of the non-Hodgkin's type occur in the Waldeyer's ring area. They present as unilateral submucosal masses that may have focal ulcerations. Histologically, all types of lymphoma may be seen in these regions. Leukemic infiltrations of Waldeyer's ring tend to be of chronic lymphocytic or acute lymphocytic type.

PARAPHARYNGEAL MASSES

Most parapharyngeal masses are schwannomas or pleomorphic adenomas. The parapharyngeal pleomorphic adenomas arise from the deep lobe of the parotid gland, and the relation to the parotid may be difficult to establish. Schwannomas may arise from myelinated nerves in any location. Schwannomas tend to be encapsulated, with easy separation from the surrounding tissues. The vascularity of the schwannoma usually differentiates it from the pleomorphic adenoma. The vascular spaces in schwannomas may develop thrombosis, resulting in areas of hemorrhagic necrosis and occasionally cystification.[141]

LARYNX/UPPER TRACHEA

Congenital Anomalies

The most common laryngeal congenital anomaly causing stridor and upper respiratory obstruction in infants is *laryngomalacia,* which accounts for about 65% to 75% of congenital laryngeal anomalies.[142, 143] The epiglottis of the neonate is softer, more pliable, and less rigid than in the adult, and there is often a relatively exaggerated infolding of its lateral edges, as well as a longer, more tubular shape.[144, 145] Excessive flaccidity of the soft epiglottis and the loose aryepiglottic folds cause these structures to collapse on inspiration, causing stridor. Histologically, edematous aryepiglottic folds have been noted.[143] These changes are aggravated with crying and agitation, because the inspiratory effort, and hence the collapse of the soft and flabby supraglottic structures, is greater. Interestingly, on induction of general anesthesia with a mask, the decreased agitation and less forceful respiratory movements lead to a decrease in the stridor, a significant differential diagnostic point.[146] As the child grows, the epiglottis stiffens, flaccidity lessens, and the laryngomalacia disappears; therefore, aggressive therapy is rarely indicated.

Congenital vocal cord paralysis or paresis may be unilateral or bilateral. Bilateral paralysis usually is caused by a disorder of the central nervous system, such as hydrocephalus, fourth ventricle lesions, intracerebral hemorrhage, cerebral agenesis, meningoencephalocele, or Arnold-Chiari malformation.[142, 146, 147] The position of the paralyzed cords, in abduction or adduction, contributes to the relative severity of aspiration or respiratory obstruction, respectively. Fortunately, unilateral cord paralysis is more common, especially on the left,[142, 147] the side of the longer recurrent laryngeal nerve. Left-sided paralysis may be associated with congenital cardiovascular anomalies or, in older individuals, mediastinal cysts or tumors. Unilateral paralysis is more commonly idiopathic, however, and often is temporary, with spontaneous improvement.[142] Bilateral paralysis is the more serious disorder.

Congenital subglottic stenosis may be caused by abnormalities of the soft tissues or cricoid cartilage.[147, 148] A histologically studied example of congenital soft-tissue subglottic stenosis showed hyperplasia of normal structures (seromucinous glands and fibrofatty tissue) without inflammation. Cricoid abnormalities, such as a more ovoid shape than normal, can narrow the subglottic space. Acquired subglottic stenosis, such as after intubation injury, is discussed later.

Congenital *laryngeal webs* (Fig. 2–1) are most commonly glottic, but may be subglottic or supraglottic as well. They are caused by

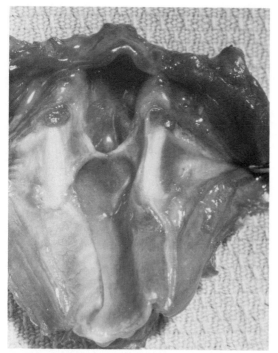

Figure 2–1. Laryngeal web at approximately the level of the true cords, the most common location for congenital laryngeal webs.

various degrees of failure of recanalization of the embryonic larynx,[142, 147] and thus may be thin or thick.

A defect in posterior fusion of the embryologic cricoid lamina or tracheoesophageal septum causes a *laryngeal* or *laryngotracheal cleft*.[149] There may be associated anomalies such as tracheoesophageal fistula or absence of various tracheal rings. Histologically, there is a defect in the posterior cricoid lamina, with a corresponding defect in the overlying mucosa; thus, a direct continuity exists between the respiratory laryngeal mucosa and squamous postcricoid mucosa. A corresponding hypoplasia of the interarytenoid muscle has been reported.[149]

Saccular cysts are cystic enlargements of the laryngeal saccule, an appendiceal outpouching at the end of the laryngeal ventricle. The cysts are fluid filled and do not communicate with the laryngeal lumen, as do *laryngoceles,* air-filled dilatations of the saccule. Saccular cysts may be congenital or acquired (Fig. 2–2). When large and congenital, they can present as rare, large, submucosal cystic supraglottic masses, often in the aryepiglottic fold region,[147] and can produce significant airway obstruction. With such large cysts, aspiration of cyst fluid is rarely curative, and marsupialization is gen-

erally required.[146] Acquired saccular cysts can become infected, and may very rarely be associated with carcinoma.[150, 151] Laryngoceles are usually acquired lesions. They may be related to repeated increases in intralaryngeal pressure, as in wind instrument players,[152] but this relation is not universally accepted.[150] Laryngoceles may be external, protruding laterally into the neck through an opening in the thyrohyoid membrane; internal, protruding into the region of the false cord and aryepiglottic fold; or combined.[151] The lining of laryngoceles and saccular cysts is the lining of the normal saccule (ie, respiratory epithelium and subepithelial seromucinous glands).

Infantile subglottic hemangioma usually presents before 6 months of age. The frequently eccentric subglottic mass often produces stridor and severe respiratory embarrassment. In about half the patients, cutaneous hemangiomas are present.[142, 146, 153] A soft subglottic mass, bluish in color, on direct laryngoscopy is generally diagnostic.[142] Biopsy usually does not result in severe hemorrhagic complications.[153] Histologically, the tumor is almost always a capillary hemangioma of infantile type, a hemangioendotheliomatous lesion that is more cellular and solid appearing than adult capillary hemangiomas (Fig. 2–3). The vascular spaces infiltrate and surround normal struc-

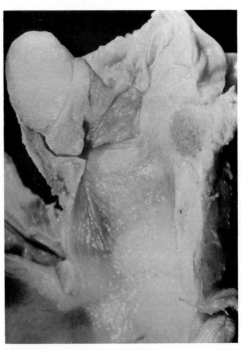

Figure 2–2. Saccular cyst filled with mucus, located at the tip of the laryngeal ventricle.

Figure 2–3. Subglottic hemangioma. A cellular proliferation of plump endothelial cells with small inconspicuous vascular lumina. An uninvolved central glandular structure is surrounded by tumor. (From Shapshay SM, Aretz HT. Benign Lesions of the Larynx. Alexandria, VA: American Academy of Otolaryngology Head and Neck Surgery Foundation, Inc.; copyright 1984, with permission.)

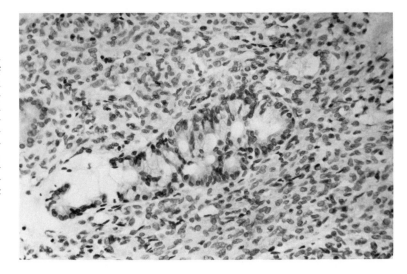

tures, such as seromucinous glands. Infantile subglottic hemangiomas usually regress spontaneously as the child grows older.[142, 147, 154]

Inflammatory Conditions

Acute bacterial epiglottis (supraglottitis) is an important cause of upper airway obstruction in children and, less commonly, in adults as well.[155, 156] The offending organism in children is usually *Hemophilus influenzae.* The condition causes a redness and swelling of the epiglottis and other supraglottic structures (ie, the aryepiglottic folds) (Fig. 2–4), presenting, in children, as a "cherry red" epiglottis. Histologically, one sees marked edema and extensive neutrophilic infiltration of the loose supraglottic mucosa, with focal abscess formation in severe cases (Fig. 2–5).

Allergic laryngitis may also cause respiratory obstruction via swelling of the supraglottic structures, as in epiglottitis. However, in laryngeal angioedema, both of the urticarial type (associated with cutaneous urticariae) and the hereditary, nonurticarial type, the mechanism is most likely marked edema of the supraglottic structures without an associated prominent neutrophilic infiltrate.[157]

Granulomatous Disorders. Granulomatous disorders make up the other major segment of laryngeal inflammatory disease.

Tuberculosis of the larynx, once a common disorder in patients with far-advanced pulmonary tuberculosis, occurs much more rarely now in Western societies. When it does occur, it often presents as a mass lesion in patients who are relatively healthy (albeit usually with some pulmonary manifestations of tuberculosis) and thus mimics carcinoma of the larynx clinically.[158–161] Histologically, the characteristic necrotizing granulomas with multinucleated histiocytic giant cells are seen, and acid-fast bacilli may be found (Fig. 2–6). Response to

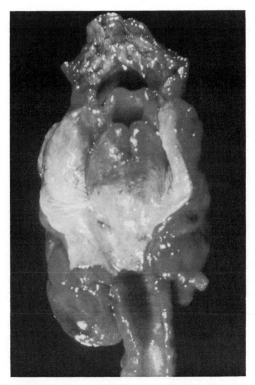

Figure 2–4. Acute epiglottitis (supraglottitis). The supraglottic structures are markedly edematous and erythematous. (Reprinted by permission of the New England Journal of Medicine 276:924, 1967.)

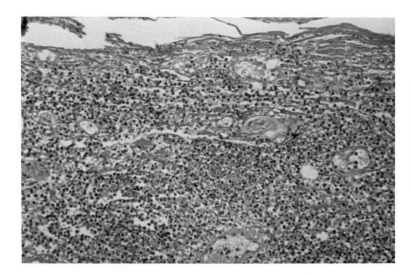

Figure 2–5. Acute epiglottitis (supraglottitis): Deep to the epiglottic perichondrium is a florid inflammatory infiltrate composed predominately of polymorphonuclear leukocytes. (Reprinted by permission of the New England Journal of Medicine 276:881, 1967.)

appropriate chemotherapy is generally excellent, and infectivity appears to be low.[158]

Histoplasmosis may initially present in the upper respiratory tract in about 30% of cases of disseminated disease.[162] As in tuberculosis, laryngeal histoplasmosis may mimic carcinoma. Histologically, granulomatous inflammation is present, and *Histoplasma* yeast forms may be present in macrophages.[162]

Other specific granulomatous infections of the larynx have been reported but are rare, such as blastomycosis,[163] coccidioidomycosis,[164, 165] actinomycosis,[166] leprosy,[167] and syphilis.[162]

Noninfectious granulomatous disorders can also rarely involve the larynx. *Wegener's granulomatosis* may contribute to subglottic stenosis and cause respiratory embarrassment.[168–171]

Sarcoidosis may occasionally involve the larynx,[172] and may produce upper airway obstruction.[173] The histologic findings on biopsy specimens include the presence of tightly compact, noncaseating epithelioid granulomas characteristic of sarcoidosis. A rare case of granulomatous laryngitis in a patient with Crohn's disease has been reported,[174] as has a case of chronic granulomatous laryngitis of obscure cause.[175]

Degenerative Conditions

Vocal cord polyps are generally small, nodular masses on the vocal cord. They are thought to arise as a result of a reactive change in response to vocal abuse or "phonotrauma,"[176] and perhaps also as a reaction to industrial exposure to airborne irritants.[157, 177] Interestingly, smoking was not found to be a significant etiologic factor.[177] The noxious stimuli stimulate increased blood flow and vascular permeability to produce edema of Reinke's space, the area between the vocal cord mucosal epithelium and the vocal ligament. This space is thought to be poor in lymphatics, and this may result in a tendency for fluid to accumulate locally.[157] Exudation of edema fluid and fibrin occurs, along with occasional hemorrhage. The fibrin may organize, much as an intravascular thrombus, resulting in endothelial vascularization and eventual fibrosis. Thus, polyps morphologically may consist of a loose, myxoid edematous subepithelial accumulation with scattered spindled or stellate cells; dilated proliferating vascular channels with intravascular and extravascular fibrin deposition; or a com-

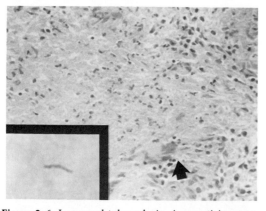

Figure 2–6. Laryngeal tuberculosis. A necrotizing granuloma has a necrotic center rimmed by epithelioid histiocytes. A Langhans' type giant cell is present *(arrow)*. *Inset,* An acid-fast, beaded, *Mycobacterium* bacillus present in the tuberculous lesion.

bination of these patterns (Fig. 2–7).[156, 176, 177] There appears to be little morphologic or pathogenetic basis for distinguishing vocal cord "polyps" from "nodules."[177]

Trauma to the thin mucosa covering the vocal process of the arytenoid cartilage in the posterior vocal cord region, either due to mechanical injury (eg, secondary to intubation) or chemical injury (eg, reflux of acid gastric contents), can result in so-called *"contact" ulcers and granulomas* (postintubation granuloma). Intubation can cause mechanical abrasion to the thin mucosa that overlies the vocal

processes. In addition, prolonged intubation can lead to a pressure necrosis of this mucosa. Such intubation-related injuries are usually minor and self-healing. With excessive trauma, movement, or friction between tube and mucosa, the injury may become more severe and a perichondritis may occur.[178, 179] Tissue necrosis, ulceration, and perichondritis lead to a "contact" ulcer, and if exuberant granulation tissue as a reparative process supervenes, which not uncommonly occurs, a "contact granuloma" results. The pathology of the contact granuloma is that of polypoid granulation

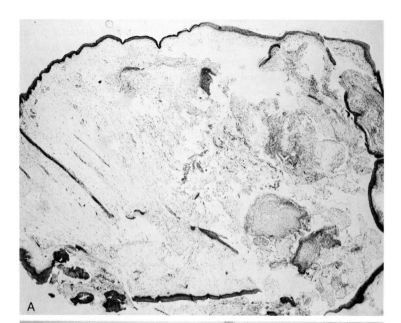

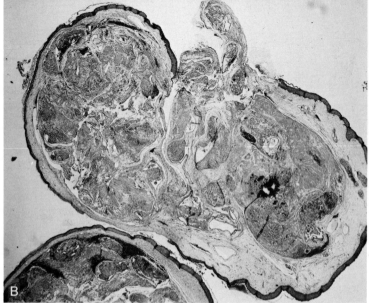

Figure 2–7. Vocal cord polyp. *A,* Myxoid type: the subepithelial space of the vocal cord is expanded by loose myxoid tissue. *B,* Vascular type: dilated vascular channels, blood, and fibrin deposition are prominent.

tissue, usually with a focally ulcerated surface, with superimposed acute and chronic inflammation, and often with fibrosis and hemosiderin deposition at the base (Fig. 2–8). There may be squamous epithelial hyperplasia at the ulcer's edge. Although such lesions have erroneously been called pyogenic granulomas in the past, true pyogenic granulomas are spontaneously arising capillary hemangiomas with a lobular architecture that occur in the nasal and oral cavities, as opposed to the trauma-induced, radially oriented capillaries of the contact granuloma.[180, 181]

The histologic appearance of contact ulcers and granulomas that occur in the absence of prior intubation is similarly one of ulceration, granulation tissue, and inflammation.[157] It was classically thought that these nonintubation-associated contact granulomas were the result of vocal abuse, habitual throat clearing, and coughing.[182] Recently, however, such contact ulcers and granulomas have been found to be associated with gastric reflux due to hiatus hernia.[183, 184] The coughing and throat clearing may be secondary to the granulomas, rather than their cause.[185] A recent paper has, in fact, advocated the term "peptic granuloma" as a replacement for "contact granuloma," to reflect this new concept of pathogenesis.[185]

More serious intubation-related injury occurs in the subglottic area and trachea, where ulceration, infection, and necrosis of soft tissue and cartilage can result in fibrosis and significant, therapeutically refractory subglottic and tracheal stenosis.[179, 186, 187]

The larynx and trachea may be sites of either systemic or localized *amyloidosis*. Although

commonly involved in systemic amyloidosis,[188] the larynx is usually the site of clinically significant amyloid deposition in localized rather than systemic cases.[188–190] The amyloid may present as isolated, subepithelial tumor-like nodules, or as a diffuse submucosal infiltrate, often in a subglottic location. Significant airway compromise may, although does not usually, occur, especially with the diffuse infiltrative form.

Histologically, amyloid is an eosinophilic, amorphous, homogeneous, extracellular, proteinaceous deposit. It tends to concentrate in vessel walls or around seromucinous gland structures, eventually causing atrophy and disappearance of the glands. The diagnostic hallmark of amyloid deposition is a characteristic apple-green birefringence when the amyloid is stained with Congo red stain and viewed under polarized light.

The intrinsic joints of the larynx are involved in a surprisingly high percentage of cases of *rheumatoid arthritis,* possibly 50% to 80%.[191] Both the cricoarytenoid and cricothyroid joints may be involved, the cricoarytenoid being clinically the more significant. Pathologically, early lesions show a chronic hypertrophic synovitis, with synovial thickening and a lymphoplasmacytic infiltrate.[157, 191] Later in the disease, a fibrous pannus may cover the articulating surface, and joint destruction with fibrous ankylosis occurs.[192] If this occurs such that both vocal cords are fixed in adduction, stridor and significant respiratory obstruction may result. Rheumatoid nodules may rarely occur in laryngeal soft tissue in cases of rheumatoid arthritis.[157, 191]

The cricoarytenoid joint rarely can be involved in cases of severe *gout,* and tophaceous gouty arthritis of the cricoarytenoid joint can lead to symptoms such as hoarseness, dysphonia, and aspiration.[193] A case of a gouty tophus of the vocal cord that caused hoarseness also has been described.[194]

Benign Neoplasms

Squamous papillomas of the larynx are often multiple and recurrent, and thus can cause substantial morbidity and respiratory obstruction, particularly in the small airways of children. These lesions have a history of controversy regarding occurrence, classification, and behavior. Laryngeal papillomas have traditionally been divided into juvenile and adult varieties, but current opinion is that the nonker-

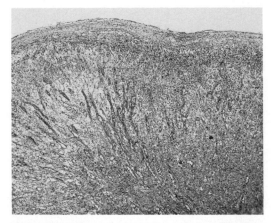

Figure 2–8. Laryngeal contact "granuloma." The lesion has an ulcerated surface with fibrin deposition, and underlying granulation tissue with radially oriented capillaries.

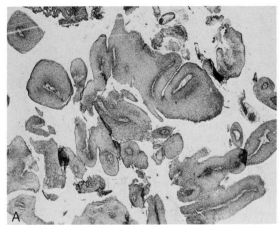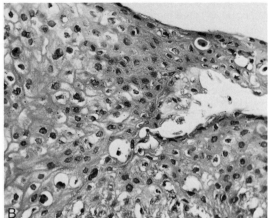

Figure 2–9. Laryngeal squamous papilloma. *A,* Thickened squamous epithelial mucosa is thrown up into papillary fronds that contain central fibrovascular cores. *B,* Koilocytosis is manifested by perinuclear clearing, hyperchromatic nuclei, and occasional multinucleated epithelial cells.

atinizing, often multiple, true squamous papilloma, especially when associated with human papilloma virus (HPV), is an identical entity, whether manifesting in children or adults.[157, 195, 196] The so-called "keratinizing papilloma," usually a solitary lesion of adults, is considered an exophytic hyperplastic/keratotic, occasionally dysplastic squamous epithelial lesion, a papillary "leukoplakia," distinct from the viral-associated multiple papillomas.[195]

It is now generally accepted that multiple laryngeal papillomas are related to infection by HPV[196–198] in an analogous fashion to condylomas of the genital tract. In fact, a relation between juvenile laryngeal papillomatosis and the presence of maternal genital condylomas has been established.[199] Improved molecular biologic techniques have allowed subtyping laryngeal papilloma-associated viruses such as HPV types 6 and 11.[196]

Laryngeal squamous papillomas commonly occur on the true vocal cord, but the false cord and anterior commissure are also common sites,[195] and papillomas may extend supraglottically or subglottically into the trachea. Rarely, papillomatosis may be very extensive and involve the entire tracheobronchial tree, even down to the level of the alveoli, causing obstruction and abscess formation. This is an extremely grave complication of laryngeal papillomatosis and may lead to the death of the patient. Such seeding of the lower respiratory tract has been noted to occur after tracheostomy.[200, 201]

The histopathologic appearance of laryngeal squamous papillomas is that of a thickening of the squamous epithelial mucosal layer that is thrown up into papillary fronds containing fibrovascular cores (Fig. 2–9*A*). First- and second-degree branching of the papillae may occur. The surface layers may often have many squamous cells with perinuclear clearing and an enlarged, dark, wrinkled nucleus, so-called "koilocytosis" (Fig. 2–9*B*), a finding strongly correlated with HPV infection and described extensively in the uterine cervix. When papillomas extend to areas normally lined by respiratory epithelium, a ciliated layer of cells may cover the papillomatous projections.[157]

Laryngeal papillomas are notorious for their persistence and recurrence, often requiring multiple endoscopic surgical procedures, and this tendency has been positively correlated with the intensity of staining for HPV types 6 and 11 by in situ hybridization.[196] The once widely held notion that laryngeal papillomas regress or disappear at puberty has been largely abandoned.[202] Laryngeal papillomas rarely undergo malignant transformation to squamous cell carcinoma. When they do, this is usually related to some inciting event, such as radiotherapy. This may be related to the fact that HPV types 6 and 11, found in the laryngeal papillomas, are the types of HPV generally found not to be associated with carcinoma of the uterine cervix, in contrast to HPV types 16 and 18, which are carcinoma-associated viral types.

Treatment of squamous papillomas consists of repeated surgical removal as needed, with the CO_2 laser emerging as a useful therapeutic tool. Tracheostomy and radiation are avoided if at all possible.

Granular cell tumors (granular cell "myoblastomas") are uncommon, usually benign tumors of characteristic morphology and controversial histogenesis. They occur most commonly in the skin and subcutaneous tissues, but a distinct minority are present in the larynx, usually in the posterior portion,[203, 204] and the tumor rarely has been reported in the trachea.[205] The laryngotracheal tumors generally do not cause significant airway obstruction. Histologically, the tumor is composed of large, polygonal, rarely spindled cells with eosinophilic cytoplasm that displays a striking and characteristic granularity. The granules are periodic acid-Schiff (PAS) positive and diastase resistant. The lesions are poorly circumscribed, and granular cells infiltrate into the surrounding tissue. Nuclear anaplasia and mitotic activity is generally minimal, and the vast majority of tumors are benign. A striking pseudoepitheliomatous hyperplasia of the overlying squamous epithelium in lingual and laryngeal lesions is often seen, and care must be taken not to misinterpret this reactive phenomenon as squamous cell carcinoma (Fig. 2–10). The cell of origin is controversial, and current opinion is that although many granular cell tumors are likely of neurogenic Schwann cell origin, some may be derived from other cell types, possibly histiocytic.[206]

Malignant Neoplasms

Squamous cell carcinoma is by far the most common laryngeal malignancy. Lesions of the true vocal cord are often diagnosed early, because hoarseness occurs when the tumors are still of small size. Supraglottic tumors can become rather bulky before causing significant respiratory embarrassment, and hypopharyngeal neoplasms of the pyriform sinus (traditionally, a clinically "silent" area) may attain considerable size and even metastasize to cervical lymph nodes before being diagnosed.

Laryngeal carcinomas may appear grossly as exophytic plaque-like or nodular masses[157] that may be focally ulcerated or papillary and shaggy (Fig. 2–11A). Alternatively, they may be ulceroinfiltrative and burrow deeply into laryngeal tissues without the presence of a large bulky surface mass (Fig. 2–11B).[207] Verrucous carcinoma, a relatively rare, locally aggressive, but virtually nonmetastasizing variant of laryngeal squamous cell carcinoma, exhibits a broad-based, warty exophytic pattern of growth.[207]

Histologically, squamous cell carcinoma consists of a neoplastic proliferation of epithelial cells that retains some properties of squamous differentiation (ie, keratinization or presence of prominent intercellular junctions or "bridges") and that has penetrated beyond the confines of the mucosal epithelial layer and its contiguous ducts and into the surrounding connective tissue stroma. In general, the extent to which the neoplasm histologically resembles the parent squamous epithelium determines its degree of differentiation, with well-differentiated tumors closely resembling stratified

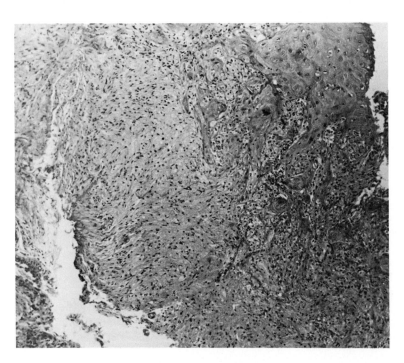

Figure 2–10. Laryngeal granular cell tumor. There is a subepithelial proliferation of large ill-defined cells with ample granular cytoplasm. Note the overlying mucosal pseudoepitheliomatous hyperplasia in the upper right of the figure that simulates squamous cell carcinoma. (From Shapshay SM, Aretz HT. Benign Lesions of the Larynx. Alexandria, VA: American Academy of Otolaryngology Head and Neck Surgery Foundation, Inc.; copyright 1984, with permission.)

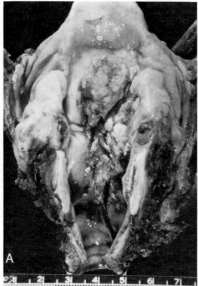
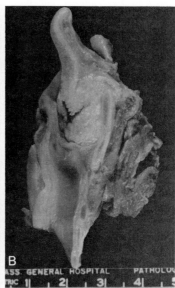

Figure 2–11. Laryngeal squamous cell carcinoma. *A*, Exophytic shaggy transglottic tumor involving the right true and false cords. *B*, Cross section of an ulceroinfiltrative supraglottic cancer, with a minimal surface component, invading deeply to the perichondrium of the thyroid cartilage.

squamous epithelium, usually with prominent keratinization, and with poorly differentiated tumors manifesting increased cellular pleomorphism and nuclear anaplasia and less obvious keratinization or intercellular bridge formation (Fig. 2–12). Poorly differentiated carcinomas also may exhibit focal necrosis and raggedly infiltrating, rather than rounded, pushing borders. Attempts to correlate histologic differentiation with biologic behavior have not been uniformly successful.[207] Carcinomas can invade lymphatics, bone and cartilage, soft tissue and muscle, and vascular structures, usually veins.

Large, bulky tumors, especially glottic or subglottic lesions, may produce airway obstruction that at times may require emergency intervention.[208]

Cartilaginous tumors are rare lesions of the larynx and are even rarer in the trachea.[207, 209]

They occur most commonly in the cricoid cartilage, followed in frequency by the thyroid cartilage. Cartilaginous laryngeal tumors are slowly growing lesions that usually project anteriorly into the airway from the cricoid lamina, and can significantly narrow the airway (Fig. 2–13*A*). Because these lesions may be difficult to diagnose on conventional chest radiography, some patients with respiratory embarrassment and wheezing secondary to these lesions may be erroneously diagnosed as asthmatics. The radiographic picture is characteristic, with a laryngeal, cartilage-based mass that contains the punctate calcifications characteristic of cartilage.[209]

Histologically, the tumors are generally low-grade cartilaginous neoplasms, and have a morphology analogous to low-grade chondrosarcomas of the skeleton (Fig. 2–13*B*). Despite

Figure 2–12. Laryngeal squamous cell carcinoma. Nests of malignant squamous epithelium, with focal keratinization, invade desmoplastic stromal tissue.

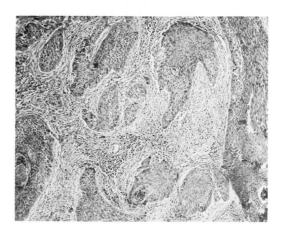

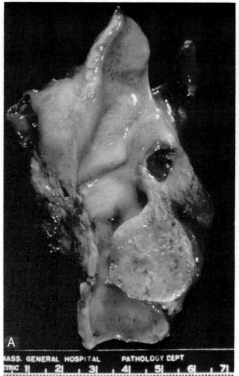

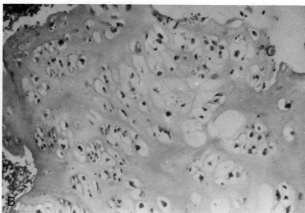

Figure 2–13. Laryngeal cartilaginous tumor. *A,* A cartilaginous neoplasm arising from the lamina of the cricoid cartilage posteriorly penetrates anteriorly into the laryngeal lumen, significantly narrowing the airway. (From Shapshay SM, Aretz HT. Benign Lesions of the Larynx. Alexandria, VA: American Academy of Otolaryngology Head and Neck Surgery Foundation, Inc.; copyright 1984, with permission.) *B,* Histologically, a moderately cellular proliferation of chondrocytes with enlarged nuclei is present, corresponding to the morphology of a low-grade skeletal chondrosarcoma.

exhibiting the histologic features seen in low-grade sarcomas, the laryngeal tumors are slow growing, very rarely metastasize, and generally may be adequately treated by conservative, larynx-sparing surgery.

References

1. Bouquot JE. Common oral lesions found during a mass screening examination. J Am Dent Assoc 112:50–57, 1986.
2. Bouquot JE, Gundlach KKH. Oral exophytic lesions in 23,616 white Americans over 35 years of age. Oral Surg Oral Med Oral Pathol 62:284–291, 1986.
3. Bouquot JE. Epidemiology. In Gnepp DR (ed). Pathology of the Head and Neck. New York: Churchill Livingstone, 1988; pp. 263–304.
4. Jones WB. Weight gain and feeding in the neonate with cleft: A three year study. Cleft Palate J 25:379–384, 1988.
5. Strauss RP, Broder H, Helms RW. Perceptions of appearance and speech by adolescent patients with cleft lip and palate and by their parents. Cleft Palate J 25:335–342, 1988.
6. Kolas S, Halperin V, Jefferies K, et al. The occurrence of torus palatinus and torus mandibularis in 2,478 dental patients. Oral Surg 6:1134–1141, 1953.
7. Shklar G, Meyer I. Vascular tumors of the mouth and jaws. Oral Surg 19:335–358, 1965.
8. Osler W. On multiple hereditary teleangiectases with recurrent hemorrhages. Q J Med (Oxford) 1:53–58, 1907.
9. Sturge WA. A case of partial epilepsy apparently due to a lesion of one of the vasomotor centers of the brain. Clin Soc TR 12–162, 1879.
10. Weber FP. Right-sided hemi-hypertrophy resulting from right-sided congenital spastic hemiplegia with a morbid condition of the left side of the brain, revealed by radiogram. J Neuro Psychopath London 37:301–311, 1922.
11. Maffucci A. Di un caso encondroma ed angioma multiple. Mov Med Chir 3:399, 1881.
12. Abbey LM. The clinical and histopathologic features of a series of 464 oral sqamous cell papillomas. Oral Surg 49:419–428, 1980.
13. Jenson AB, Lancaster WD, Hartmann D, et al. Frequency and distribution of papilloma virus structural antigens in verruca, multiple papilloma, and condylomata of the oral cavity. Am J Pathol 107:212–218, 1982.
14. Eversole LR. Oral sialocysts. Arch Otolaryngol Head Neck Surg 113:51–56, 1987.
15. Roediger WEW, Kay S. Pathogenesis and treatment of plunging ranulas. Surg Gynecol Obstet 144:862–864, 1977.
16. Catone GA, Merrill RG, Henny FA. Sublingual gland mucous escape phenomenon: Treatment by excision of sublingual gland. J Oral Maxillofac Surg 27:774–786, 1969.
17. Gibson WS Jr, Fenton NA. Congenital sublingual dermoid cyst. Arch Otolaryngol 108:745–748, 1982.
18. Mirchandan R, Sciubba J, Gloster ES. Congenital oral cyst with heterotopic gastrointestinal and respiratory mucosa. Arch Pathol Lab Med 113:1301–1302, 1989.
19. Mickel RA, Calcaterra TC. Management of recurrent thyroglossal duct cysts. Arch Otolaryngol 109:34–36, 1983.
20. deMello DE, Lima JA, Liapis H. Midline cervical cysts in children: Thyroglossal anomalies. Arch Otolaryngol Head Neck Surg 113:418–420, 1987.
21. Harris M, Toller P. The pathogenesis of dental cysts. Br Med Bull 31:159–163, 1975.

22. Browne RM. The odontogenic keratocyst: Clinical aspects. Br Dent J 128:225–231, 1970.

23. Shteyer A, Lustmann J, Lewin-Epstein J. The mural ameloblastoma: A review of the literature. J Oral Surg 36:866–872, 1978.

24. Sehdeu MK, Huvos AC, Strong EW, et al. Ameloblastoma of maxilla and mandible. Cancer 33:324–333, 1974.

25. Gardner DG. Peripheral ameloblastoma: A study of 21 cases, including 5 reported as basal cell carcinoma of the gingiva. Cancer 39:1625–1633, 1977.

26. Guralnick W, Chuong R, Goodman M. Peripheral ameloblastoma of the gingiva. J Oral Maxillofac Surg 41:536–539, 1983.

27. Gardner DG, Pecak AMJ. The treatment of ameloblastoma based on pathologic and anatomic principles. Cancer 46:2514–2519, 1980.

28. Ascenzi A, Marinozzi V. Biophysical study of Von Recklinghausen's disease of bone. Arch Pathol 72:297–309, 1961.

29. Rosenberg EH, Guralnick WC. Hyperparathyroidism: A review of 220 proved cases with special emphasis on findings in the jaws. Oral Surg 15 (Suppl 2):84–94, 1962.

30. Shannon E, Rapoport Y. Giant cell tumor of the palate in hyperparathyroidism. Laryngoscope 82:425–429, 1972.

31. Dehner LP. Tumors of the mandible and maxilla in children. I: Clinicopathologic study of 46 histologically benign lesions. Cancer 31:364–384, 1973.

32. Austin LT, Dahlin DC, Roger RQ. Giant cell reparative granuloma and related conditions affecting the jaw bones. Oral Surg 12:1285–1295, 1959.

33. Cares HL, Bakay L. Giant cell lesions of the skull. Acta Neurochir 25:1–18, 1971.

34. Mnaymneh WA, Dudley HR, Mnaymneh LG. Giant cell tumor of bone; an analysis and follow-up study of the forty-one cases observed at the Massachusetts General Hospital between 1925 and 1960. J Bone Joint Surg [Am] 46:63–75, 1964.

35. Harris H, Dudley HR, Barry RJ. The natural history of fibrous dysplasia: An orthopedic, pathological, and roentgenographic study. J Bone Joint Surg [Am] 44:207–233, 1962.

36. Van Hoan PE Jr, Dahlin DC, Bickel WH. Fibrous dysplasia: A clinical pathologic study of orthopedic surgical cases. Proc Mayo Clin 38:175–189, 1963.

37. Fu YS, Perzin KH. Non-epithelial tumors of the nasal cavity, paranasal sinuses, and nasopharynx: A clinical pathologic study. II: Osseous and fibro-osseous lesions, including osteoma, fibrous dysplasia, ossifying fibroma, osteoblastoma, giant cell tumor, and osteosarcoma. Cancer 33:1289–1305, 1974.

38. Langdon JD, Rapidis AD, Patel MF. Ossifying fibroma—one disease or six? An analysis of 39 fibro-osseous lesions of the jaws. Br J Oral Surg 14:1–11, 1976.

39. Waldron CA, Giansanti JS. Benign fibro-osseous lesions of periodontal ligament origin. Oral Surg 35:340–349, 1973.

40. Kristensen S, Tueteras K. Aggressive cementifying fibroma of the maxilla. Arch Otorhinolaryngol 243:102–105, 1986.

41. Wu PC, Leung PK, Mak M. Recurrent cementifying fibroma. J Oral Maxillofac Surg 44:229–234, 1986.

42. Jones WA. Familial multilocular cystic disease of the jaws. Am J Cancer 17:946–950, 1933.

43. Faircloth WJ, Edwards RC, Farhood VW. Cherubism involving a mother and daughter: Case report and review of the literature. J Oral Maxillofac Surg 49:535–542, 1991.

44. Hames MJ. Cherubism and its orbital manifestations. Ophthalmic Plastic and Reconstructive Surg 5:133–140, 1989.

45. Vaillant JM, Romain P, Divaris M. Cherubism findings in three cases in the same family. J Craniomaxillofac Surg 17:345–349, 1989.

46. Deuxchaisnes CN de, Krane SM. Paget's disease of bone: Clinical and metabolic observations. Medicine 43:233–266, 1964.

47. Eisman JA, Martin TJ. Osteolytic Paget's disease: Recognition and risks of biopsy. J Bone Joint Surg [Am] 68:112–117, 1986.

48. Smith BJ, Eveson JW. Paget's disease of bone with particular reference to dentistry. J Oral Pathol 10:233–247, 1981.

49. Cawson RA. Premalignant lesions in the mouth. Br Med Bull 31:164–169, 1975.

50. Bouquot JE, Gorlin RJ. Leukoplakia, lichen planus, and other oral keratoses in 23,616 white Americans over the age of 35 years. Oral Surg 61:373–381, 1986.

51. Waldron CA, Shafer WG. Leukoplakia revisited: A clinicopathologic study of 3256 oral leukoplakias. Cancer 36:1386–1392, 1975.

52. Barone R, Ficarra G, Gaglioti D, et al. Prevalence of oral lesions among HIV infected intravenous drug abusers and other risk groups. Oral Surg 69:169–173, 1990.

53. Eversole LR, Jacobsen P, Stone CE, et al. Oral condyloma planus (hairy leukoplakia) among homosexual men: A clinicopathologic study of thirty-six cases. Oral Surg 61:249–255, 1986.

54. Pindborg JJ. Classification of oral lesions associated with HIV infection. Oral Surg 67:292–295, 1989.

55. Lindberg R. Distribution of cervical lymph node metastases from squamous cell carcinoma of the upper respiratory and digestive tracts. Cancer 29:1446–1452, 1972.

56. Sloan D, Goepfert H. Conventional therapy of head and neck cancer. Hematol Oncol Clin North Am 5:601–625, 1991.

57. Wang CC (ed). Radiation Therapy for Head and Neck Neoplasms, 2nd ed. Chicago: Year Book Medical, 1990; pp. 110–185.

58. Dreyfus AI, Clark JR. Analysis of prognostic factors in squamous cell carcinomas of the head and neck. Hematol Oncol Clin North Am 5:701–712, 1991.

59. Medina JE, Dichtel W, Luna MA. Verrucous squamous carcinomas of the oral cavity: A clinicopathologic study of 104 cases. Arch Otolaryngol 110:437–440, 1984.

60. Fonts EA, Greenlaw RH, Rush BF, et al. Verrucous squamous cell carcinoma of the oral cavity. Cancer 23:152–160, 1969.

61. Eisenberg E, Rosenberg B, Krutchkoff DJ. Verrucous carcinoma: A possible viral pathogenesis. Oral Surg 59:52–57, 1985.

62. Mark RJ, Sercarz JA, Tran L, et al. Osteogenic sarcoma of the head and neck: The UCLA experience. Arch Otolaryngol Head Neck Surg 117:761–766, 1991.

63. Clark L, Uni KK, Dahlin DC. Osteosarcoma of the jaw. Cancer 51:2311–2316, 1983.

64. Ficarra G, Berson AM, Silverman S Jr, et al. Kaposi's sarcoma of the oral cavity: A study of 134 patients with a review of pathogenesis, epidemiology, clinical aspects and treatment. Oral Surg 66:543–550, 1988.

65. Willis RA. Pathology of Tumors, 3rd ed. Washington, D.C.: Butterworth, 1960; pp. 321–349.

66. Waldron CA, El-Mofty SK, Gnepp DR. Tumors of

the intraoral minor salivary glands: A demographic and histologic study of 426 cases. Oral Surg 66:323–333, 1988.

67. Eveson JW, Cawson RA. Salivary gland tumors: A review of 2410 cases with particular reference to histological types, site, age and sex distribution. J Pathol 146:51–58, 1985.

68. Spiro RH. Salivary neoplasms: Overview of a 35-year experience with 2,807 patients. Head Neck Surg 8:177–184, 1986.

69. Erlandson RA, Cardon-Cardo C, Higgins PJ. Histogenesis of benign pleomorphic adenoma (mixed tumor) of the major salivary glands. An ultrastructural and immunohistochemical study. Am J Surg Pathol 8:803–820, 1984.

70. Takeuchi J, Sobue M, Katoh Y, et al. Morphologic and biologic characteristics of adenoid cystic carcinoma cells of the salivary gland. Cancer 38:2349–2356, 1976.

71. Moran JJ, Becker SM, Brady LW, et al. Adenoid cystic carcinoma: A clinicopathological study. Cancer 14:1235–1250, 1961.

72. Perzin KH, Gullane P, Clairmont AC. Adenoid cystic carcinomas arising in salivary glands: A correlation of histologic features and clinical course. Cancer 42:265–282, 1978.

73. Kadish SP, Goodman ML, Wang CC. Treatment of minor salivary gland malignancies of upper food and air passage epithelium: A review of 87 cases. Cancer 29:1021–1026, 1972.

74. Matsuba HM, Spector GJ, Thawley SE, et al. Adenoid cystic salivary gland carcinoma: A histopathologic review of treatment failure patterns. Cancer 57:519–524, 1986.

75. Batsakis JG, Pinkston GR, Luna MA, et al. Adenocarcinomas of the oral cavity: A clinicopathologic study of terminal duct carcinomas. J Laryngol Otol 97:825–835, 1983.

76. Evans HL, Batsakis JG. Polymorphous low-grade adenocarcinoma of minor salivary glands: A study of 14 cases of a distinctive neoplasm. Cancer 53:935–942, 1984.

77. Aberle AM, Abrams AA, Bowe R, et al. Lobular (polymorphous low-grade) carcinoma of minor salivary glands. Oral Surg 60:387–395, 1985.

78. Gnepp DR, Chen JC, Warren C. Polymorphus low-grade adenocarcinoma of minor salivary gland. Am J Surg Pathol 12:461–468, 1988.

79. Bhaskar SN, Bernier JL. Mucoepidermoid tumors of major and minor salivary glands: Clinical features, histology, variations, natural history, and results of treatment for 144 cases. Cancer 15:801–817, 1962.

80. Healey WV, Perzin KH, Smith L. Mucoepidermoid carcinoma of salivary gland origin: Classification, clinical-pathology correlation and result of treatment. Cancer 26:368–388, 1970.

81. Spiro RH, Huvos AG, Berk R, et al. Mucoepidermoid carcinoma of salivary gland origin: A clinicopathologic study of 367 cases. Am J Surg 136:461–468, 1978.

82. Abrams AM, Melrose RJ, Howell FV. Necrotizing sialometaplasia: A disease simulating malignancy. Cancer 32:130–135, 1973.

83. Grillon GL, Lally ET. Necrotizing sialometaplasia: Literature review and presentation of five cases. J Oral Surg 39:747–753, 1981.

84. Granick MS, Pilch BZ. Necrotizing sialometaplasia in the setting of acute and chronic sinusitis. Laryngoscope 91:1532–1535, 1981.

85. Bloch KJ, Buchanan WW, Wohl MJ, et al. Sjögren's syndrome: A clinical pathological and serological study of sixty-two cases. Medicine 44:187–231, 1965.

86. Anderson LG, Talal N. The spectrum of benign to malignant lymphoproliferations in Sjögren's syndrome. Clin Immunol 9:199–221, 1971.

87. Daniels TE. Labial salivary gland biopsy in Sjögren's syndrome: Assessment as a diagnostic criterion in 362 suspected cases. Arthritis Rheum 27:147–156, 1984.

88. Hyjek E, Smith WJ, Isaacson PG. Primary B-cell lymphoma of salivary glands and its relationship to myoepithelial sialadenitis. Hum Pathol 19:766–776, 1988.

89. Fishleder A, Tubbs R, Hesse B, et al. Uniform detection of immunoglobulin gene rearrangement in benign lymphoepithelial lesions. N Engl J Med 316:1118–1122, 1987.

90. Kisileusky R. Amyloid and amyloidosis: Differences, common themes and practical considerations. Mod Pathol 4:514–518, 1991.

91. Glenner CG, Terry WD, Isersky C. Amyloidosis: Its nature and pathogenesis. Semin Hematol 10:65–86, 1973.

92. Blumstein GI. Nasal polyps. Arch Otolaryngol 83:266–269, 1966.

93. Holpainen E, Makinen J, Paauolainen M, et al. Nasal polyposis. Acta Otolaryngol 87:330–334, 1979.

94. Clement PAR, VanderVeken P, Verstraelen J, et al. Some remarks on nasal polyposis. Acta Otorhinolaryngol Belg 43:267–278, 1989.

95. Levine HL. Functional endoscopic sinus surgery: Evaluation, surgery, and follow-up of 250 patients. Laryngoscope 100:79–84, 1990.

96. Giltator E. Tertiary syphilis of the nasal fossa and pharynx. Acta Otorhinolaryngologica Iberio-Am 22:366–384, 1971.

97. Gordon WN, Cohn AM, Greenberg SD, et al. Nasal sarcoidosis. Arch Otolaryngol 102:11–14, 1976.

98. Waldman SR, Levine HL, Sebek BA, et al. Nasal tuberculosis: A forgotten entity. Laryngoscope 91:11–16, 1981.

99. Berger SA, Pollock AA, Richmond AS. Isolation of *Klebsiella rhinoscleromatis* in a general hospital. Am J Clin Pathol 67:499–502, 1977.

100. Fauci AS, Haynes BF, Katz P, et al. Wegener's granulomatosis: Prospective clinical and therapeutic experience with 85 patients for 21 years. Ann Intern Med 98:76–85, 1983.

101. Arkin CR, Masi AT. Relapsing polychondritis: A review of current status case report. Semin Arthritis Rheum 5:41–61, 1975.

102. Kassel SH, Echevarria RA, Gusso FP. Midline malignant reticulosis (so-called lethal midline granuloma). Cancer 23:920–935, 1969.

103. Warder FR, Chikes PG, Hudson WR. Aspergillosis of the paranasal sinuses. Arch Otolaryngol 101:683–685, 1975.

104. Yanagisawa E, Friedman S, Kundargi RS, et al. Rhinocerebral phycomycosis. Laryngoscope 87:1319–1335, 1977.

105. McDonald TJ, DeRemee RA. Wegener's granulomatosis. Laryngoscope 93:220–230, 1983.

106. Feinberg R. The protracted superficial phenomenon in pathergic (Wegener's) granulomatosis. Hum Pathol 12:458–467, 1980.

107. DelBuono EA, Flint A. Diagnostic usefulness of nasal biopsy in Wegener's granulomatosis. Hum Pathol 22:107–110, 1991.

108. Specks U, Wheatley CL, McDonald TJ, et al. Anticytoplasmic autoantibodies in the diagnosis and fol-

low-up of Wegener's granulomatosis. Mayo Clin Proc 64:28–36, 1989.

109. Michaels L, Gregory MM. Pathology of non-healing (midline) granuloma. J Clin Pathol 30:317–327, 1977.

110. Ishii Y, Yamanaka N, Ogawa K, et al. Nasal T-cell lymphoma as a type of so-called "lethal midline granuloma." Cancer 50:2236–2244, 1982.

111. Chan JFC, Ng CS, Lau WH, et al. Most nasal/nasopharyngeal lymphomas are peripheral T-cell neoplasms. Am J Surg Pathol 11:418–429, 1987.

112. Lipford EH, Margolich JB, Longo DL, et al. Angiocentric immunoproliferative lesions: A clinicopathologic spectrum of post-thymic T-cell proliferations. Blood 5:1674–1681, 1988.

113. Hyams VJ, Batsakis JG, Michaels L. Tumors of the upper respiratory tract and ear; 2nd series, fascicle 25. Washington, D.C.: Armed Forces Institute of Pathology, 1988; pp. 134–149.

114. Economou TS, Abemayor E, Ward PH. Juvenile nasopharyngeal angiofibroma: An update of the UCLA experience, 1960–1985. Laryngoscope 98:170–175, 1988.

115. Duvall AJ III, Moreano AE. Juvenile nasopharyngeal angiofibroma: Diagnosis and treatment. Otolaryngol Head Neck Surg 97:534–540, 1987.

116. Amedee R, Klaeyel D, Geyer H. Juvenile angiofibromas: A 40-year experience. ORL 51:56–61, 1989.

117. Snyder RN, Perzin KH. Papillomatosis of nasal cavity and paranasal sinuses (inverted papilloma, squamous papilloma): A clinicopathologic study. Cancer 30:668–690, 1972.

118. Weissler MC, Montgomery WW, Turner P, et al. Inverted papilloma. Ann Otol Rhinol Laryngol 95:215–221, 1986.

119. Hyams VJ. Papillomas of the nasal cavity and paranasal sinuses: A clinicopathologic study of 315 cases. Ann Otol Rhinol Laryngol 80:192–206, 1971.

120. Ishibashi T, Tsunokawa Y, Matsushima S, et al. Presence of human papilloma virus type-6-related sequences in inverted nasal papillomas. Eur Arch Otorhinolaryngol 247:296–299, 1990.

121. Gadeberg CC, Hjelm-Hansen M, Sogaard H, et al. Malignant tumors of the paranasal sinuses and nasal cavity: A series of 180 patients. Acta Radiologica Oncology 23:181–187, 1984.

122. Lund VJ. Malignant tumors of the nasal cavity and paranasal sinuses. ORL 45:1–12, 1983.

123. Robin PE, Powell DJ, Stansbie JM. Carcinoma of the nasal cavity and paranasal sinuses: Incidence and presentation of different histological types. Clin Otolaryngol 4:431–456, 1979.

124. Hopkin N, McNicoll W, Dalley VM, et al. Cancer of the paranasal sinuses and nasal cavities: I. Clinical features. J Laryngol Otol 98:585–595, 1984.

125. Lund V. Malignant melanoma of the nasal cavity and paranasal sinuses. J Laryngol Otol 96:347–355, 1982.

126. Panje WR, Moran WJ. Melanoma of the upper aerodigestive tract: A review of 21 cases. Head Neck Surg 8:309–312, 1986.

127. Appleblatt NH, McClatchey KD. Olfactory neuroblastoma: A retrospective clinicopathologic study. Head Neck Surg 5:108–113, 1982.

128. Mills SE, Frierson HF Jr. Olfactory neuroblastoma: A clinicopathologic study of 21 cases. Am J Surg Pathol 9:317–327, 1985.

129. Klintenberg C, Olofsson J, Hellquist H, et al. Adenocarcinoma of the ethmoid sinuses: A review of 28 cases with special reference to wood dust exposure. Cancer 54:482–488, 1984.

130. Barnes L. Intestinal-type adenocarcinoma of the nasal cavity and paranasal sinuses. Am J Surg Pathol 10:192–202, 1986.

131. Heffner D, Hyams VJ, Hauck KW, et al. Low-grade adenocarcinoma of the nasal cavity and paranasal sinuses. Cancer 50:312–322, 1982.

132. Whittshaw E. The natural history of extramedullary plasmacystoma and its relation to solitary myeloma of bone and myelomatosis. Medicine 55:217–228, 1976.

133. Medini E, Rao Y, Levitt SH. Solitary extramedullary plasmacytoma of the upper respiratory and digestive tract. Cancer 45:2893–2896, 1980.

134. Fu YS, Perzin KH. Non-epithelial tumors of the nasal cavity, paranasal sinuses and nasopharynx: A clinicopathologic study. IX: Plasmacytomas. Cancer 42:2399–2406, 1978.

135. Robbins KT, Fuller LM, Valsak M, et al. Primary lymphomas of the nasal cavity and paranasal sinuses. Cancer 56:814–819, 1985.

136. Brook I. Aerobic and anaerobic bacteriology of adenoids in children: A comparison between patients with chronic adenotonsillitis and adenoid hypertrophy. Laryngoscope 91:377–382, 1981.

137. Kornblut AD (ed). Otolaryngol Clin North Am 20:259–390, 1987.

138. Beeden AG, Evans JNG. Quinsy tonsillectomy: A further report. J Laryngol Otol 84:443–448, 1973.

139. Herbild O, Bonding P. Peritonsillar abscess. Arch Otolaryngol 107:540–542, 1981.

140. Cvitkovic E, Bachouci M, Armand JP. Nasopharyngeal carcinoma. Biology, natural history and therapeutic implications. Hematol Oncol Head Neck Cancer 5:821–838, 1991.

141. Shoss SM, Donovan DT, Alford BR. Tumors of the parapharyngeal space. Arch Otolaryngol 111:753–757, 1985.

142. Cotton RT, Richardson MA. Congenital laryngeal anomalies. Otolaryngol Clin North Am 14:203–218, 1981.

143. Tucker JA, Tucker G, Vidic B. Clinical correlation of anomalies of the supraglottic larynx with the staged sequence of normal human laryngeal development. Ann Otol 37:636–644, 1978.

144. Birrell JF. Paediatric Otolaryngology. Chicago: Year Book Medical, 1978; pp. 157–166.

145. Fishman RA. Developmental anatomy and physiology of the airway. In Balkany TJ, Pashley NRT (eds). Clinical Pediatric Otolaryngology. St. Louis: C.V. Mosby, 1986; pp. 329–334.

146. Pashley NRT. Congenital anomalies of the upper airway. In Balkany TJ, Pashley NRT (eds). Clinical Pediatric Otolaryngology. St. Louis: C.V. Mosby, 1986; pp. 365–368.

147. McGill TJI, Healey GB. Congenital and acquired lesions of the infant larynx. Clin Pediatr 17:584–589, 1978.

148. Tucker GF, Ossoff RH, Newman AN, et al. Histopathology of congenital subglottic stenosis. Laryngoscope 89:866–876, 1979.

149. Lim TA, Spanier SS, Kohut RI. Laryngeal clefts: A histopathologic study and review. Ann Otol Rhinol Laryngol 88:837–845, 1979.

150. Harrison DFN. Saccular mucocele and laryngeal cancer. Arch Otolaryngol 103:232–234, 1977.

151. Holinger LD, Barnes DR, Smid LJ. Laryngocele and saccular cysts. Ann Otol 87:675–685, 1978.

152. Macfie DD. Asymptomatic laryngoceles in wind-instrument bandsmen. Arch Otolaryngol 83:268–275, 1966.

153. Shikhani AH, Marsh BR, Jones MM, et al. Infantile subglottic hemangiomas. Ann Otol Rhinol Laryngol 95:336–347, 1986.
154. Jokinen K, Palva A, Karja J. Cryocauterization in the treatment of subglottic hemangioma in infants. Laryngoscope 91:78–82, 1981.
155. Case records. Case 42. N Engl J Med. 297:878–883, 1977.
156. Gorfinkel HJ, Brown R, Kabins SA. Acute infectious epiglottitis in adults. Ann Intern Med 70:289–294, 1969.
157. Michaels L. Pathology of the Larynx. Berlin: Springer Verlag, 1984.
158. Thaller SR, Gross JR, Pilch BZ, et al. Laryngeal tuberculosis as manifested in the decades 1963–1983. Laryngoscope 97:848–850, 1987.
159. Case records. Case 51. N Engl J Med 309:1569–1574, 1983.
160. Bull TR. Tuberculosis of the larynx. Br Med J 2:991–992, 1966.
161. Yarnal JR, Golish JA, Van der Kuypt F. Laryngeal tuberculosis presenting as carcinoma. Arch Otolaryngol 107:503–505, 1981.
162. Caldarelli DD, Friedberg SA, Harris AA. Medical and surgical aspects of the granulomatous disease of the larynx. Otolaryngol Clin North Am 12:767–781, 1979.
163. Blair PA, Gnepp DR, Riley RS, et al. Blastomycosis of the larynx. South Med J 74:880–882, 1981.
164. Platt MA. Laryngeal coccidioidomycosis. JAMA 237:1234–1235, 1977.
165. Ward PH, Morledge D, Berci G, et al. Coccidioidomycosis of the larynx in infants and adults. Ann Otol 86:655–660, 1977.
166. Brandenburg JH, Finch WW, Kirkham WR. Actinomycosis of the larynx and pharynx. Trans Am Acad Opthalmol Otolaryngol 86:739–742, 1978.
167. Gupta JC, Gandagule VN, Nigam JP, et al. A clinicopathological study of laryngeal lesions in 30 cases of leprosy. Leprosy in India 52:557–564, 1980.
168. Case records. Case 31. N Engl J Med 315:378–387, 1986.
169. Talerman A, Wright D. Laryngeal obstruction due to Wegener's granulomatosis. Arch Otolaryngol 96:376–379, 1972.
170. Thomas K. Laryngeal manifestations of Wegener's granuloma. J Laryngol Otol 84:101–106, 1970.
171. Hoare TJ, Jayne D, Evans PR, et al. Wegener's granulomatosis, subglottic stenosis and antineutrophil cytoplasm antibodies. J Laryngol Otol 103:1187–1191, 1989.
172. Neel HB III, MacDonald TJ. Laryngeal sarcoidosis. Ann Otol Rhinol Laryngol 91:359–362, 1982.
173. Weisman RA, Canalis RF, Powell WJ. Laryngeal sarcoidosis with airway obstruction. Ann Otol Rhinol Laryngol 89:58–61, 1980.
174. Case records. Case 35. N Engl J Med 299:538–544, 1978.
175. Haar JG, Chaudhry AP, Kaplan HM, et al. Granulomatous laryngitis of unknown etiology. Laryngoscope 90:1225–1229, 1980.
176. Kleinsasser O. Pathogenesis of vocal cord polyps. Ann Otol Rhinol Laryngol 91:378–381, 1982.
177. Kambic V, Radsel Z, Zargi M, et al. Vocal cord polyps: Incidence, histology and pathogenesis. J Laryngol Otol 15:609–618, 1981.
178. Barton RT. Observation on the pathogenesis of laryngeal granuloma due to endotracheal anesthesia. N Engl J Med 248:1097–1099, 1953.
179. Gould SJ, Howard S. The histopathology of the larynx in the neonate following endotracheal intubation. J Pathol 146:301–311, 1985.
180. Mills SE, Cooper PH, Fechner RE. Lobular capillary hemangioma: The underlying lesion of pyogenic granuloma. Am J Surg Pathol 4:471–479, 1980.
181. Fechner RE, Cooper PH, Mills SE. Pyogenic granuloma of the larynx and trachea. Arch Otolaryngol 107:30–32, 1981.
182. Holinger PH, Johnston KC. Contact ulcer of the larynx. JAMA 172:511–515, 1960.
183. Goldberg M, Noyek AM, Pritzker KP. Laryngeal granuloma secondary to gastro-esophageal reflux. J Otolaryngol 7:196–202, 1978.
184. Ward PH, Zwitman D, Hanson D, et al. Contact ulcers and granulomas of the larynx: New insights into their etiology as a basis for more rational treatment. Otolaryngol Head Neck Surg 88:262–269, 1980.
185. Miko TL. Peptic (contact ulcer) granuloma of the larynx. J Clin Pathol 42:800–804, 1989.
186. Bryce DP, Briant TDR, Pearson FG. Laryngeal and tracheal complications of intubation. Ann Otol Rhinol Laryngol 77:442–461, 1968.
187. Quiney RE, Gould SJ. Subglottic stenosis: A clinicopathological study. Clin Otolaryngol 10:315–327, 1985.
188. Simpson GT, Skinner M, Strong MS, et al. Localized amyloidosis of the head and neck and upper aerodigestive and lower respiratory tracts. Ann Otol Rhinol Laryngol 93:374–379, 1984.
189. Hellquist H, Olofsson J, Sokjer H, et al. Amyloidosis of the larynx. Acta Otolaryngol 88:443–450, 1979.
190. Ryan RE, Pearson BW, Weiland LH. Laryngeal amyloidosis. Trans Am Acad Ophthalmol Otolaryngol 84:872–877, 1977.
191. Bridger MWM, Jahn AF, van Nostrand AWP. Laryngeal rheumatoid arthritis. Laryngoscope 90:296–303, 1980.
192. Montgomery WW. Pathology of cricoarytenoid arthritis. N Engl J Med 260:66–69, 1959.
193. Goodman ML, Montgomery WW, Minette L. Pathologic findings in gouty cricoarytenoid arthritis. Arch Otolaryngol 102:27–29, 1976.
194. Marion RB, Alperin JE, Maloney WH. Gouty tophus of the true vocal cord. Arch Otolaryngol 96:161–162, 1972.
195. Batsakis JG, Raymond AK, Rice DH. The pathology of head and neck tumors: Papillomas of the upper aerodigestive tracts, part 18. Head Neck Surg 5:332–344, 1983.
196. Quiney RE, Wells M, Lewis FA, et al. Laryngeal papillomatosis: Correlation between severity of disease and presence of HPV 6 and 11 detected by in situ DNA hybridisation. J Clin Pathol 42:694–698, 1989.
197. Costa J, Howley PM, Bowling MC, et al. Presence of human papilloma viral antigens in juvenile multiple laryngeal papilloma. Am J Clin Pathol 75:194–197, 1981.
198. Braun L, Kashima H, Eggleston J, et al. Demonstration of papillomavirus antigen in paraffin sections of laryngeal papillomas. Laryngoscope 92:640–643, 1982.
199. Quick CA, Krzyzek RA, Watts SL, et al. Relationship between condylomata and laryngeal papillomata. Ann Otol Rhinol Laryngol 89:467–471, 1980.
200. Cohen SR, Seltzer S, Geller KA, et al. Papilloma of the larynx and tracheobronchial tree in children. Ann Otol Rhinol Laryngol 89:497–503, 1980.
201. Brach BB, Klein RC, Mathews AJ, et al. Papillo-

matosis of the respiratory tract. Arch Otolaryngol 104:413–416, 1978.

202. Lindeberg H, Elbrond O. Laryngeal papillomas: Clinical aspects in a series of 231 patients. Clin Otolaryngol 14:333–342, 1989.

203. Stanley RJ, Scheithauer BW, Weiland LH, et al. Neural and neuroendocrine tumors of the larynx. Ann Otol Rhinol Laryngol 96:630–638, 1987.

204. Agarwal RK, Dorl MS, Blitzer A, et al. Granular cell tumors of the larynx. Otolaryngol Head Neck Surg 87:807–814, 1979.

205. Mikaelian DO, Cohn H, Israel H, et al. Granular cell tumor of the trachea. Ann Otol Rhinol Laryngol 93:457–459, 1984.

206. Nathrath WBJ, Remberger K. Immunohistochemical study of granular cell tumours. Virchows Arch [A] 408:421–434, 1986.

207. Pilch BZ, Brodsky GL, Goodman ML. Pathology of laryngeal malignancies. In Fried MP (ed). The Larynx: A Multidisciplinary Approach. Boston: Little Brown, 1988; pp. 421–452.

208. Fried MP. Carcinoma of the glottis and subglottis. In Fried MP (ed). The Larynx: A Multidisciplinary Approach. Boston: Little Brown, 1988; pp. 471–490.

209. Weber AL, Shortsleeve M, Goodman ML, et al. Cartilaginous tumors of the larynx and trachea. Radiol Clin North Am 16:261–271, 1978.

EVALUATING THE AIRWAY

CHAPTER 3

Radiology of the Upper Airway

Alfred L. Weber, M.D., and Reginald E. Greene, M.D.

The upper airway is composed of the nasal cavity, oral cavity, oropharynx, larynx, and trachea. A wide spectrum of different entities occur in these respective locations and can be investigated by various radiologic techniques. The indications for these different radiologic examinations depend on the clinical problems to be investigated. Their judicious application requires an understanding of the value and limitations of these various radiologic modalities.

This chapter enumerates and discusses the different radiologic methods in the examination of the upper airway, their indications, and interpretation of the roentgenographic findings. Evaluation of the patient's symptoms, physical examination, and indirect and direct laryngoscopy and bronchoscopy form the basis for selection of the radiologic studies. Table 3–1 lists the techniques that are available for radiologic assessment of the upper airway.

RADIOLOGIC TECHNIQUES FOR THE ASSESSMENT OF THE UPPER AIRWAY

Radiologic Evaluation of the Nasal Cavity, Oral Cavity, and Oropharynx

Routine sinus films are essential for the evaluation of the nasal cavity and oral cavity. They demonstrate the nasal passages and provide a survey view of the choanal area and adjacent nasopharynx and oropharynx. In addition, they outline the mandible, tongue, and remaining structures in the oral cavity. Depending on the clinical question and findings on the conventional films, additional studies may be needed, such as conventional tomography, computed tomography (CT), or magnetic resonance imaging (MRI).

Radiologic Evaluation of the Larynx

Routine radiologic investigation of the larynx is composed of *anteroposterior (AP) and*

Table 3–1. RADIOLOGIC TECHNIQUES IN EVALUATION OF THE UPPER AIRWAY

A. Sinus films
B. Conventional films of the neck
   1. Anteroposterior (AP) and lateral soft-tissue films of the neck
   2. Single-emulsion films
   3. Xeroradiography
C. Tomography
D. Fluoroscopy of the larynx and barium swallow
E. Contrast laryngography
F. Computed tomography (CT)
G. Magnetic resonance imaging (MRI)

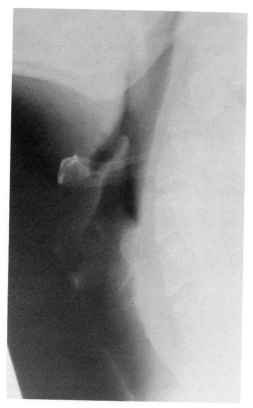

Figure 3–1. Lateral film of the neck demonstrates the larynx, trachea, pharynx, and precervical soft tissues.

"swallowing film" also allows visualization of a foreign body in the upper esophagus that has been obscured by the soft-tissue structures of the superimposed shoulders. One to 2 cm of the trachea and esophagus ascend out of the mediastinum during swallowing.

Xeroradiography is characterized by a wider exposure latitude with edge enhancement, thereby producing higher contrast and increased image resolution.[5] This technique allows delineation of structures that have a roentgenographic density similar to that of the surrounding tissue, such as small calcifications, soft-tissue masses, cartilage abnormalities (fracture, erosion), and foreign bodies.

Tomography of the larynx is carried out in a linear mode, with a 40-degree tube arc and a 0.63-second exposure time.[6] The examination consists of a series of AP views made in

lateral films[1, 2] (Figs. 3–1 and 3–2). The lateral view of the neck provides useful information about the base of tongue, vallecular area, thyroid and cricoid cartilages, posterior pharyngeal wall, precervical soft tissues, and intralaryngeal structures, which include the epiglottis, aryepiglottic folds, arytenoids, false cords, ventricles, true cords, and subglottic space. Diseases that arise or spread in the sagittal plane, including the posterior pharyngeal wall, are readily visible. The use of a *single-emulsion film* permits better visualization of the structures of different densities because of the wider exposure latitude of the film. The AP view (frontal) of the larynx is obtained by using a high-kilovoltage technique (120 kV) and placing a 1-mm copper filter in front of the x-ray tube.[3, 4] This technique enhances the air–soft tissue interface by obscuring bone shadows. The frontal projection aids in lateralizing disease processes and supplements the lateral view. In cases of a suspected foreign body, a lateral view during swallowing is added to distinguish a foreign body from the cartilaginous structures, which move upward. This

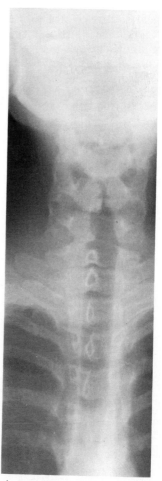

Figure 3–2. Anteroposterior view with high-kilovoltage technique demonstrates the larynx and trachea in the frontal view. High kilovoltage diminishes density of superimposed structures of the spine.

contiguous, 5-mm intervals, extending from the anterior cervical spine to the anterior part of the thyroid cartilage (Fig. 3–3). The 5-mm-thick sections are made during different phonation maneuvers, including quiet inspiration, phonation of E, reverse E (phonation of E during inspiration), and the modified Valsalva maneuver. The reverse E documents the laryngeal ventricles to the best advantage and thereby separates the true from the false cords. The Valsalva maneuver, in which the cheeks are blown out and the lips are closed, distends the pyriform sinuses. The upper trachea is routinely included in the frontal examination of the larynx. Because of delineation of the anatomy in sections, tomography is a useful tool to outline any soft-tissue thickening or mass secondary to inflammation, benign or malignant tumors, or cysts (including laryngoceles). The disadvantage of conventional tomography is the failure to demonstrate the paralaryngeal soft-tissue structures, including the pre-epiglottic space. Also, the anterior and posterior commissures are poorly seen on the frontal coronal sections. Conventional tomography is superior to CT in outlining the laryngeal ventricles, as well as in detecting superficial lesions of the true and false cords.[7] Conventional tomography is equally good as CT for assessing the subglottic space.

Fluoroscopy of the larynx and barium swallow is indicated in the assessment of the dynamics of the larynx.[1] This examination is performed with the patient in the sitting position. It supplements all other radiologic studies of the larynx, including CT. Assessment of vocal cord motion is important in the staging of malignant tumors of the larynx.[8] Fixation of the vocal cords or paralysis of the cords from other causes can be assessed easily with phonation maneuvers, such as phonation of E and inspiration. Opening of the ventricles can be accomplished by having the patient phonate E during inspiration (reverse E). In order to test the distensibility of the pyriform sinus, predominantly the medial and lateral wall and the apex, puffing of the cheek with the mouth closed is performed.

Examination of the pyriform sinus should be carried out in the frontal and both oblique projections, especially if the apex of the pyriform sinus has to be evaluated for tumor. The examination also should be supplemented with a view of the pyriform sinus completely distended by barium and by an air contrast study of the barium-coated pyriform sinus mucosa. If barium coating is insufficient, barium paste (Esophotrast) may be used. The postcricoid portion of the hypopharynx may be secondarily involved by large supraglottic laryngeal and pyriform sinus neoplasms. This area can be examined in the lateral projection by adequate distention with barium (Fig. 3–4). In this manner, transgression of the laryngeal tumor to the postcricoid portion of the hypopharynx and the esophagus can be assessed easily.

In the fluoroscopic study of the larynx, visualization of the air–soft tissue interface can be easily increased by mounting a 1-mm copper filter on the tabletop into the field of the x-ray beam. This is especially useful in studying the infant larynx in the frontal view for assessment of the vocal cord and subglottic space.

Contrast laryngography allows good dem-

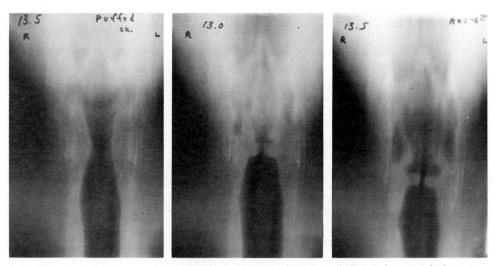

Figure 3–3. Anteroposterior tomographic section in inspiration, phonation of "E," and reversed phonation of "E" demonstrates the intralaryngeal structures in great detail and evaluates the mobility of cords.

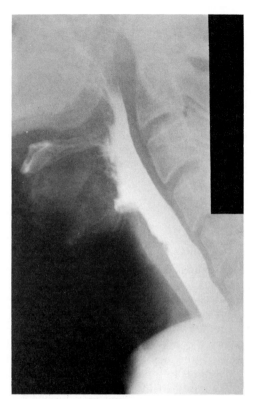

Figure 3–4. Lateral fluoroscopic spot film during swallow demonstrates barium in the pharynx and cervical esophagus. The relation of the postcricoid segment of the hypopharynx is well demonstrated.

onstration of the tomographic anatomy and a clear assessment of the functional dynamics of the larynx and hypopharynx. The value of its practical application is limited, because it cannot be used to demonstrate tumor extension into the deeper structures of the larynx. It has been replaced by CT in the evaluation of laryngeal tumors. This procedure occasionally is applied to determine the extent and configuration of laryngeal stenosis and to simultaneously assess functional alteration of the larynx. This examination should not, however, be undertaken in a severely compromised airway. Under such circumstances, a mild tissue reaction to the media used may be sufficient to precipitate severe respiratory distress.

In recent years, CT has found wide application in the assessment of laryngeal abormalities.[7, 9–12] The standard technique for CT evaluation of the larynx consists of 4- to 5-mm contiguous axial sections (Fig. 3–5). Those slices encompass the entire larynx from the hyoid bone to the second tracheal ring. The patient's head is slightly extended so that the axial sections are parallel with the horizontal

structures within the larynx, such as the vocal cords. In order to carry out a complete examination, 10 to 12 axial sections are usually necessary for assessment of the entire larynx from the hyoid bone to the second tracheal ring. The transaxial scans can be supplemented by coronal and sagittal reformatted images produced from contiguous 1.5-mm transaxial sections.

CT allows more accurate assessment of the paracordal, para-arytenoidal, and pre-epiglottic spaces, as well as the anterior and posterior commissures. In addition, CT demonstrates changes in the laryngeal cartilages, especially in laryngeal injuries or the destruction caused by malignant tumors.[13, 14] An added advantage of CT is the evaluation of soft-tissue structures in the neck, especially for metastatic lymph nodes.

MRI[15, 16] is a new modality that can be used in the assessment of the upper airway, including larynx. The examination is performed with a T1 sequence in the axial, coronal, and sagittal planes, supplemented by an axial T2 sequence. A major advantage of MRI over CT is the acquisition of coronal, oblique, and sagittal sections that encompass the various segments of the upper airway. This is especially helpful to delimit the superoinferior extent of laryngotracheal stenosis and tumors. In addition, vessels of the neck and mediastinum are visualized by their flow voids.

Contrast resolution, which is slightly better than CT, has made significant contributions in

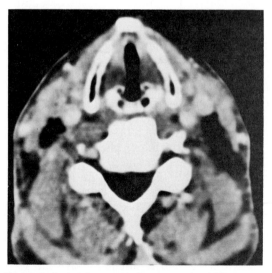

Figure 3–5. Axial computed tomography (CT) section through the larynx at the level of the cords demonstrates the thyroid cartilage, cricoid cartilage, processes of the arytenoids, and vocal cords.

the definition of the various abnormalities, such as stenosis, cysts, and benign and malignant tumors.

Radiologic Evaluation of the Trachea

The radiologic work-up of the trachea[17-20] consists of a lateral neck film, which reveals the larynx and cervical trachea. This is followed by an AP high-kilovoltage film (over 120 kV) with a 1-mm copper filter attached to the overhead tubes. These films demonstrate the air–soft tissue interface to the best advantage. They are supplemented by oblique views of the trachea with the patient in a 45- to 60-degree rotation. Fluoroscopy is performed to check for vocal cord motion and to simultaneously secure spot films of the trachea with different degrees of rotation.

For further assessment, linear tomography in the AP, lateral, and oblique projections can be used. Sections are obtained 0.5 cm apart with linear motion and a 40-degree arc. Lesions arising from the anterior and posterior walls are optimally seen in the oblique and lateral tomographic sections. Lateral wall lesions are best depicted on the AP tomographic sections.

For detailed assessment, including circumferential evaluation of tracheal lesions, CT and MRI can be performed. A survey of the trachea is performed with 5- to 8-mm axial CT sections using the mediastinal technique. A disadvantage of CT, however, is the limitation to axial sections.

For depiction of the trachea in the axial, coronal, sagittal, and oblique planes, MRI is the method of choice. The examination is carried out with a T1-weighted sequence in these various projections, depending on the type of lesion, and supplemented by T2 axial images, especially in benign and malignant tumors and cysts.

Collapsibility of the trachea is age-dependent and more pronounced in the younger individual. With the loss of the supporting structures, mainly cartilage, extreme collapsibility of the trachea takes place, including obliteration of air space; this is referred to as tracheomalacia. The most fixed point is in the area of the aortic arch, which crosses anterior to the trachea and is situated above the left mainstem bronchus. The remaining parts of the trachea can be moved vertically in relation to the surrounding anatomic structures. In the young individual, more than half of the trachea can be positioned above the suprasternal notch in the hyperextended position. In the adult, about 1 to 2.5 cm of the trachea moves above the suprasternal notch in hyperextension of the neck. This is age-dependent and decreases progressively in older patients, especially if they suffer from chronic obstructive pulmonary disease (COPD). In the lateral position, the trachea assumes an oblique course from superoanterior to inferoposterior.

ROENTGENOGRAPHIC ANATOMY

The roentgenographic interpretation of abnormal findings requires a good knowledge of the normal roentgenographic anatomy of the upper airway. The oral cavity is made up of the floor of the mouth, tongue, and hard and soft palate, with the lateral boundaries composed of the mandible. The nasal cavity is divided by the nasal septum, which extends from the nares to the choanal area. Each nasal cavity contains an inferior and middle turbinate with the respective inferior, middle, and superior meati. The upper portion of the nasal cavity is slit-like and bounded laterally by the ethmoid labyrinth and superiorly by the cribriform plate region. The nasal cavity is delimited posteriorly by the choanal areas, which communicate with the nasopharynx.

The oral cavity is bounded posteriorly by the oropharynx and is separated from the larynx by the vallecular areas. The larynx is composed of the aryepiglottic folds, arytenoids, true and false cords, and ventricles, which are usually symmetrical. The subglottic space is tubular and is delimited superiorly by symmetrical cords that form a right angle with the lateral wall of the subglottic space. Posterior to the larynx and the continuation of the oropharynx is the hypopharynx, which is composed of the pyriform sinuses, a lateral and posterior wall. The trachea is anatomically delimited superiorly by the inferior margin of the cricoid cartilage and inferiorly by the carinal spur. Its length ranges from 10 to 13 cm, averaging approximately 11 cm, according to the size of the individual. The airway is roughly elliptical in shape where the lumen is maintained by cartilaginous rings, which form a C with an open membrane posteriorly. The tracheal lumen remains open even in the extreme circumstances of coughing and forced expiration. There is a marked posterior collapsibility of the membranous trachea during coughing.

Pathologic Conditions

When interpreting an abnormal roentgenogram, one should follow a sequence in the description that allows a detailed and complete analysis of the pathologic process. The following parameters of lesions should be determined: the structures involved, size, character, margin, presence of calcification, upper and lower limits, airway compromise, cartilaginous abnormalities, invasion of adjacent structures, ability of the true and false cords including the epiglottis during swallowing, displacement of structures, and abnormal vessels that exert pressure on the airway externally.

Oral Cavity and Nasal Cavity

Significant airway obstruction in the oral cavity or nasal cavity is usually found in newborns. In the oral cavity, there may be marked enlargement of the tongue, such as hemangioma, lymphangioma, amyloidosis, cysts, and in patients with myxedema. Relative enlargement of the tongue is found in Pierre Robin syndrome, which is accentuated by underdevelopment of the mandible. The most important entity in the nasal cavity that causes severe airway obstruction after birth is choanal atresia (Fig. 3–6). Choanal atresia results from a persistence of the nasal buccal membrane; the atresia may be caused by bone or a membranous osseous wall in 80% to 90% and, in the remainder, is membranous. One third of choanal atresias are bilateral, whereas two thirds are unilateral. When bilateral, the condition causes airway obstruction in neonates, who are obligate nasal breathers for up to several weeks. The atresia plate and the adjacent airway can be demonstrated on axial CT sections. Additional information can be obtained by introducing a catheter into both nasal cavities with selective injection of barium. This is done in conjunction with fluoroscopy. Lateral spot films are obtained following the injection of barium in the supine position.

Larynx

Pathologic conditions in the larynx[21–23] can be subdivided into inflammatory, cystic, and

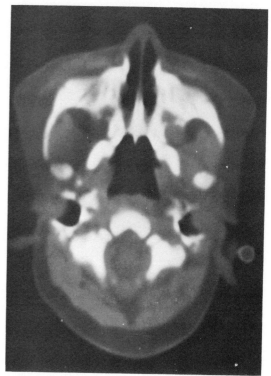

Figure 3–6. Choanal atresia. Axial computed tomography (CT) section (bone window setting) through the nasal cavities demonstrates marked narrowing of the choanal areas, especially on the left.

benign and malignant tumors. The surface contour of the endolarynx is smooth and symmetrical. Inflammatory lesions cause smooth thickening with preservation of mobility of the intralaryngeal structures. In acute supraglottitis, the epiglottis is diffusely swollen, along with the aryepiglottic folds. The edema often encroaches on the valleculae.

In children, the hypopharynx, including the pyriform sinuses, is often distended because air is prevented from entering the vestibule of the larynx. In laryngotracheal bronchitis, also known as croup, edema is noted in the subglottic portion of the larynx and trachea. On the frontal view of the larynx, the subglottic airway is seen to be tapered up to the cords; whereas on the lateral view, the subglottic airway shows a generalized increase in density.

Diffuse airway obstruction may be encountered in patients with severe radiation edema. Radiation edema usually subsides 1 to 3 months after completion of radiation therapy. There often is associated swelling of the precervical soft tissue, which may provide a clue to the underlying cause if a history is not available.

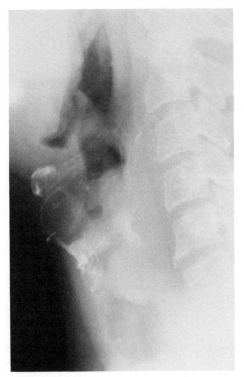

Figure 3–7. Chondroma of the subglottic larynx. Lateral neck film demonstrates a hemispherical-shaped mass in the subglottic larynx that arises from the lamina of the cricoid cartilage. The larynx is deformed as a result of previous surgical procedures for removal of chondroma.

Chronic granulomatous diseases of the larynx may be caused by tuberculosis, fungal disease, and sarcoidosis. They may manifest as diffuse or localized soft-tissue thickening. If irregularity is associated with the thickening, a malignant tumor cannot be differentiated from the granulomatous process.

Benign tumors manifest as sharply defined masses that have no invasive features. They often are homogeneous, and the majority have no characteristic features to differentiate them by radiologic means. A vocal cord polyp is frequently on a stalk and flips up and down with inspiration and expiration. This polyp usually causes no airway obstruction. Papillomas, however, if extensive, may lead to significant airway problems. They are usually irregular soft-tissue excrescences around the glottic and subglottic larynx. In a small number of cases, they spread to the trachea, bronchi, and lung.

Subglottic hemangioma is a lesion seen in the first 6 months of life. This lesion produces an asymmetrical soft-tissue density in the subglottic space and often is associated with stridor and respiratory distress.

Lesions that contain mottled calcification and that often are sharply defined represent the chondroma or low-grade chondrosarcoma (Fig. 3–7). Phleboliths may be encountered in the rare supraglottic cavernous hemangioma.

Laryngoceles arise from the laryngeal ventricle and extend superiorly within the aryepiglottic folds. They are endo- or exolaryngeal and are characterized by an air-filled, cystic structure. If the cyst is filled with fluid, differentiation from a benign tumor is not possible by radiographic means (Fig. 3–8). Differentiation, however, can often be ascertained by CT, where water density is demonstrated, or by MRI, where low-signal intensity is noted on the T1-weighted images and high-signal intensity on the T2-weighted images.

Malignant tumors may arise from any portion of the larynx, but most commonly arise from the true vocal cords. Next in frequency are supraglottic lesions that occur in the larynx above the cords. Most vocal cord lesions do not cause airway obstruction. Large supraglottic tumors, however, are often advanced when the diagnosis is established because of the vague and often nonspecific symptomatology. These lesions often are bulky and project into the supraglottic larynx. The lumen may be

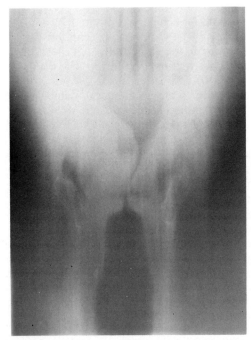

Figure 3–8. Fluid-filled laryngocele. Anteroposterior tomographic section reveals an oval-shaped mass arising from the right aryepiglottic fold, with a bulge into the supraglottic larynx and pyriform sinus. A small air-fluid level is demonstrated in the mid portion of the laryngocele medially.

significantly compromised and airway obstruction may be so severe that an emergency tracheotomy has to be carried out. Again, CT and MRI are the preferred modalities in the assessment of these lesions, especially with respect to location, extent, and the pathognomonic irregularity of the margins.

Laryngeal stenosis is not an uncommon complication which, in most instances, results from iatrogenic trauma or intubation (Fig. 3–9). The stenosis may involve the supraglottic, glottic, or subglottic larynx. Insult of the larynx after intubation may be followed by granuloma formation. If the granuloma is small, no significant airway obstruction is encountered. However, in some cases, especially if it arises in the subglottic larynx, severe airway obstruction may occur (Fig. 3–10). Also, adhesions may form in the anterior and posterior commissure and cause significant limitation in abduction of the vocal cords, with consequent narrowing of the laryngeal lumen at the glottic level. In these instances, fluoroscopy is valuable in defining the remaining lumen with spot radiography and in simultaneously assessing vocal cord mobility, specifically limitation in adduction and abduction.

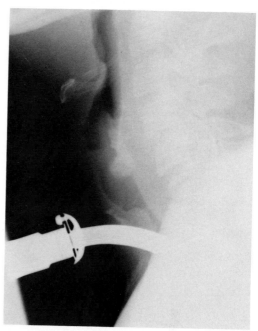

Figure 3–10. Granulomas in the larynx and trachea. Lateral film of the neck reveals a granuloma arising from the lamina of the cricoid cartilage and projecting into the lumen of the subglottic larynx. A second granuloma is visible in the upper anterior trachea, above the tracheotomy tube.

Trachea

Tracheal Stenosis

Post-tracheotomy and intubation lesions occur primarily at two sites: (1) the tracheotomy opening or stoma, and (2) in the area of the balloon cuff.[24–26] In a small percentage of cases, a combination of lesions at these two sites

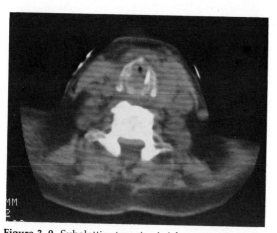

Figure 3–9. Subglottic stenosis. Axial computed tomography (CT) section (bone window setting) demonstrates marked stenosis in the subglottic space, with a small remaining airway anteriorly.

occurs. The lesion at the tracheotomy stoma involves the anterior and lateral tracheal walls and forms a triangular-shaped area of narrowing (Fig. 3–11). Changes in the tracheal wall consist of fibrosis and are often associated with granulation tissue (Fig. 3–12). Another complication seen at the tracheotomy site is the formation of an anterior wall flap from the anterior wall of the trachea above the stoma. The anterior wall flap is displaced into the lumen from extrinsic pressure by the tracheotomy tube. Granulation tissue forming on the flap may increase the severity of the obstruction. When the tracheotomy tube is removed, the flap may act as a ball-valve mechanism and obstruct the tracheal lumen. Lesions at the cuff site are approximately 1 to 1.5 cm below the inferior margin of the tracheotomy stoma and usually involve a segment of trachea from 1 to 4 cm in length (Fig. 3–13A and B). The stenosis is usually circumferential and results from healing of the damaged tracheal wall. If cartilaginous support is lost at this level, tracheomalacia may ensue at the stenosis or in a segment of the trachea above the cuff stenosis. In its fully developed stage, the lesion at the cuff site may vary in appearance from a cir-

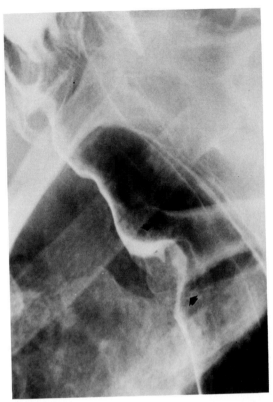

Figure 3–11. Stenosis at the tracheotomy site. Lateral view of a tracheogram obtained following introduction of contrast material reveals detraction of the anterior wall posteriorly, with simultaneous narrowing of the lumen *(arrows)*.

for malacia by having the patient inspire and expire forcefully, followed by coughing. A malacic segment demonstrates marked collapsibility of the trachea, especially the lateral and anterior walls. For detailed assessment of the wall thickness, metaplastic ossification and calcification (a frequent finding in the tracheal wall), the exact length of the stenosis, and the remaining luminal diameter are best assessed with linear tomography. Tomographic sections should be acquired in the AP position and in about 60 to 80 degrees of obliquity, preferably the left anterior oblique position.

CT has contributed significantly to the accurate assessment of the luminal diameter and the exact thickness of the tracheal wall. CT, however, can only be carried out in the axial projection; therefore, the superoinferior extent and the distance from the inferior margin of the cricoid cartilage (beginning of the trachea) and the bifurcation are often difficult to relate.

MRI is a useful modality because of its multiplanar capability. However, due to the cost involved, and often to the unavailability prior to surgery, this radiologic technique has not been used extensively. AP, oblique, and

cumferential diaphragm of fresh granulation tissue to a dense ring of mature fibrous tissue, often covered by metaplastic squamous epithelium. The configuration length of the stenotic segment and obstruction of the lumen cover a wide spectrum of findings.

Anteroposterior and oblique conventional films frequently outline the stenotic lesion, especially the superoinferior dimension. For detailed assessment of the wall thickness and the compromise of the lumen, linear tomography in the AP and oblique projections is used (see Fig. 3–13*B*). The obliquity of the trachea during the examination varies from about 45 to 80 degrees. Most of the stenotic lesions are close to the thoracic inlets, and lateral projections cannot be ascertained because of the overlying shoulders. The appropriate obliquity is, therefore, important for a successful study. In addition to the overhead oblique films, fluoroscopic spot films can be obtained after the patient has been placed into the proper oblique projection during fluoroscopy. The trachea is simultaneously evaluated

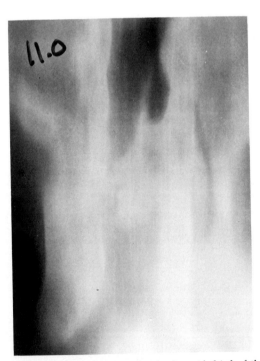

Figure 3–12. Granulation tissue in the mid third of the trachea. Anteroposterior tomographic section through the trachea and proximal mainstem bronchi reveals an irregularly shaped density within the lumen of the trachea, reflecting extensive granulation tissue.

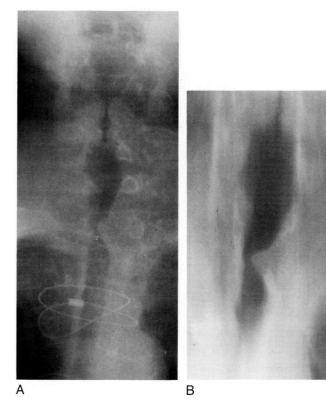

Figure 3–13. Tracheal stenosis. *A,* Anteroposterior high-kilovoltage conventional view of the trachea reveals funnel-shaped narrowing in the mid to upper third of the trachea. *B,* Anteroposterior tomographic section demonstrates a narrowing of the trachea with thickening of the wall.

A   B

lateral views can be obtained in conjunction with coronal and axial sections. Because of the greater contrast resolution, this modality provides considerably more detail than conventional tomography, which is still used extensively in the assessment of tracheal stenosis.

Tracheal Tumors

Tumors of the trachea[27] are relatively rare. They often present late in the course of the patient's disease, and frequently present as obstructive airway disease. The majority of benign lesions are encountered in the pediatric age group, whereas the majority of malignant lesions occur after age 40 years. The most common malignant lesions are squamous cell carcinoma and adenoid cystic carcinoma. Sarcomas and other, rarer malignant lesions are considerably less frequent.

On radiologic examinations, benign lesions are well circumscribed, sometimes lobulated, and are frequently under 2 cm in size. They may be broad based or circumferential, arising from the tracheal wall. Calcification is demonstrated in cartilaginous lesions, such as chondroma, chondroblastoma, and hamartoma.

Most malignant lesions have an irregular surface, with variable extension within the wall of the trachea (Fig. 3–14). They may be flat or bulky with irregular margins (Fig. 3–15). The average length of these tumors is about 2 to 4 cm. Not infrequently, especially the adenoid cystic carcinoma, they may be as long as 10 cm. Irregularity of the surface may be a reflection of ulceration of the tumor. Because of late diagnosis, extratracheal extension into the mediastinum and esophagus may be encountered. The modalities of choice for assessment of the location and extent of the tumor are CT with intravenous contrast infusion and MRI. As mentioned previously, CT can only perform axial sections and therefore lacks the ability to determine the superoinferior extent of the lesion. MRI provides this capability and quite accurately determines the extent of the lesion cranially and caudally. In addition, MRI depicts, by virtue of different signal intensities, the extratracheal tumor component. Because of flow void of fast-flowing blood, vessel invasion, such as into the superior vena cava and pulmonary artery, can be seen. The signal characteristics on the variable imaging parameters, such as T1, proton-density, and T2-weighted images, have no specificity with respect to the histologic type of the lesion. As

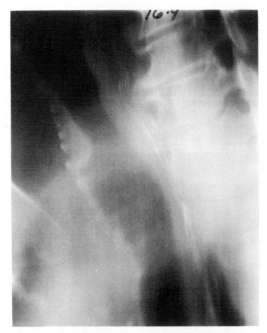

Figure 3–14. Squamous cell carcinoma of the trachea. Oblique tomographic study of the trachea slightly above the thoracic inlet reveals diffuse thickening of the anterior wall of the trachea secondary to tumor.

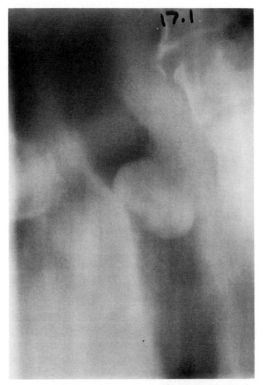

Figure 3–15. Adenoid cystic carcinoma of the trachea. Oblique tomographic section of the trachea reveals an oval-shaped, fairly well demarcated mass arising from the posterior wall of the trachea. There is marked airway compromise, which is caused by the bulky lesion.

mentioned previously, many of these lesions cause airway obstruction as one of the initial symptoms manifested by the patient.

Miscellaneous Lesions of the Trachea

A large variety of miscellaneous lesions affect the trachea, some of which are relapsing polychondritis, rhinoscleroma, amyloidosis, and vascular rings.

Relapsing polychondritis is a systemic disease that is characterized by necrosis of the cartilaginous structures. This is followed by tracheal narrowing with or without malacia.

Rhinoscleroma is a bacterial disease and most commonly involves the larynx but, on occasion, may extend into the trachea. The granulation tissue causes polypoid, irregular masses and narrowing of the lumen secondary to marked fibrosis of the tracheal wall with the consequent stricture.

Amyloidosis is most frequently deposited as a primary form in the larynx. Rarely, amyloidosis is demonstrated within the tracheal wall and causes diffuse narrowing with consequent airway obstruction.

A large variety of *vascular rings* are encountered. The form causing severe airway obstruction is encountered in conjunction with the double aortic arch. In this instance, the trachea is indented anteriorly. A barium swallow is mandatory to demonstrate the posterior segment of the double aortic arch. The posterior segment causes indentation of the esophagus posteriorly. An aberrant left pulmonary artery arising from the right pulmonary artery usually extends between the trachea and esophagus and causes posterior indentation of the trachea and anterior indentation of the esophagus. If the indentation is moderate to severe, airway obstruction of the lower trachea may ensue. On the barium swallow film, there is indentation of the anterior wall of the esophagus at the level of the aberrant left pulmonary artery.

References

1. Weber AL. Radiology of the larynx. Otolaryngol Clin North Am 17:13–28, 1984.
2. Hemmingsson A, Lofroth PO. Xeroradiography and conventional radiography in examination of the larynx. Acta Radiol (Diagn) 17:723–732, 1976.
3. Samuel E, Lloyd GAS. Clinical Radiology of the Ears, Nose and Throat. Philadelphia: W. B. Saunders, 1978.
4. Maguire GH. The larynx: Simplified radiological examination using heavy filtration and high voltage radiography. Radiology 87:102–109, 1966.
5. Doust BD, Ting YML. Xeroradiography of the larynx. Radiology 110:727–730, 1974.
6. Ardran GM, Ebrys Roberts E. Tomography of the larynx. Clin Radiol 16:369, 1965.
7. Gregor RT, Lloyd GAS, Michaels L. Computed tomography of the larynx: A clinical and pathologic study. Head Neck Surg 3:284–296, 1981.
8. Kirchner JA, Som PM. Clinical significance of the fixed vocal cord. Laryngoscope 81:1029, 1971.
9. Mafee MF. CT of the normal larynx. Radiol Clin North Am 22:251–264, 1984.
10. Mancuso AA, Calcaterra TC, Hanafee WN. Computed tomography of the larynx. Radiol Clin North Am 16:195–208, 1978.
11. Silverman PM, Korobkin M, Thompson WM, Johnson GA, Cole TB, Fisher SR. High-resolution, thin-section computed tomography of the larynx. Radiology 145:723, 1982.
12. Mafee MF, Schild JA, Valvassori GE, Capek V. Computed tomography of the larynx: Correlation with anatomic and pathologic studies in cases of laryngeal carcinoma. Radiology 147:123, 1983.
13. Mancuso AA, Hanafee WN. Computed tomography of the injured larynx. Radiology 133:139–144, 1979.
14. Lloyd GAS, Michael I, Phelps PD. The demonstration of cartilaginous involvement in laryngeal carcinoma by computerized tomography. Clin Otolaryngol 6:171–175, 1981.
15. Teresi LM, Lufkin RN, Hanafee WN. Magnetic resonance imaging of the larynx. J Comp Assist Tomogr 11:134, 1987.
16. Curtin HD. Imaging of the larynx: Current concepts. Radiology 173:1, 1989.
17. Felson B, Wiot JF (eds). The trachea. Semin Roentgenol 18:51–60, 1983.
18. Gamsu G, Webb WR. Computed tomography of the trachea and mainstem bronchi. Semin Roentgenol 18:51–60, 1983.
19. Gamsu G, Webb WR. Computed tomography of the trachea: Normal and abnormal. AJR 139:321–326, 1982.
20. Momase KJ, MacMillan AS. Roentgenologic investigations of the larynx and trachea. In Weber AL (ed). The larynx and trachea [symposium]. Radiol Clin North Am 16:321–341, 1978.
21. Kushner DC, Harris BGC. Obstructing lesions of the larynx and trachea in infants and children. Radiol Clin North Am 16:181–194, 1978.
22. Jing BS. Roentgenographic diagnosis of diseases of the larynx. CRC Crit Rev Clin Radiol 401–455, 1973.
23. Weber AL, Shortsleeve M, Goodman M, Montgomery W, Grillo H. Cartilaginous tumors of the larynx and trachea. Radiol Clin North Am 16:261–272, 1978.
24. Weber AL, Grillo HC. Tracheal stenosis: An analysis of 151 cases. Radiol Clin North Am 16:291–308, 1978.
25. Cooper JD, Grillo HC. The evolution of tracheal injury due to ventilatory assistance through cuffed tubes: A pathologic study. Ann Surg 169:334, 1969.
26. Grillo HC, Mathisen DJ, Wain JC. Laryngotracheal resection and reconstruction for subglottic stenosis. Ann Thorac Surg (in press).
27. Weber AL, Grillo HC. Tracheal tumors: A radiological, clinical, and pathological evaluation of 84 cases. Radiol Clin North Am 16:227–246, 1978.

CHAPTER 4

Pulmonary Function Tests to Evaluate the Airway

Carl G. W. Dahlberg, M.D.,* and Charles A. Hales, M.D.

Basic tests of pulmonary function are easily obtained and can be very useful in evaluating a patient whose upper airway is suspected to be compromised. For purposes of this discussion, the "upper airway" is defined as that portion of the respiratory tree from the mouth to the carina, encompassing the mouth, pharynx, larynx, and trachea. Although the presence of upper airway compromise may already be known or may become apparent on the patient's presentation or during the course of a routine history and physical examination, a condition such as upper airway obstruction (UAO) frequently may be unrecognized or may be misdiagnosed as another condition involving obstruction of the smaller airways, such as chronic obstructive airways disease or asthma. Basic spirometry can offer valuable, reliable, and quick information concerning both the location (intrathoracic versus extrathoracic) as well as the nature (fixed versus dynamic) of the lesion. Pulmonary function testing is further valuable in this group of patients because a large number also have coexisting pulmonary parenchymal disease, the quantitation of which may become important

in the subsequent medical or surgical management of the patient's airway compromise.

The physiologic characteristics of UAO in adults were first classified by Miller and Hyatt in 1969,[1] who, through the use of simple volume displacement spirometry, were able to recognize distinct forms of UAO by anatomic location as well as physiologic behavior. Although the methods by which spirometry is obtained have become more sophisticated with time, the same physiologic principles relating to dynamic airflow through the large airways still holds true in the evaluation of the patient in whom UAO is suspected. This chapter focuses on those aspects of clinical pulmonary function testing that may help the clinician properly assess the location, nature, and severity of a UAO.

PHYSIOLOGY

Understanding the physiology of airflow in the large airways is essential to the accurate interpretation of spirometric testing in the patient with acute or chronic obstruction of the upper airway. Clearly, the consequences of any obstruction of the upper airways depends on several variables, which include (1) the

*Support provided under NIH Training Grant HL-07354.

anatomic location of the obstruction; (2) the diameter of the airway at the site of the obstruction; (3) the nature of the lesion (fixed versus dynamic); and (4) the point in the respiratory cycle during which the obstruction is detected.[2] Indeed, whether or not a lesion even causes symptoms depends on the severity of the obstruction, as well as on the performance status of the patient. For example, Geffin and associates[3] demonstrated that, in a patient at rest, an intratracheal lesion must obstruct the airway to a 5-mm diameter to produce inspiratory stridor at rest; Al-Bazzaz and colleagues[4] showed that a lesser degree of tracheal obstruction (to an 8-mm tracheal diameter) would cause symptoms with exercise. The occurrence of stridor with lesser degrees of tracheal obstruction during exercise is thought to be secondary to increased turbulence in the upper airway, as seen with increased airflow during exertion; lesser degrees of UAO therefore may be more readily apparent in the more active patient, who has a higher performance status.

A knowledge of the transmural pressures across the large central airways during both inspiratory and expiratory phases of the respiratory cycle is key to understanding the effects of obstructing lesions of the central airways on those flows. The extrathoracic upper airway is surrounded by atmospheric pressure, whereas the intrathoracic upper airway is surrounded by pleural pressure. The exact anatomic site of this transition between the intra- and extrathoracic airway is not well defined and may vary with longitudinal movement of the trachea, as occurs with extension of the neck. Thus, there is a zone in the region of the thoracic inlet where varying effects may be seen. The difference between the intraluminal pressure of the upper airway and the external (atmospheric) pressure is the transmural pressure. This concept can be confusing unless one remembers that transmural pressure is calculated by subtracting the pressure outside the object of interest from that inside it. Therefore

$$P_{inside} - P_{outside} = \text{transmural pressure}$$

For the airway, this means that transluminal pressure equals intraluminal minus extraluminal pressure, or

$$P_{trans} = P_{IL} - P_{EL}$$

where P_{trans} is transmural pressure, P_{IL} is intraluminal pressure, and P_{EL} is extraluminal pressure. Remembering this convention will help one understand the nature of tracheal transmural pressure inside or outside the thorax,

because extraluminal airway pressure changes from negative inside the thorax to positive outside. Clearly, if the extraluminal pressure exceeds the intraluminal pressure, the lumen of the airway tends to collapse. Conversely, if the intraluminal pressure exceeds the external pressure, the airway remains open. Therefore, a negative transmural pressure tends to collapse the airway, whereas a positive transmural pressure tends to open, or "splint," the airway. Figure 4–1 diagrammatically illustrates the different pressures present in the intra- and extrathoracic airway. With normal inspiration, the chest cage expands and the diaphragm descends, increasing intrathoracic volume and creating a negative intrathoracic pressure due to decompression of gases within the thorax. This creates a pressure gradient compared to atmospheric pressure outside the chest, so that opening the mouth allows air to rush in and expand the lungs. During normal inspiration, there is a negative pressure inside the extrathoracic airway at the same time that there is relative positive pressure, which is caused by normal atmospheric pressure outside the airway. Thus, there is a normal tendency of the extrathoracic airway to collapse during inspiration; this tendency is countered by the relative rigidity of the airway in the neck, as well as the neural innervation of the pharynx, which keeps the pharynx taut in order to prevent upper airway collapse.

The nature of the airway obstruction is equally as important as its anatomic location. An obstruction that differs with the phase and duration of the respiratory cycle is termed a variable obstruction. In extrathoracic variable obstruction, the degree of obstruction is increased during inspiration. As a patient in-

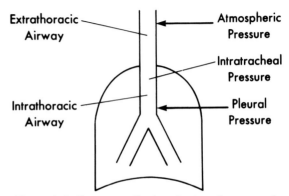

Figure 4–1. Pressures affecting the intrathoracic and extrathoracic upper airway. (From Acres JC, Kryger MH. Upper airway obstruction. Chest 80:207–211, 1981; with permission.)

spires, the pressure within the trachea falls, whereas the external pressure around the trachea (barometric pressure) remains unchanged. A decrease in intraluminal pressure results in a decrease in the transmural pressure, causing the trachea to collapse and worsening the obstruction. With expiration, the intraluminal pressure of the trachea rises, causing a relative increase in the transmural pressure and lessening the degree of obstruction with concomitant improvement of airflow (Fig. 4–2).

In the presence of a variable intrathoracic obstruction, the physiology of airflow around or through the obstruction is the reverse of the case of variable extrathoracic obstruction. In intrathoracic obstruction, the positive pleural pressure generated on forced expiration may exceed the intraluminal pressure, causing a decrease in the transmural pressure and consequent collapse of the airway, thus worsening the obstruction. On inspiration, the pleural pressure becomes more negative than the intraluminal pressure, causing an increase in the transmural pressure, thereby lessening the obstruction and improving flow (Fig. 4–3).

A fixed obstruction does not change with the phase or frequency of respiration and therefore is unaffected by the location of the obstruction. In other words, a fixed extrathoracic obstruction has the same effects as a fixed intrathoracic obstruction.

FLOW–VOLUME CHARACTERISTICS

As noted previously, the flow–volume loop can impart a great deal of information con-

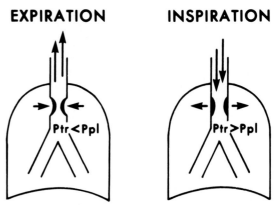

Figure 4–3. Behavior of an intrathoracic upper airway obstruction during the respiratory cycle. Note that intratracheal pressure (Ptr) increases with inspiration, decreasing the magnitude of the obstruction. (From Acres JC, Kryger MH. Upper airway obstruction. Chest 80:207–211, 1981; with permission.)

cerning the nature and location of a UAO. To this end, a brief description of the physiology of a normal flow–volume loop is essential to understand the pathophysiology demonstrated by a flow–volume loop in a patient with UAO.

Normally, the flow rate of the first 25% of the expired forced vital capacity is directly dependent on effort and inversely dependent on resistance. As an example, if a wrestler applies a bear hug to your chest during this initial phase of expiration, air flow at the mouth will rise even beyond your best forced expiratory effort. The remaining 75% of the loop is termed the "effort-independent" portion. This designation is somewhat of a misnomer, because a good expiratory effort is still necessary, but "super" efforts or training (or assistance from Hulk Hogan) will not augment airflow in addition to that which can be achieved with a good effort. Flow is limited in such a way that an increase in expiratory effort with an associated increase in pleural pressure does not result in increased flow.[2] During a forced exhalation from total lung capacity (TLC), the first 25% of flow reflects the emptying of air from the central as well as the peripheral airways. It is this "effort-dependent" portion of the flow–volume curve that assumes particular importance in the diagnosis of UAO. In the presence of UAO, flow in the effort-dependent portion of the curve may be limited by two factors: the presence of an upper airway obstruction or the collapse of the airway itself under negative transmural pressure, as noted previously. This phenomenon was first recognized by Miller and Hyatt in

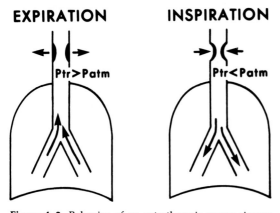

Figure 4–2. Behavior of an extrathoracic upper airway obstruction throughout the respiratory cycle. Note that the magnitude of the obstruction increases with forced inspiration. Ptr, intratracheal pressure. (From Acres JC, Kryger MH. Upper airway obstruction. Chest 80:207–211, 1981; with permission.)

1969,[1] when they simulated the effect of central airway obstruction by having normal subjects breathe through fixed resistances at the mouth while they measured the resulting flow–volume loops. They discovered that the flow rate increased to a certain level early in both inspiration and expiration and then plateaued. The flow rate at which the plateau was reached was inversely related to the magnitude of the resistance employed[1] (Fig. 4–4).

As an extension of this concept, limitation of airflow in the effort-dependent portion of the curve is recognized by the presence of a plateau in either the inspiratory or expiratory arm (or both) of the flow–volume loop. As might be expected, the lower (the last 25% to 50%), more effort-independent portion of the curve is unaffected by a central obstruction, because at lower volumes flow is limited as a result of dynamic compression of the small airways, rather than by a central mechanism.[5] In the case of an extrathoracic variable obstruction, one would expect to see a plateau in the inspiratory portion of the flow–volume loop (due to the decrease in transmural pressure during inspiration), whereas the expiratory portion of the curve would appear closer to normal (Fig. 4–5A). Conversely, an intrathoracic variable obstruction would manifest as a plateau in the expiratory portion of the flow–volume loop due to a negative transmural pressure during that portion of the respiratory cycle, whereas the inspiratory portion of the curve would appear less abnormal (Fig. 4–5B). The character of these flow–volume loops underscores the importance of carefully obtaining high-quality inspiratory as well as expiratory loops on any patient in whom an upper or central airway obstruction is suspected. It can readily be seen that poor patient effort may mimic UAO. A good set of pulmonary function tests should contain at least three reproducible flow–volume curves in order to minimize the occurrence of a false-positive test. Anatomic disease is likely to be readily reproducible; poor effort is rarely so.

A plateau is present in the early portion of both the inspiratory and expiratory flow–volume loops in the presence of a fixed upper airway obstruction, regardless of whether the obstruction is intra- or extrathoracic. A fixed obstruction demonstrates little variability in

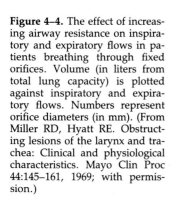

Figure 4–4. The effect of increasing airway resistance on inspiratory and expiratory flows in patients breathing through fixed orifices. Volume (in liters from total lung capacity) is plotted against inspiratory and expiratory flows. Numbers represent orifice diameters (in mm). (From Miller RD, Hyatt RE. Obstructing lesions of the larynx and trachea: Clinical and physiological characteristics. Mayo Clin Proc 44:145–161, 1969; with permission.)

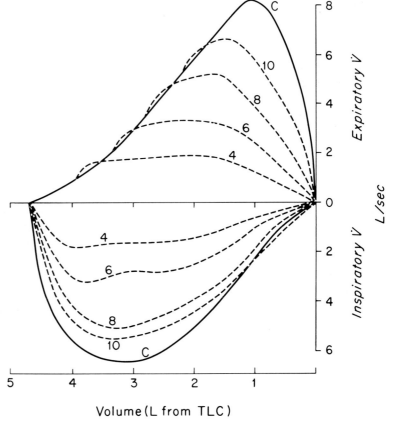

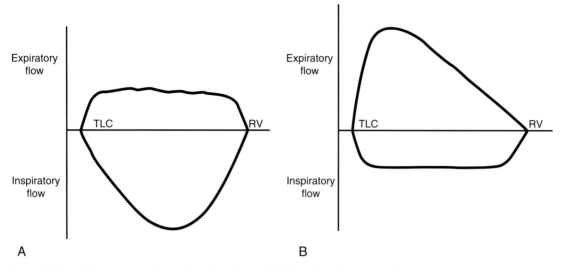

Figure 4–5. *A,* Characteristic flow–volume loop in variable intrathoracic airway obstruction. *B,* Characteristic flow–volume loop in variable extrathoracic airway obstruction.

changing transmural pressures, as noted previously; therefore, limitation to flow will be equally demonstrated in both phases of the respiratory cycle (Fig. 4–6).

SPIROMETRY

Although the shape of flow–volume curves can provide valuable insight into the nature and location of a UAO, spirometric testing, which generates flow–volume curves, may not always be available. Several clues to UAO may be obtained from a spirometric program that only calculates standard variables, such as the forced expiratory volume in one second (FEV_1), the forced vital capacity (FVC), the peak expiratory flow (PEFR), forced inspiratory and expiratory flows at 50% of vital capacity (FIF 50% and FEF 50%), without the production of a flow–volume loop. For example, the presence of a peak expiratory flow that is reduced out of proportion to the FEV_1 may be highly indicative of some form of UAO. Several investigators have used these various pulmonary function tests to compare patients with UAO to normals. Rotman and colleagues[6] compared patients with documented tracheal obstruction with normals as well as with those with chronic obstructive pulmonary disease (COPD). They identified four variables that reliably served to separate the individuals with UAO from those with chronic obstructive lung disease; these variables are presented in Table 4–1. The first two

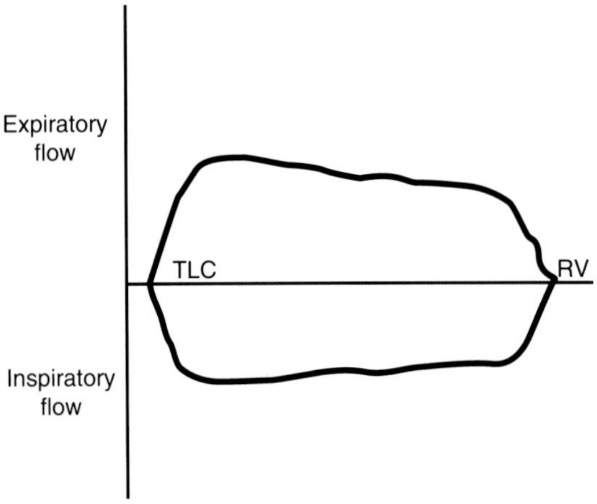

Figure 4–6. Characteristic flow–volume loop in fixed intra- or extrathoracic upper airway obstruction.

Table 4–1. SPIROMETRIC CRITERIA OF ROTMAN FOR DIFFERENTIATION OF PATIENTS WITH UPPER AIRWAY OBSTRUCTION FROM THOSE WITH CHRONIC AIRWAYS OBSTRUCTION

1. FIF 50% $\leq$ 100 L/min
2. FEF 50%/FIF 50% $\geq$ 1
3. FEV_1/PEFR $\geq$ 10 mL/L/min
4. FEV_1/$FEV_{0.5}$ $\geq$ 1.5

50%, forced inspiratory flow at 50% of the vital capacity; FEF 50%, forced expiratory flow at 50% of the vital capacity; PEFR, peak expiratory flow rate in L/min; FEV_1, forced expiratory volume in 1 second in mL; $FEV_{0.5}$, forced expiratory volume in 0.5 second in mL.

criteria are absolute and are clearly related to the reduction of airflow that one would expect around the obstruction. (Note that the first of these criteria identifies a decrement in the forced inspiratory flow at 50% of the vital capacity in the patient with UAO, a criterion that is seldom used today.) The third criterion relates to the fact that the PEFR is proportionately more reduced by the UAO compared to the FEV_1. This concept is more easily grasped if one remembers that the peak flow in normals occurs at the very beginning of forced exhalation and is sustained only very briefly. Modern spirometers are often unable to respond quickly enough to represent this peak graphically in a flow–volume loop, but record the peak flow numerically in a separate format from the spirometric tracing. A patient with true UAO is unable to produce this initial sharp "peak" in the expiratory arm of the flow–volume loop that is coincident with a normal peak flow. Instead, there is a decrement in the peak flow that is out of proportion to that decrement seen in the FEV_1, because it is this initial "explosive" high flow rate at the beginning of exhalation that is most affected by the presence of an UAO. The only caveat here is that the clinician must also remember that the PEFR is directly dependent on patient effort. Therefore, if a patient is consistently providing maximal efforts on forced expiration yet cannot generate a PEFR in a predicted range similar to that obtained for the FEV_1, the diagnosis of UAO should be suspected.

Similarly, the $FEV_{0.5}$ is reduced disproportionately to the FEV_1 in UAO, further describing the plateau in expiratory flow rates at high lung volumes seen on the flow–volume loop, as noted previously. These values are readily available from most pulmonary function laboratories and may serve to alert the physician to an unsuspected case of UAO. Additionally, in patients with known obstruction, these indices can be used to follow the severity or progression of disease. If available, however, a flow–volume loop is preferable, because inspection of the flow–volume loop allows more ready assessment of patient effort and because the flow–volume system is more sensitive to transients in flow rate.

MIXED UPPER AND LOWER AIRWAY OBSTRUCTION

Although rare, the combination of chronic airway obstruction and UAO can coexist in the same patient. As an example, a patient with severe asthma might develop tracheal stenosis after endotracheal intubation for respiratory failure. By taking advantage of the differences in the properties of airflow between the larger upper airways and the smaller peripheral airways and by using special maneuvers that employ a mixture of helium and oxygen, the presence of UAO can be detected in those patients who otherwise appear to demonstrate chronic diffuse airways obstruction.

In the upper, larger airways, flow is turbulent and depends on the density of the gas being measured, whereas in smaller, peripheral airways, flow is laminar and less dependent on gas density.[7] Breathing a mixture of helium and oxygen, which is less dense than air, increases the flow of the gas in density-dependent portions of the lung. This effect is magnified in the presence of a UAO, which increases turbulence in the upper airway. By contrast, in the peripheral airways the flow of air is laminar, and laminar flow is not increased when breathing a helium–oxygen mixture. This principle was illustrated by Lavelle and colleagues,[8] who examined three patients with chronic airflow obstruction, seven patients with documented UAO, and six normals by having them perform basic spirometry while breathing room air and while breathing a mixture of 80% helium and 20% oxygen. They demonstrated that the patients with documented tracheal obstruction were able to increase their expiratory flow rates at peak flow, 75% of ventilatory capacity (VC), and 50% of VC while breathing the helium–oxygen mixture, presumably due to a decrease in turbulent airflow in the upper airways as a result of the decreased density of the gas mixture. The patients with chronic airway obstruction showed no significant change in their expiratory flows at any lung volume, because the dominant site of airflow obstruction in advanced chronic obstructive pulmonary disease is the small airways.[8] Although not often employed, observance of changes in flow rates after inhalation of helium–oxygen mixtures can help differentiate between patients with UAO and patients with chronic obstruction of the smaller airways. In particular, this test may be useful in detecting UAO in patients with COPD.

Another approach that has been used to help detect the presence of UAO when it occurs concomitantly with chronic airways obstruction is to apply other measures of distribution of ventilation, such as the nitrogen washout method. In the nitrogen washout test, the patient breathes 100% oxygen for several minutes to wash the nitrogen from the lungs. Normally, all but 1% to 2% of the nitrogen is washed out in 2 to 3 minutes. In patients with COPD, however, the maldistribution of ventilation may be so pronounced that breathing 100% oxygen for as long as 20 minutes may be necessary to obtain an end-expired concentration of nitrogen of 1% to 2%. In patients with UAO but without chronic airways obstruction, the nitrogen washout test is normal.[9, 10] An increase in airways resistance that is unresponsive to bronchodilators also is seen in patients with UAO. Therefore, the combination of a normal nitrogen washout test in the presence of increased airways resistance that is resistant to bronchodilators should lead one to suspect the presence of UAO.

OTHER TESTS OF SPIROMETRIC FUNCTION

The maximum voluntary ventilation (MVV) maneuver may be used to distinguish the presence of UAO. The MVV maneuver is performed by having a subject ventilate as vigorously as possible for a period of 15 or 30 seconds, measuring the volume expired, and then multiplying that number by 4 or 2 to obtain the volume expired per minute. In normals, the MVV (L/min) will be 35 to 40 times the value obtained for the FEV_1 (L). The patient's ability to perform the MVV maneuver relies in great part on the resistance encountered across the upper airway. In adults, this resistance is approximately 1 cm $H_2O/L/sec$, whereas patients with symptomatic UAO may have a resistance between 4 and 15 cm $H_2O/L/sec$. The resistance across the upper airway is not constant; with increasing flow (such as during exercise), this resistance increases disproportionately with flow.[3] This increase in airways resistance is reflected in the performance of the MVV maneuver; patients with UAO exhibit increasing airway resistance as they attempt to augment their ventilation and increase flow. The result is a reduction in MVV that is out of proportion to the patient's decrement in FEV_1. In patients with COPD, the decrement noted in the performance of the MVV maneuver is more proportional to the decrement in the FEV_1 because the principal site of obstruction in these patients is the small airways.

SUMMARY

The physician confronted with the challenge of a possible partial obstruction of the upper or central airway may be faced with a situation in which rapid clinical and diagnostic assessment may be necessary to prevent significant morbidity. The judicious use of simple spirometric maneuvers may help quickly define the anatomy as well as physiology of the obstructing lesion, giving the physician valuable insight into the subsequent management necessary to provide the best outcome possible. Pulmonary function tests may also alert the physician to a mixed lesion in which severe COPD may make postoperative respiratory management of the patient difficult. Although the performance of basic pulmonary function tests may be possible in an acute setting, it is also important to remember that patients with severe UAO may not be able to cooperate with even the simplest flow–volume maneuvers; in such cases, other diagnostic procedures, such as flexible endoscopy, may be necessary. In less acute settings, studies of pulmonary function as outlined above are valuable as a screening tool to alert the physician to the presence of previously unrecognized, possibly severe upper airway pathology.

References

1. Miller RD, Hyatt RE. Obstructing lesions of the larynx and trachea: Clinical and physiologic characteristics. Mayo Clin Proc 44:145–161, 1969.
2. Acres JC, Kryger MH. Upper airway obstruction. Chest 80:207–211, 1981.
3. Geffin B, Grillo HC, Cooper JD, Pontoppidan H. Stenosis following tracheostomy for respiratory care. JAMA 216:1, 1971.
4. Al-Bazzaz F, Grillo H, Kazemi H. Responses to exercise in upper airway obstruction. Am Rev Respir Dis 111:631–640, 1975.
5. Miller RD, Hyatt RE. Evaluation of obstructing lesions of the trachea and larynx by flow-volume loops. Am Rev Respir Dis 108:475–481, 1973.
6. Rotman HH, Liss HP, Weg JG. Diagnosis of upper airway obstruction by pulmonary function testing. Chest 68:796, 1975.
7. Gold M, Marks A, Bocles JS. Effects of reduction in air density on dynamic function in obstructive airways disease. Am Rev Respir Dis 90:316, 1964.
8. Lavelle TF Jr, Rotman HH, Weg JG. Isoflow-volume curves in the diagnosis of upper airway obstruction. Am Rev Respir Dis 117:845–852, 1978.
9. Sackner MA. Physiologic features of upper airway obstruction. Chest 62:414–417, 1972.
10. Simonsson BG, Malmberg R. Differentiation between localized and generalized airway obstruction. Thorax 19:416–419, 1964.
11. Kryger M, Bode F, Antic R, Anthonisen N. Diagnosis of obstruction of the upper and central airways. Am J Med 61:85–93.

CHAPTER 5

Bedside Evaluation of the Pediatric Airway

James T. Roberts M.D., M.A., and
Ronald D. Eavey, M.D., F.A.A.P., F.A.C.S.

The general location of a partial airway obstruction may often be obtained at the patient's bedside. Common sites of obstruction in the pediatric patient and the usual sounds associated with each are illustrated in Figure 5–1 and Table 5–1.

HISTORY

The history of the patient should include details about respiration, aspiration, phonation, and cough.

Respiration. Is the breathing noisy? Is there stridor? Is the stridor inspiratory or expiratory? Is the stridor to and fro? Is there a "wet" sound in the chest with respiration? If apnea is present, is it a central pattern or an obstructive pattern? Is there cyanosis? What degree of respiratory distress is present? Is the respiratory distress related to feedings or position? Is there a prior history of respiratory distress, perhaps associated with intubation, prematurity, or the need for an apnea monitor? Is there arching of the back?

Aspiration. Is there a feeding pattern of choking, coughing, or vomiting? Is this associated immediately with swallowing, or does it occur later on? Is there a difference between how the child handles liquids and solids? Has the child gained weight from birth? Does the

child overeat or undereat? In what position does the child prefer to feed? Is there nasal reflux?

Phonation. Is the voice projection robust, with a lusty cry and strong voice, or is the voice hoarse, weak, and muffled? Is there aphonia? What is the intubation history?

Cough. Is the cough normal, croupy, or brassy? Is it ever associated with swallowing?

VISUAL EXAMINATION

General Appearance. What is the patient's general appearance? Are there gross neurologic or dysmorphic features?

Respiratory Rate. Is the respiratory rate within normal limits, regular or irregular? Look for tachypnea.

Color. Are the nail beds cyanotic?

Skin Retractions. Is there nasal flare, suprasternal retraction, intercostal or subcostal retraction?

Position. Is the child arched back or leaning forward?

Mouth. Is the mouth open or closed?

Drooling. Is there drooling?

Oral Intake. Examine the infant with a pacifier or bottle.

Neck Appearance. Is there distention of the

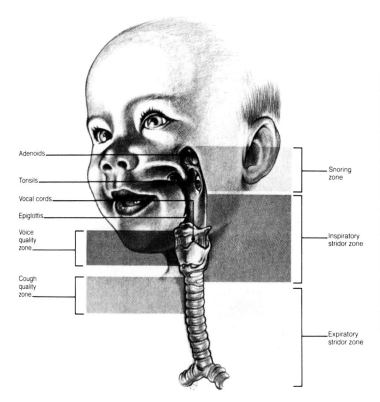

Adenoids

Tonsils

Vocal cords

Epiglottis

Voice quality zone

Cough quality zone

Snoring zone

Inspiratory stridor zone

Expiratory stridor zone

Figure 5–1. Sounds and sites of pediatric airway obstruction. Listening can help locate the site of airway obstruction. A loud, gasping snore suggests that tonsils or adenoids are enlarged. Inspiratory stridor occurs when the airway is compromised at the level of the supraglottic larynx, vocal cords, subglottic region, or upper trachea. Expiratory stridor results from a foreign body or vascular ring in the lower trachea or bronchi. Hoarseness or a weak cry is a byproduct of obstruction at the level of the vocal cords. When the cough is croupy, suspect constriction below the vocal cords; when it is also low pitched, the trachea probably is constricted. (Reprinted with permission from PATIENT CARE, March 30, 1986, copyright © Medical Economics Publishing, Inc., Montvale, New Jersey 07645. All rights reserved.)

neck veins? Look for discoloration or edema as signs of trauma.

AUDITORY EXAMINATION

Stridor. Is the stridor inspiratory or expiratory? Is the stridor to and fro?

Voice. What is the voice quality?

Cough. What is the cough quality? Is it

Table 5–1. USUAL SOUNDS INDICATING COMMON SITES OF PEDIATRIC AIRWAY OBSTRUCTION

1. *Snoring that is loud and gasping* is associated with enlarged adenoids and tonsils.
2. *Inspiratory stridor* suggests partial obstruction at the supraglottic, vocal cord, or subglottic level.
3. *Expiratory stridor* suggests a foreign body or vascular ring in the lower trachea or larger bronchi.
4. *Hoarseness* or a weak cry may imply vocal cord disturbances.
5. *Croupy cough* indicates obstruction below the level of the vocal cords.
6. *Croupy cough that is low pitched* probably implies that the trachea is also involved.

croupy, suggesting subglottic narrowing, or is it brassy, suggesting tracheal narrowing?

Wet Respirations. Are there pooled secretions?

PALPATION

Anterior Thyroid Cartilage. Is there fremitus with bilateral abductor vocal cord paralysis associated with light palpation of the anterior thyroid cartilage?

Chest Palpation. Is there fremitus with significant tracheal compression?

AUSCULTATION

Listen over the nose, face, neck, chest, and heart if cor pulmonale is suspected.

COMMON CAUSES OF PARTIAL AIRWAY OBSTRUCTION IN THE CHILD

Enlarged Tonsils or Adenoids

When airway obstruction is suspected due

to enlarged tonsils or adenoids, inquire about the child's sleeping and eating habits, as well as any history of nasal congestion. Snoring is commonly associated with enlarged adenoids or enlarged tonsils, whereas stridor is associated with partial laryngeal or tracheal obstruction. Quiet, rhythmic snoring is of little concern, but loud, choppy, intermittent snoring, where the child is straining for air, should be a red flag. Inquire whether sleep is disturbed. An elevated PCO_2 secondary to inadequate ventilation may induce nocturnal sweating. Mouth breathing is common. Drooling may also occur. Usually, the child with enlarged tonsils or adenoids eats with his or her mouth open, gulps his or her food, and talks as if his or her mouth were full of cotton. A history that the child chokes, gags, or feeds without taking intermittent breaths is a sign of airway obstruction. Nasal congestion may also be a significant event in the history. Nasal stuffiness without rhinorrhea and an impaired sense of smell are consistent with enlarged adenoids. With enlarged tonsils, examination of the nasal passages may demonstrate a clear pathway between nasal septum and turbinates in the presence of obstructed nasal ventilation. Hyponasal speech is common.

Laryngomalacia

Laryngomalacia is characterized by collapse of the supraglottic structures during inspiration. The epiglottis may be furled and admit air through only a small slit. Laryngomalacia may also be complicated by enlarged arytenoids that approximate the midline. Obstruction at this level induces hoarseness or diminished cry.

Partial Obstruction at the Level of the Vocal Cords

Subtotal obstruction at the level of the vocal cords produces hoarseness and is characterized by the ability to cry, but prevents adequate ventilation. Vocal cord paralysis may be acquired or congenital.

During indirect examination of the vocal cords, have the child keep the tongue inside his or her mouth (not protruded), and have the child pant (not say "Ah") while the tongue is depressed with a tongue blade placed parallel to the floor.

Examination of the vocal cords may be easily obtained with a headlamp and mirror or perhaps more easily with a flexible fiberoptic laryngoscope. During inspiration, the vocal cords are abducted; during expiration, the vocal cords tend to approximate one another. Paralysis of a single vocal cord allows ventilation to occur, but the patient's voice quality is changed and diminished. Paralysis of both vocal cords that results from injury of both recurrent laryngeal nerves causes ventilatory obstruction. This type of vocal cord paralysis occurs infrequently after surgery of the thyroid gland, as well as after blunt trauma to the neck.

Subglottic Stenosis

Subglottic stenosis (where the airway within the cricoid ring is constricted) usually produces either a high- or low-pitched croupy cough. Subglottic stenosis in infants most commonly follows intubation. A pertinent history, when airway compromise involving the larynx or trachea is suspected, should include whether the respiratory stridor is inspiratory or expiratory. Inspiratory stridor results from airway obstruction at or above the level of the upper trachea. Expiratory stridor implies obstruction at the midtracheal to bronchial level. Situations leading to stridor include not only laryngeal or tracheal swelling during the postintubation period, but also trauma to the larynx or neck, aspiration of a foreign body, and upper respiratory burns.

CHAPTER 6

Rigid and Flexible Bronchoscopy

John Wain, M.D.

Bronchoscopy is the technique for direct visualization of the airway from the glottic region to the fifth-order bronchi via an instrument that allows both inspection and instrumentation of the tracheobronchial tree. Two types of instruments are used for this procedure: *rigid* bronchoscopes and *flexible* bronchoscopes. The construction and techniques for use of these differ greatly, but both have overlapping clinical applications, as well as advantages unique to each instrument. Problems of airway management, particularly ones of a complex nature, are optimally handled with the concerted use of both types of bronchoscopes, as dictated by clinical circumstances.

HISTORICAL BACKGROUND

The ability to perform *endoscopy* (from the Greek, to examine within) was limited until the late 19th century. Although optical science was well developed prior to that time, attempts at inspection of body cavities were hampered by the available light sources (primarily open flames) and the cooperation of the patient. The invention of the carbon incandescent electric lamp in 1879 and the discovery and characterization of local anesthetic agents in 1880 allowed further advancement of endoscopic techniques. Mikulicz[1] pioneered the use of incandescent light with rigid endoscopes to view the esophagus. In 1897, Killian[2] made use of a Mikulicz-type esophagoscope, combined with topical application of cocaine to the tracheobronchial tree, to extract a bronchial foreign body under direct visualization and became "the father of bronchoscopy." He subsequently designed a rigid tube illuminated by reflected light from an incandescent lamp specifically for visualization of the tracheobronchial tree—the first rigid bronchoscope. The incorporation of an auxiliary tube serving as a light carrier within the lumen of the bronchoscope by Jackson in 1904 perfected the rigid instrument. Later developments included the addition of a side arm to allow for administration of gaseous agents via the bronchoscopic lumen and the development of a telescopic rod–lens system. Ikeda and others[3] applied fiberoptic technology (as described by Hopkins and Kapany[4]) to bronchoscopy and demonstrated the first flexible fiberoptic bronchoscope, using a "cold" light source for illumination. Recent advances include refinement of the fiberoptics to allow instruments with as small as a 1.8-mm outer diameter to be available and clinically useful.

ANATOMY AND PHYSIOLOGY

The methods of insertion of the rigid and flexible bronchoscopes differ widely, but once through the glottic opening, the disposition of the tracheobronchial tree can be consistently identified by either instrument. Bronchoscopy, rigid or flexible, mandates observation of (1) tracheobronchial anatomy, (2) respiratory alterations in the airway, (3) mucosal characteristics, and (4) pathologic lesions. The normal structural and functional characteristics of the tracheobronchial tree must be familiar to the bronchoscopist in order to interpret the findings visualized in the airway.

Subglottic Region and Trachea

The *subglottic region* is a dome-like area circumscribed intraluminally by the conus elasticus and externally by the signet-ring shaped cricoid cartilage and cricothyroid membrane. The proximal limit of the subglottic space is defined by the undersurface of the true cords; distally, it continues as the tracheal airway.

The *trachea* is a flexible tube extending from the subglottic region to the right and left main bronchi. It is composed of conjoined horseshoe arches of cartilage anterolaterally that are spanned by a membranous wall of smooth muscle (the trachealis muscle) posteriorly. This construction forms a semicircular cross section and allows for motion in longitudinal, transverse, and anteroposterior axes. During spontaneous tidal respiration, with inspiration the trachea lengthens longitudinally, the cartilages become more circular, and the membranous wall expands slightly posteriorly; the trachealis muscle actually contracts on inspiration via a parasympathetic pathway that closely parallels activity in the phrenic nerve.[5] During expiration, the trachea shortens, the cartilages become more elliptical, and the membranous wall moves anteriorly. These motions, which are also identifiable in the mainstem and lobar bronchi, become more pronounced as the extremes of lung volumes are approached, and may be diminished or accentuated by pathologic states. At its terminus, the trachea divides into the right and left mainstem bronchi, with the *carina* (from the Latin for keel) forming a thin, mobile septum that divides the two airways distally.

Right Tracheobronchial Tree

The *right mainstem bronchus* continues from the carina at a 30-degree angle from the longitudinal axis of the trachea, with a similar arrangement of cartilaginous arches and smooth muscle and similar conformational change during respiration. It extends to the take-off of the *right upper lobe bronchus,* which has three segmental bronchi *(anterior, apical,* and *posterior).* The airway continues as the *bronchus intermedius,* from which originates the *middle lobe bronchus,* leading to *lateral* and *medial* segmental bronchi. The *right lower lobe bronchus* continues beyond this and distributes a *superior* segmental bronchus prior to terminating in four basilar segmental bronchi *(medial basal, anterior basal, lateral basal,* and *posterior basal).*

Left Tracheobronchial Tree

The *left mainstem bronchus* originates at a 50-degree angle from the longitudinal tracheal axis, travels beneath the aortic arch (whose pulsations can be visualized), and terminally bifurcates. The *left upper lobe bronchus* divides into an *upper division,* including *apical-posterior* and *anterior* segmental bronchi, and a *lingular division* (almost directly aligned with the longitudinal axis of the left main bronchus), with *superior* and *inferior* segmental bronchi. The *left lower lobe bronchus* gives off a proximal *superior* segmental bronchus, and ends distally in three basilar segmental bronchi *(anteromedial basal, lateral basal,* and *posterior basal).*

Bronchopulmonary Segments

The individual anatomic units that make up the lung are the bronchopulmonary segments, pyramid-shaped elements of pulmonary parenchyma that contain a single pulmonary arterial and venous branch, with a discrete airway— the *segmental bronchus.* The right lung is composed of 10 segments and the left lung of eight, as described previously.[6] The segmental (or third-order) bronchus typically divides several times within a segment, forming fourth-, fifth-, and sixth-order bronchi that lead to the terminal bronchi. Each terminal bronchus is the origin of 20 to 30 bronchioles and their associated respiratory units. As the segmental bronchi originate and then bifurcate, the anterior cartilaginous arches become less well defined, the relative amount of smooth muscle increases and becomes more evenly distributed about the circumference, and the airway becomes more circular in cross section. Respiratory alterations along longitudinal and transverse axes, similar to those of the larger airways, are apparent to the level of the fourth- and fifth-order bronchi.

Bronchial Mucosa

The mucosa of the tracheobronchial tree to the level of the fourth-order bronchi (ie, from subglottic space through segmental bronchi) is a pseudostratified columnar epithelium made up of ciliated cells, brush cells, and goblet cells. The epithelium rests on a basement membrane that overlies a vascular tunica propria and is covered by a thin (<15 μ) layer of fluid. The fluid is composed of a continuous, nonviscous periciliary layer (a sol) surmounted by a discontinuous layer of mucus (a gel), the latter secreted by goblet cells and submucosal glands. In concert with the uniform pattern of ciliary motion, this layer acts to transport particulate matter from the peripheral airways cephalad to the larynx, at rates of 2 to 20 nm/min.[7, 8] Macroscopically, the normal mucosa is pale, glistening, nearly white, with few accumulated secretions except at points of bronchial confluence. In the more peripheral airways, the underlying vascular plexus is relatively larger and the surface fluid layer is thinner, resulting in a more erythematous appearance to the mucosa.

Vagal and thoracic sympathetic nerves provide afferent and efferent nerve fibers to the tracheobronchial tree. The vagal nerves appear to predominate, establishing a resting bronchial tone.[9] Stimulation of vagal fibers results in bronchoconstriction and an increase in the normal secretions of the mucosa and submucosal glands. Sympathetic stimulation (beta-adrenergic) causes bronchodilation and an increase in the viscosity of mucosal secretions. Alpha-adrenergic stimulation alone results in a decreased viscosity of secretions.[10, 11] Cough, in which increased mucosal secretion and strong contraction of airway muscles occur simultaneously, is mediated via a parasympathetic, atropine-sensitive reflex arc initiated by stimulation of the airway mucosa.[12] The receptors involved appear to fatigue easily and become fewer approaching the bronchiole level. Direct application of topical anesthetic agents succeeds in abolishing this reflex arc, facilitating the performance of bronchoscopy or other airway manipulations.

INDICATIONS FOR BRONCHOSCOPY

Bronchoscopy is indicated for *all* patients with symptoms of (1) hemoptysis, (2) persistent cough, and (3) airway obstruction. Bronchoscopy is indicated for asymptomatic patients with (1) roentgenographic studies that demonstrate intrathoracic pathologic changes of a nonphysiologic nature, (2) cytologic or bacteriologic abnormalities of the sputum, (3) a history of aspiration or inhalation injury, (4) trauma (penetrating or blunt) to the cervicothoracic region, (5) a necessity for neoplastic surveillance (eg, prior neoplasm or high-risk environmental exposure), (6) prior reconstructive surgery of the airway, or (7) an impending thoracotomy.

Bronchoscopy may be diagnostic, therapeutic, or both, depending on the clinical circumstances and indications for the procedure. The rigid and flexible instruments each have specific advantages, but either may be used for most indications. A routine for inspection of the tracheobronchial anatomy, observing respiratory changes and mucosal characteristics, followed by identification of pathologic lesions and, finally, biopsy or other interventions, should be used with both types of bronchoscopes.

RIGID BRONCHOSCOPY

Equipment

A rigid bronchoscope consists of a nonflexible, tapered tube with a flared and beveled distal tip, which contains an eccentrically placed inner cannula for conduction of light to its end. The typical "light-carrier" is a thin glass rod that is connected to a proximal incandescent source (usually by a fiberoptic cable). Most also have a side arm that originates from the proximal end for the instillation of gases (oxygen or anesthetic agents); perforations in the wall of the tube distally assist in the egress of these substances. Ventilatory assistance for the patient during bronchoscopy can be provided by occlusion of the proximal end of the bronchoscope (eg, by a removable lens or a digit), and positive-pressure ventilation can be provided via the side arm or by a modified Venturi apparatus attached to the side arm with the proximal end open.

Nominal size for a rigid bronchoscope is determined by the smallest internal diameter of the tube (which may be 3 to 4 mm less than its external diameter), which ranges from 2.5 to 10 mm. The length of the rigid broncho-scope is graduated in sizes 2.5 to 6 mm. Adult rigid bronchoscopes are 40 cm in length, and a standard set includes 7, 8, and 9 mm nominal sizes. The standard set also includes a side arm adapter for ventilatory assistance, a removable lens for the proximal end of the bronchoscope, a rigid suction catheter, and a set of grasping and biopsy forceps for instrumentation.

An invaluable adjunct to the standard rigid bronchoscope is a set of telescopic rods, pos-sessing 0-, 30-, and 90-degree lenses at their tips, which improve distal resolution and allow visualization of those lobar and segmental bronchi with acute take-offs from the main bronchus. A recent development is the incor-poration of glass rods between the lenses of these telescopes, improving the transmission of light and widening the angle of field from approximately 40 degrees to nearly 70 de-grees.[13] These telescopes are passed via dia-phragms on the proximal end of the broncho-scope in order to preserve the capability for ventilatory assistance. The resulting images, as compared to standard rigid bronchoscopes or flexible bronchoscopes, are unsurpassed for their degree of resolution and field of vision. Accurate determination of anatomic relation-ships and mucosal details are identifiable to the level of the segmental bronchi, a limit imposed by the inflexibility of the rigid instru-ment. Forceps specifically designed for use with these telescopes, maintaining the illumi-nation and visual field of the telescope during their manipulation, are useful, particularly in pediatric patients.[14]

Anesthesia and Patient Preparation

Rigid bronchoscopy can be performed equally well with either topical or general anesthesia. Attaining an adequate level of an-esthesia is crucial to the success of either method. Because of its innate advantages, in-cluding its size and larger lumen for instru-mentation, the rigid bronchoscope is fre-quently employed in clinical situations that require an interventional instrument. Topical anesthesia has the advantage of an awake, spontaneously breathing patient who may ac-tively assist in maintaining the patency of the airway. However, the necessary explanatory preparation and topical anesthetic application may unwisely lengthen the prebronchoscopy period when rapid interventions are necessary (eg, massive hemoptysis). Some degree of se-dation is also required, which may be undesir-able in clinical situations where the airway is acutely or severely compromised. General an-esthesia can provide rapid attainment of an adequate anesthetic level, but requires some degree of muscle relaxation to allow for inser-tion of the rigid bronchoscope, considering the reflexive nature of the patient. Active main-tenance of the airway by the patient and spon-taneous ventilation is lost, making the ability to identify the airway and insert the broncho-scope critical. A slow induction with a general inhalational agent, coupled with topical anes-thetic application to the proximal airway, is ideal when maintenance of spontaneous ven-tilation with gradual abolition of the normal airway reflexes is required (eg, inflammatory or neoplastic tracheal stenosis). In general, the choice of anesthesia for rigid bronchoscopy is best tailored to the clinical circumstances, the capabilities of the bronchoscopist, and the skill and experience of the anesthesiologist.

As an adequate level of anesthesia is ob-tained, the patient should be ventilated with 100% O_2. Monitoring equipment varies ac-cording to the patient's status, but should always include a continuous-display electrocar-diogram monitor, continuous transcutaneous O_2 saturation monitor, and blood pressure determinations. The procedure should only be performed in a facility with full equipment for cardiopulmonary resuscitation.

Proper positioning of the patient is crucial to successful insertion of the bronchoscope. The occiput should be supported, flexing the lower neck at the *cervicothoracic* region; the head is then rotated dorsally, extending the upper neck at the *atlanto-occipital* level. The longitudinal axis of the larynx and proximal trachea approximates the open oral cavity in this position. Longer necks require more cer-vicothoracic flexion, and shorter necks require more atlanto-occipital extension. Cervical spine disease that prevents positioning of the neck is the only absolute contraindication to rigid bronchoscopy. The eyes should be ade-quately protected, and a cushioning support must be placed over the incisors or superior alveolar ridge to protect these structures.

Technique and Complications

The bronchoscope, with light carrier in place and light source functioning, is grasped at its proximal end between the thumb and index finger of the right hand, resting on the middle finger much like a writing implement. The flared distal tip of the scope is directed toward the patient's feet. The left hand is positioned in the midline over the maxilla, with the thumb extended parallel to and above the patient's upper lip. The left thumb serves as a rest for the bronchoscope during further manipulations, and the left fingers can assist in stabilizing and guiding the scope through the oropharynx. The tip of the scope is introduced through the oral cavity from the right and directed toward the posterior pharyngeal wall. Viewing through the proximal end, the median furrow of the tongue and uvula are identified, and the tip of the scope is positioned in the midline as it is passed into the oropharynx. As the bronchoscope is advanced through the pharynx, it is gently rotated from a sagittal position toward a coronal plane, with the left thumb serving as the center of the arc of rotation. The superior margin and ventral surface of the epiglottis are brought into view and the midline position of the instrument should be ascertained. The tip of the bronchoscope is advanced 3 to 4 mm further into the hypopharynx, beyond the tip of the epiglottis. Further advancement is discontinued and the left thumb, on which the bronchoscope is resting, is elevated from the maxilla as the rotation of the instrument is continued. The tip of the bronchoscope is applied to the dorsal surface of the epiglottis by this maneuver, and elevation of this structure anteriorly brings the larynx into the longitudinal axis of the instrument. The glottic opening is identified and observed. The cords, posterior arytenoid prominences, and usually some of the distal airway (subglottic space or tracheal rings) are seen. The scope is rotated 90 degrees, positioning the widest part of the tip parallel to the cords, and advanced through the glottis into the proximal trachea. Support beneath the occiput is removed, and the side arm of the bronchoscope is connected to the ventilatory apparatus. Observation is made of tracheobronchial anatomy, respiratory variations in the airway, mucosal characteristics, and any pathologic lesions. The bronchoscope is advanced by the right hand to the carina, always supported by the left thumb. Intubation of the right or left mainstem bronchi is aided by rotating the patient's head to the contralateral side, making the tracheobronchial angles less acute. The 0-degree telescopic rod can be used to inspect the trachea, carina, and mainstem bronchi to their lobar bifurcations. The 30-degree telescope improves visualization of the right middle lobe and lingular division orifices, as well as of the basilar segmental bronchi bilaterally. The 90-degree telescope is used for the right upper lobe and left upper division bronchi, and for the superior segmental bronchi on either side. When the bronchoscope is removed, inspection of the subglottic region, cords, and supraglottic area should be performed with the 0-degree telescope. The bronchoscope is withdrawn in a manner opposite to its insertion.

The possible need for rapid reinsertion of the bronchoscope or other intubation of the patient always exists, and facilities should be available for such an occasion. Subglottic edema is the most common complication following rigid bronchoscopy and can usually be managed conservatively (ie, without reintubation) using humidification, oxygen, and aerosolized racemic epinephrine (0.2 to 0.5 mL of a 2% solution every 1 to 2 hours); systemic steroids (methylprednisolone, 100 to 250 mg, or dexamethasone, 4 to 10 mg intravenously) have been used, but their efficacy has not been conclusively demonstrated. After the procedure, all patients should have a chest roentgenogram to identify any alteration from the preoperative radiograph, including improvement or complications such as pneumothorax or atelectasis from obstruction of distal bronchi.

Advantages and Limitations

The innate characteristics of the rigid bronchoscope, including its contour, stiffness, and intraluminal size, are uniquely suited to interventional maneuvers involving the proximal airways. *Securing a stenotic airway* is one of the maneuvers a rigid bronchoscope does best. The instrument is specifically designed for accurate identification of the opening to the airway in the midst of the soft-tissue structures of the oropharynx. Its rigidity allows displacement of these structures for visualization of the glottis, and the firm, beveled tip is ideal for insinuation through a small, noncircular opening. Once in the airway, the bronchoscope can be used to dilate stenotic airways with a gentle corkscrew motion of the tip, removing and replacing bronchoscopes of increasing nominal size until an adequate luminal diameter is achieved. At times, a laryngoscope (eg, Jackson type) is used to maintain visualization of the glottic opening while the bronchoscopes are being exchanged. Insertion of a rigid bronchoscope past a malacic segment or across a tracheal disruption will stent the lumen prior to further assessment of the distal airway or definitive surgical repair. The capacity to provide positive-pressure ventilation with the rigid bronchoscope during any of these maneuvers assures control of the patient's respiratory status once the airway has been secured.

Rapid aspiration of inspissated material in the airway (secretions, aspirated substances, or blood) is allowed by the large diameter lumen of the instrument (identified by the nominal size). The rigid bronchoscope is especially helpful if large amounts of material are encountered or ongoing contamination is occurring (eg, active bleeding).

The lumen of the rigid bronchoscope also accommodates forceps (grasping or biopsy type) capable of opening to the size of the cross-sectional diameter of the trachea and main bronchi. *Foreign body removal* from the major airways often requires forceps of this size, making the rigid bronchoscope the instrument of choice. Practice using the forceps within a bronchoscope with a replica of the foreign body prior to insertion of the bronchoscope in the patient is helpful. When the object is firmly grasped, the forceps are held against the tip of the bronchoscope, and the instrument, forceps, and foreign body are withdrawn as a unit.

Neoplastic obstruction of the airway to the level of the main bronchi may be removed completely with the rigid bronchoscope. Large pieces of tissue are obtained with standard rigid biopsy forceps. A neoplastic obstruction can be excised with such biopsy forceps or by positioning the tip of the bronchoscope between the wall of the airway and the tumor and applying a gentle rotatory motion to "core out" the malignancy. The tumor is then extracted from the lumen of the bronchoscope. Hemorrhage from these manipulations, an infrequent complication, but more common with primary tumors than metastatic lesions, is controlled with topical application of 1:10,000 epinephrine-soaked swabs or by direct pressure of the wall of the bronchoscope over the region for 3 to 5 minutes. Violation of the wall of the trachea or main bronchi by these maneuvers is possible, but infrequent in skilled hands.[15] For tears within the mediastinum less than 1 cm in size in spontaneously breathing patients, cautious observation is indicated. Other lacerations are best dealt with by passing the bronchoscope beyond the injury in order to stabilize the airway and then proceeding directly to surgical repair.

The very characteristics that make the rigid bronchoscope uniquely useful (contour, stiffness, size) also limit visualization by the instrument to the segmental bronchial orifices. A role for the rigid bronchoscope in a diagnostic or therapeutic manner beyond the segmental bronchi is very limited. As a diagnostic instrument in the proximal airways, however, the rigid bronchoscope, combined with the telescopic rod–lens, is entirely satisfactory. The ability to use the rigid bronchoscope in therapeutic situations in the trachea and main bronchi, moreover, depends on an adequate facility with it, "obtained only by educating the eye and the fingers in repeated exercise."[16] The necessary skill and experience can be gained only by frequent use of the instrument for diagnostic indications in the airway proximal to the segmental bronchial level.

FLEXIBLE BRONCHOSCOPY

Equipment

A flexible bronchoscope consists of a flexible shaft with an objective lens at one end and an eyepiece at the other. Within the shaft are three bundles of fiberoptic cables, two for illumination and one for image transmission. These bundles are composed of several thousand coherent glass fibers of 10 μ in diameter with precisely assorted ends. Light passage occurs through these glass fibers by internal reflection, conducting rays from one end of the bundle to the other. The eyepiece image is composed of several thousand points of light, with a consequent limit of resolution imposed by the number and size of fibers. The remainder of the sheath contains a pair of control cables, which allow directioning of the tip of the device from a control at the eyepiece in one plane only (ie, up or down). A common channel for aspiration, instillation, or instrumentation completes the contents; a double-lumen device exists for separation of aspiration and other functions, but is limited in its application. A self-contained fiberoptic cable that originates at the eyepiece provides connection to a light source. The device is essentially solid in cross section, requiring ventilation around it, rather than through its lumen, as for the rigid bronchoscope.

Nominal size for flexible bronchoscopes refers to the outer diameter of the sheath and

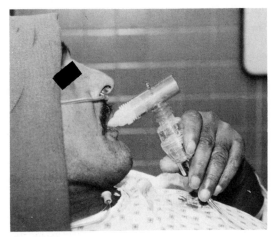

Figure 6–1. Aerosol device to topically anesthetize the airway. Typically, 2% lidocaine is used as the anesthetic.

ranges from 3.5 mm (pediatric size) to 4.7 to 6.3 mm (adult sizes). The size of the enclosed common channel varies with the outside diameter, from 1.2 mm (pediatric size) to 1.8 to 2.6 mm (adult sizes). Flexible devices with an outer diameter as small as 1.8 mm have been developed, but are limited by a lack of an enclosed suction channel or directional control, or both. Adult flexible bronchoscopes are about 60 cm long. A standard set includes an adult instrument, sources for illumination and suction, and a set of flexible instruments, including brushes, biopsy forceps, curettes, and aspirating needles. These instruments should be thoroughly cleaned at the end of each procedure with solutions capable of germicidal decontamination and of clearing the common channel without residue (eg, glutaraldehyde and sterile water).

Anesthesia and Patient Preparation

Flexible bronchoscopy can be performed with either general or topical anesthesia. Because of the flexible bronchoscope's solid construction, general anesthesia mandates endotracheal intubation prior to the procedure in order to maintain patient ventilation. The relative size of the bronchoscope within the lumen of the endotracheal tube must be considered, in terms of the ability to adequately exchange gases around the instrument and in terms of the ability to easily manipulate it within the tube. For the standard adult flexible bronchoscope, a 7.5-mm tube is limiting, whereas a pediatric bronchoscope can pass

through a tube of 4.5-mm internal diameter. General anesthesia is useful if the bronchoscopy is prolonged or if the patient's status is not amenable to a local anesthetic.

Under topical anesthesia (Fig. 6–1), the bronchoscope can be inserted either nasotracheally or orotracheally. Nasotracheal insertion allows inspection of the most proximal airway passages, usually requires less anesthetic solution, and is unencumbered by deglutition or closure of the mouth. Orotracheal insertion limits examination of the nasopharynx, may require a greater volume of anesthetic, and necessitates a bite block (Fig. 6–2), but it has the advantage of allowing easy introduction of an orotracheal tube with the subsequent capability for ventilation or general anesthesia (if necessary) and for ease of removal and reinsertion of the bronchoscope. Topical cocaine (4%) for the nasal passages, and lidocaine (2% or 4%) for the oral cavity, pharynx, and larynx are most commonly used after the initial administration of mild sedative. In an adult patient, about 200 mg of lidocaine is usually needed. Further direct application of lidocaine (2%) to the tracheobronchial tree is performed after insertion of the bronchoscope through the glottic opening. As with rigid bronchoscopy, an adequate level of anesthesia is critical for accurate bronchoscopic visualization.

The ease of insertion of the flexible bronchoscope, related to its small size and easy maneuverability, belies the potential physiologic insult imposed by the instrument. All patients who undergo flexible bronchoscopy

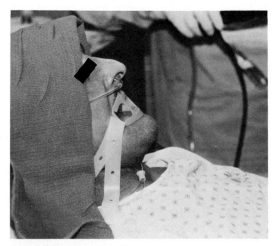

Figure 6–2. Oral bite block to allow easy introduction of an orotracheal tube or easy introduction and withdrawal of a bronchoscope.

have some diminution in Pa_{O_2} (probably related to V/Q [ventilation/perfusion] abnormalities), which may persist for several hours following the procedure.[17] This hypoxia has been correlated with major cardiac arrhythmias in 10% of patients.[18] Reflex sympathetic stimulation by mechanical irritation of the larynx and bronchi results in increases in mean arterial pressure, heart rate, cardiac index, and pulmonary capillary wedge pressure, with higher values noted in patients with preexisting pulmonary disease.[19] The topical anesthetic agents alone elicit increases in airway resistance and diminish expiratory flow.[20] The performance of flexible bronchoscopy, therefore, demands no less monitoring and attention to the patient's physiologic status than rigid bronchoscopy. Supplemental oxygen should always be administered and continued for several hours after the procedure, until any V/Q abnormalities have resolved. Continuous monitoring of the electrocardiogram and transcutaneous O_2 saturation, as well as intermittent blood pressure measurements, are needed. All such procedures should be performed only in facilities with full capability for intubation (including rigid bronchoscopy) and cardiopulmonary resuscitation. With these appropriate measures, a mortality rate of 0.1% has been reported in a prospective study.[21]

Technique and Complications

Under topical anesthesia, the patient is in the sitting or semierect position and the flexible bronchoscope is inserted by the chosen route, following the upper air passages down to the glottis. Passage through the nose may be facilitated by occluding the opposite nostril and asking the patient to sniff, enlarging the appropriate passage and depressing the soft palate. Visualization of the supraglottic region and cords may be enhanced by having the patient protrude his or her tongue, and topical anesthetic may be applied directly to and through the opening. After traversing the glottic space, topical anesthetic is then applied in 2- to 4-mL aliquots to the distal trachea, carina, and mainstem bronchi, allowing sufficient time (3 to 5 min) for anesthetic effect. If an orotracheal tube is to be inserted, the bronchoscope may be threaded through it prior to passing into the airway; once in the distal trachea, the tube may then be advanced over the bronchoscope and positioned appropriately. When the patient has an indwelling endotracheal tube, an inline adapter with a port to accommodate the bronchoscope is used to maintain ventilation during the procedure. Topical anesthetic is applied to the tracheobronchial tree, as described previously, when the tube is negotiated. Once in the airway and having established proper orientation, flexible bronchoscopy proceeds in a systematic fashion. One hand, at the eyepiece, provides tip deflection and rotation; the other hand, at the point of insertion of the bronchoscope, provides axial control and rotational assistance. Tracheobronchial anatomy is assessed, respiratory motion and mucosal characteristics are observed, and any pathologic findings are identified. The flexible bronchoscope provides the maximal visualization possible of the tracheobronchial tree, with the capability of visualizing all fourth-order bronchi, the majority of fifth-order bronchi, and up to half of the sixth-order bronchi.[22]

The possibility of airway obstruction and the need for rapid reintubation following the procedure exists, but is much less common than with rigid bronchoscopy. Hypoxia of some degree is the most common complication of flexible bronchoscopy, but is usually overcome by supplemental O_2 administered during and after the procedure. As with rigid bronchoscopy, all patients should have a chest roentgenogram following the procedure to assess any change or complication. Up to 16% of patients may develop fever (T>101°F) following the procedure, likely due to obstructive atelectasis and contamination of the lower airways with oropharyngeal flora. The incidence of this is correlated with increasing age of the patient, findings of tracheobronchial pathology, and instrumentation (especially bronchial brushing). Pneumonia or bacteremia following flexible bronchoscopy is extremely rare (<1%).[23]

Advantages and Limitations

The primary goal of bronchoscopy is to provide direct visualization of the tracheobronchial tree. The greater the number of airways visible, the greater the number of abnormalities that can be identified. Flexible bronchoscopy, therefore, has greatly advanced the field by increasing the amount of information obtained from the procedure. The flexible scope can be applied to any patient with an inadequately understood pulmonary problem, of the airway or parenchyma, with minimal morbidity and a high degree of accuracy in skilled hands. In addition, because of its relative ease of insertion, it has allowed application of the technique to a wider spectrum of patients than was possible with rigid bronchoscopy. Particularly for patients with a compromised pulmonary status who require mechanical ventilation, the flexible instrument can be used diagnostically and therapeutically without jeopardizing the patient's status by transport or extubation.[24]

Instrumentation through the flexible bronchoscope is a valuable adjunct to the increased visualization provided. Most of the devices adapted to the instrument relate to diagnostic indications; these include brushes, biopsy forceps, curettes, and aspirating needles. A feature common to all of these is the small size of specimens obtained, necessitating accurate positioning of the instrument, multiple sampling, and close coordination of specimen preparation with the cytopathologic and bacteriologic services. If an abnormality can be seen, these instruments are employed at that site. If a lesion is beyond the level of direct visualization, fluoroscopic guidance is used to maneuver the flexible bronchoscope into the appropriate subsegmental bronchus prior to instrumentation (Fig. 6–3). Sequential use is made of the instruments, generally brushing, followed by biopsy or curettage, then needle aspiration, and finally local washings with 10 to 20 mL of sterile saline that are collected for study.

Bronchial brushings are performed by directing the brush into the appropriate site by the bronchoscope and vigorously agitating it within the confines of the bronchus. The brush is not retracted into the bronchoscope, which would strip it of its contents, but is removed with the bronchoscope as a unit, and applied to slides that are to be placed in cytologic fixative. For bacteriologic diagnosis, a brush within a wax-plugged sheath is used, with the brush being withdrawn into the sheath prior to its removal, protecting its contents from contamination by other tracheobronchial flora.[25]

Biopsy forceps (ranging from 1.8 to 2.2 mm in size) are effective in obtaining mucosal or parenchymal specimens, but less efficacious for cartilaginous specimens (eg, carina or lobar spurs). Fluoroscopic guidance allows transbronchial biopsy of distant parenchymal lesions. The forceps are advanced to the lesion and the jaws are opened; then the forceps are withdrawn 1 cm to ensure complete opening prior to re-advancing to the lesion and then closing the forceps. Withdrawal should not require excessive force and, in the awake patient, should not elicit pain, which may indicate pleural transgression. The subsegmental bronchus should be observed for bleeding after biopsy; if seen, the tip of the bronchoscope should be wedged in the orifice for 5 minutes with intermittent application of suction. Endobronchial lesions have a high diagnostic yield (near 100%) with three to four biopsy specimens,[26] whereas parenchymal neoplastic lesions have a lower yield (60%) with four to eight biopsy specimens, which is improved (80% to 90%) when combined with brushing and washings.[27] The yield for transbronchial biopsy is better for parenchymal lesions greater than 2 cm in diameter. For interstitial lung disease, transbronchial biopsy has a high yield in sarcoidosis (>90%),[28] but is less useful in idiopathic interstitial fibrosis, other interstitial pneumopathies (desquamative interstitial pneumonitis [DIP], usual interstitial pneumonitis [UIP], lymphocytic interstitial pneumonia [LIP]), as well as vasculitides. In these instances, open-lung biopsy more commonly provides diagnostic information.[29] Finally, patients with documented positive human immunodeficiency virus (HIV) titers and new pulmonary infiltrates are best evaluated by staining of induced sputum or subsequent flexible bronchoscopy and lavage when attempting to identify *Pneumocystis carinii.*[30]

Curettes have an advantage over biopsy forceps, which by their construction are inflexible over the length of the hinge and jaws, in

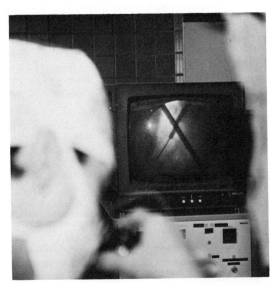

Figure 6–3. Fluoroscopy helps to guide the bronchoscope into the appropriate subsegmental bronchus.

flexibility and greater control of the tip. The curette is passed beyond the area of interest and scraped proximally to an uninvolved region several times in order to improve the diagnostic yield. Results are similar to bronchial biopsy.

Aspirating needles enclosed in plastic sheaths are available in both metal and more flexible plastic forms. They range in size from 21 guage to 18 guage and from 0.5 to 1 cm in length. They are used by insertion into the area of interest, protrusion of the needle, application of suction, agitation of the needle, gentle release of suction, and withdrawal of the needle into the sheath. The needle and sheath are removed, and the aspirated contents are flushed onto a slide. Centrally, they may be useful to assess submucosal (oblique insertion) and peribronchial (perpendicular insertion) involvement of the airway by tumor, as well as in the assessment of vascular endobronchial lesions without the excessive bleeding of biopsy. Peripherally, with fluoroscopic guidance, aspirating needles provide similar results to transbronchial biopsy, although they may be easier to position in lesions of the superior and apical segments than forceps. In general, the incidence of pneumothorax and bleeding is less with aspirating needles than with transbronchial biopsy.[31]

Bronchial washing or lavage involves the instillation of various volumes of buffered saline into segmental or subsegmental bronchi, with retrieval of the injected volume (usually about 50% to 60%) for bacteriologic and cytologic examination. Washing is best used in conjunction with the other methods described in order to improve their diagnostic accuracy. Future uses, such as in following ongoing pulmonary pathology and responses to treatment (especially in sarcoidosis and idiopathic pulmonary fibrosis), are less well defined. For alveolar proteinosis, however, *whole-lung* lavage is the treatment of choice.[32]

The flexible bronchoscope is limited in the realm of interventional capabilities, at which the rigid bronchoscope is so useful, by the very characteristics—size and maneuverability—that make it such a useful diagnostic tool. The physics of the fiberoptic bundles limits the level of resolution and necessarily fragments the conducted image when compared to the telescopic rodlens. The optics also result in a distortion of size at the periphery of the field, with larger bronchi appearing similar in size to smaller ones. In a stenotic airway, the solid nature of the instrument may occlude the airway completely, hampering its usefulness in evaluating the responsible pathology. The size of the common channel, determined by the size of the instrument, limits the amount of material that may be handled by aspiration or instrumentation to a critical diameter of 2.6 mm or less. Multiple attempts at aspiration of secretions, assisted by saline lavage, or multiple instrumentations are necessary (Fig. 6–4). With ongoing contamination of the airway, as in massive hemoptysis, the aspirating capabilities of the instrument may be quickly overwhelmed, requiring a resort to rigid bronchoscopy or other methods. Recent development of collapsible forceps has improved the capability of the flexible bronchoscope for foreign body retrieval, but the rigid instrument, for reasons of optics, maneuverability, and ventilatory capabilities, remains the instrument of choice, especially in the pediatric population.[33] Finally, because of the attendant smaller amounts of tissue obtained, the flexible instrument is of little benefit in the excision of the large amounts of tissue seen in neoplastic obstruction of the airways, although adaptation of the laser to this device allows for sequential vaporization of such lesions. This modification, however, offers no practical advantage in the large airways over the rigid bronchoscope, is significantly more expensive, and is more time consuming.

In summary, flexible bronchoscopy is the ultimate diagnostic tool for pulmonary disease against which other methods must be judged. Its role as a therapeutic tool, however, is less effective than the rigid bronchoscope for most applications in the airway proximal to the

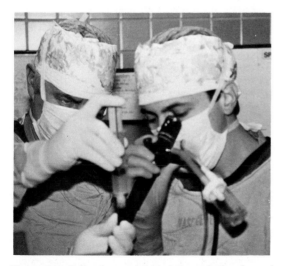

Figure 6–4. Saline lavage injected through the channel of the bronchoscope.

segmental bronchi. As with the rigid broncho-scope, however, repetitive use is the key to gaining the skill needed to maximize the ca-pabilities of the flexible bronchoscope for both diagnostic and therapeutic indications.

CONCLUSIONS

Rigid and flexible bronchoscopy are the two techniques available for visualization of the tracheobronchial tree. Both are invasive pro-cedures that can be performed under either topical or general anesthesia, and both require appropriate cardiopulmonary monitoring and a fully equipped endoscopy suite. The rigid bronchoscope is limited in visualization to the level of the segmental bronchial orifices. It provides, however, superior visualization to that level when applied with the telescopic rod–lens system. In addition, its construction makes it the interventional instrument of choice for the proximal airway, especially in securing a stenotic airway, rapidly aspirating large volumes of secretions, and removing for-eign bodies or neoplastic obstructions. The flexible bronchoscope, because of its size and maneuverability, is easier to insert in a wider spectrum of patients than the rigid instrument, with a much larger proportion of the tracheo-bronchial tree (to fifth- and sixth-order bron-chi) visualized. The more of the airways seen, the greater the possibility of identifying abnor-malities; the flexible bronchoscope, with ap-propriate instrumentation, is unequalled in di-agnostic accuracy. Its application in the proximal airways, especially for therapeutic interventions, is, however, much more limited. Both rigid and flexible techniques should be familiar to the bronchoscopist and employed in appropriate instances. Judicious application, diligent observation, and persistent practice of the necessary technical skills ensures the max-imum clinical benefit from bronchoscopy.

References

1. Mikulicz J. Ueber Gastroskopie un Oesophagoskopie. Wiener Med Press 12:1405–1577, 1881.
2. Killian G. Ein vier Jahre lang in der rechten Lunge steckendes Knochenstuck auf naturlichem Wege ent-fernt. Dtsch Med Wochenschr 26:161–163, 1900.
3. Ikeda S, Yanai N, Ishikawa S. Flexible bronchofiber-scope. Keio J Med 17:1–16, 1968.
4. Hopkins HH, Kapany NS. A flexible fiberscope. Na-ture 173:39–41, 1954.
5. Mitchell RA, Herbert DA, Baker DG. Inspiratory

rhythm in airway smooth muscle tone. J Appl Physiol 58:911–920, 1985.
6. Jackson CL, Huber JF. Correlated applied anatomy of bronchial tree and lungs with system of nomencla-ture. Dis Chest 9:319–326, 1943.
7. Van As A. Pulmonary airway clearance mechanisms: A reappraisal. Am Rev Respir Dis 115:721–726, 1977.
8. Yeates DB, Pitt BR, Spektor DM, et al. Coordination of mucociliary transport in human trachea and intra-pulmonary airways. J Appl Physiol 51:1057–1064, 1981.
9. Gross NJ, Skorodin MS. Role of the parsympathetic system in airway obstruction due to emphysema. N Engl J Med 311:421–425, 1984.
10. Leikauf GD, Ueki IF, Nadel JA. Autonomic regula-tion of viscoelasticity of cat tracheal gland secretions. J Appl Physiol 56:426–430, 1984.
11. Ueki I, German VF, Nadel J. Micropipette measure-ment of airway submucosal gland secretion: Auto-nomic effects. Am Rev Respir Dis 121:351–357, 1980.
12. Paintal AS. Vagal sensory receptors and their reflex effects. Physiol Rev 53:159–227, 1973.
13. Hopkins HH. Optical principles of the endoscope. In Berci G (ed). Endoscopy. New York: Appleton-Cen-tury-Crofts, 1976; pp. 3–26.
14. Berci G. Analysis of new optical systems in broncho-esophagology. Ann Otol Rhinol Laryngol 87:451, 1978.
15. Mathisen DJ, Grillo HC. Endoscopic relief of neo-plastic airway obstruction. (In press).
16. Jackson C. TracheoBronchoscopy, Esophagoscopy and Gastroscopy. St. Louis: The Laryngoscope Co., 1907.
17. Salisbury BG, Metzger LF, Altose MD, et al. Effect of fiberoptic bronchoscopy on respiratory performance in patients with chronic airways obstruction. Thorax 30:441–446, 1975.
18. Shrader DL, Lakshminarayan S. The effect of fiber-optic bronchoscopy on cardiac rhythm. Chest 73:821–824, 1978.
19. Lundgren R, Haggmark S, Reiz S. Hemodynamic effects of flexible fiberoptic bronchoscopy performed under topical anesthesia. Chest 82:295–299, 1982.
20. Miller WC, Awe R. Effect of nebulized lidocaine on reactive airways. Am Rev Respir Dis 111:739–741, 1975.
21. Periera W, Kovnat DM, Snider GL. A prospective cooperative study of complications following flexible fiberoptic bronchoscopy. Chest 73:813–816, 1978.
22. Kovnat DM, Rath GS, Anderson WM, et al. Maximal extent of visualization of bronchial tree by flexible fiberoptic bronchoscopy. Am Rev Respir Dis 110:88–90, 1974.
23. Periera W, Kovnat DM, Khan MA, et al. Fever and pneumonia after flexible fiberoptic bronchoscopy. Am Rev Respir Dis 112:59–64, 1975.
24. Snow N, Lucas AE. Bronchoscopy in the critically ill surgical patient. Am Surg 50:441–445, 1984.
25. Wimberly N, Faling J, Bartlett JG. A fiberoptic bron-choscopy technique to obtain uncontaminated lower airway secretions for bacterial culture. Am Rev Respir Dis 119:337–343, 1979.
26. Shure D, Astarita RW. Bronchogenic carcinoma pre-senting as an endobronchial mass. Chest 83:865–867, 1983.
27. Popovich J, Kvale PA, Eichenhorn MS. Diagnostic accuracy of multiple biopsies from flexible fiberoptic bronchoscopy: A comparison of central versus periph-eral carcinoma. Am Rev Respir Dis 125:521–523, 1982.

28. Gilman MJ, Wang KP. Transbronchial lung biopsy in sarcoidosis: An approach to determine the optimal number of biopsies. Am Rev Respir Dis 122:721–724, 1980.

29. Wall CP, Gaensler EA, Carrington CB, et al. Comparison of transbronchial and open biopsies in chronic infiltrative lung diseases. Am Rev Respir Dis 123:280–285, 1981.

30. Walzer PD. Diagnosis of *Pneumocystis carinii* pneumonia. J Infect Dis 157:629–632, 1988.

31. Wang KP, Haponik EF, Gupta PK, et al. Flexible transbronchial needle aspiration: Technical considerations. Ann Otol Rhinol Laryngol 93:233–236, 1984.

32. DuBuois RM, McAllister WAC, Branthwaite MA. Alveolar proteinosis: Diagnosis and treatment over a ten-year period. Thorax 38:360–363, 1983.

33. Wood RE, Potsma D. Endoscopy of the airway in infants and children. J Pediatr 112:1–6, 1988.

CHAPTER 7

Acoustic Response Measurements of the Airway

Victor Hoffstein, M.D., and Jeffrey J. Fredberg, M.D.

The acoustic reflection method for assessment of upper airway structure and function has been developed during the last 13 years[1, 2] and is slowly gaining popularity in North America and Europe. This method is based on measurements of sound waves reflected from the upper airway in response to an incident sound wave. It permits one to construct a plot of airway cross-sectional area as a function of distance from the mouth. In this chapter, we describe the theoretic foundations of the acoustic method, discuss its validation, point out how it contributed to our understanding of the structure and function of the upper airway, and review its clinical applications and future directions.

THEORETIC BACKGROUND

Principles of the Acoustic Method

If a sound wave is emitted at the opening of a tube, it travels through the tube without any reflections as long as the tube is of constant diameter, is filled with gas that has a uniform density, and has walls that are of uniform stiffness. If these conditions are not satisfied, the incident wave is partially reflected back toward the tube opening. The amplitude of the reflected wave depends, among other things, on the changes in the cross-sectional area along the length of the tube. The travel time of the reflected wave from its site of origination to the point of reflection and back to the tube opening is determined by the length of the tube and by the wave speed; the wave speed is usually constant and depends on the composition of the gas that fills the tube. Consequently, provided we can measure the amplitude of the reflected wave and its time of arrival to the tube opening, it is possible to determine the cross-sectional area of the tube and its length.

The above example illustrates the general principle. Geometric information about a duct may be obtained from the analysis of sound waves reflected from it. This principle is at the heart of the acoustic reflection method.

The mathematic techniques for computing the dimensions of each layer were developed by Ware and Aki[3]; their algorithm forms the basis for converting the amplitudes and arrival times of reflections to areas and distances. This

Supported in part by Grant No. HL33009 from the National Institutes of Health.

algorithm is general enough to be applicable to a wide range of problems, from geology (oil exploration) to medicine (measurement of airway areas).

Although conceptually simple, the actual application of this principle to the calculation of the cross-sectional area of the human airway as a function of distance along the airway is quite complex, due to asymmetrical branching, nonuniform gas composition, and varying properties of the airway walls, as well as other variables. Certain assumptions and idealizations are necessary in order to infer airway cross-sectional area from the measurements of the reflected sound waves, and these are discussed below. For a full discussion of the underlying assumptions and approximations of the acoustic method, the reader is referred to a review by Fredberg.[4]

Assumptions and Approximations

One-Dimensional Wave Propagation

One-dimensional wave propagation is a fundamental assumption of the acoustic reflection method, and means that the phase and amplitude of pressure waves are constant across the tube diameter. If this is not the case, the algorithm of Ware and Aki[3] for converting measured amplitudes of reflected waves and their arrival times to areas and distances is no longer applicable.

In order for this assumption to be satisfied, the wavelength of the sound wave that propagates along a tube must not be smaller than twice the diameter of the tube. Because the product of the wavelength and the frequency is constant and equal to the wave speed, this limitation on the minimum wavelength places a restriction on the maximum frequency of sound waves that may be used for measurements. In the human airway, the greatest diameter occurs between the cheeks (about 5 cm), which limits the maximum frequency of sound to about 3.5 kHz. In this frequency range, human airway walls are not rigid, and acoustic energy couples into wall motion. In the case of compliant walls, the reflected waves have lower amplitude than in the case of perfectly rigid walls, and this may lead to the overestimation of airway area.

Airway Wall Rigidity

To avoid the problem of compliant airway walls, Fredberg and colleagues[2] suggested the use of a helium–oxygen mixture instead of air when measuring airway cross-sectional area in humans during breathing. Because the wave speed of sound is approximately two times higher in an 80% helium–20% oxygen mixture than in air, it is possible to double the bandwidth without altering the wavelength and therefore without violating the assumption of one-dimensional wave propagation. At these higher frequencies, the airway walls are thought to be stiffened by virtue of their inertia. The amplitude of the reflected sound waves would then be determined solely by the changes in the cross-sectional area of the airway. It has been shown[2] that using air instead of a helium–oxygen mixture results in overestimating airway areas by as much as 500%, particularly in the distal airway, near the carina.

The above considerations of bandwidth versus accuracy also place a theoretic limit on the spatial resolution of the acoustic reflection technique. The spatial resolution is the distance between two points along the airway whose areas may be distinctly resolved by the acoustic technique. This resolution is determined by the wavelength of the highest frequency sound waves and is approximately equal to 0.8 cm.

Branching

The algorithm used for computing areas from the amplitudes of the reflected waves assumes that the sound propagates along a single duct. If there are parallel pathways, as in the case of symmetrical branching, then, provided the properties of all parallel pathways are identical, the algorithm computes total cross-sectional area across all parallel pathways. If the pathways are not identical, or if the branching is asymmetrical, then the algorithm cannot be expected to yield anatomically correct total cross-sectional area.[4] This poses a problem if we want to measure airway cross-sectional areas past the carina, or if the nasopharyngeal velum is open during measurements, or if we attempt to measure upper airway area beginning at the nares. Theoretically, we would not expect the acoustic method to provide anatomically correct areas under those circumstances. However, Jackson and Olson[5] demonstrated in dried excised canine lung that the acoustic method is capable of measuring airway areas up to 6 cm distal to the carina.

Opening of the nasopharyngeal velum is

usually easily detected by the very abnormal appearance of the area–distance function. Usually, removal of the nose clips and instructing the subject to breathe through the mouth results in closure of the velum.

Nasal area–distance functions could presumably still be measured, provided we obliterate the parallel pathway (second nostril) by filling one of the nostrils with water. No such measurements have been performed to date.

Nonuniform Gas Composition

Accurate measurement of airway areas and distances assumes that the speed of sound is constant within the airway. One of the important determinants of the wave speed is gas composition within the airway. During measurements, the gas composition changes due to accumulation of carbon dioxide. This decreases the wave speed, causing overestimation of areas and distances. Although theoretically important, in practice this does not seem to pose a significant problem. D'Urzo and associates[6] found that for CO_2 concentrations of up to 10%, the overestimate in area was no more than 6%, whereas the distance was systematically shifted chestward by up to 2.5 cm. Under normal measurement conditions accumulation of carbon dioxide does not exceed 5%, and the chestward shift in the area–distance function is well within the expected variability of the technique.

Validation of the Acoustic Method

Here we summarize the available results comparing the acoustic cross-sectional areas[7–10] with those obtained by other techniques. The description of specific results is organized in an anatomic fashion, starting with the pharynx and moving toward the peripheral airways.

Pharynx

Despite the fact that the pharynx constitutes an important site of pathology in such diverse conditions as tonsillar hypertrophy causing upper airways obstruction, oropharyngeal malignancy, or obstructive sleep apnea, no validation measurements for this structure have been performed to date, presumably because the pharynx is a difficult structure to study. Composed primarily of muscle tissue and the mucosa, the pharynx is very compliant; its cross-sectional area is influenced by several factors,

including neural regulation of pharyngeal constrictors, dilators, and other upper airway muscles that influence pharyngeal size, muscle tone, posture, and phase of respiration. It is difficult to control for all these factors when comparing the acoustic areas with those obtained by other means, such as computed tomography (CT) scans or magnetic resonance imaging (MRI). Although there are several studies comparing pharyngeal structure and function in normal subjects and patients with sleep apnea (discussed below), in all of them only the acoustic areas were measured.

Brooks and colleagues[7] simulated pharynx, larynx, and trachea by a system of glass tubes of varying cross-sectional areas and compared the acoustic data with the radiographic ones. They found that, for pharyngeal areas of up to 5.5 cm², acoustic and radiographic areas were virtually identical; for larger pharyngeal areas, approximately 10 cm², acoustic areas underestimated the radiographic ones by as much as 15%.

Glottis

D'Urzo and associates[8] studied 11 patients with laryngeal pathology (mainly laryngeal carcinoma) and compared the acoustic glottic areas with those obtained by CT. All measurements were performed during quiet tidal breathing in supine posture with patients awake. Both methods correlated well with each other, with a correlation coefficient of 0.95. There was an excellent quantitative agreement between the acoustic and CT areas: 1.8 ± 0.8 cm² for the acoustic method versus 1.7 ± 0.9 cm² for the CT method. Some patients had a very small laryngeal area (0.4 cm²), which was still adequately resolved by the acoustic technique.

In vitro measurements by Brooks and colleagues[7] showed that, over the range of areas studied by these authors (0.5 to 2.0 cm²), the acoustic areas were virtually identical to the radiographic ones.

Trachea

Most of the validation of the acoustic method was performed for the trachea. Jackson and Olson[5] measured acoustic area in two rigid casts of human central airways and found very close agreement between the acoustic and direct areas for up to 6 cm distal to the carina. The authors concluded that many of the assumptions of the acoustic method, such as branching asymmetry and internal energy losses, introduce negligible errors in acoustic inferences of cross-sectional areas. In a subsequent study, Jackson and Krevans[9] studied tracheostomized dogs and found that the ratio of acoustic to radiographic area ranged from 0.91 to 1.03.

The results of simulation studies using glass tubes[7] indicate that the acoustic method may overestimate radiographic tracheal area by up to 40%, depending primarily on the glottic area. The greatest overestimate occurs when the glottic area is less than 0.5 cm². For glottic areas greater than 1.0 cm², tracheal area is independent of the glottic size, and overestimates the radiographic area by about 10%.

There are three in vivo studies in humans where acoustic tracheal areas were compared to the radiographic ones. Fredberg and colleagues[2] performed acoustic and radiographic (using posterior–anterior and lateral radiographs of the airway) measurements of the tracheal area in six normal human volunteers and found close correlation between the radiographic and acoustic measurements, as well as close direct agreement between the areas measured by both methods. In a subsequent study,[7] the authors performed similar measurements in 10 normal volunteers and once again found close correspondance between the radiographic and acoustic areas, with an acoustic/radiographic area ratio of 1.06 ± 0.13. Furthermore, these authors studied the variability of the method, examining the reproducibility of the area measurements by performing many measurements in rapid succession, performing measurements on separate days, or by using different mouthpieces. The results indicate that the maximum coefficient of variation for any of the above protocols is approximately 10%.

D'Urzo and colleagues[10] employed CT to measure tracheal area in seven subjects, all of whom had a history of upper airway abnormalities. CT measurements were performed in 1-cm increments beginning at the glottis and extending up to 13 cm distally in some subjects. The results indicate a close correspondence between the two methods (correlation coefficient of 0.92, acoustic/radiographic area ratio of 0.96).

Peripheral Airways

The assumptions of the acoustic method break down for the subcarinal airways, and therefore this method is not expected to reproduce the anatomic areas of these airways. However, in vitro measurements by Jackson and Olson[5] suggest that the equivalence between the acoustic and the anatomic areas may extend for up to 6 cm distal to the carina. Jackson and associates[11] found that although the anatomic areas of the peripheral airways are not reproduced by the acoustic areas, the *changes* in the anatomic cross-sectional area of peripheral airways are accurately represented by the *changes* in the acoustic areas. This implies that the acoustic technique may be useful for measuring the relative changes in the cross-sectional areas of peripheral airways in response to various interventions.

Nose

The most recent application of the acoustic method is assessment of the nasal cavity. The results are still preliminary. Only one study[12] described a direct comparison between the acoustic and CT areas; this was performed in a cadaver and the results showed that the correlation between the two methods was high, with a correlation coefficient of 0.94. No direct comparison of acoustic and radiographic areas were performed in humans, but the indirect comparisons, using anterior rhinomanometry or water displacement method, indicate high correlation between these indirect measurements of area and the acoustic results. Clearly, further studies are necessary in order to validate the applicability of this technique to measurement of nasal cavity, but the preliminary results certainly are promising.

EQUIPMENT AND MEASUREMENT TECHNIQUES

The apparatus for measurement of airway area by acoustic reflection is quite simple (Fig. 7–1). It consists of a wave tube, a microphone, and a sound source. An audio amplifier and filter are used to enhance and condition the reflected intensities, and a computer equipped with an analog-to-digital converter is necessary to coordinate the timing of measurements of the incident and reflected sound waves, as well as to analyze and process the data.

The wave tube is 2 m long and has an internal diameter of about 2.0 cm². The sound source (loudspeaker) is mounted in the middle of the tube. The pressure sensor (microphone) is mounted near the subject's end of the tube.

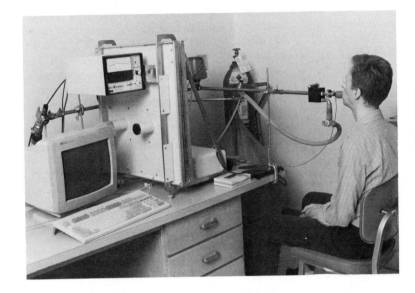

Figure 7–1. Acoustic reflection apparatus. Note that the wave tube is shaped in a 90-degree angle, with the loudspeaker mounted in the middle, spirometer mounted at the distal end, and the microphone near the proximal end.

If required, a spirometer, pneumotachygraph, and pressure transducers may be mounted at the distal or proximal ends of the wave tube to permit simultaneous measurements of lung volume, flow rate, and airway pressure. The subject is connected to the wave tube by means of an ordinary pulmonary function mouthpiece and must breathe an 80% helium–20% oxygen mixture during area measurements. Initially, it was thought that a special mouthpiece might be required in order to smooth out the transition between the relatively narrow wave tube and the relatively wide area between the cheeks; however, measurements by Rubinstein and associates[13] indicate that, provided the subject holds his or her lips tightly around the mouthpiece and does not balloon out the cheeks, ordinary mouthpieces may be used.

The existing computer software allows us to perform a maximum of 256 uninterrupted measurements of airway area. The measurements may be performed either automatically, as fast as every 0.2 second, or manually, adjusting the time delay between measurements as required for a particular protocol. Upper airway areas may be measured in this manner during various respiratory maneuvers, such as quiet tidal breathing, or during slow or forced vital capacity maneuvers. The data processing is performed on-line and the area–distance function is displayed on the computer screen. It takes approximately 132 seconds to acquire and plot 256 area functions.

This capability of measuring many area functions repetitively provides a convenient means to ensure the quality of the measurements. Area functions measured under nearly identical conditions look similar, and an occasional unphysiologic measurement is easily recognized and can be rejected from the data analysis. Such unphysiologic measurements usually result from the failure to close the nasopharyngeal velum during measurements or from the involuntary closure of the glottis. The artifacts in acoustic area measurements due to various causes have been discussed by Rubinstein and colleagues[13] and Molfino and associates.[14]

An example of 256 area functions obtained during slow vital capacity expiration and inspiration is shown in Figure 7–2. We note (Fig. 7–2 A) that the airway is a dynamic structure whose area changes during quiet breathing. One of the important contributions of the acoustic technique to the study of upper airway has been to emphasize this dynamic nature of the airway. The distance scale refers to the distance from the microphone. The gross anatomic structures (pharynx, glottis, and trachea) are easily identified. The glottic minimum provides a convenient point of reference for the area plot: the structure proximal to the glottic minimum is the pharynx, whereas the distal structure is the trachea.

The computer software is capable of computing and plotting the average (and standard deviation or standard error) of the entire area–distance function (Fig. 7–2B). Furthermore, the average area of any segment of the area–distance function may also be computed and plotted versus lung volume (Fig. 7–2C), flow, or pressure.

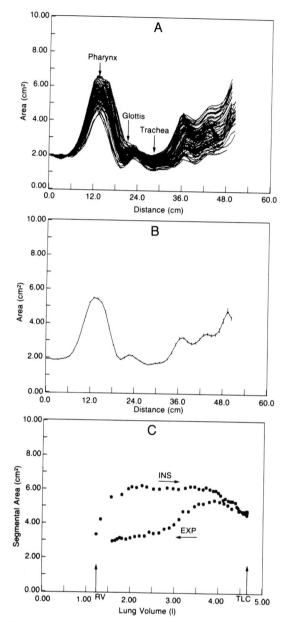

Figure 7–2. *A*, Area–distance functions measured during quiet expiration from total lung capacity to residual volume, followed by quiet inspiration to total lung capacity; anatomic landmarks are indicated; the origin of the distance axis corresponds to the position of the microphone. *B*, Average ± SD area–distance function. *C*, Average area of the pharyngeal segment contained between 7 and 18 cm (panel *A*) plotted versus lung volume during expiration (EXP) and inspiration (INS).

APPLICATIONS

Being a relatively new technique, there are only a few specific applications so far. Most of the applications described in the literature originated from two or three laboratories. In what follows, we describe only the applications dealing with human airways. The discussion is organized anatomically, rather than by disease category.

Nose

This is the newest application of the acoustic technique, described by a group from Denmark.[12, 15, 16] Having previously validated acoustic reflection in humans in vivo by comparing acoustic nasal areas with the results of anterior rhinomanometry and water displacement, the authors used the technique to evaluate the nasal cavity in patients with septal deviation undergoing septoplasty.[16] They determined the location of maximal narrowing, studied its displacements after nasal decongestant, and compared the nasal areas before and after surgery. Improvement in nasal patency objectively documented by acoustic rhinometry correlated well with subjective improvement expressed by the patients. The authors concluded that the acoustic technique is useful for pre- and postoperative evaluation of patients undergoing septoplasty or turbinoplasty.

Better understanding of the nasal physiology can be achieved if direct, repeated measurements of nasal volume are available. Yamagiwa and associates[15] used acoustic reflections to examine changes in nasal volume due to fluctuations in nasal blood flow induced by cooling of the skin. The authors found marked minute-to-minute fluctuations in nasal volume and concluded that nasal vascular changes cannot be reliably studied based on single measurements. Acoustic rhinometry, which provides rapid and reproducible measurements of nasal area, appears to be uniquely suitable for this problem.

Pharynx

Most of the clinical applications of the acoustic method were directed toward study of pharyngeal structure and function. Measurements of pharyngeal cross-sectional area and pharyngeal distensibility have been performed in normal subjects and patients with sleep-related respiratory disorders, such as snoring and sleep apnea. The major contribution of the acoustic technique has been to point out that patients with idiopathic obstructive sleep apnea have subtle abnormalities in pharyngeal structure and function. The structural abnormalities consist of reduction in pharyngeal cross-sectional area[17] as compared to nonapneic controls. Pharyngeal function is assessed by measuring changes in pharyngeal area in response to applied pressure (ie, pharyngeal distensibility) or in response to changes in lung volume. Hoffstein and colleagues,[18] Brown and associates,[19] and Bradley and coworkers[20] found that patients with obstructive sleep apnea have higher pharyngeal distensibility and larger changes in pharyngeal area with lung volume than nonapneic controls. It is now thought that increased pharyngeal distensibility and small pharyngeal area, further reduced by virtue of reduction in functional residual capacity in supine posture, are important factors promoting complete pharyngeal collapse during sleep in patients with sleep apnea.[21–27]

Several other factors that influence pharyngeal mechanics have been investigated with the help of acoustic technique. It was found that pharyngeal area and its lung volume-related changes are affected by body weight,[28] posture,[29, 30] and pharyngeal surgery.[31]

An important contribution of the acoustic method was to recognize that snoring, which is considered to be a precursor of sleep apnea, is also associated with abnormalities in pharyngeal mechanics. Bradley and coworkers[20] showed that nonapneic snorers have smaller lung volume-related changes in pharyngeal area than apneic snorers; their pharyngeal area at functional residual capacity is similar to that of patients with sleep apnea, but at residual volume it is higher than in apneic patients.

Patients with central sleep apnea, who are usually thought to have abnormal control of breathing rather than disordered airway function, have also been shown to have abnormal pharyngeal mechanics. Their pharyngeal area is normal, but pharyngeal distensibility is increased above that of patients with obstructive sleep apnea.[32]

The major drawback of the acoustic technique as applied to the study of pharyngeal mechanics in patients with sleep apnea is that all measurements were performed in awake patients. The technique in its present form is not amenable to measurements during sleep, although it may be possible to modify the wave tube and the mouthpiece to permit measurements of pharyngeal area during sleep.

Glottis

Glottic structure and function have been studied in normals and in patients with sleep apnea. Rubinstein and colleagues[33] found that glottic movements during breathing are variable, even in normal subjects. Although most normal subjects exhibit inspiratory descent of the glottis accompanied by increase in its cross-sectional area, there are subjects whose glottis remains relatively fixed during breathing, sometimes paradoxically narrowing during inspiration.

Rivlin and coworkers[17] noted that patients with obstructive sleep apnea have reduced glottic cross-sectional area. Subsequent observations by Rubinstein and associates[34] indicated that not only glottic structure, but also glottic function, may be abnormal in such patients. These authors described a subset of patients with severe obstructive sleep apnea and seemingly normal pharyngeal function who demonstrated glottic paradox even in the awake state. Instead of the normal widening of the glottis on inspiration, these patients had paradoxical inspiratory narrowing of the glottis. This abnormality, if present also during sleep, would predispose such patients to complete upper airway obstruction at the level of the larynx.

Trachea

Several investigators employed the acoustic reflection technique to study tracheal function in normal subjects and in patients with tracheal stenosis, asthma, cystic fibrosis, and sleep apnea.

Several studies in normal subjects included measurements of tracheal distensibility, hysteresis, and the relationship between tracheal size and lung size.[35–39] These studies provided new insight into the physiology of the normal trachea. Some of the major findings obtained using acoustic area measurements are (1) the area of tracheal and bronchial segments increases with increasing lung volume and transpulmonary pressure; (2) trachea and bronchi exhibit hysteresis, which may be greater or smaller than that of the lung parenchyma, depending on the location of the airway segment; (3) classic distinction between the extrathoracic and intrathoracic tracheal segments may not be appropriate, because both segments behave as if they were subjected to similar transmural pressure; (4) lung parenchyma grows independently of the airways; and (5) bronchomotor tone along the trachea is not uniform, causing different tracheal segments to respond differently to similar stimuli.

The results of these studies may be useful in modeling flow limitation, assessing tracheal muscle tone, and explaining the variability in maximum expiratory flow–volume curves. The reader is referred to the original articles[35–39] for the details of these investigations.

The first clinical application of the acoustic technique was to patients with radiographically or endoscopically proven tracheal stenosis, comparing the acoustic method with the only other noninvasive method—maximum inspiratory and expiratory flow–volume loop.[40] Despite the fact that the majority of patients had normal flow–volume curves, the acoustic technique was able to demonstrate the stenosis and measure the length of the stenotic segment, as well as measure its minimum cross-sectional area.

It is commonly accepted that in patients with exercise-induced asthma, bronchoconstriction that follows exercise is relatively uniform, involving the entire airway. However, acoustic measurements of airway area in asthmatics following exercise demonstrated dichotomous airway response to exercise, with bronchi undergoing reduction in area, whereas the proximal and middle tracheal segments undergo an increase in area.[41] This observation points out that control of bronchomotor tone in asthmatics is complex and nonuniform.

An original finding, made possible only because of the availability of the acoustic reflection technique, relates to abnormality of tracheal function and structure in sleep apnea. It was commonly thought that airway abnormalities in sleep apnea are confined to the supraglottic and glottic region. However, Rubinstein and associates[42] found that reduction in airway area in patients with sleep apnea does not stop at the level of the glottis, but in fact descends more distally, to the level of the proximal trachea. Not only tracheal structure, but also tracheal function, is abnormal in patients with sleep apnea. Katz and colleagues[43] measured the relative hysteresis of the trachea in patients with sleep apnea and found that it is smaller than that of the lung parenchyma, implying a reduction in tracheal muscle tone. Although patients with sleep apnea have a local site of airway obstruction during sleep, the disease itself appears to be systemic, characterized by disordered control of upper airway muscle tone.

Brooks[44] carried out a study of tracheal structure and function in patients with cystic fibrosis. Previous indirect measurements of tracheal area in these patients suggested that they may have tracheomegaly. However, Brooks did not find any differences in tracheal area in cystic fibrosis patients as compared to normal controls, but demonstrated increased tracheal distensibility.

CONCLUSIONS

Although the acoustic reflection technique for measuring upper airway areas is still relatively new and unexplored, it offers many potential advantages over other techniques. It is noninvasive, rapid, reproducible, and may be performed repeatedly in the same patients on different occasions. More work needs to be done regarding its validation, particularly for the pharynx. Comparison of acoustic areas with those obtained using MRI may provide a better and more convincing demonstration of the validity of this technique than those done to date. It may be uniquely suited to the study of several problems of airway management, such as assessment of upper airway prior to intubation in patients with suspected abnormal airway anatomy and the effect of long- and short-term intubation on upper airway structure and function. It is hoped that recent technical improvements in the use of this technique will make it more accessible for routine use.

References

1. Jackson AC, Butler JP, Millet EJ, Hoppin FG Jr, Dawson SV. Airway geometry by analysis of acoustic pulse response measurements. J Appl Physiol 43:523–536, 1977.
2. Fredberg JJ, Wohl MEB, Glass GM, Dorkin HL. Airway area by acoustic reflections measured at the mouth. J Appl Physiol 48:749–758, 1980.
3. Ware JA, Aki K. Continuous and discrete inverse scattering problems in a stratified elastic medium. I: Plane waves at normal incidence. J Acoust Soc Am 54:911–921, 1969.
4. Fredberg JJ. Acoustic determinants of respiratory system properties. Ann Biomed Eng 9:463–473, 1981.
5. Jackson AC, Olson DE. Comparison of direct and acoustical area measurements in physical models of human central airways. J Appl Physiol 48:896–902, 1980.
6. D'Urzo T, Rebuck AS, Lawson V, Hoffstein V. Effect of CO_2 concentrations on acoustic inferences of airway area. J Appl Physiol 60:398–401, 1986.
7. Brooks LJ, Castile RG, Glass GM, Griscom NT, Wohl MEB, Fredberg JJ. Reproducibility and accuracy of airway areas by acoustic reflections. J Appl Physiol 57:777–787, 1984.
8. D'Urzo AD, Rubinstein I, Lawson V, Vassal KP, Rebuck AS, Slutsky AS, Hoffstein V. Comparison of glottic areas measured by acoustic reflections vs. com-

puterized tomography. J Appl Physiol 64:367–370, 1988.

9. Jackson AC, Krevans JR Jr. Tracheal cross-sectional areas from acoustic reflections in dogs. J Appl Physiol 57:351–353, 1984.

10. D'Urzo AD, Lawson V, Vassal K, Rebuck AS, Slutsky AS, Hoffstein V. Airway area by acoustic response measurements and computerized tomography. Am Rev Respir Dis 135:392–395, 1987.

11. Jackson AC, Loring SH, Drazen JM. Serial distribution of bronchoconstriction induced by vagal stimulation or histamine. J Appl Physiol 50:1286–1292, 1981.

12. Hilberg O, Jackson AC, Swift DL, Pedersen OF. Acoustic rhinometry: Evaluation of nasal cavity by acoustic reflection. J Appl Physiol 66:295–303, 1989.

13. Rubinstein I, McClean PA, Boucher R, Zamel N, Fredberg JJ, Hoffstein V. Effect of mouthpiece, nose clips, and head position on airway area measured by acoustic reflections. J Appl Physiol 63:1469–1474, 1987.

14. Molfino N, Zamel N, Fredberg J, Hoffstein V. Artefacts in measuring airway areas by acoustic reflections. Am Rev Respir Dis 142:1465, 1990.

15. Yamagiwa M, Hilberg O, Pedersen O, Lundqvist GR. Evaluation of the effect of localized skin cooling on nasal airway volume by acoustic rhinometry. Am Rev Respir Dis 141:1050–1054, 1990.

16. Grymer LF, Hilberg O, Elbrond O, Pedersen O. Acoustic rhinometry: Evaluation of the nasal cavity with septal deviations, before and after septoplasty. Laryngoscope 99:1180–1187, 1989.

17. Rivlin J, Hoffstein V, Kalbfleish J, McNicholas W, Zamel N, Bryan AC. Upper airway morphology in patients with obstructive sleep apnea. Am Rev Respir Dis 129:355, 1984.

18. Hoffstein V, Phillipson EA, Zamel N. Lung volume dependence of pharyngeal cross-section in patients with obstructive sleep apnea. Am Rev Respir Dis 130:175, 1984.

19. Brown I, Bradley D, Zamel N, Phillipson E, Hoffstein V. Pharyngeal compliance in snoring subjects with and without obstructive sleep apnea. Am Rev Respir Dis 132:211–214, 1985.

20. Bradley D, Brown I, Grossman R, Zamel N, Phillipson E, Hoffstein V. Pharynx in snorers, non-snorers, and patients with obstructive sleep apnea. N Engl J Med 315:1327–1331, 1986.

21. Remmers JE, De Groot WJ, Sauerland EK, Anch AM. Pathophysiology of upper airway occlusion during sleep. J Appl Physiol 44:931–938, 1978.

22. Issa FG, Sullivan CE. Upper airway closing pressures in obstructive sleep apnea. J Appl Physiol 57:520–527, 1984.

23. Suratt PM, Wilhoit SC, Cooper K. Induction of airway collapse with subatmospheric pressure in awake patients with sleep apnea. J Appl Physiol 57:140–146, 1984.

24. Strohl KP, Olson LG. Concerning the importance of pharyngeal muscles in the maintenance of upper airway patency during sleep: An opinion. Chest 92:918–920, 1987.

25. Smith PL, Wise RA, Gold AR, Schwartz AB, Permutt S. Upper airway pressure-flow relationships in obstructive sleep apnea. J Appl Physiol 64:789–795, 1988.

26. Hudgel DW, Hendricks C, Hamilton HB. Characteristics of the upper airway pressure-flow relationship during sleep. J Appl Physiol 64:1930–1935, 1988.

27. Hoffstein V, Zamel N. Sleep apnea and the upper airways. Br J Anaesth 65:139–150, 1990.

28. Rubinstein I, Colapinto N, Rotstein LE, Brown IG, Hoffstein V. Improvement in pharyngeal properties after weight loss in patients with obstructive sleep apnea. Am Rev Respir Dis 138:1192–1195, 1988.

29. Brown I, McClean P, Boucher R, Zamel N, Hoffstein V. Changes in pharyngeal size with posture and application of continuous positive airway pressure in patients with obstructive sleep apnea. Am Rev Respir Dis 136:628–632, 1987.

30. Fouke JM, Strohl KP. Effect of position and lung volume on upper airway geometry. J Appl Physiol 63:375–380, 1987.

31. Wright S, Haight J, Zamel N, Hoffstein V. Changes in pharyngeal properties after uvulopalatopharyngoplasty. Laryngoscope 99:62–69, 1989.

32. Bradley TD, Brown IG, Zamel N, Phillipson EA, Hoffstein V. Differences in pharyngeal properties between snorers with predominantly central sleep apnea and those without sleep apnea. Am Rev Respir Dis 135:387–391, 1987.

33. Rubinstein I, England SJ, Zamel N, Hoffstein V. Glottic dimensions and movements during vital capacity maneuvres in normal males and females. Respir Physiol 77:263–267, 1989.

34. Rubinstein I, Slutsky AS, Zamel N, Hoffstein V. Paradoxical glottic narrowing in patients with severe obstructive sleep apnea. J Clin Invest 81:1051–1055, 1988.

35. Brown I, Zamel N, Webster P, Hoffstein V. Changes in tracheal cross-sectional area during Mueller and Valsalva maneuvers in humans. J Appl Physiol 60:1865–1870, 1986.

36. Hoffstein V. Relationship between lung volume, maximum expiratory flow, FEV_1, and tracheal area in normal men and women. Am Rev Respir Dis 134:956–961, 1986.

37. Hoffstein V, Castile R, O'Donnell CR, Glass GM, Strieder DS, Wohl MEB, Fredberg JJ. In vivo estimation of tracheal distensibility and hysteresis in normal adults. J Appl Physiol 63:1469–1474, 1987.

38. Brooks LJ, Byard PJ, Helms RC, Fouke JM, Strohl KP. Relationship between lung volume and tracheal area as assessed by acoustic reflection. J Appl Physiol 64:1050–1054, 1988.

39. Katz I, Zamel N, Rebuck AS, Slutsky AS, Hoffstein V. Relative hysteresis of the airways and lung parenchyma in normal subjects. J Appl Physiol 65:2390–2394, 1988.

40. Hoffstein V, Zamel N. Tracheal stenosis measured by acoustic reflection technique. Am Rev Respir Dis 130:355, 1984.

41. Rubinstein I, Zamel N, Rebuck AS, Hoffstein V, D'Urzo AD, Slutsky AS. Dichotomous airway response to exercise in asthmatic patients. Am Rev Respir Dis 138:1164–1168, 1988.

42. Rubinstein I, Bradley TD, Zamel N, Hoffstein V. Graded narrowing of the upper airway areas in patients with obstructive sleep apnea. J Appl Physiol 67:2427–2431, 1989.

43. Katz I, Zamel N, Rebuck AS, Slutsky AS, Hoffstein V. Tracheal hysteresis in sleep apnea. J Appl Physiol 67:1349–1353, 1989.

44. Brooks LJ. Tracheal size and distensibility in patients with cystic fibrosis. Am Rev Respir Dis 141:513–516, 1990.

CHAPTER 8

Airway Sound Transmission Analysis

George R. Wodicka, Ph.D., and Daniel C. Shannon, M.D.

The use of sound to noninvasively evaluate the structural integrity of a system is a commonly employed engineering technique. Since the invention of the stethoscope by Laennec[1] in the early 19th century, clinicians have listened to transmitted voice or breath sounds on the chest wall as indices of regional lung function and disease. More recently, physicians and engineers have begun to develop more sophisticated techniques to probe the respiratory system with sounds of known quality and to accurately measure their transmission to the chest wall. These techniques allow regional acoustic properties to be determined without the confounding effects of variations in the sound source. Sophisticated signal-processing algorithms can then be employed to extract information concerning alterations in the underlying structure of the lungs in a reproducible manner. Also, physiologic information may be derived from a knowledge of the exact mechanisms and attributes of transmission, so that auscultatory techniques may be used more successfully in the diagnosis or monitoring of patients.

Recent investigations indicate that the acoustic properties of the respiratory system are quite complex, due to its heterogeneous anatomy. Sound generated within or intro-duced into the airways propagates in a number of different media, such as air, parenchyma, and chest wall, all of which have significantly different acoustic characteristics. Also, these characteristics and the exact pathways of the propagation are a strong function of the sonic frequency. For example, at low frequencies within the audible range, the large airway walls vibrate significantly in response to intra-airway sonic perturbations, whereas at higher frequencies the walls become effectively rigid and thereby affect the propagation pathways to the chest wall. It is a challenge for investigators to elucidate the mechanisms of transmission over the entire audible frequency range and to elicit the key relationships between the structure of the system and acoustic measurements.

The topic of airway sound transmission analysis is covered in this chapter through an overview of recent physiologic, engineering, and clinical investigations. The acoustic characteristics of the respiratory system, particularly the relationships between chest wall measurements and underlying lung structure, are emphasized. Wherever possible, experimental findings that permit advances in the use of auscultatory techniques for diagnosis and monitoring of patients with lung disease are noted. Because most audible sonic energy that readily passes through the lungs does so at low frequencies, the response of the respiratory system to perturbations within the low-frequency range is discussed in detail.

THEORY AND MODELING

For sound to travel from the mouth or the large airways to the chest wall, it must propagate within the airways, through the parenchyma, and into the chest wall. As previously noted, the acoustic properties of these individual structures, as determined by their composition and geometry, are a strong function of the frequency of the perturbing sound wave. The audible frequency range extends from roughly 20 to 20,000 cycles per second, units commonly described as Hertz (Hz). As a reference, the fundamental frequency of middle C on a piano is 256 Hz. Each component of the respiratory system has a unique frequency-dependent response that not only affects measurements performed on the chest wall, but which also determines the dominant pathways of propagation from the airways to the chest wall. These factors suggest that the optimal detection of altered structure using acoustic techniques must be performed over a frequency range where the transmission is strongly affected by the particular system structure (large and small airways, parenchyma, chest wall) of interest.

Propagation of Sound Within Airways

A sound wave that is propagating down the airways below the vocal folds encounters an ever-changing environment. The airways, although roughly cylindrical in shape, have non-rigid walls and form a highly complex branching structure that terminates in the alveoli. This branching network has been modeled from an acoustic perspective by a number of investigators,[2-5] primarily to assess the structural determinants of input acoustic impedance measurements. Acoustic impedance is defined as the ratio of acoustic pressure to volume velocity (analogous to electrical impedance, which is the ratio of voltage to current). It is a parameter that is, in general, a function of the sonic frequency. These models suggest that the airways possess a number of interesting acoustic properties at frequencies below

roughly 1000 Hz: the large airway walls vibrate significantly (ie, the airways cannot be assumed to be rigid) and have a strong effect on the overall acoustic response of the system; the entire branching network behaves to a first approximation in a manner similar to a single nonrigid tube that opens into the large volume of gas contained within the small airways and alveoli. This behavior results in part from the total cross-sectional area of the branching network being roughly constant for the first few airways generations and then increasing rapidly thereafter, as indicated in Figure 8–1. It also stems from the relatively long sonic wavelengths at these low frequencies, as compared to the airway segment lengths. In a homogeneous and elastic medium, the sonic frequency f and the wavelength λ are related to the sound speed in the media c by

$$c = f\lambda$$

Because c is determined by physical properties (density and compliance) of the media, f is inversely related to λ. As a reference, c in air is roughly 35,000 cm/s; thus, at f = 100 Hz, λ is 350 cm. If f is increased to 1000 Hz, λ is reduced to 35 cm. It should be noted that the exact c for airway propagation is also a function of the airway wall properties (and thus a function of frequency), but that the inverse relationship between f and λ still holds true.

A single-tube model of the airways at low frequencies was first applied by Gupta and colleagues in 1973,[6] yet only the compliant properties of the airway walls were included in the model. More recently, Wodicka and associates[7] included the effects of the wall mass and surrounding lung parenchyma. This model was employed not only to estimate the amount of sonic energy coupled from the large airways into the surrounding parenchyma via wall motion (which is discussed in more detail later in this chapter), but to provide a geometrically simple first approach toward understanding the recent input impedance measurements by Jackson and coworkers in human subjects.[8]

The respiratory tract behaves as an air-filled cylindrical conduit for sonic propagation. The airway wall properties are such that at frequencies below roughly 1000 Hz, they vibrate and allow some sonic energy to be coupled directly into the surrounding parenchyma, by-passing the smaller airways. At higher frequencies, the airway walls become essentially rigid due to their mass[9] and allow a higher percentage of energy to remain within the airway lumen and travel down the branching airways. Quantitative information concerning

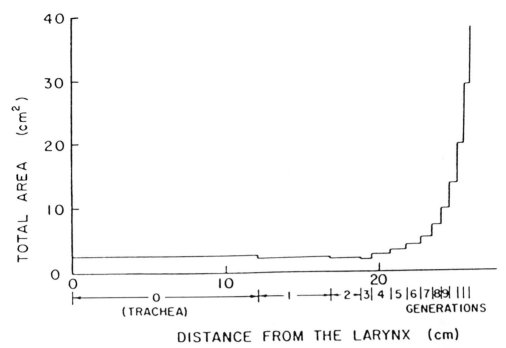

Figure 8–1. Total cross-sectional area of the branching airways as a function of the distance from the larynx. (From Gupta V, Wilson TA, Beavers GS. A model for vocal cord excitation. J Acoust Soc Am 54:1607–1617, 1973; with permission.)

the frequency-dependent nature of these propagation modes is not known and is currently being investigated.[9a] For example, it would be invaluable to know for each sonic frequency of interest the exact spatial and temporal distribution of its propagation through the airways and into the parenchyma and chest wall.

Propagation Within the Parenchyma to the Chest Wall

The parenchyma that surrounds the large airways consists primarily of alveoli, small airways, capillaries, and supporting lung tissue. In 1983, Rice proposed that, from an acoustic perspective, the parenchyma acts as a homogeneous mixture of tissue and gas at audible frequencies below approximately 10,000 Hz.[10] In this frequency range, as will be discussed in more detail, the sound wavelengths in the parenchyma are significantly longer than the alveolar radii, which have an average value in adult humans of roughly 0.015 cm. This approach assumes that the forces required to move air between adjacent alveoli are large and that therefore no gas exchange occurs due to the acoustic wave propagation. This assumption is clearly invalid at the very low

frequencies associated with high-frequency ventilation, as reported by Butler and associates in 1987.[11]

In the model of the parenchyma, the composite density ρ and volumetric compliance K of the mixture was estimated based on the relative proportions of tissue t (composed primarily of water) and gas g (air)

$$\rho = (1 - h)\rho_g + h\rho_t$$
$$K = (1 - h)K_g + hK_t$$

where h is the volumetric proportion of the tissue and thus $(1 - h)$ is the volumetric proportion of the gas. As one may have guessed, ρ is dominated by the ρ_t term due to the more dense tissue, where K is dominated by K_g, due to the greater gas compliance. The resulting predicted sound speed in the parenchyma is estimated by

$$c = \sqrt{\frac{1}{\rho K}}$$

and ranges from roughly 2000 to 6000 cm/s, values significantly less than the free field speeds in either air (35,000 cm/s) or tissue (150,000 cm/s). These relatively low parenchymal sound speeds, which compared well with in vitro measurements, indicate that the corresponding λs at a given frequency are small when compared to propagation purely within

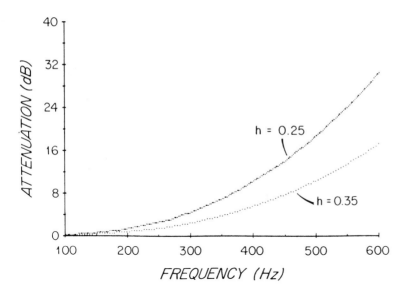

Figure 8–2. Attenuation of a sound pressure wave after propagation through 10 cm of model parenchyma. h = the volumetric proportion of tissue in the model parenchyma. (From Wodicka GR, Stevens KN, Golub HL, Cravalho EG, Shannon DC. A model of acoustic transmission in the respiratory system. IEEE Trans Biomed Eng 36:925–934, 1989; with permission; © 1989 IEEE.)

air or tissue. These smaller wavelengths make the application of models that lump the acoustic characteristics of the parenchyma into single elements inappropriate,[12] and suggest the need for more distributed approaches. It does suggest that, due to the shorter wavelengths, one may be able to obtain more regional information from sound transmission measurements at lower frequencies than initially expected. The model also suggests that the characteristics of parenchymal propagation are a function of the relative proportions of tissue and gas, which is altered in lung pathologies.

To estimate the losses associated with propagation through the parenchyma, Wodicka and coworkers[7] represented the parenchymal mixture in the geometric form of spherical air bubbles (alveoli) in water (lung tissue). This representation allowed theories that describe the effects of ships' wakes on sonar[13] to be extended and adapted toward parenchymal transmission. At frequencies less than a few thousand Hz, where the sonic wavelengths are significantly longer than the alveolar diameters, the thermal losses are predicted to dominate over either viscous or scattering effects. These thermal losses arise as the wave propagates within the parenchyma, because the compressions and expansions of the alveoli are polytropic; they are more adiabatic at the center of the alveolar bubble and more isothermal where the bubble is in contact with the surrounding water-filled tissue. Thus, the work performed by the sound wave in bubble compression is greater than that performed by the bubble in expansion, resulting in a net flow of heat into the lung tissue. Although the effect

of a single alveolar bubble is negligible, the composite effect of the large number of alveoli per unit volume is quite pronounced.

Figure 8–2 depicts the estimated attenuation of a sound wave as a function of frequency when it is transmitted through 10 cm of model parenchyma at resting lung volume where h, the volumetric proportion of tissue, is increased from 0.25 to 0.35 by the addition of roughly 300 mL of fluid distributed uniformly. The attenuation is plotted in the logarithmic units of decibels (dB)

$$dB = 20 \log_{10} \frac{\text{measured amplitude}}{\text{initial amplitude}}$$

and thus an attenuation of 20 dB represents an order of magnitude reduction in amplitude. For the normal case, the magnitude of the attenuation is negligible at a frequency of 100 Hz, but increases rapidly to roughly 30 dB at 600 Hz. This strong frequency dependence qualitatively explains previous auscultatory and experimental observations by Kraman[14] and Wodicka and colleagues[15] of poor sound transmission to the chest wall above 400 Hz in human subjects. It is also consistent with the hypothesis that the transmission of sound at frequencies below 250 Hz, where the attenuation is small in magnitude, is dominated by airway and chest wall effects, as suggested by Kraman and Bohadana[16] and Wodicka and Shannon.[17]

The interface between the lung parenchyma and the chest wall is an important structure affecting sound transmission. Because the chest wall is significantly more massive and less compliant per unit volume than the parenchyma, a significant amount of the energy in a wave reaching this interface is reflected back toward the airways, rather than transmitted to the surface. The relative mismatch between these two structures has been used to explain a number of clinical findings, such as the increase in breath sound intensity over the congested lung.[18] However, theories that describe the acoustic behavior that occurs at the interface between two homogeneous media may be applied to the lung–chest wall only with a number of simplifying assumptions.

The need for simplification arises, at least in part, from the heterogeneous structure of the chest wall and its relatively large sound speed as compared to the parenchyma. Because the ribs lie within the chest wall, there exist additional acoustic interfaces between bone and soft tissue. Even if one assumes that the sound speed in the entire chest wall is that of soft tissue, roughly 150,000 cm/s, the resulting wavelengths at frequencies less than 1000 Hz are greater than 150 cm—considerably longer than the chest wall thickness. This indicates that the chest wall vibrates as a single, lumped structure in response to low-frequency sonic perturbations and that wave motion does not arise within it. These complex issues necessitate further investigation into the interaction between these structures in order to elucidate their composite acoustical behavior and thereby better understand the relationships between sound detected on the chest wall and the underlying sound pressure in the pleural space.

An Integrated Model of Sound Transmission

The transmission of sound from within the airways to the chest wall due to large airway wall motion was modeled by Wodicka and colleagues in 1989.[7] As previously noted, in this approach the airways were represented as a single, effective tube with non-rigid walls (Figure 8–3). The coupling of sonic energy from within the airways into the surrounding parenchyma due to wall motion was modeled as the source of an outgoing cylindrical wave because of the roughly cylindrical airway geometry. The parenchyma was represented as a homogeneous mixture of gas and tissue in the form of air bubbles in water, and the effects of thermal losses were incorporated (see the previous section for details of this representation). The chest wall was considered to be a

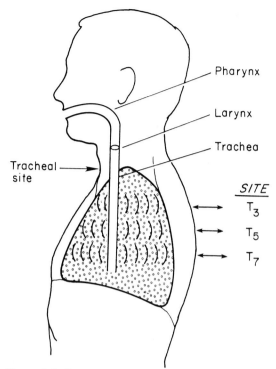

Figure 8–3. Diagram of a model respiratory system at low frequencies. (From Wodicka GR, Stevens KN, Golub HL, Cravalho EG, Shannon DC. A model of acoustic transmission in the respiratory system. IEEE Trans Biomed Eng 36:925–934, 1989; with permission; © 1989 IEEE.)

primarily massive boundary to the wave propagation that vibrated as a single, lumped structure. The model predicted the magnitude of the acceleration over the extrathoracic trachea and three locations on the midposterior chest wall corresponding to the levels of the third, fifth, and seventh thoracic vertebrae (designated T3, T5, and T7, respectively), for a sonic perturbation introduced at the mouth.

The predicted magnitude of acceleration as a function of frequency between 100 and 600 Hz for an ideal sound source placed at the mouth is depicted in Figure 8–4. The peaks in the spectra of transmission are determined by the model respiratory tract, which exhibits resonance behavior roughly analogous to that which is observed in organ pipes. The difference in magnitude between the chest wall measurements and the tracheal one at low frequencies is predicted by two factors of roughly equal magnitude: the loss in acoustic pressure as the cylindrical wave propagates outward within the parenchyma, and the relatively more massive chest wall as compared to the tissue that overlies the extrathoracic tra-

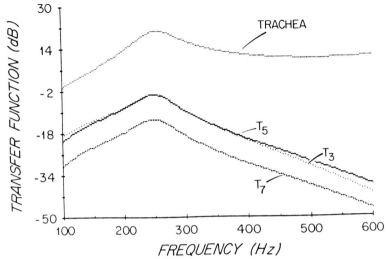

Figure 8–4. Acceleration at the trachea and three model chest wall locations as a function of frequency for sound (noise) introduced into the mouth. (From Wodicka GR, Stevens KN, Golub HL, Cravalho EG, Shannon DC. A model of acoustic transmission in the respiratory system. IEEE Trans Biomed Eng 36:925–934, 1989; with permission; © 1989 IEEE.)

chea. The decrease in transmission to the chest wall at higher frequencies in this range is due primarily to the frequency-dependent attenuation in the model parenchyma.

Effects of changes in the structure of the respiratory system on sound transmission may be estimated using this modeling approach. Figure 8–5 depicts the predicted spectrum of acceleration at the T5 site for a volumetric proportion of tissue h increased to 0.35 by the homogeneous addition of 300 mL of water to the lung. The predicted increase in acceleration is significant at higher frequencies for this magnitude of an increase in h. This prediction is consistent with previous clinical observations of increased transmission of voice sounds through the lung in pulmonary congestion, especially at higher frequencies.[19] It is also qualitatively consistent with the increased amplitude of transmission that was observed by Donnerberg and associates[20] in dogs after the induction of pulmonary edema. Conversely, the model suggests that in diseases in which h is decreased, such as asthma or emphysema, the magnitude of transmission would decrease due to the increased attenuation of the sound wave in the parenchyma.

MEASUREMENTS OF SOUND TRANSMISSION

There have been a number of investigations that focused on the transmission of sound

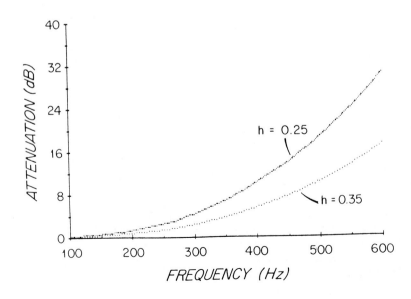

Figure 8–5. The effect of changing the volumetric proportion of tissue h in the parenchyma on the predicted acceleration of the chest wall at the T5 site. (From Wodicka GR, Stevens KN, Golub HL, Cravalho EG, Shannon DC. A model of acoustic transmission in the respiratory system. IEEE Trans Biomed Eng 36:925–934, 1989; with permission; © 1989 IEEE.)

through the respiratory systems of healthy human subjects at frequencies below approximately 1000 Hz. In general, the goal of these studies was to assess the effects of the respiratory system on a sound of known quality introduced into the mouth and measured on the chest wall. In some cases, the observations were studied in an empirical fashion only, and in others they were analyzed in order to test a particular hypothesis regarding transmission or to validate a model of the system's acoustic properties.

The two most widely measured acoustic variables are the transit time and the amplitude change of transmission from the mouth to the chest wall. Kraman[14] measured the effect of inhaled gas composition and measurement site on the propagation time of sound between detection at a site over the extrathoracic trachea and sites on the posterior chest wall of adult subjects. Cross-correlation techniques were employed to estimate the propagation times for input noise with significant energy between 125 and 500 Hz. The estimated times ranged from approximately 2 ms on the upper chest to 5 ms on the lower chest. Assuming that the sound travels the vertical distance to a site within the airway and then propagates through 10 cm of parenchyma, the estimated parenchyma sound speed ranges from approximately 2000 to 6000 cm/s. Changing the inhaled gas from air to a mixture of 80% helium and 20% oxygen resulted in less than a 10% decrease in the measured propagation times. The predicted increase in sound speed if the propagation were through the gas alone would be greater than 100%. This observation is consistent with the modeling approaches of Rice,[10] which treat the parenchyma as a homogeneous mixture, and suggests that low-frequency sound spends a considerable amount of its propagation time within the parenchyma.

The effect of the sonic frequency on the propagation time from mouth to chest wall was investigated by Rice in 1984.[21] Narrow-band pulses were directed into the mouths of healthy subjects, and it was observed that the propagation times decreased from roughly 5 to 2.5 ms as frequency increased from 255 to 640 Hz. These observations suggest that the point where the majority of the energy couples from the airways to the parenchyma is frequency dependent and moves toward smaller airways with increasing frequency. Thus, more information about the small airways may be available from higher frequency measurements; for example, those performed by Jacobs in 1982[22] and Goncharoff and colleagues in 1989.[23]

A number of investigators have measured the amplitude of sound transmission in the respiratory system as a function of various physiologic parameters. Ploysongsang and associates[24, 25] employed the overall amplitude of transmission at a given chest wall site in an attempt to compensate for the transmission characteristics of the system and thereby use breath sounds more optimally as indices of regional ventilation. Kraman[26] observed that the amplitude of transmission to sites overlying the right lung was significantly greater than that measured at corresponding locations over the left lung. These observations suggest that preferential coupling of sound to the right lung occurs due to the effects of the massive mediastinum (primarily the heart), which lies to the left of the major airways.

The spectral characteristics of sound transmission from the mouth to the chest wall between 100 and 600 Hz were determined by Wodicka and colleagues[15] (Figure 8–6). Kraman[14] had noted significant effects of the sound source and introduction system on his overall transmission measurements. Thus, Wodicka and colleagues included these effects in the integrated model of the acoustic properties of the respiratory system. This inclusion allowed direct comparisons to be made between sound transmission measurements performed on healthy adults at resting lung volume and model predictions. In this manner, the strength and weakness of the modeling approach were assessed and the key structures that affect transmission were suggested.

Figure 8–7 depicts a direct comparison between the amplitude of sound transmission as a function of frequency and the model predictions for measurements performed on the posterior chest wall at the level of the sixth thoracic vertebra. The experimental spectra are an average of those estimated from eight subjects, and the dotted lines demarcate the 95% confidence intervals of the estimates. There exists reasonable agreement between the measurements and the predictions at both of the measurement sites. The absolute transmitted power, the location and sharpness of the spectral peaks, and the overall difference in magnitude between the chest wall and tracheal measurements are all predicted with a fair degree of accuracy. The transmission to the chest wall at higher frequencies is significantly less than predicted, however, and indicates a deviation of the parenchymal acoustic properties from those of air bubbles in water. The overall agreement suggests that this model provides a framework upon which to investi-

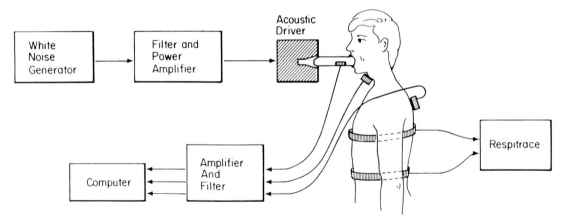

Figure 8–6. Experimental apparatus employed to perform acoustic transmission measurements on adult subjects. (From Wodicka GR, Stevens KN, Golub HL, Shannon DC. Spectral characteristics of sound transmission in the respiratory system. IEEE Trans Biomed Eng 37:1130–1135, 1990; with permission; © 1990 IEEE.)

gate and better understand the acoustic properties of this complex system. The approach also puts forth a number of testable hypotheses concerning the mechanisms of transmission, which are the focus of current investigations.

In order to reduce the effects of the sonic delivery system on the acoustic measurements, Wodicka and Shannon[17] estimated the transfer function of sound transmission between the chest wall and the tracheal site. In this manner, the chest wall measurements are analyzed relative to their tracheal counterpart, and information concerning transmission through the subglottal respiratory system is emphasized. Figure 8–8 depicts the average magnitude of the transfer functions (ie, frequency response) estimated from measurements performed on eight subjects at chest wall sites corresponding to the level of the third and sixth (T3, T6) thoracic vertebrae. The spectra exhibited a

single peak at low frequencies (roughly 135 Hz) and a strong decrease in magnitude with increasing frequency above the peak location. This frequency-dependent attenuation is qualitatively consistent with that measured by Shioya and associates,[27] who noted that the system behaved as a low-pass acoustic filter.

Although the observed increase in sonic attenuation with frequency can be attributed to the frequency-dependent parenchymal absorption, the structural determinant of the observed resonance is probably not due to the airways, because the fundamental resonance of the subglottal airways was measured in human subjects to be roughly 640 Hz by Ishizaka and associates.[3] This fact led Wodicka and Shannon[17] to suggest that the lower frequency resonance could be due to thoracic cavity effects. Because the magnitude of the parenchymal attenuation is predicted to be

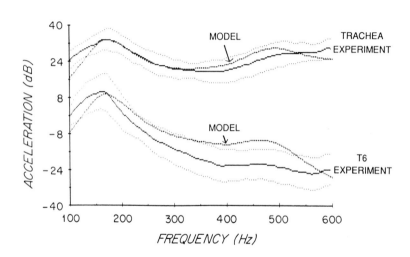

Figure 8–7. A direct comparison between the average magnitude spectra of acceleration and the model predictions at the trachea and T6 chest wall site. The dotted lines demarcate the 95% confidence intervals of the estimates for the study group. (From Wodicka GR, Stevens KN, Golub HL, Shannon DC. Spectral characteristics of sound transmission in the respiratory system. IEEE Trans Biomed Eng 37:1130–1135, 1990; with permission; © 1990 IEEE.)

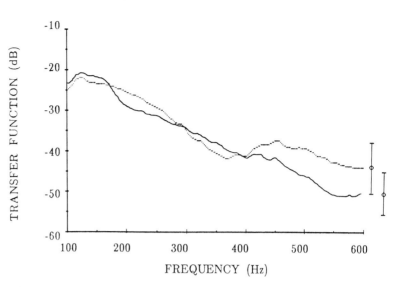

Figure 8–8. Average acoustical transfer functions derived from measurements performed on eight subjects at the T3 *(dashed line)* and T6 *(solid line)* chest wall sites, both relative to the tracheal site. (From Wodicka GR, Shannon DC. The transfer function of sound transmission in the subglottal human respiratory system at low frequencies. J Appl Physiol 69:2126–2130, 1990; with permission.)

small at frequencies below 250 Hz, sound waves that reach the lung–chest wall interface may be nearly as large in amplitude as when they were generated at the airway wall. At resonance, the combined effects of the incident and reflected waves are additive in amplitude and result in an increase in the parenchymal sound pressure and chest wall acceleration. If one represents the thoracic cavity as a large rigid cylinder with a radius of 11 cm that is filled with lossless lung tissue and estimates the location of its fundamental resonance, it occurs at approximately 130 Hz. This is in reasonable agreement with the experimental findings and gives support to the hypothesis that the chest wall has important effects on sound transmission at frequencies below 250 Hz. This hypothesis is also consistent with the conclusion of Kraman and Bohadana,[16] who proposed that the thoracic cavity effects dominate the overall transmission characteristics in this range, yielding measurements that are a relatively weak function of parenchymal structure. Thus, the parenchyma may affect sound transmission predominantly at frequencies above roughly 250 Hz, where its absorptive properties appear to become significant in magnitude.

MEASUREMENTS OF SOUND TRANSMISSION IN DISEASE

Auscultation provides diagnostic information in diseases as different as asthma and pneumonia. Clearly, the changes in structure that occur in these diseases affect the acoustic properties and alter the characteristics of sound transmission from the airways to the chest wall. Surprisingly, there have been few formal transmission studies performed to quantitate these changes and understand these phenomena better.

Bohme and Bohme[28] measured the transmission of sound in the 50 to 600 Hz frequency range from the mouth to the chest wall in patients with emphysema. In comparison to measurements performed on healthy subjects, decreased transmission was observed in the patients, predominantly at the higher frequencies (250 to 600 Hz). These findings are qualitatively consistent with the common clinical finding of decreased breath sound amplitude in patients with this disease. The investigators believed that the decrease in amplitude was due to an increase in absorption in the more air-filled parenchyma—a preliminary hypothesis that is consistent with the model predictions of Wodicka and colleagues.[7] Ploysongsang and associates[24, 29] measured the overall intensity of sound transmission up to 700 Hz in patients with emphysema. A large spatial variability in the measurements was found, much larger than that which was observed in healthy subjects. It is likely that this finding is indicative of the heterogeneous structural alterations in this disease, which results in regional disturbances in the sound transmission patterns.

The effect of cardiogenic pulmonary edema on the intensity of sound transmitted from the trachea to the chest wall in dogs over the 50 to 2000 Hz range was investigated by Donnerberg and colleagues.[20] The measured intensity was compared to postmortem wet-to-dry lung ratios, and a reasonably linear relationship was observed over a wide range of edema. The observation that an increase in lung water and concurrent decrease in air volume led to increased transmitted sound intensity is again consistent with the mechanisms of parenchymal transport proposed by Wodicka and colleagues.[7] The investigators stated that the bulk of the intensity change was observed at higher frequencies, but no frequency distribution was reported.

CONCLUSIONS

The characteristics of sound transmission through the respiratory system depend on the acoustic properties of the various structures between the sound source and the site of recording or auscultation. The large airways become effectively rigid at higher frequencies, so that sounds are not predominantly transmitted in a radial direction to parenchyma, but rather in a longitudinal direction to smaller airways. Conversely, sounds at lower frequencies appear to be better transmitted radially via large airway motion to parenchyma and hence to the chest wall. Chest wall structures further affect the sound waves by reflection at the lung–chest wall interface, resulting in the complex sounds heard through a stethoscope.

Parenchyma exhibits increased attenuation at frequencies above roughly 250 Hz, so that sounds above 600 Hz are not easily distinguishable from background noise through auscultation. Sounds below 250 Hz are readily transmitted from the airways to the chest wall, especially at approximately 135 Hz. This latter observation may indicate a natural acoustic resonance effect of the thorax. The effects of airways, parenchyma, and chest wall act in concert to determine the quality of sounds detected at the chest wall surface. Each individual effect can be altered by disease and should be explainable both qualitatively and quantitatively once a better understanding of the acoustic characteristics and interactions of diseased tissues is obtained. For example, a model of the lung parenchyma as homogeneous bubbles of air in water appears to be qualitatively satisfactory and predicts both experimental and clinical observations, but it underestimates the extent of attenuation at higher frequencies. Clinically, many diseases can be considered to change the relative proportions of air and water in various regions, so that sounds above roughly 250 Hz are either

more or less attenuated. However, this information could not be interpreted in isolation from the distance that sound waves travel from the source or from the effects of overlying chest wall structures. More complete understanding that will permit enhanced clinical use of this information requires further characterization of these important interactions.

References

1. Laennec RTH. De L'Auscultation Mediate. Paris: Brosson & Chande, 1819.
2. Van den Berg J. An electrical analogue of the trachea, lungs and tissues. Acta Physiol Pharmacol Neerlandica 9:361–385, 1960.
3. Ishizaka K, Matsudaira M, Kaneko T. Input acoustic-impedance measurement of the subglottal system. J Acoust Soc Am 60:190–197, 1976.
4. Fredberg JJ, Hoenig A. Mechanical response of the lungs at high frequencies. J Biomech Eng 100:57–66, 1978.
5. Fredberg JJ. Spatial considerations in oscillation mechanics of the lung. Fed Proc 39:2747–2754, 1980.
6. Gupta V, Wilson TA, Beavers GS. A model for vocal cord excitation. J Acoust Soc Am 54:1607–1617, 1973.
7. Wodicka GR, Stevens KN, Golub HL, Cravalho EG, Shannon DC. A model of acoustic transmission in the respiratory system. IEEE Trans Biomed Eng 36:925–934, 1989.
8. Jackson AC, Giurdanella CA, Dorkin HL. Density dependence of respiratory system impedances between 5 and 320 Hz in humans. J Appl Physiol 67:2323–2330, 1989.
9. Rice DA. Sound speed in the upper airways. J Appl Physiol 49:326–336, 1980.
9a. Rice DA, Rice JC. Central to peripheral sound propagation in excised lung. J Acoust Soc Am 82:1139–1144, 1987.
10. Rice DA. Sound speed in pulmonary parenchyma. J Appl Physiol 54:304–308, 1983.
11. Butler JP, Lehr JL, Drazen JM. Longitudinal elastic wave propagation in pulmonary parenchyma. J Appl Physiol 62:1349–1355, 1987.
12. Bohme HR. An attempt at physical characterization of the passive response of the lungs to sound waves in a model. Z Inn Med 29:401, 1974.
13. Prosperetti A. Thermal effects and damping mechanisms in the forced radial oscillations of gas bubbles in liquids. J Acoust Soc Am 61:17–27, 1977.
14. Kraman SS. Speed of low-frequency sound through the lungs of normal men. J Appl Physiol 55:1862–1867, 1983.
15. Wodicka GR, Stevens KN, Golub HL, Shannon DC. Spectral characteristics of sound transmission in the respiratory system. IEEE Trans Biomed Eng 37:1130–1135, 1990.
16. Kraman SS, Bohadana AB. Transmission to the chest of sound introduced at the mouth. J Appl Physiol 66:278–281, 1989.
17. Wodicka GR, Shannon DC. The transfer function of sound transmission in the subglottal human respiratory system at low frequencies. J Appl Physiol 69:2126–2130, 1990.
18. Rice DA. Transmission of lung sounds. Semin Resp Med 6:166–170, 1985.

19. Bates B. A Guide to Physical Examination. Philadelphia: J. B. Lippincott, 1979.
20. Donnerberg RL, Druzgalski CK, Hamlin RL, Davis GL, Campbell RM, Rice DA. Sound transfer function of the congested canine lung. Br J Dis Chest 74:23–31, 1980.
21. Rice DA. Dispersion in pulmonary sound transmission. Proc. 37th Annual Conference of Engineering in Medicine and Biology, Los Angeles, 1984, p. 75.
22. Jacobs JE. Wideband acoustic energy studies of pulmonary airways. Bioelectromagnetics 3:167–177, 1982.
23. Goncharoff V, Jacobs JE, Cugell DW. Wideband acoustic transmission of human lungs. Med Biol Eng Comput 27:513–519, 1989.
24. Ploysongsang Y, Martin RR, Ross WRD, Loudon RG, Macklem PT. Breath sounds and regional ventilation. Am Rev Respir Dis 116:187–199, 1977.
25. Ploysongsang Y, Pare JAP, Macklem PT. Correlation of regional breath sounds with regional ventilation in emphysema. Am Rev Respir Dis 126:526–529, 1982.
26. Kraman SS. Comparison of lung sound and transmitted sound amplitude in normal men. Am Rev Respir Dis 128:451–454, 1983.
27. Shioya N, Takezawa Y, Mikami R, Kudoh S, Shibuya A. Acoustic transmission of the respiratory system using sinusoidal sound waves introduced orally. Nippon Kyobu Shikkan Gakkai Zasshi 22:125–130, 1984.
28. Bohme HR, Bohme H. Variable low-frequency sound conduction through the lungs in pulmonary emphysema. Z Inn Med 27:765–770, 1972.
29. Ploysongsang Y, Pare JAP, Macklem PT. Lung sounds in patients with emphysema. Am Rev Respir Dis 124:45–49, 1982.

SECURING THE AIRWAY

CHAPTER 9

Managing the Airway Outside of the Operating Room

Reid Rubsamen, M.D.

The health care professional frequently is called to assist in airway management in the hospital but outside of the operating room. Ideally, an optimal set of equipment should be available during such a situation. This chapter outlines the contents of a recommended emergency airway management kit (Table 9–1). The realities of airway management in hostile environments where all appropriate equipment may not be available also is discussed.

FUNDAMENTALS

Management of the airway is the essential first step in the evaluation of the acutely ill patient. In its most basic form, emergency airway management is a low-technology skill involving proper initial positioning and subsequent manipulation of the head, neck, and jaw. In the absence of suspected neck injury, the head should be placed in the occiput forward "sniffing" position to facilitate establishing a patent airway, positive pressure ventilation, and subsequent endotracheal intubation.

A critical tool for emergency airway management therefore is a firm, adjustable platform on which to place the patient's head. A set of at least three folded blankets serves well

for this purpose (Fig. 9–1). From one to three of these blankets can be placed under the head to lift the occiput forward into the sniffing position, depending on the patient's size. Folded blankets may seem an unlikely component of an emergency airway management set; however, as with the other items discussed here, their availability at the scene of the emergency cannot be ensured unless they are explicitly provided by the airway management team.

After the head and neck have been properly

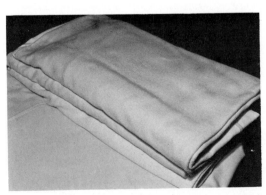

Figure 9–1. Blankets to facilitate head and neck positioning.

Table 9–1. BASIC EMERGENCY AIRWAY
MANAGEMENT KIT CONTENTS

Suction
    Suction tubing, regulators, and valves required for
      establishing continuity with hospital wall suction
      system
    Portable suction system (if wall suction is not
      commonly available)
    Yankauer suction tip
    Flexible suction catheter tip
Airway Support
    Three folded blankets for head support
    Oral airways (#3–#5)
    Nasal airways (#28–#34)
Surgical Lubricant
    5% lidocaine ointment
Ventilation
    Oxygen tank
    Green oxygen mask and tubing
    Ambu bag with infant, pediatric, and adult (small,
      medium, and large) masks
Intubation
    Laryngoscopes
      Miller 0–4 blades
      Macintosh 1–4 blades
      Two standard handles
      Datta (short) handle
    Endotracheal tubes (#0–#7 uncuffed; #4–#9 cuffed)
    Magill forceps
    Lighted stylet
    Plastic adhesive tape
    Benzoin solution
    Gauze squares (for application of benzoin)
Cricothyrotomy Kit
    #12 gauge catheter
    Oxygen jet valve device
    Emergency cricothyrotomy set
    3-mL plastic, Luer-Lok syringe with #7.0
      endotracheal tube adaptor in barrel end
Monitors
    Pulse oximeter
    Pulse oximeter probes
    End-tidal CO_2 monitor
    End-tidal CO_2 colorimetric detecter
Field Airway Management Tools
    Pocket mask

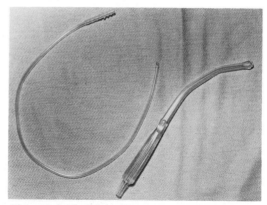

Figure 9–2. Flexible and Yankauer suction catheters.

Oral (Fig. 9–3) and nasal airways should
also be available as tools to aid in opening the
airway. Nasal airways may be especially important if the patient's mouth cannot be
opened. These airways are easier to use if
lubricated with surgical jelly or lidocaine ointment prior to their insertion. The use of oral
or nasal airways is a critical part of emergency
airway management, because the institution of
positive pressure ventilation by mask is the
critical first task of the emergency airway management team. Although endotracheal intubation is a laudable goal of emergency airway
management, 100% oxygen should almost always be administered via Ambu bag or a
similar device prior to the first intubation attempt. This typically raises the hemoglobin
oxygen saturation to a level compatible with
life, even if optimal ventilation cannot be attained without the use of an endotracheal tube.

The importance of positive pressure by mask
prior to attempted endotracheal intubation

positioned, a patent airway must be established. The importance of adequate suction
cannot be overemphasized. If gastric contents
have migrated into the pharynx, this debris
must be rapidly evacuated early in the course
of emergency airway management. The only
really effective way to do this is through the
use of suction, preferably supplied by a high-
vacuum central source. The burden lies with
the emergency airway management team to
ensure that (1) all proper regulators, fittings,
tubing, and suction tips (Fig. 9–2) are available; and (2) if central "wall suction" is unlikely to be available, that an appropriate
portable suction apparatus is part of the airway
management equipment set.

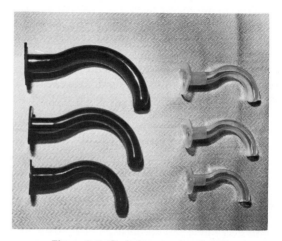

Figure 9–3. Oral airways, sizes 0 to 5.

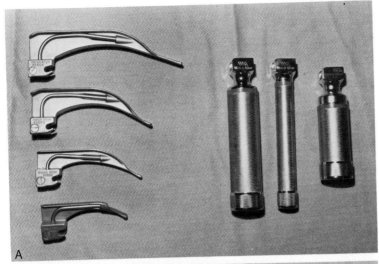

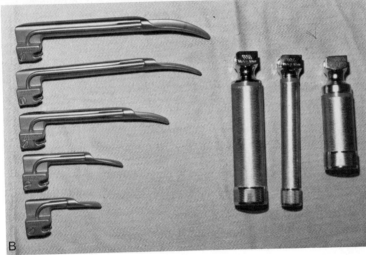

Figure 9–4. Laryngoscopes. *A,* Fiberoptic Macintosh blades 1 to 4, shown with standard, pediatric, and short quartz-halogen handles. *B,* Fiberoptic Miller blades 0 to 4, shown with standard, pediatric, and short quartz-halogen handles.

cannot be overemphasized. When the emergency airway management team arrives on the scene of an apneic patient, the crucial initial goal is to supply at least some oxygen to the tissues. Rapid initial airway management should allow positive pressure ventilation within 30 seconds. After several breaths have been given in this fashion, endotracheal intubation can be attempted and the degree of difficulty of the intubation procedure assessed. If a difficult intubation is encountered, the team can proceed with positive pressure ventilation by mask between intubation attempts.

The endotracheal intubation set should consist of a wide variety of blades and handles, including the Datta short handle popular in obstetrics. The amount of high-quality light emitted by the laryngoscope blade is crucial and may make the difference between an easy intubation and a difficult one. Consideration

should be given to the newer, quartz-halogen bulb laryngoscopes, which convey the bright light of a halogen lamp, located in the handle, up to the blade via a fiberoptic guide (Fig. 9–4).

A complete set of endotracheal tubes should be provided, with stylets available for each (Fig. 9–5). Pediatric tubes should be included, with both cuffed and uncuffed types in the intermediate size range. A superior adhesive tape applied to skin that has been pretreated with benzoin solution ensures that the placed endotracheal tube will not be dislodged during ventilation and transport.

IMPORTANT ADDITIONAL EQUIPMENT

The Ambu bag serves as an excellent tool for positive pressure ventilation by mask of

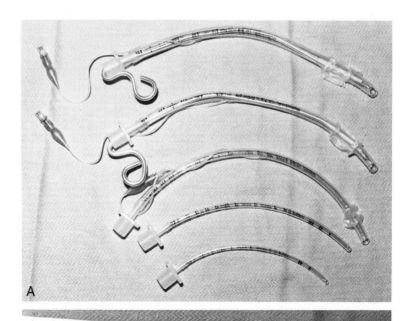

Figure 9–5. *A,* Endotracheal tubes, sizes 3, 4, 6, 7, and 8. Size 8.0 is shown with inserted stylet. *B,* Lighted stylet for blind oral or nasal endotracheal intubation. *C,* Magill forceps.

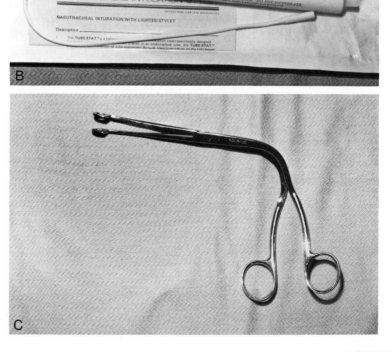

the apneic patient. It is a suboptimal choice, however, for assisted ventilation of the spontaneously breathing patient. The relatively noncompliant bag of the Ambu resuscitator will not contract with patient inspiration, thus making assessment of adequate mask seal and patient inspiratory effort difficult during spontaneous breaths. In addition, the instantaneous inspiratory flow requirement of the spontaneously breathing patient may be higher than can be accommodated by the oxygen reservoir tubing attached to the Ambu unit.

The Mapleson-D circuit, available as a self-contained mask, valve, and bag device, serves well for the assisted ventilation of the spontaneously breathing patient. Oxygen flows

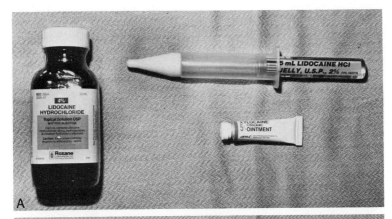

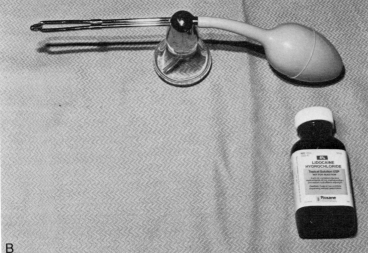

Figure 9–6. *A,* Lidocaine preparations for oral or nasal topicalization; *B,* 4% lidocaine solution with aerosolizer for pharyngeal topicalization.

through the device, however, must be high if controlled ventilation is attempted using this system, or significant rebreathing will occur.

Compromised patients who are awake and spontaneously breathing frequently require endotracheal intubation for proper ventilatory support. Direct, awake laryngoscopy frequently is the method of choice for definitive airway management in this patient population. Proper topicalization of the tongue and pharynx can be accomplished via insertion of successively larger oral airways coated with 5% lidocaine ointment. Adequate pharyngeal anesthesia can usually be established in a few minutes with this technique.

The tip of a laryngoscope blade can also be coated with the 5% lidocaine ointment to further blunt the response to direct laryngoscopy. As a general rule, the more compromised the patient, the less topicalization required.

Magill forceps (see Fig. 9–5C) can be useful to help guide the endotracheal tube through the cords during direct laryngoscopy, and should be optionally included.

Two percent lidocaine jelly, available in a syringe-style injector, is useful for nasal topicalization prior to nasal intubation. Four percent xylocaine solution, suitable for aerosol spray delivery, is effective for pharyngeal topicalization prior to awake laryngoscopy. Lidocaine preparations are shown in Figure 9–6.

The possibility that the patient cannot be intubated or positive pressure ventilated by mask must always be considered and prepared for. In this case, the emergency airway management team must perform an emergency cricothyrotomy. The simplest way to accomplish this is with a 12-gauge intravenous cannula that is advanced through the cricothyroid membrane and subsequently connected to an oxygen jet-valve device (Fig. 9–7A). This technique is not designed to optimally ventilate the patient; the partial pressure of carbon dioxide typically continues to increase after successful

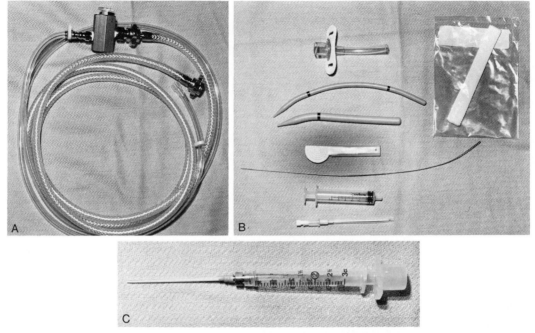

Figure 9–7. Emergency cricothyroid management set. *A,* A 12-gauge intravenous catheter connected to a 3-mL syringe with a #7.0 endotracheal tube adaptor in barrel. *B,* Jet ventilator. *C,* Percutaneous cricothyrotomy endotracheal tube placement kit.

administration of oxygen as described via the cricothyroid catheter. Rather, the method is meant as a stop-gap measure to administer enough oxygen to the patient until a formal cricothyrotomy can be performed and an endotracheal tube can be securely placed through the incision (see Chap. 10). This surgical therapy should ideally take place within a few minutes after placement of the transcricothyroid 12-gauge cannula.

Percutaneous cricothyrotomy sets are available that allow insertion of a full-sized tube into the trachea through the use of a wire/dilator technique (Fig. 9–7B). Although use of this set typically takes longer than placement of the 12-gauge catheter described above, the patient can be fully ventilated once the large tube has been placed.

If a positive pressure oxygen jet ventilation valve is not available, oxygen can be administered through the cannula using an alternate technique (Fig. 9–7). A common, 3-mL plastic syringe with the plunger removed, preferably with a Luer-Lok tip, frequently accommodates a #7.0 endotracheal tube adaptor in its barrel end (Fig. 9–7C). This syringe, with the endotracheal tube adaptor attached, can be fitted to the 12-gauge catheter after the catheter has been inserted into the cricothyroid membrane. An Ambu bag can then be attached to the

endotracheal tube adaptor and used to administer positive pressure oxygen.

Difficult intubations in the field can sometimes be simplified through the use of a lighted stylet that allows blind introduction of the endotracheal tube via oral or nasal approach. The disposable device does not require an external light source or power supply and is therefore well suited for the portable emergency airway management kit (Fig. 9–5B). The tube is positioned by following the lighted stylet tip as it glows through the neck on its way through the larynx.

IN THE FIELD

The health care professional occasionally needs to manage the airway in patients encountered outside of the health care delivery setting. A reasonable piece of equipment to always carry is the Ambu Rescue Key (Fig. 9–8). This device allows a positive pressure seal to be established around the patient's mouth, thereby allowing subsequent mouth-to-mask ventilation of the apneic patient.

Health care professionals traveling on U.S. domestic airlines should realize that the required emergency medical kit aboard U.S. carriers (Table 9–2) does not include a mech-

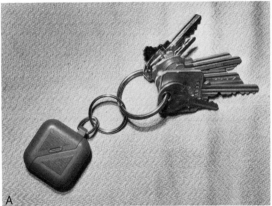

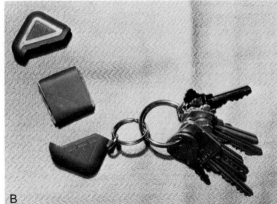

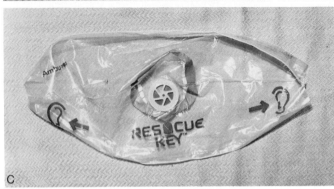

Figure 9–8. Ambu Rescue Key. *A,* Attached to key chain. *B,* With plastic case open, revealing contents. *C,* Rescue Key mask unfolded. Note that mouth diagram represents *rescuer* mouth.

anism for positive pressure ventilation. Although oral airways are provided, an Ambu bag or similar device is not. This author routinely carries an Ambu bag in his carry-on luggage in case positive pressure ventilation of a passenger en route becomes necessary. It is against federal law to carry compressed gas (including oxygen) without approval aboard commercial airline flights. However, a standard Ambu bag device can be connected to stand-alone in-flight oxygen tanks, available on all flights.

MONITORING

Adequate ventilation of the patient, defined as adequate oxygenation and carbon dioxide exchange, is the goal of emergency airway management. Pulse oximetry and end-tidal carbon dioxide measurement are very appropriate additions to the emergency airway management kit.

Ventilation of the apneic patient by positive pressure mask prior to endotracheal intubation may cause a sufficiently high P_{O_2} to produce a hemoglobin oxygen saturation of 100% several minutes after a subsequent esophageal intu-

bation. The prompt measurement of end-tidal carbon dioxide after placement of the endotracheal tube provides the best protection against inadvertent esophageal intubation.

End-tidal carbon dioxide monitors typically are bulky and may be impractical for the emergency airway management kit. An alternative is afforded by disposable, qualitative end-tidal CO_2 analyzers, which are self-contained plastic chambers placed between the endotracheal tube and ventilation device. A chemically impregnated disc within the clear chamber changes color when in contact with carbon dioxide. This color change does not take place immediately. A few breaths must be given before correct placement can be de-

Table 9–2. CONTENTS OF U.S. DOMESTIC AIRLINE EMERGENCY MEDICAL KIT

Oral airways
One vial of epinephrine
One intravenous cannula with heparin lock
One stethoscope
One vial of diphenhydramine hydrochloride (Benadryl)
One ampule of 50% dextrose
One bottle of nitroglycerine sublingual tablets
One pair of latex gloves
One sphygmomanometer

termined by this method. As always, auscultation over the fundus of the stomach and chest must serve as the initial check of correct placement of the endotracheal tube.

CAVEATS

The goal of emergency airway management outside of the operating room should be to establish adequate ventilation of the patient by whatever means necessary until more definitive therapy, if required, is available. Therefore, the emergency airway management team should not attempt to perform airway management maneuvers more appropriate for the operating room setting. Specifically, endotracheal tube changes in severely compromised patients or in patients who are known or suspected to be difficult intubations should be considered carefully before they are performed outside of the operating room. If the patient is being adequately ventilated, although perhaps suboptimally, these procedures in the patients described are usually better performed in the operating room, with a surgical team standing by to perform emergency cricothyrotomy.

CHAPTER 10

Cricothyrotomy and Tracheostomy

Ashby C. Moncure, M.D.

GENERAL CONSIDERATIONS

This chapter describes the technique of cricothyrotomy and conventional tracheostomy. The initial priority in every clinical situation is assurance of an adequate airway and that effective ventilation is occurring. Usually, oral endotracheal or nasotracheal intubation can be accomplished and a secure satisfactory airway established. A ventilating bronchoscope may allow ventilation until a more carefully considered procedure may be done. Under some circumstances, these procedures may not be possible, and an alternative technique, such as cricothyrotomy or tracheostomy, may be necessary to establish and maintain an adequate airway.

Some of the clinical situations that may require cricothyrotomy or tracheostomy because of inability to intubate the trachea via the oral or nasal route are massive facial trauma; severe cervical spine deformity, either acutely secondary to trauma or chronically secondary to ankylosing spondylitis; the presence of temporomandibular joint disease, such as seen in rheumatoid arthritis; and in acute laryngotracheal trauma, where attempted oral intubation may precipitate a total obstruction. The burned hypopharynx, retropharyngeal swelling, or the presence of a foreign body or other obstructing mechanical factor may also prevent intubation from above.

The need for an adequate and secure airway in these circumstances is usually initially best met by cricothyrotomy, which is more rapidly accomplished than conventional tracheostomy, in that the anatomic landmarks are fixed, thereby simplifying the approach, and the thyroid isthmus, the usual cause for hemorrhage in conventional tracheostomy, is not within the operative field. However, in the circumstance of acute laryngeal trauma, if partial airway obstruction is present, it is preferable to proceed directly to tracheostomy. If the trachea is partially divided, the tracheostomy may be established through the area of division if a primary repair is not done. If totally divided, the trachea usually retracts into the mediastinum and, by digital exploration, the divided end of the distal trachea may be identified and thereafter elevated into the operative field with Allis clamps and an endotracheal tube placed into it to provide a controlled airway. If primary repair is not done, the trachea is secured to the skin as an end stoma. Conservation of trachea to allow later repair is of utmost importance.

Because tracheostomy can be a complex procedure, it is not commonly performed for acute emergent relief of airway obstruction when endotracheal intubation cannot be accomplished and when cricothyrotomy is an equally available alternative, the exception being the circumstance of laryngotracheal trauma. Tracheostomy is commonly performed electively, with an indwelling endotracheal tube in place to relieve airway obstruction, to provide for prolonged mechanical ventilation, and to reduce dead space.

TECHNIQUE OF CRICOTHYROTOMY

Figure 10–1 diagrams the anatomic relationships of importance in performing cricothyrotomy. The midline, fixed, anatomic relationship of the lower border of the thyroid cartilage and the upper border of the cricoid cartilage can be easily and accurately located by palpation, even in an agitated, restless patient; hence, accurate placement of the transverse incision (dotted line) to accomplish cricothyrotomy can be executed. A roll or pillow beneath the shoulders to hyperextend the neck may facilitate the procedure, after infiltrating with a local anesthetic. The skin incision is carried directly through the more deeply located platysma muscle, and thereafter through the cricothyroid membrane (Fig. 10–2). After spreading scissors widely to enlarge the opening transversely, a small metal tracheostomy tube, if available, is placed through the opening. A patent, small cylinder of any rigid material can be placed as a temporary airway if a tracheostomy tube is not available.

A small artery (cricothyroid artery) may cross the cricothyroid membrane, and it may be necessary to control this vessel, if bleeding, with ligature or cautery. Any instrument placed into the airway and spread to facilitate passage of a tracheostomy tube should be pointed down the trachea in order to avoid injury to the larynx. A 6-mm tracheostomy tube can usually be placed in an adult with relative ease.

A major disadvantage of cricothyrotomy relates to the anatomic circumstance that a tube placed in this location passes through the most narrow portion of the subglottic airway; hence, inflammation related to the tube may produce a chronic subglottic stenosis. This stenosis may be extremely difficult to subsequently repair, in that the recurrent laryngeal nerves penetrate the posterior cricoid plate at approximately the level of the stenosis. Therefore, many surgeons advise conventional tracheostomy in an elective setting, allowing removal of the tube previously placed through the cricothyrotomy incision in order to avoid this potential complication.[1–3]

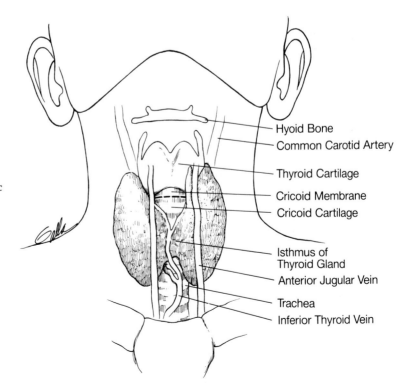

Figure 10–1. Important anatomic relations for cricothyrotomy.

- Hyoid Bone
- Common Carotid Artery
- Thyroid Cartilage
- Cricoid Membrane
- Cricoid Cartilage
- Isthmus of Thyroid Gland
- Anterior Jugular Vein
- Trachea
- Inferior Thyroid Vein

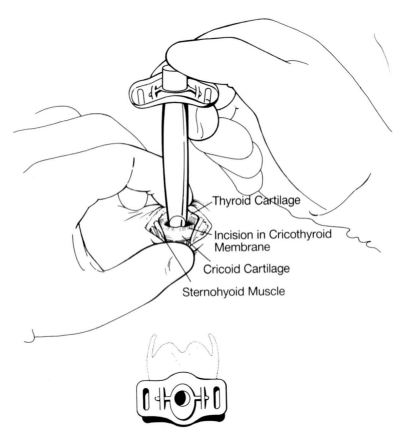

Thyroid Cartilage

Incision in Cricothyroid
Membrane

Cricoid Cartilage

Sternohyoid Muscle

Figure 10–2. Enlarge the opening through the cricothyroid membrane, then insert a small tracheostomy tube.

TECHNIQUE OF TRACHEOSTOMY

Figure 10–3 diagrams the anatomic relationships of importance in performing tracheostomy. The procedure is more complex than cricothyrotomy and, with the exception of airway obstruction in the setting of laryngotracheal trauma, it is usually performed with an endotracheal tube in place.

Hyperextension of the neck usually elevates the trachea into the neck, more so in the young, and variably in the aged patient. After routine preparation of the skin and placement of sterile drapes, the skin is infiltrated with a local anesthetic and either a vertical (dotted line) or transverse incision is made, centered approximately 2 cm below the cricoid cartilage, which is the most important landmark for performing both cricothyrotomy or tracheostomy. The vertical incision is probably best done for emergency tracheostomy and the transverse incision for elective tracheostomy, and need not be more than 4 cm in length.

After incision through the platysma, the midline is identified by palpating the trachea, and the fascia overlying it is incised (Fig. 10–4A). The surgeon again palpates the cricoid

cartilage, and is thus able to identify the location of the anterior trachea between the second and third tracheal rings. An assessment of the need to incise the thyroid isthmus is made and, if the isthmus cannot be retracted to allow exposure of this area, a hemostat is passed posterior to the thyroid isthmus (Fig. 10–4B) and the isthmus is divided between the hemostats (Fig. 10–4C) and suture ligated with absorbable sutures. A tracheal hook is placed above the site of planned stoma (Fig. 10–4D), a cruciate incision is made centered at the third tracheal cartilage (Fig. 10–4E) and, after the balloon of the endotracheal tube is deflated and the endotracheal tube is elevated above the stoma, a tracheostomy tube with obturator is placed through the stoma (Fig. 10–4F). The obturator is removed and the low-pressure tracheostomy tube cuff is inflated until no air leak is detectable by positive pressure ventilation. The tracheostomy tube is thereafter flagged to the skin, but the wound is not closed. Hemostasis is assured before the final dressing is applied.

The importance of the level of the placement of the tracheal stoma cannot be overemphasized. Incisions into the cricoid cartilage or first tracheal ring can produce subglottic ste-

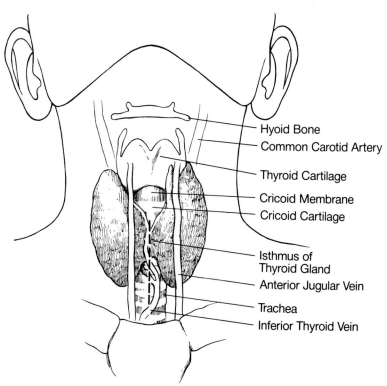

- Hyoid Bone
- Common Carotid Artery
- Thyroid Cartilage
- Cricoid Membrane
- Cricoid Cartilage
- Isthmus of Thyroid Gland
- Anterior Jugular Vein
- Trachea
- Inferior Thyroid Vein

Figure 10–3. Anatomic relationships of importance in performing tracheostomy.

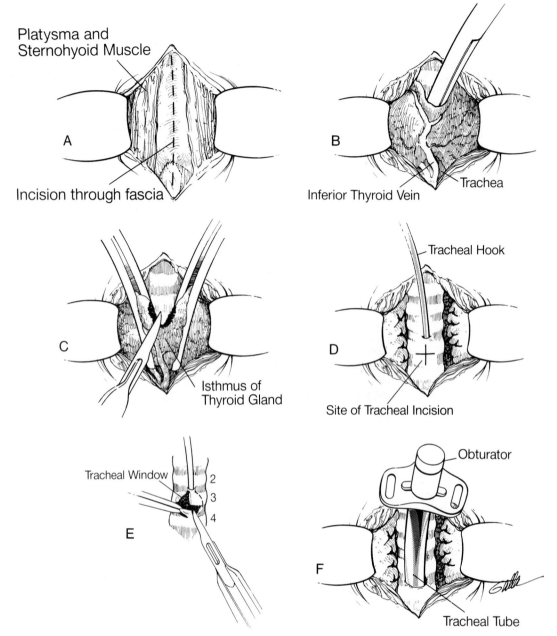

Figure 10–4. *A,* After the incision through the platysma, the midline is identified by palpating the trachea. The fascia overlying it is then incised. *B,* If the isthmus cannot be retracted to allow exposure of this area, a hemostat is passed posterior to the thyroid isthmus. *C,* The isthmus is divided between two hemostats and suture ligated with absorbable sutures. *D,* A tracheal hook is placed above the site of the planned stoma. *E,* A cruciate incision is centered at the third tracheal cartilage. *F,* A tracheostomy tube with obturator is placed through the stoma.

nosis secondary to inflammation, and subsequent reconstruction at this level can be extremely difficult. Furthermore, an incision at or below the fifth tracheal ring may produce dislodgement of the tracheostomy tube, or impingement on the innominate artery as it courses anteriorly to the trachea, with subsequent erosion with hemorrhage.

It is wise to carefully inspect the neck prior to performing tracheostomy and to consider the appropriate length of the tracheostomy tube necessary to comfortably rest within the trachea. An obese or emphysematous patient may require a longer tube than normally required, and the appropriate tube must be at hand when the procedure is undertaken.[4–6]

References

1. Boyd AD, Conlan AA. Emergency cricothyroidotomy: Is its use justified? Surg Rounds 1:19–23, 1979.
2. Boyd AD, Romita MC, Conlan AA, Fink SD, Spencer FC. A clinical evaluation of cricothyroidotomy. Surg Gynecol Obstet 149:365, 1979.
3. Moncure AC. Cricothyrotomy. In Wilkins EW (ed). Emergency Medicine, 3rd ed. Baltimore: Williams & Wilkins, 1989; pp. 997–998.
4. Grillo HC. Tracheostomy and its complications. In Sabiston DC Jr (ed). Textbook of Surgery, 13th ed. Philadelphia: W. B. Saunders, 1986; pp. 2000–2007.
5. Golden GT, Fox JW, Edlich RF, Edgerton MT. Emergency tracheostomy. Am J Surg 131:766, 1976.
6. Mathisen DJ, Grillo H. Laryngotracheal trauma. Ann Thorac Surg 43:254–262, 1987.

CHAPTER 11

Overview of the Intubation Process

James T. Roberts, M.D., M.A.

Intubation is "the introduction of a tube into a hollow organ to keep the latter open or to restore its patency if obstructed."[1] Endotracheal intubation is "the insertion of a tube into the trachea for administration of anesthesia, maintenance of an airway, aspiration of secretions, ventilation of the lungs, or prevention of entrance of foreign material into the tracheobronchial tree."[2]

JUSTIFICATION FOR INTUBATION

For our purposes, the need for endotracheal intubation emanates from a malfunction or disruption of ventilation, oxygenation, or protective mechanisms of the larynx, or as a route for diagnostic or therapeutic measures (Table 11–1).

Failure of Ventilation

Ventilatory failure may result from a disruption of the central nervous system respiratory center, loss of ventilatory muscle power, trauma to the bellows mechanism, airway obstruction, or intrinsic lung disease.

Direct brain injury, asphyxia secondary to cardiac arrest or, for example, hanging as a suicide attempt, can radically alter the rhythmicity of the respiratory center function of the central nervous system.

Power for the bellows mechanism arises from the intercostal muscles and the diaphragm. Muscular relaxation induced for surgery, neuromuscular blockade from insecticide poisoning, Guillain-Barré, myasthenia gravis, and phrenic nerve injury all reduce ventilatory muscle power. The most common of these, prolonged effect of anesthetic neuromuscular blockade, affects the anesthetist's daily practice.

Damage to the bellows mechanism may arise prior to hospitalization, as in flail chest injuries or congenital chest wall abnormalities. Pneumothorax may occur at any time. Foreign bodies, infection, trauma, or tumors may obstruct the airway. In addition, coma or semicoma can allow the tongue to fall back in the pharynx, reducing airway flow. Tracheal stenosis and bilateral recurrent laryngeal nerve injury after thyroid surgery must also be included as causes of airway obstruction. Finally, intrinsic lung disease (asthma, chronic obstructive pulmonary disease [COPD]) frequently disrupts ventilation.

Inadequate Oxygenation

Inadequate tissue oxygenation may be indicated by low arterial oxygen pressure (Pa_{O_2}).

Table 11–1. JUSTIFICATION FOR INTUBATION

Failure of Ventilation
  Removal of CNS drive may result from CNS trauma,
    cardiac arrest, or as the result of hanging
  Removal of ventilatory power may result from
    muscular relaxation for surgery, insecticide
    poisoning, or Guillain-Barré syndrome
  Damage to the bellows mechanism due to flail chest,
    pneumothorax, or chest wall abnormalities
  Obstruction of airway patency may be due to a
    foreign body, infections such as Ludwig's angina
    and epiglottitis, trauma, tumors, coma, tracheal
    stenosis, or bilateral recurrent laryngeal nerve
    injury
  Intrinsic lung disease
Inadequate Oxygenation due to
  Pneumothorax
  Drowning
  Trauma
  Postoperative atelectasis
  Postoperative splinting from chest surgery or upper
    abdominal surgery
  Pulmonary embolus
  Carbon monoxide poisoning
Failure of Protective Mechanisms of the Larynx
  Drug overdose
  Stroke
  Tracheo-esophageal fistula
  Partial paralysis
  Coma
Diagnostic or Therapeutic Measures

CNS, central nervous system.
(From Roberts JT. Fundamentals of Tracheal Intubation. New York: Grune & Stratton, 1983, p. 51.)

Inadequate oxygenation may be caused by (1) abnormal delivery of oxygen to the alveoli (hypoventilation) secondary to pneumothorax, atelectasis, postoperative splinting, multiple trauma, flail chest injury, loss of airway patency, ventilation-perfusion (V-Q) abnormalities secondary to COPD, adult respiratory distress syndrome (ARDS), or restrictive lung disease; (2) poor transfer of oxygen across the alveoli (diffusion abnormality) due to pulmonary edema, both cardiogenic and noncardiogenic, pneumonia, or pulmonary fibrosis; (3) circulation of blood through the lungs without oxygenation (shunting) caused by pulmonary emboli, fat emboli, or congenital shunts; (4) decreased binding of oxygen to hemoglobin due to carbon monoxide poisoning or abnormal hemoglobin species; or (5) deficient delivery of oxygen to the tissues from impaired circulation. Even if delivery of oxygen to the tissues is within normal limits, thyroid storm, malignant hyperthermia, and other hypermetabolic states can increase tissue demand for oxygen beyond the transfer capacity of the lungs.

Intubation, although it does not affect the underlying cause of tissue hypoxia, does provide undisturbed access to the pulmonary tree and may improve ventilation while measures to treat the underlying cause of tissue hypoxia proceed.

Failure of Protective Mechanisms of the Larynx

The epiglottis normally folds over the laryngeal entrance in order to protect the airway during swallowing. Stimulation of the pharynx initiates the reflex arc, which results in folding. An airway burn may destroy sensory receptors critical to this reflex and leave the airway vulnerable. Drug overdose, stroke, and coma can interfere with the reflex arc, and partial paralysis may prevent mechanical execution of the reflex. Intubation eliminates the need for the protective mechanisms, buying time to allow recovery of the damaged reflex.

A tracheo-esophageal fistula (TEF) bypasses the protective mechanisms entirely. The fistulous tract may shunt gastric contents directly to the trachea, completely bypassing the protective effect of the epiglottis.

Diagnostic or Therapeutic Measures

In addition to providing a means for improving deficient ventilation, oxygenation, or defunct protective reflexes, intubation may aid in the diagnosis of certain pulmonary problems by serving as a guide for the fiberoptic bronchoscope or a bronchogram. Therapeutically, an endotracheal tube provides access for pulmonary lavage.

APPROACHES TO INTUBATION

There exists a multiplicity of specific indications for intubation in modern medical practice. Consider the historic methods and instruments that have proven useful for endotracheal intubation. Tactile blind, nontactile blind, indirect laryngoscopy, direct laryngoscopy, and a percutaneous retrograde catheter have all served as methods of guiding a tube into the trachea.

Tactile Blind

Historically the oldest method of intubation, tactile blind was practiced by Kite in the 18th

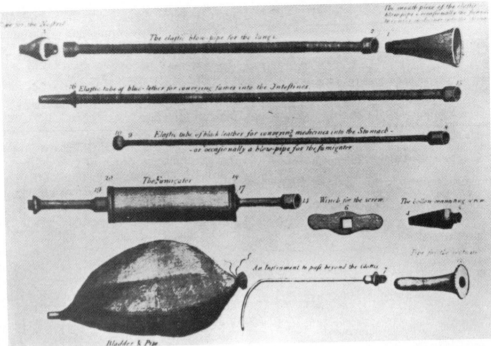

Figure 11–1. A rigid endotracheal tube used by Kite in the 18th century. The tube was introduced and guided digitally into the trachea. (From Sykes WS. Essays on the First Hundred Years of Anaesthesia. Huntington, NY: Robert E. Krieger, 1972, p. 98.)

century. The rigid endotracheal tube (Fig. 11–1), used for resuscitation of drowning victims, was guided into the trachea digitally. This method may still aid in the reintubation of patients inadvertently extubated in the operating room in awkward positions that hinder direct laryngoscopy.

Nontactile Blind

Blind nasal intubation was originally described by Desault in 1814. It still holds a respected place in the physician's armamentarium, primarily for intubating agitated patients in whom direct laryngoscopy proves difficult. See Chapter 17 for details of a technique for blind nasal intubation.

Indirect Laryngoscopy

Indirect laryngoscopy originated with the investigations of Garcia in 1855. Garcia, professor of singing at the Paris Conservatoire, read a paper before the Royal Society entitled "Observations on the Human Voice." He had, with great patience, examined his own vocal cords with the aid of a dental mirror.

The history of indirect laryngoscopes began with the Labordette speculum, and includes the Siker blade, Huffman prism, and various fiberoptic instruments, including rigid, malleable, and flexible laryngoscopes.

The Labordette laryngoscopy speculum (1866) incorporated a mirrored surface to view the laryngeal opening (Fig. 11–2). The mirrored surface on a Siker laryngoscope blade (Fig. 11–3) allows indirect visualization of an inverted image for difficult intubations, ie, where direct laryngoscopy proves impossible.

The Huffman prism clips to a standard, #3 Macintosh blade, permitting indirect visualization; the image is upright, in contrast to the inverted image of the Siker blade (Fig. 11–4).

Recent advances in indirect laryngoscopy use fiberoptic bundles to transmit an upright image, direct light to the field, and guide the endotracheal tube to the laryngeal entrance. Fiberoptic laryngoscopy was critical to intubating the patient in Figure 11–5. Use of the Storz rigid fiberoptic laryngoscope is described in Chapter 13, whereas use of the flexible fiberoptic laryngoscope is described in Chapters 21, 22, and 25.

Direct Laryngoscopy

Portable laryngoscopes for direct laryngoscopic examination of the epiglottis and laryn-

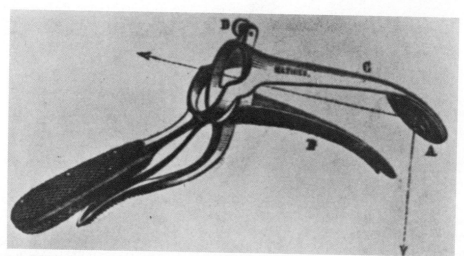

Figure 11–2. Labordette laryngoscope used a mirrored surface to view the glottic opening. (From Sykes WS. Essays on the First Hundred Years of Anaesthesia. Huntington, NY: Robert E. Krieger, 1972, p. 97.)

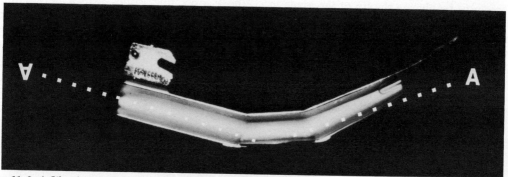

Figure 11–3. A Siker laryngoscope blade also used a mirrored surface to indirectly view the laryngeal opening. Note how the image is inverted, which may lead to confusion in inexperienced hands. (From Roberts JT. Fundamentals of Tracheal Intubation. New York: Grune & Stratton, 1983, p. 51.)

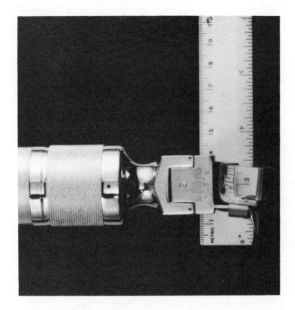

Figure 11–4. The Huffman prism clips to a #3 Macintosh blade. With the Huffman prism, the image of the larynx is not inverted, as it is with the Siker blade. (From Roberts JT. Fundamentals of Tracheal Intubation. New York: Grune & Stratton, 1983, p. 58.)

geal opening (to guide the endotracheal tube home) were developed at the beginning of the 20th century. Jackson pioneered direct laryngoscopy. An updated version of his original laryngoscope appears in Figure 13–2. The design of this laryngoscope diverts force away from the upper teeth.

In 1941, Miller described his laryngoscope, a modified straight blade (see Fig. 13–4).[1] In 1943, Macintosh developed a curved laryngoscope blade (see Fig. 13–4), designed to lift the epiglottis by placing the tip of the blade in the vallecula.[2] The left-sided ridge on both blades removes the tongue from the visual path, but also may be forcibly pressed against the upper teeth by the careless. Countless

modifications of these blades have been constructed, and some of the more interesting ones are discussed in Chapter 13.

Recently, several rigid laryngoscopes have incorporated coherent fiberoptic bundles to indirectly view the larynx during *oral* intubation. These include the Bullard, Upsher, and Storz laryngoscopes. Although these instruments are somewhat awkward to use, they basically still force the patient's anatomy to conform to the laryngoscope, in contrast to the flexible fiberscopes, which permit the fiberscope to conform to the patient's anatomy. The rigid scopes are limited to oral use, whereas the flexible scopes may be used nasally as well as orally.

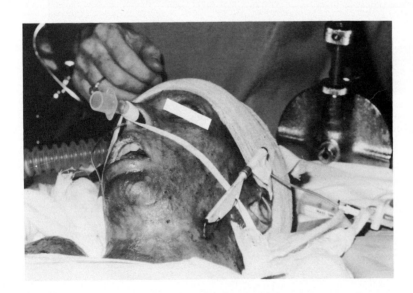

Figure 11–5. Fiberoptic laryngoscopy was critical to intubating this patient.

DIFFICULT INTUBATION RECORD

Date _____   Patient's name _____ Unit number _____

Person performing intubation _____ Ht. _____ Wgt. _____

Sex _____

Ease of ventilation by mask ___ Denitrogenation: %O_2 _____ Duration: min _____
Description of laryngoscopy
   Prelaryngoscopy examination
     Mandibular mobility _____
     Teeth _____
     Neck _____

Laryngoscope: Type _____   Blade No. _____
Other mechanical aids _____
Ease of visualization _____
   Description of: N = Normal   N.V. = not visualized   A = Abnormal
     Teeth _____   Epiglottis _____   False cords _____
     Cords _____   Arytenoids _____   Tonsils _____
     How abnormal _____
Endotracheal tube: Type _____   Size _____
   Depth of insertion from upper teeth _____
   Cuff air requirement to seal to 30 mm Hg _____
Drugs used to supplement intubation:
   Local anesthetic _____
     % _____   Amt. _____   Where applied _____
   Sedatives _____

Complications: _____

Figure 11–6. Difficult intubation record sheet. (From Roberts JT. Fundamentals of Tracheal Intubation. New York: Grune & Stratton, 1983, p. 7.)

Percutaneous Retrograde Catheter

When other attempts at intubation fail, a catheter or guidewire may be inserted percutaneously through the cricothyroid membrane and threaded up through and out the mouth to guide an endotracheal tube.

NECESSARY BACKGROUND INFORMATION

To become skilled at airway management, one must know airway structure and innervation in detail (Chap. 1); know the equipment (Chaps. 12, 13, and 21); prepare the patient psychologically and with drugs (Chaps. 14 and 31); be familiar with oral (Chap. 16) and nasal (Chap. 17) intubation techniques; and understand the physiologic consequences of prolonged apnea, hypoxia, hypercarbia, and ventilation attempts against a closed glottis, as well as have predetermined alternatives when initial attempts at intubation fail (Chap. 19). Needless to say, one should keep a record of difficult intubations. Figure 11–6 suggests a format for such a record. Once the problem that required intubation resolves, perhaps as difficult a problem is faced: extubation (Chap. 25). Finally, avoid or recognize and treat complications (Chap. 24).

References

1. Miller R. A new laryngoscope. Anesthesiology 2:318, 1941.
2. Macintosh R. A new laryngoscope. Lancet Feb 13:914, 1943.

CHAPTER 12

Endotracheal Tubes

James T. Roberts, M.D., M.A., William T. Denman, M.D., and Paul H. Alfille, M.D.

In 1543, 1 year after the publication of *De Fabrica Corporis Humani,* which signaled the onset of modern anatomy, Andreas Vesalius, the renowned anatomist of Brussels, first described endotracheal intubation. In *Humani Corporis Fabrica Libri Septem,* he reported successful artificial ventilation of a pig through a tube inserted into its windpipe.

Two hundred and forty-two years later, Kite designed an endotracheal tube for resuscitation of drowning victims at the Dumfries and Galloway Royal Infirmary. He blindly guided a curved metal tube through the mouth into the trachea. In 1796, Herholdt and Rafn developed life-saving measures for drowning victims, including intubation with an endotracheal tube and mouth-to-mouth resuscitation. In 1814, nasotracheal intubation was first described by Desault, and in 1880 Macewen first administered anesthesia (chloroform) via an oral endotracheal tube. Historical events in the development of endotracheal tubes are summarized in Table 12–1.

GENERAL CHARACTERISTICS OF ENDOTRACHEAL TUBES

Use of endotracheal tubes is now ubiquitous in medical practice. The usual scenarios involve intensive care, general anesthesia, and severe respiratory or cerebral compromise.

Tube Composition

Endotracheal tube design has evolved since the early metal tubes. Rubber tubes were popular, but suffered from cuff properties that caused tracheal injuries in prolonged intubations. Furthermore, the composition of red rubber tubes, obtained from any of a number of rubber plantations, varied because rubber, as a natural product, varied in composition.[1] Almost all endotracheal tubes are now made of plastic, which has many advantages over the older red rubber tubes. Plastic cuffs, if not overinflated, will seal at low transmural pressures, protecting the tracheal mucosa. Extensive testing ensures minimal antigenic stimulation to the host. Finally, thermoplastic conforms to the recipient's anatomy once it is in place and warmed to body temperature.

Disposable, single-lumen plastic tubes may be cut to any length and allow nasal as well as oral intubation. Shortening a tube decreases the dead space of ventilation. The tube may be cut before intubation is attempted or it may be cut more accurately after the tube is introduced and taped in place.

Red rubber double-lumen endotracheal tubes are now seldom used, except for those double-lumen tubes remaining in circulation. Double-lumen tubes are not cut because of their more complex design. Details to check prior to using an endotracheal tube are provided in Table 12–2.

Table 12–1. HISTORY OF ENDOTRACHEAL TUBE DEVELOPMENT

Year	Developer	Development
1543	Vesalius	Kept pig alive by intubation and ventilation
1667	Hooke	Ventilated a dissected dog
1705	Kite	Invented device for resuscitating drowning victims
1796	Herholdt & Rafn	Blind intubation for drowning
1814	Desault	Nasotracheal intubation
1826	Bretonean	Silver cannula for intubation
1878	Macewen	First intubation for anesthesia
1880	O'Dwyer	Laryngeal stent for croup
1890	Hailes	Tube needed introducer but no extractor
1893	Eisenmenger	First cuffed oral tracheal tube
1897	Fisher	Introducer allowed immediate ventilation through the tube
1905	Kuhn	Laryngeal stent extended outside the mouth; suggested placing cuff on tube
1909	Jackson	Put bronchoscopy on firm ground
1912	Feroud	Feroud tube needed introducer and extractor
1943	Grum & Knight	Used thin cuff to allow placement of tube through nose
1970	Guess	Implant testing Double-lumen tube for isolated lung ventilation Endotracheal tube with blocker

Tube Diameter

The guidelines listed in Table 12–3 estimate single-lumen endotracheal tube size; however, one should keep a variety of tubes, both larger and smaller than that recommended, to allow proper selection of size after viewing the larynx. Millimeter sizes are listed. Double-lumen endotracheal tube sizes are usually described in French units.

Tube Tip Configuration

Single-lumen endotracheal tubes come with the older Magill tip or the newer Murphy tip (Fig. 12–1). The Murphy tip has an eye to allow ventilation of the right upper lobe bron-

chus. The bronchial tips of the right-sided double-lumen endotracheal tubes vary with the manufacturer, but invariably have an opening in the bronchial limb for ventilation of the right upper lobe bronchus.

Tube Cuff Design

In 1893, Eisenmenger introduced the first cuffed endotracheal tube.[2] In the 1950s and 1960s, Europe and the United States provided the proving ground for the cuffed tracheostomy tube for prolonged ventilation during the poliomyelitis epidemics. Problems with early cuffs, such as tracheal necrosis, stenosis, and tracheoesophageal fistula, were all reported during this widespread use of controlled ven-

Table 12–2. ENDOTRACHEAL TUBE CHECKLIST

Know the composition of the tube (potential fire hazard, etc)
Assure sterility
Select correct diameter tube
Modify length of tube if necessary
Ensure patency of lumen—no foreign bodies present
Lubricate distal end of tube and cuff
Test pilot balloon and cuff(s)
Have proper size stylet immediately available
Have syringe available to inflate balloon
Make sure ventilating apparatus has adapter that properly fits endotracheal tube
Use appropriate tube for given procedure; ie, double-lumen tube
Have a selection of back-up tubes immediately available
Know how to correctly insert and position the tube

Table 12–3. ESTIMATING PROPER ENDOTRACHEAL TUBE SIZE FOR ORAL INTUBATION

Age	Endotracheal Tube Inner Diameter (mm)
Newborn	3.0
6 mo	3.5
18 mo	4.0
3 yr	4.5
5 yr	5.0
6 yr	5.5
8 yr	6.0
12 yr	6.5
16 yr	7.0
Adult (female)	7.5–8.0
Adult (male)	8.0–8.5

Modified from Standards for cardiopulmonary resuscitation (CPR) and emergency cardiac care (ECC). JAMA 1992; 268:2262–2275. Copyright 1992, American Medical Association

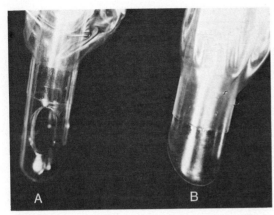

Figure 12–1. *A*, Magill and *B*, Murphy tipped endotracheal tubes.

tilation. Double-walled cuffs and replacement of the narrow, high-pressure cuff with the low-pressure balloon have helped to minimize morbidity from endotracheal intubation.[3-12] All cuffs are permeable to nitrous oxide over time. When exposed to nitrous oxide, they increase in cuff volume and pressure. Remember, pressures above 30 cm H_2O compromise circulation to the tracheal mucosa. The cuffs on the bronchial portion of four right-sided double-lumen tubes are compared later in this chapter.

SINGLE-LUMEN ENDOTRACHEAL TUBES

Single-lumen endotracheal tubes are available, both cuffed and uncuffed (for pediatric use), in a variety of sizes. Single-lumen tubes are manufactured with a radius close to the curvature of the oropharynx (Fig. 12–2).

The MLT (microlaryngeal-tracheal) tube with a Murphy eye is designed for microlaryngeal surgical procedures (Fig. 12–3). The MLT tube has a standard length and cuff size, but a small diameter, allowing greater access to the surgical field. An uncuffed tracheal tube with a monitoring lumen is designed primarily for pediatric use, and is available with or without a Murphy eye[13] (Fig. 12–4).

A jet ventilation tube, such as the tube shown in Figure 12–5, has three tubing ports: one for cuff inflation, one for jet ventilation, and one for pressure monitoring.

A protective steel spring coiled the length of an armored tube prevents collapse of the tube from a point pressure source such as teeth (Fig. 12–6). Tube length varies with size. An acutely bent armored tube will not kink and thereby close the airway, making it ideal for neurosurgical procedures in which access to the endotracheal tube may be difficult once the procedure begins. A significant problem occurs with this tube, despite adequate taping (or perhaps because of adequate taping): it coils in the mouth and inadvertently extubates the patient. A standard curved tube will not coil, but may kink if allowed to protrude a distance from the mouth. Cutting the standard tube to length minimizes this risk. Two other examples of an armored endotracheal tube include the uncuffed, reinforced tracheal tube shown in Figure 12–7 and the double-cuffed Laserflex reinforced tracheal tube shown in Figure 12–8, which is designed for intraoral laser surgery.

Figure 12–9 shows a single-lumen endotracheal tube with a Lanz pressure-regulating valve, designed to prevent overinflation of the cuff and subsequent tracheal damage.

Preformed endotracheal tubes, such as the cuffed laryngectomy tube (Fig. 12–10), the oral RAE tube (Fig. 12–11), and the nasal RAE tube (Fig. 12–12), each have a molded angle at the point where they emerge from the mouth or the nose. This permits a Y connector to the circle system of an anesthesia machine

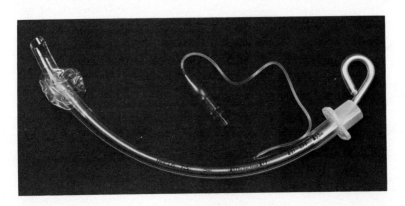

Figure 12–2. Disposable, precut, intermediate Hi-Lo tracheal tube with stylet. Available in sizes of 6.0, 7.0, 7.5, 8.0, 8.5, and 9.0 mm inner diameter. Manufactured by Mallinckrodt Critical Care (Glens Falls, NY).

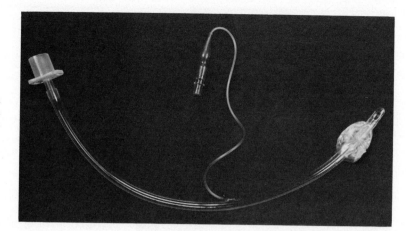

Figure 12–3. MLT tube (6.9-mm size shown). Also available in sizes 4.0, 4.5, 5.0, and 6.6 mm inner diameter.

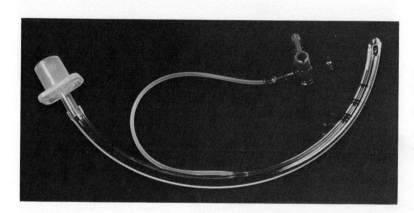

Figure 12–4. Uncuffed tracheal tube with a monitoring lumen (4.5 mm inner diameter, 6.6 mm outer diameter). Available in sizes of 2.5, 3.0, 3.5, 4.0, 4.5, 5.0, and 5.5 inner diameter. Also available with a Murphy eye.

Figure 12–5. Hi-Lo Jet tracheal tube with a Magill tip, designed for high-frequency jet ventilation. Note the triple lumens for cuff inflation, jet ventilation, and pressure monitoring. Manufactured by Mallinckrodt Critical Care (Glens Falls, NY). Available in sizes of 6.0, 7.0, 8.0, and 9.0 mm inner diameter.

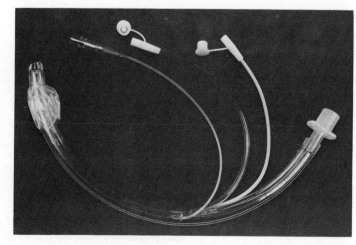

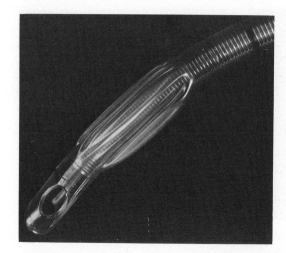

Figure 12–6. Cuffed, reinforced tracheal tube with a Murphy eye (7.5 mm size shown). Manufactured by Mallinckrodt Critical Care (Glens Falls, NY). Available in sizes of 6.0, 6.5, 7.0, 7.5, 8.0, 8.5, 9.0, and 9.5 mm inner diameter.

Figure 12–7. Uncuffed, reinforced tracheal tube (4.0 mm inner diameter shown). Manufactured by Mallinckrodt Critical Care (Glens Falls, NY). Available in sizes of 2.5, 3.0, 3.5, 4.0, 4.5, 5.0, and 5.5 mm inner diameter.

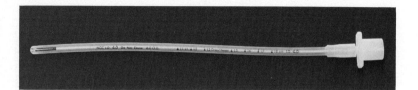

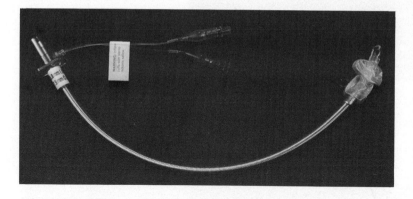

Figure 12–8. Double-cuffed, Laserflex reinforced endotracheal tube designed for use during intraoral laser surgery. Cuffs are designed for filling with sterile isotonic saline. Available in sizes of 4.5, 5.0, 5.5, and 6.0 mm inner diameter. Uncuffed Laserflex endotracheal tubes are also available in sizes of 3.0, 3.5, and 4.0 mm inner diameter.

Figure 12–9. Single-lumen endotracheal tube with a Lanz pressure-regulating valve. Available in sizes of 5.0, 5.5, 6.0, 6.5, 7.0, 7.5, 8.0, 8.5, and 9.0 mm inner diameter.

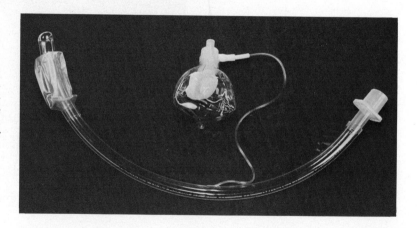

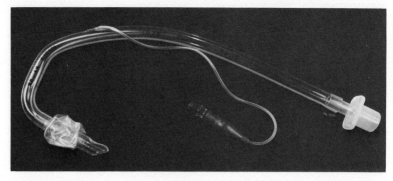

Figure 12–10. Preformed, cuffed laryngectomy tube (LGT) with Murphy eye (7.0 mm inner diameter, 9.6 mm outer diameter shown). Also available in 8.0 mm inner diameter.

to be placed conveniently away from the surgical field. A standard tube bent at a similar angle may kink and obstruct the lumen.

A guidable-tip endotracheal tube (Endotrol tube) facilitates blind nasotracheal intubation or intubation of the patient with difficult airway anatomy (Fig. 12–13). Placing traction on the ring decreases the radius of curvature of the distal end of the tube. This bend facilitates advancing the tube around the posterior nasopharyngeal wall and guiding the tip toward the laryngeal entrance. This tube is particularly useful for fiberoptic intubation in a patient with ankylosing spondylitis, because ankylosing spondylitis may cause an exaggerated cervical flexure, pushing the epiglottis against the posterior pharyngeal wall. When this occurs, one advances the fiberscope into the trachea, only to be unable to advance the endotracheal tube through the vocal cords because the tube tip hangs up on the laryngeal entrance. Flexing the tube tip of the Endotrol tube facilitates passage through the vocal cords.

Verification of Single-Lumen Tube Placement

It is necessary to establish quickly and accurately the position of an endotracheal tube after intubation, because an unrecognized esophageal intubation will result in catastrophe.[14] Tube placement verification is a daily task of anesthetists, but is still one of the most common mistakes that is associated with a fatal outcome.[15] There is no absolute gold standard to determine proper tube placement; therefore, extreme vigilance is required. Confirmation of the tube position within the trachea has been assessed by a myriad of tests.[16, 17] The literature includes as means of confirming tube position auscultation of the thorax, the sensation of normal ventilation, gastric and thoracic movement, condensation of water vapor in the tube, palpation of the tube cuff, pulse oximetry, and radiographs of the thorax.[18] The reliability of the above tests, however, is not sufficient. To achieve a reasonable degree of

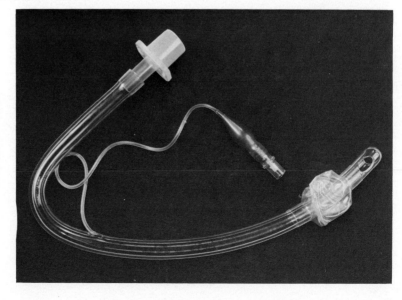

Figure 12–11. Preformed oral RAE cuffed endotracheal tube (7.0 mm inner diameter shown). Available in sizes of 4.0, 4.5, 5.0, 5.5, 6.0, 6.5, 7.0, 7.5, 8.0, 8.5, and 9.0 mm inner diameter. Also available uncuffed in sizes of 3.0, 3.5, 4.0, 4.5, 5.0, 5.5, 6.0, 6.5, and 7.0 mm inner diameter.

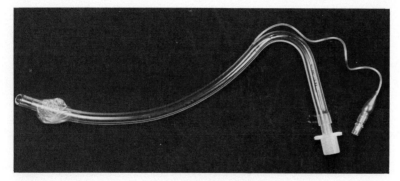

Figure 12–12. Preformed nasal RAE cuffed endotracheal tube (8.0 mm inner diameter shown). Available in sizes of 6.0, 6.5, 7.0, 7.5, and 8.0 mm inner diameter. Also available in uncuffed sizes of 3.0, 3.5, 4.0, 4.5, 5.0, 5.5, 6.0, 6.5, and 7.0 mm inner diameter.

accuracy, the following maneuvers have been demonstrated to be reliable: repeat laryngoscopy and direct visualization of the tube passing between the vocal cords; fiberoptic bronchoscopy[19]; suction on the endotracheal tube with a 60-mL syringe[20–23]; auscultation of the upper abdomen and the lungs, particularly in the axillae; and the presence of end-tidal carbon dioxide.[24–26]

In all of these verification tests, there may be uncertainty. In emergency situations,[27–30] the presence of a low end-tidal carbon dioxide may signify a misplaced tube or inadequate resuscitation efforts. Therefore, further clarification of tube position is needed.

Other tests for tube position have been advocated: acoustic properties of tracheal and esophageal tube placement,[31] a magnetic field interference-sensing technique,[32] the use of a lighted stylet,[33] and measuring volume and temperature of expired gas.[34]

Esophageal intubations continue to occur; hence the vast array of tests to detect misplaced endotracheal tubes. The number of tests is evidence that no one method is foolproof. Consequently, the following aphorism is still valid: if in doubt, take it out.

Single-Lumen Endotracheal Tube With a Bronchial Blocker

The Univent tube is designed for one-lung anesthesia and is available from Fuji Systems Corporation in sizes of 6.0, 7.0, 8.0, and 9.0 mm inner diameter (Fig. 12–14).

The bronchial blocker may be inserted into either the left or right mainstem bronchus. The bronchial blocker is advanced and positioned with the aid of a fiberscope. A channel through the blocker allows the blocked lung to be deflated by applying suction, or the channel may be used for jet ventilation. At the end of anesthesia, one need only to deflate and withdraw the blocker to use the tube for long-term ventilation. The blocker of the Univent tube has both a central lumen and a cuff. Administering gas under pressure through this lumen without a means of escape can cause overinflation, barotrauma, and circulatory compromise.

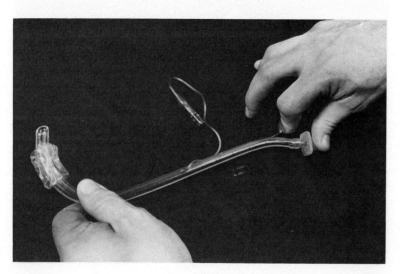

Figure 12–13. Guidable Endotrol tracheal tube, cuffed with Murphy eye tip (7.0 mm inner diameter shown). Available in sizes of 6.0, 7.0, 8.0, and 9.0 mm inner diameter.

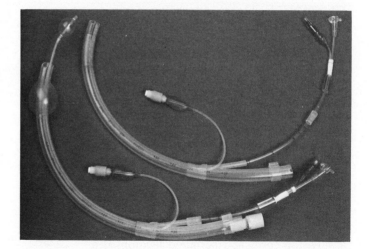

Figure 12–14. Univent endotracheal tubes. The upper tube is shown with the bronchial blocker retracted; the lower tube is shown with the endobronchial blocker extended and the tracheal and bronchial cuffs inflated.

To deflate the blocked lung, the blocker cuff must be inflated.

Several methods of positioning the blocker have been described. It has been suggested that a fiberscope be inserted into the mainstem bronchus and the Univent tube advanced over the fiberscope into the bronchus. Once the Univent tube is in the bronchus, the blocker is advanced and the tube withdrawn, leaving the blocker in place. A problem occurs when a larger-sized Univent tube will not advance into the appropriate bronchus because of its larger diameter.

Another method suggests that the tip of the Univent tube be placed above the carina, and the blocker advanced into either the left or right mainstem bronchus by twisting the blocker to guide it toward the appropriate bronchus. The blocker easily advances into the right mainstem bronchus, but guiding it toward the left mainstem bronchus by merely twisting the blocker is seldom successful in our hands.

The most successful technique in our hands is to rotate the entire Univent tube, placing the point where the blocker exits the larger tube next to the desired bronchial orifice. The blocker then easily enters the appropriate bronchus. This maneuver is preferably done with the aid of fiberscope, but may also be done blindly.

The Univent tube has some advantages over double-lumen tubes: the main lumen is larger, allowing larger fiberscopes; the tube can be used for postoperative ventilation; and the blocker may be easier to place in the presence of distorted bronchial anatomy. There are some disadvantages to the Univent design, however. The tube material is a silicone polymer, which binds to suction catheters, does not soften or conform with body heat, and adheres poorly to tape. The blocker has only a small central lumen, which is easily clogged by secretions, so deflation of the blocked lung may be slow. The blocker must be placed in the bronchus of the operative lung and may interfere with surgery on that bronchus. Finally, differential ventilation of the two lungs is not possible. For these reasons, the competent anesthetist should be familiar with both Univent and double-lumen tubes.

Single-Lumen Endobronchial Tubes

Single-lumen endobronchial tubes are mentioned because of their historical interest. Their use in current medical practice essentially has been abandoned and replaced with the Univent tube or the various double-lumen tubes. In an emergency, or in children, an appropriately sized single-lumen tube can be advanced into a mainstem bronchus.

DOUBLE-LUMEN ENDOTRACHEAL TUBES

Historically, three types of double-lumen tubes—the Carlens, White, and Robertshaw—were designed for specialized anesthesia use, principally in thoracic surgery. The Carlens tube,[35] the first double-lumen tube suitable for the administration of anesthesia, was originally intended for bronchospirometry. It provides control of ventilation as well as a route for removal of secretions from one or both lungs. The Carlens tube, made of soft rubber or plastic, with two cuffs (tracheal and bronchial), two pilot bags, and a left-sided bronchial lumen, uses a carinal hook to help judge depth of insertion (Fig. 12–15). A technique for using this tube is described in Chapter 22.

The White tube,[36] a right-sided Carlens tube, allows ventilation of the right lung and collapse of the left lung, or vice versa. A slotted cuff facilitates ventilation of the right upper lung.

Robertshaw enlarged the lumen of his tube to lower resistance to air flow.[37] Both right-sided and left-sided Robertshaw tubes are available. The slotted tip in the cuff of the right-sided model allows ventilation of the right upper lobe.[38] Robertshaw tubes came in three sizes (large, medium, and small) with outer diameters of 11, 9.5, and 8 mm—all too large for use in children. The absence of a carinal hook facilitated insertion of the tube through the cords and permitted ligation of a mainstem bronchus close to the carina for pneumonectomy.[39] Figure 12–16 shows a 37 Fr left-sided Mallinckrodt double-lumen endotracheal tube modeled after the original Robertshaw tubes. A beveled bronchial orifice on the left-sided model, with restricted bronchial cuff inflation on the medial side, minimizes interference with right lung ventilation.

The most commonly used right-sided double-lumen endotracheal tubes are shown in Figures 12–17 through 12–21. They are all modifications of the original Robertshaw double-lumen tube. They differ primarily in the design of the bronchial segment and cuffs (tracheal and bronchial), as well as in the composition of the tube itself. The designs are obvious, but the exact composition of the tubes are often trade secrets.

The Mallinckrodt right-sided double-lumen endotracheal tube, the Broncho-Cath, is characterized by a clever design of the bronchial cuff and a useful difference in the color of the tracheal (white) and bronchial (light blue) cuffs (Figs. 12–17 and 12–21A). On the outside, a black line (and on the inside, a white line) delineates the beginning of the tracheal and bronchial cuffs. The tip of the endobronchial limb is rather flat.

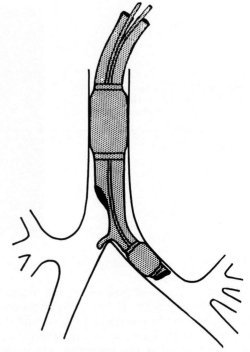

Figure 12–15. The carinal hook on the Carlens tube. (From Mushin WW. Thoracic Anesthesia. Oxford: Blackwell Scientific, 1963.)

The Portex double-lumen endotracheal tube does not differentiate the tracheal from the bronchial cuff by color (both cuffs are a light blue) (Figs. 12–18 and 12–21B). The proximal part of the bronchial cuff surrounds the bronchial limb, whereas the distal part of the cuff does not surround it, but lies opposite the opening of the right upper lobe bronchus.

The Sheridan right-sided double-lumen endotracheal tube, the Sher-i-Bronch (Figs. 12–19 and 12–21C), has a unique double bronchial cuff and slotted eye for the right upper lobe.

The right-sided Rüsch double-lumen endotracheal tube is manufactured in a size 28 Fr, suitable for smaller individuals (Figs. 12–20 and 12–21D).

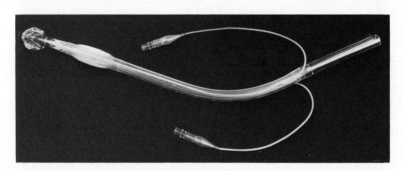

Figure 12–16. Disposable, plastic Broncho-Cath endobronchial tube, 37 Fr left. Manufactured by Mallinckrodt Critical Care (Glens Falls, NY). Available in sizes of 28, 35, 37, 39, and 41 Fr. Also available with a left carinal hook in sizes of 35, 37, 39, and 41 Fr, and in sizes of 35, 37, 39, and 41 Fr in the right-sided model.

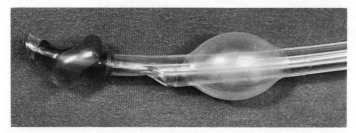

Figure 12–17. Endobronchial portion of the right-sided Broncho-Cath double-lumen endotracheal tube, illustrating the asymmetrical bronchial cuff, which allows ventilation of the right upper lobe bronchus.

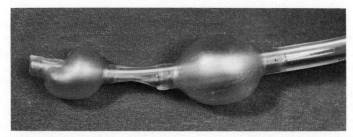

Figure 12–18. Close-up view of the bronchial portion of the right-sided Portex double-lumen endotracheal tube. The endobronchial and tracheal balloons are not differentiated by color; this makes them difficult to differentiate with a fiberscope from the inside of the tube.

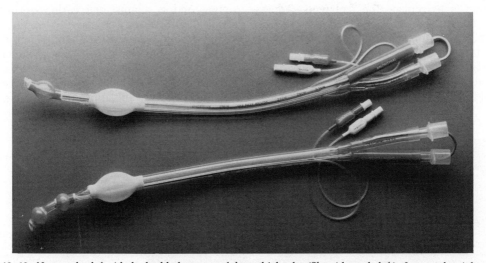

Figure 12–19. *Upper tube:* left-sided, double-lumen endobronchial tube (Sher-i-bronch left). *Lower tube:* right-sided, double-lumen endobronchial tube (Sher-i-bronch right). There is a large eye on the endobronchial portion for ventilation of the right upper lobe. The bronchial cuff is dark blue, whereas the tracheal cuff is light blue.

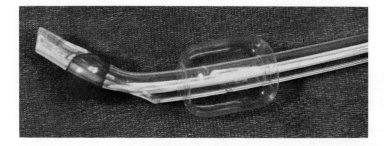

Figure 12–20. Right-sided Rusch double-lumen endotracheal tube in size 28 Fr, suitable for smaller individuals and children. The tip of the bronchial portion has a nice, flat configuration. The bronchial cuff is asymmetrical and dark blue, whereas the tracheal cuff is symmetrical and white colored.

Verifying Placement of a Double-Lumen Endotracheal Tube

Once the double-lumen endotracheal tube is presumably inserted into the trachea, an algorithm based on three questions may be started (Table 12–4). The first question is **are you in the trachea?** You should initially inflate only the tracheal cuff, then attempt to ventilate both sides. Potential responses include (1) a large leak of air, (2) the stomach inflates, (3) poor compliance, or (4) both lungs ventilate well.

A large air leak may be indicative of a disconnection of the endotracheal tube; the valve on the anesthesia machine may be open; or the lumen may be uncapped. These causes of a leak are easily remedied once they are identified. A fourth reason for a large leak is a broken cuff on the endotracheal tube; this may not be as easily remedied. The preferred solution is to replace the damaged endotracheal tube.

When the stomach inflates, the double-lumen tube should be immediately withdrawn, the patient oxygenated, and intubation reattempted. At an appropriate time, the stomach should be decompressed with a nasogastric tube.

Poor compliance may be due to a kinked tube or bronchospasm. The first response should be to check for and correct a kinked tube. Other appropriate responses may include deepening the anesthetic, giving a bronchodilator, or applying positive end-expiratory pressure when bronchospasm is the culprit.

In the event that both lungs ventilate well, one should proceed to the second question: **are you in the correct bronchus?**

To test whether the bronchial limb is in the correct bronchus, one should first clamp the tracheal lumen, uncap the tracheal port distal to the clamp, and ventilate via the bronchial limb. Potential responses to these maneuvers include (1) poor compliance, (2) the wrong side ventilates, (3) both sides ventilate, (4) there is no isolation, or (5) the correct side isolates.

Poor compliance may indicate that the bronchial end is against the carina or bronchial wall. The tube may be inserted too far, so that only a single lobe or segment is being ventilated. Another cause of poor compliance in this situation is kinking or folding of the bronchial lumen. This may be easily checked with a fiberscope and the appropriate repairs made. When the wrong side ventilates, the bronchial

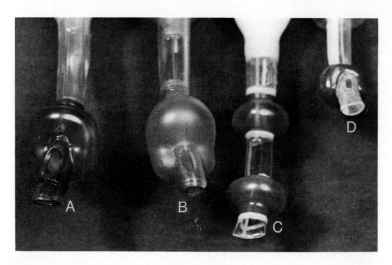

Figure 12–21. Distal portions of four right-sided, double-lumen tubes. *A*, Mallinckrodt; *B*, Portex; *C*, Sheridan; and *D*, Rusch. Note the shapes of the bronchial cuffs, each designed to optimize ventilation of the right upper lobe.

Table 12–4. POSITIONING DOUBLE-LUMEN TUBES ALGORITHM

1. Are you in the trachea?
    Test as a single-lumen tube
        Procedure
            Inflate tracheal cuff (only)
            Ventilate via both lumens
        Question
            Can you ventilate both lungs?
        Responses
            Ventilates well: go to *Test by Isolating*
            Stomach inflates
                Esophageal intubation
                Tracheoesophageal fistula
            Poor compliance
                Tube kinked
                Bronchospasm
            Large leak
                Lumen uncapped
                Cuff broken
                Valve on anesthesia machine open
                Tube disconnected
2. Are you in the bronchus?
    Test by isolating
        Procedure
            Clamp tracheal lumen
            Uncap tracheal port distal to clamp
            Ventilate via bronchial lumen
        Question
            Can you isolate by inflating bronchial cuff?
        Responses
            Correct side isolates: go to *Test After Isolating*

2. Are you in the bronchus? *Continued*
    No isolation
        Tube cuff too small
        Cuff not in bronchus
        Cuff broken
    Poor compliance
        Bronchial end against carina or bronchial wall
        Tube too distal, ventilating single lobe or segment
        Bronchial lumen kinked or folded
    Wrong side ventilates
        Tube in wrong side
        Wrong side clamped
    Both sides ventilate
        Bronchial cuff above carina
Test after isolating
    Procedure
        Unclamp tracheal lumen
        Recap tracheal side
        Ventilate via both lumens
    Question
        Can you ventilate both lungs?
    Responses
        Both sides ventilate: *success!*
        Only one side ventilates
            Bronchial cuff herniating, blocking carina
            Tube too distal
            Tracheal opening in bronchus
            Secretions or tumor

Courtesy of Paul H. Alfiller, Laurie E. Shapiro, and James T. Roberts; Massachusetts General Hospital, Boston, MA.

portion has been inserted in the opposite bronchus, or the wrong side of the double-lumen tube has been clamped. If both sides ventilate, the bronchial cuff is positioned above the carina. Cuff position can be easily checked with a fiberscope. When there is no isolation, the bronchial cuff may be too small, the cuff may not be in the bronchus, or the cuff may be broken. The pilot balloon should be tested, and bronchial limb position checked with a fiberscope. A transparent double-lumen tube also aids in checking cuff placement by viewing airway anatomy through the wall of the tube itself. The carina may usually be identified in this manner. In the event that the correct side ventilates, you should proceed to the third question: **with both cuffs inflated, can you ventilate both sides?**

To answer this question, you should unclamp the tracheal lumen, recap the tracheal side, and ventilate both lumens. It may be that only one side ventilates. This may indicate that the bronchial cuff is herniating and blocking the carina, that the tube is distal to the tracheal opening in the bronchus, or that secretions or a tumor prevent ventilation of both sides. When both sides ventilate appropriately, proceed to next step; ie, positioning the patient on the operating table. Once the patient is positioned for surgery, again verify correct placement of the tube.

BRONCHIAL BLOCKERS

The Magill balloon-tipped bronchial blocker (Fig. 12–22) is a double-lumen rubber catheter designed in 1936. It has two channels; one to inflate the balloon, and one to allow suctioning and degassing of the lung distal to the blocker. After the blocker is placed (under fiberoptic control), the endotracheal tube is inserted. The inflated cuff of the endotracheal tube helps to maintain the position of the blocker. Embolectomy catheters and urinary catheters can also be used to block the bronchus. The Univent tube (described previously) is usually used for elective bronchial blocking. A separate blocker is used if a single-lumen tube is in place, and reintubation is risky.

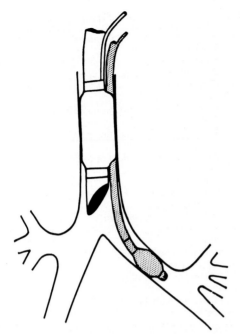

Figure 12–22. Illustration of a Magill balloon-tipped bronchial blocker. (From Mushin WW. Thoracic Anesthesia. Oxford: Blackwell Scientific, 1963.)

THE ENDOTRACHEAL TUBE AS A DRUG ROUTE

Recently, there have been an increasing number of papers dealing with the administration of drugs through an endotracheal tube. For years, drugs have been used to treat bronchoconstriction (epinephrine, metaproterenol, ipratropium bromide), but other drugs, such as lidocaine, insulin, midazolam, theophylline, tobramycin, and gentamicin, have recently been examined for systemic absorption via the endotracheal route.

Using the Endotracheal Tube to Monitor a Circulating Drug Level

Blood alcohol concentrations may be inferred by measurements of exhaled alcohol levels using an infrared or a fuel cell analyzer. These measurements are commonly made by police to check for drunken drivers. In the past few years, reports have appeared using ethanol as a tag to estimate absorption of irrigation fluid during a transurethral prostatectomy (TURP). Exhaled ethanol may be measured directly from the anesthetic circuit.

The presence of exhaled ethanol indicates and is proportional to the systemic absorption of irrigation fluid.

An alcohol analyzer for expired air may also be used to estimate blood ethanol levels in patients being treated by sclerotherapy for large venous malformations. In these cases, large amounts (30 to 40 mL depending on body weight) of 100% ethanol may be administered directly into the malformation, and from there move to the general circulation. Monitoring circulating ethanol levels is useful to help judge the level of general anesthesia necessary for pain relief. The postanesthetic wake-up period may be prolonged to greater than an hour, depending on the blood ethanol level achieved.

References

1. Watson W. Development of the PVC endotracheal tube. Biomaterials 1:1–4, 1980.
2. Eisenmenger V. Zur Tamponade des larynx nach Prof. Maydl. Wein Med Wochenschr 43:199, 1893.
3. Carroll R. Evaluation of tracheal tube cuff designs. Crit Care Med 1:45, 1973.
4. Carrol R, Grenvik A. Proper use of large diameter, large residual volume cuffs. Crit Care Med 1:153, 1973.
5. Wu W, Arteaga M, Mlodozeniec AR, Poppers PJ. Surface ultrastructure and pressure dynamics of tracheal tube cuffs. J Biomed Mater Res 14:11–21, 1980.
6. Loeser E. Reduction of postoperative sore throat with new endotracheal tube cuffs. Anesthesiology 52:257–259, 1980.
7. Crawley B, Cross D. Tracheal cuffs—A review and dynamic pressure study. Anaesthesia 30:4–11, 1975.
8. Cooper J, Grillo H. Experimental production and prevention of injury due to cuffed tracheal tubes. Surg Gynecol Obstet 129:1235, 1969.
9. Cooper J, Grillo H. Analysis of problems related to cuffs on endotracheal tubes. Chest 62:215, 1973.
10. Geffin LB, Pontoppidan H. Reduction of tracheal damage by the prestretching of inflatable cuffs. Anesthesiology 31:462, 1969.
11. Grillo HC, Cooper JD, Geffin B, Pontoppidan H. A low pressure cuff for tracheostomy tubes to minimize tracheal injury: A comparative clinical trial. J Thorac Cardiovasc Surg 62:898–907, 1971.
12. James AE Jr, MacMillan AS Jr, Eaton SB, Grillo HC. Roentgenology of tracheal stenosis resulting from cuffed tracheostomy tubes. Am J Roetgenol Radium Ther Nucl Med 109:455, 1970.
13. Wall M. Infant endotracheal tube resistance: Effects of changing length, diameter, and gas density. Crit Care Med 8:38–40, 1980.
14. Brahams D. Anaesthesia and the law: Two cases of oesophageal intubation. Anaesthesia 14:64–65, 1989.
15. Kreienbuhl G. Verification of endotracheal tube placement. Anaesthetist 41:571–581, 1992.
16. Andesen KH. Methods for ensuring correct tracheal intubation: A review. Ugesk Laeger 153:267–269, 1991.

17. Birmingham PK, Cheney GW, Ward RJ. Esophageal intubation: A review of detection techniques. Anesth Analg 65:886–891, 1986.

18. Smith GM, Reed JC, Choplin RH. Radiographic detection of esophageal malpositioning of endotracheal tubes. AJR 154:23–26, 1990.

19. Patil VU, Stehling LC, Zauder HL. Another use for the fiberoptic bronchoscope. Anesthesiology 55:484, 1981.

20. Foutch RG, Magelssen MD, MacMillan JG. The esophageal detector device: A rapid and accurate method for assessing tracheal versus esophageal intubation in a porcine model. Ann Emerg Med 21:1073–1076, 1992.

21. Oberly D, Stein S, Hess D, Eitel D, Simmons M. An evaluation of the esophageal detector device using a cadaver model. Am J Emerg Med 10:317–320, 1992.

22. Wee MYK. The oesophageal detector device: Assessment of a new method to distinguish oesophageal from tracheal intubation. Anaesthesia 43:27–29, 1988.

23. Williams KN, Nunn JF. The oesophageal detector device: A prospective trial on 100 patients. Anaesthesia 44:412–414, 1989.

24. Denman WT, Hayes M, Higgins D, Wilkinson DJ. The Fenem CO$_2$ detector device: An apparatus to prevent unnoticed oesophageal intubation. Anaesthesia 45:465–467, 1990.

25. Kelly JS, Wilhoit RD, Brown RE, James R. Efficacy of the FEF colorimetric end-tidal carbon dioxide detector in children. Anesth Analg 75:45–50, 1992.

26. Rosenberg M, Block CS. A simple, disposable end-tidal carbon dioxide detector. Anesthesia Progress 38:24–26, 1991.

27. Higgins D, Hayes M, Denman W, Wilkinson DJ. Effectiveness of using end-tidal carbon dioxide concentration to monitor cardiopulmonary resuscitation. Br Med J 300:581, 1990.

28. Ornato JP, Shipley JB, Racht EM, Slovis CM, Wrenn KD, Pepe PE, Almeida SL, Ginger VF, Fotre TV. Multicenter study of a portable, hand-size, colorimetric end-tidal carbon dioxide detection device. Ann Emerg Med 21:518–523, 1992.

29. Bhende MD, Thompson AE, Cook DR, Saville AL. Validity of a disposable end-tidal CO$_2$ detector in verifying endotracheal tube placement in infants and children. Ann Med 21:142–145, 1992.

30. Varon AJ, Morrina J, Civetta JM. Clinical utility of a colorimetric end-tidal CO$_2$ detector in cardiopulmonary resuscitation and emergency intubation. J Clin Monit 7:289–293, 1991.

31. Mizutani AR, Ozaki G, Benumof JL, Scheller MS. Auscultation cannot distinguish esophageal from tracheal passage of tube. J Clin Monit 7:232–236, 1991.

32. Blayney M, Costello D, Perlman M, Lui K, Frank J. A new system for location of endotracheal tube in preterm and term neonates. Pediatrics 87:44–47, 1991.

33. Stewart RD, LaRosee A, Kaplan RM, Ilkhanipour K. Correct positioning of an endotracheal tube using a flexible lighted stylet. Crit Care Med 18:97–99, 1990.

34. Sum-Ping ST, Mehta MP, Anderton JM. A comparative study of methods of detection of esophageal intubation. Anesth Analg 69:627–632, 1989.

35. Carlens E. A new flexible double-lumen catheter for bronchospirometer. J Thorac Surg 18:7442, 1949.

36. White G. A new double-lumen tube. Br J Anaesth 32:232, 1960.

37. Robertshaw F. Low resistance double-lumen endobronchial tubes. Br J Anaesth 34:576–579, 1962.

38. Ryder G, Short D, Zeitlin G. The anaesthetic management of patients with bronchopleural fistula with the Robertshaw double-lumen tube. Br J Anaesth 37:861–865, 1965.

39. Zeitlin G, Short D, Ryder G. An assessment of the Robertshaw double-lumen tube. Br J Anaesth 37:858–860, 1965.

CHAPTER 13

Rigid Laryngoscopes

William H. Campbell, M.D., M.B.A., F.R.C.P.(C)

HISTORY

The first laryngoscope was invented in 1805 by Bozzini (Fig. 13–1). Since that time, many laryngoscopes have been designed. Their purpose has been to assist in the direct visualization of the larynx while minimizing damage to the teeth, temporomandibular joints, and other vulnerable structures.

The next significant development in laryngoscopy came in 1907, with the development of the Jackson laryngoscope (Fig. 13–2).[1] The U-shaped handle and blade of this instrument, although awkwardly placed, represented a quantum leap forward in the medical technology of the time. In fact, the current model continues to be used today by many bronchoscopists.

COMPONENTS OF THE LARYNGOSCOPE

A laryngoscope is made up of three basic components: a handle, a blade, and a light.

The handle permits attachment of a variety of blades to compensate for variations in oral anatomy. Blades attach to the handle by means of a hook-adapter, and a small light turns on automatically when the blade is locked into its position for use. When not in use, the blade folds in order to conserve the batteries. A standard hook-on handle uses two "C" cell batteries, whereas a pediatric laryngoscope accepts two "AA" cell batteries.

LARYNGOSCOPE BLADES

In addition to the three components of the laryngoscope, the blade itself is divisible into three parts: the spatula (S), the flange (F), and the tip (T) (Fig. 13–3). The numerous permutations and combinations of these various parts give rise to seemingly endless variations in laryngoscopes. The function of the spatula is to compress and manipulate the soft tissues and mandible so that a direct line of vision can be established to the epiglottis and larynx. The long axis of the spatula may be entirely

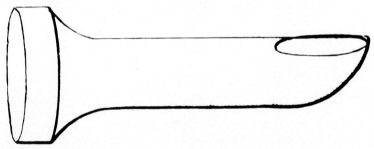

Figure 13–1. Bozzini laryngoscope. (Drawing from the Collection of the Smithsonian Institute, Washington, D.C.; with permission.)

134

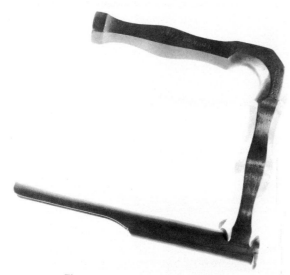

Figure 13–2. Jackson laryngoscope.

straight, or curved in a portion or all of its length.

The flange is the portion of the blade that projects from the edge of the spatula. Its function is to deflect interfering tissues and allow for unobstructed instrumentation. It is important to note that the flange is part of the cross-sectional design of the blade and may vary from a simple flat or slightly curved form to a completely closed tube.

The tip of the blade, either directly or indirectly, elevates the epiglottis and provides a clear line of vision into the larynx. To retain the epiglottis more securely, the tip has undergone a number of conformational changes. Over the years, it has been ridged, curved, slotted, and even hooked. Moreover, curved and angled blades have been fashioned to elevate the epiglottis indirectly by applying pressure on the hyoepiglottic ligament at the junction of the tongue and epiglottis (ie, the vallecula). As an additional refinement, the tip

has been blunted and thickened to prevent trauma to the soft tissues.

Curved Blades

The most popular curved blade in use today is the Macintosh (Fig. 13–4).[2] This blade was originally designed in 1941. Available sizes range from infant (87-mm #1 Macintosh) to large adult (158-mm #4 Macintosh), with a child (108-mm #2 Macintosh) and a regular adult (130-mm #3 Macintosh) in between. The regular adult size is the most useful. The tip of the Macintosh blade fits into the vallecula (see Fig. 16–5). Lifting the blade anteriorly, by virtue of its pressure on the hyoepiglottic ligament, displaces the epiglottis and exposes the vocal cords and glottic opening. The left-hand ridge keeps the tongue from obstructing the line of vision. Unfortunately, it also provides the careless and unskilled laryngoscopist with a fulcrum for leverage against the upper incisors. In order to preclude injury to the teeth, the force applied to the laryngoscope handle must be directed along the vector defined by the long axis of the handle, vector A (see Fig. 16–5). It is essential that the laryngoscopist controls the natural tendency to apply force along vector C, using the upper incisors for leverage in an effort to move the epiglottis anteriorly along vector B. Failure to do so not only results in suboptimal visualization of the desired landmarks, but may cause significant and costly dental injury.

Straight Blades

The epiglottis may also be lifted anteriorly by placing the tip of a straight blade posterior to the epiglottis. Several innovative designs of

Figure 13–3. The laryngoscope blade is divided into the spatula (S), the flange (F), and the tip (T).

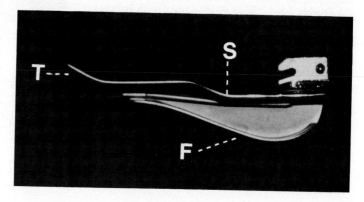

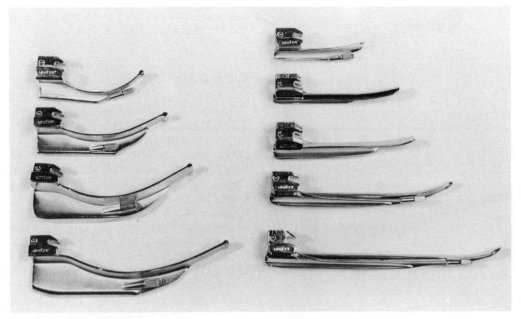

Figure 13–4. Examples of straight and curved laryngoscope blades.

the straight blade, such as the Miller[3] and Wisconsin, which have a prominent left-side ridge, prevent the visual pathway from being obstructed by the tongue. Both of these blades have a light source that is located just behind the tip of the blade (in contrast, the light on the Macintosh blade is located one third of the way back from the tip). However, the light on the Miller blade is on the right side, whereas that on the Wisconsin blade is on the left (see Fig. 13–4). One final difference between these two straight blades is that the tip of the Miller blade curves upward, whereas the tip of the Wisconsin blade does not.

The Miller blade, perhaps the most popular of the straight blades, ranges in size from premature (75-mm #0 Miller) to large adult (205-mm #3 Miller) (see Fig. 13–4). Wisconsin laryngoscope blades come in three sizes. A modification of the original blade, the Wisconsin-Hipple blade, is available for use in infants (see Fig. 13–4).

Specialized Blades

The laryngoscopist should initially master the Macintosh and Miller blades, because they serve most needs, and then develop additional skills with several of the specialized blades. The greater the skill of a clinician in performing a technical procedure, the greater the chances of success.

Specialized Curved Blades

Bizarri-Guffrida Blade. In the Bizarri-Guffrida blade, the left ridge has been removed to facilitate its use in patients with a limited mouth opening, a short neck, or an extreme "anterior" larynx (Fig. 13–5). The light is located on the mid portion of the blade.

Siker Blade. The Siker blade has a stainless steel mirrored surface. This surface frequently permits visualization of an "anterior" larynx that is inaccessible with conventional blades. However, the mirrored surface inverts the image, which makes the blade difficult to use.

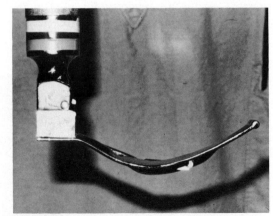

Figure 13–5. Bizarri-Guffrida blade. (From Roberts JT. Fundamentals of Tracheal Intubation, p. 51. Orlando, Grune & Stratton, 1983; with permission.)

The blade is also difficult to use in patients who have a small mouth. In order to master the use of this blade, it should be used during several routine intubations, so that its peculiarities can be learned prior to using it for a difficult laryngoscopy.

Fink Blade. Although the Fink blade retains the ridge along the left side, it is reduced in size at the proximal end. The curvature of the tip is increased and the light source also is closer to the tip. A wider spatula is intended to improve balance.

Polio Blade. During the polio era, the Macintosh blade was difficult to use on patients in tank-type respirators. Thus, the polio blade, being offset at an obtuse angle, overcame the obstructing limitation of the respirator. Fortunately, the need for this blade no longer exists.

Specialized Straight Blades

Bainton Blade. The Bainton blade is a straight blade that is partially tubular. Thus, it possesses a lumen through which numerous manipulations are possible, including the passage of an endotracheal tube.

Guedel Blade. The hook arrangement of the Guedel blade causes a 72-degree angle (rather than the usual 90 degrees) between the blade and the handle. The light source is located just behind the tip, which is curved slightly upward.

Flagg Blade. In this blade, a C-shaped flange ensures a clear visual pathway. The blade forms a 90-degree angle with the handle and has the light positioned just behind the tip.

Whitehead Blade. The Whitehead blade is a straight blade that has been modified by reducing the left-sided ridge, thus minimizing pressure against the upper incisors.

Bennett Blade. The Bennett blade has a reduced left-sided ridge and a hook arrangement similar to the Guedel blade.

Snow Blade. The Snow blade is a modified Miller blade. The tip is raised and the left-sided flange is reduced.

Eversole Blade. The Eversole blade is a straight blade with a C-shaped ridge that is reduced over the distal half of the blade.

A PROBLEM-ORIENTED APPROACH TO LARYNGOSCOPE SELECTION

McIntyre[4] has proposed a scheme for the problem-oriented approach to laryngoscope selection, which assumes that a laryngoscope or bronchoscope incorporating a fiberoptic visual device will not be used. Various laryngoscopes are classified according to the clinical problem that they specifically address.[4]

Rigid Fiberoptic Laryngoscope (Stylette)

The rigid fiberoptic laryngoscope is similar to a rigid bronchoscope with additional optics. The optics in the instrument produced by Karl Storz (Culver City, CA) are superb. As with rigid bronchoscopes, care must be taken to protect the upper teeth, because there may be a tendency to press against them with this instrument. Care must also be taken to protect the endotracheal tube cuff from tearing as it passes the teeth. The laryngoscopist can minimize this risk by raising the tongue and mandible anteriorly, either manually or with a standard laryngoscope. This facilitates introduction of the laryngoscope into the oral cavity. Because the laryngoscope is rigid, the patient must conform to the configuration of the laryngoscope, rather than vice versa. Light channels into the field via a fiberoptic bundle that is connected to a high-intensity light source.

Malleable Fiberoptic Laryngoscope

The malleable fiberoptic laryngoscope was easily molded to each patient's anatomy. This instrument is, however, no longer produced by the American Optical Company.

Bullard Laryngoscope

The Bullard laryngoscope is an instrument that combines rigid and flexible optics. It requires a minimum opening of 4 mm for insertion into the oral cavity. The blade is passed over the tongue, and the larynx is visualized. An endotracheal tube may then be inserted under direct visualization, using either a lateral approach or with the aid of the forceps that are an integral part of the laryngoscope.

Accessories for Use With Rigid Laryngoscopes

Blanket (Pillow). Aside from the laryngoscope, the most useful mechanical aid for in-

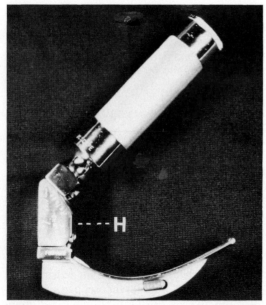

Figure 13–6. Howland adapter. (From Roberts JT. Fundamentals of Tracheal Intubation, p. 57. Orlando, Grune & Stratton, 1983; with permission.)

tubation is a blanket or pillow. Because proper patient position is the basis of good laryngoscopic technique, a blanket or pillow placed under the head flexes the cervical vertebrae, allows extension of the atlanto-occipital joint, and aligns the pharyngeal and laryngeal axes to facilitate direct laryngoscopy. This is the so-called "sniffing position."

Howland Adapter. The Howland adapter (H in Fig. 13–6) changes the angle between the handle and the blade of the standard hook-on laryngoscope. It brings the handle forward to improve exposure. Introduction of the blade into the mouth may be hindered, however,

because the top of the handle invariably presses against the patient's chest.

Huffman Prism. The plastic Huffman prism clips to the base of a #3 Macintosh blade. The leading prismatic surface bends the light rays, allowing the laryngoscopist to see the tip of the blade without reversing or inverting the image (as with the Siker blade). To prevent fogging, the prism is placed in warm water just before use. The usefulness of this accessory cannot be overstated. A disposable laryngoscope manufactured by Penlon (Riverside, CA) has a built-in prism that shifts the image laterally as well as posteriorly.

Forceps. Forceps are used with direct laryngoscopy to guide the tip of an endotracheal tube into the glottic opening. Adult Magill forceps and Aillon forceps are shown in Figure 13–7. The Aillon forceps have a spring-loaded handle and are designed to bend the tip of the endotracheal tube toward the longitudinal axis of the larynx.

The Rovenstein forceps differ from the Magill in the angle of the handle. The Magill handle is approximately 50 degrees out of alignment with the long axis of the forceps, whereas the Rovenstein handle is closer to 90 degrees. The Rovenstein forceps also have a deeper tip with which to grasp the endotracheal tube.

Stylettes. A stylette alters the shape of an endotracheal tube for easier insertion. The Foregger copper stylette is simple and malleable. The clinician must ensure that the tip of the stylette is never inserted beyond the tip of the endotracheal tube in order to avoid perforation of the trachea or esophagus. This complication can be avoided by bending the stylette acutely at the proximal end in order to prevent advancement beyond the tip of the

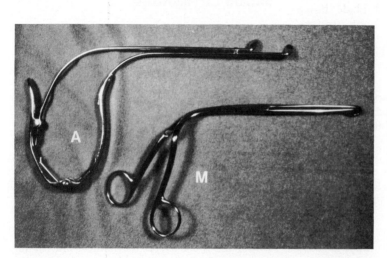

Figure 13–7. Aillon (A) and Magill (M) forceps. (From Roberts JT. Fundamentals of Tracheal Intubation, p. 58. Orlando, Grune & Stratton, 1983; with permission.)

tube. Alternatively, a Giufere tube-stop may be used in lieu of bending the copper stylette. The distal end of the copper stylette is bent to facilitate intubation of an "anterior" larynx.

A Carlens stylette is designed for use with a Carlens double-lumen endotracheal tube. The Bishop-Grillo stylette has an adjustable stop made of flexible stainless steel that is designed to prevent protrusion of the stylette beyond the tip of the tube.

Oral Airways. Oral airways can serve the following purposes: (1) to open an airway obstructed by the tongue and soft tissues of the oropharynx, (2) to provide an avenue for suctioning oral secretions, (3) to serve as a bite block, and (4) to provide a pathway for insertion of an esophageal stethoscope or or-ogastric tube. Guedel, Berman, and Cornall airways are manufactured of metal, conductive rubber, and clear or opaque plastic, respectively.

References

1. Jackson C. Thyrotomy and laryngectomy for malignant disease of the larynx. Br Med J, Nov 24:1478–1485, 1906.
2. Macintosh RR. A new laryngoscope. Lancet 1:205, 1943.
3. Miller RA. A new laryngoscope. Anesthesiology 2:318–320, 1941.
4. McIntyre JWR. Laryngoscope design and the difficult adult tracheal intubation. Can J Anaesth 36:94–98, 1989.

CHAPTER 14

Pharmacologic Aids to Intubation

James T. Roberts, M.D., M.A., and Jeffrey White, M.D.

The task of endotracheal intubation may be assisted by a variety of pharmacologic agents. For example, neuromuscular blockers produce skeletal muscle relaxation, which optimizes intubating conditions. Opiates, benzodiazepines, and barbiturates can be used to sedate a patient who will undergo intubation or to induce general anesthesia for a surgical procedure. A variety of topical agents may be used to reduce the stimulation of endotracheal intubation in the awake patient. This chapter provides an overview of the pharmacologic agents that have been proved useful aids to endotracheal intubation.

NEUROMUSCULAR BLOCKERS

Succinylcholine (Fig. 14–1) is perhaps the most widely used neuromuscular blocker because it has a rapid onset and brief duration of action. Full skeletal muscle relaxation for

$$\begin{bmatrix} CH_2COOCH_2CH_2\overset{+}{N}(CH_3)_3 \\ | \\ CH_2COOCH_2CH_2\underset{+}{N}(CH_3)_3 \end{bmatrix} 2Cl^-$$

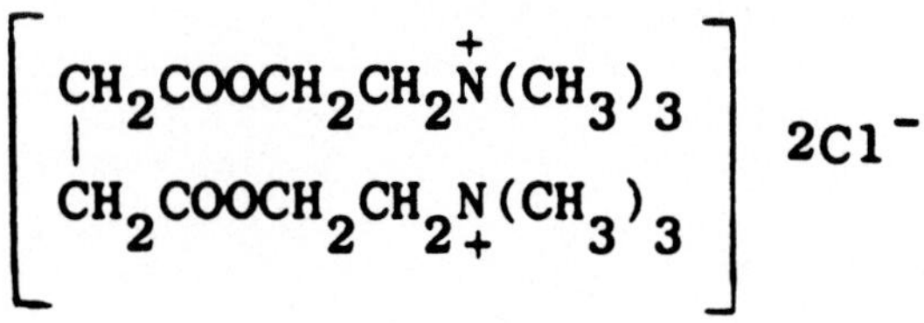

Figure 14–1. Succinylcholine.

intubation can be achieved within 1 minute after an intravenous dose of 1 mg/kg is given. Succinylcholine is a depolarizing neuromuscular blocker. It binds and opens nicotinic acetylcholine receptors at the neuromuscular junction, producing brief muscle fasciculation, followed by skeletal muscle relaxation. The open acetylcholine receptors are permeable to potassium, and there is a transient increase in serum potassium levels as intracellular potassium is released from myocytes. This transient increase in serum potassium is usually of no consequence but can lead to arrhythmias in patients with preexisting hyperkalemia (eg, renal failure). In addition, succinylcholine administration can cause severe hyperkalemia in burn patients due to increased numbers of nicotinic acetylcholine receptors in myocyte cell membranes. Therefore, succinylcholine should be avoided in burn patients. Succinylcholine should also be avoided in patients with spinal cord injuries (eg, paraplegics or quadriplegics) or in patients who have been at bed rest for lengthy periods, because denervation supersensitivity that produces an exaggerated hyperkalemic response to succinylcholine has been described.

In contrast, nondepolarizing neuromuscular blockers bind to nicotinic acetylcholine receptors at the neuromuscular junction but do not open the acetylcholine receptors. As a result, no muscle fasciculation is produced and intracellular potassium is not released from myocytes. Because serum potassium levels are stable, nondepolarizing neuromuscular blockers can be used safely in burn patients, in patients with spinal cord injuries, and in patients with preexisting hyperkalemia. Nondepolarizing neuromuscular blockers are available in two varieties. Intermediate-acting neuromuscular blockers available in the United States are atracurium (Fig. 14–2) and vecuronium (Fig. 14–3). The intubating dose of atracurium is 0.4 to 0.5 mg/kg intravenously; for vecuronium it is 0.1 mg/kg intravenously. Atracurium can cause hypotension and vasodilatation secondary to histamine release; its major advantage is that it is metabolized by nonenzymatic means (that is, its inactivation is independent of hepatic or renal function).

The long-acting neuromuscular blockers can also be used to produce skeletal muscle relaxation for intubation. Pancuronium (Fig. 14–4) at a dose of 0.1 mg/kg produces excellent skeletal muscle relaxation but can also produce a vagolytic effect. If one wishes to avoid tachycardia (eg, in a patient with significant coronary artery disease), then other neuromuscular blockers should be used. Other long-acting neuromuscular blockers are gallamine, 3 to 4 mg/kg (Fig. 14–5); metocurine, 0.4 mg/kg (Fig. 14–6); and d-tubocurarine, 0.5 mg/kg (Fig. 14–7). Both metocurine and curare liberate histamine when given by intravenous bolus and, as a result, may produce vasodilatiation and hypotension.

NARCOTICS

Opiates may be used to provide sedation for endotracheal intubation or to induce surgical anesthesia. Morphine (Fig. 14–8) and meperidine (Fig. 14–9) are useful, older narcotics, whereas fentanyl (Fig. 14–10), sufentanil (Fig. 14–11), and alfentanil (Fig. 14–12) are newer, synthetic opiate narcotics. In practice, small doses of narcotics are given intravenously and are titrated to clinical effect. This is best done by skilled clinicians who are fully prepared to manage the patient's airway should severe respiratory depression develop. Any of these drugs can cause nausea and vomiting, perhaps more so with the synthetic opiates. Also, morphine can produce histamine release with attendant vasodilation, cutaneous flushing, and hypotension. Finally, the synthetic opiates can all cause chest wall rigidity, which makes it difficult for the patient to breathe sponta-

neously and also makes it difficult to ventilate the patient by mask. Chest wall rigidity is a transient phenomenon, but one must be prepared to quickly administer neuromuscular blockers if chest wall rigidity becomes a problem. This underscores the need to limit use of these drugs to those who are skilled in airway management and who have a good working knowledge of the pharmacology of various drugs in airway management (see Chap. 31).

BARBITURATES

Barbiturates are especially useful pharmacologic aids to intubation. Barbiturates may be used to provide rapid sedation of patients for intubation (eg, in the intensive care unit) or to induce surgical anesthesia in the operating room. To produce sedation, small incremental doses can be given intravenously with dosages titrated against desired clinical effect. In the operating room, the induction dose of thiopental sodium (Fig. 14–13) and thiamylal (Fig. 14–14) are 4 to 6 mg/kg intravenously; for methohexital, 1 mg/kg intravenously (Fig. 14–15). All these drugs undergo rapid redistribution after an intravenous bolus, so that the biologic effect is rapidly terminated by drug redistribution. The induction dose should be reduced in patients who have been treated with other sedating drugs (eg, benzodiazepines, opiates), because the dose of barbiturate necessary to induce anesthesia will be reduced in the presence of other sedating drugs. Furthermore, all barbiturates produce vasodilatation and myocardial depression. Doses of these agents should be reduced or the drugs should be avoided altogether in patients with hypovolemia or marginal cardiac function. For these unstable patients, one may wish to use opiates and benzodiazepines to induce anesthesia, with judicious administration of barbiturates as needed. Another drug that has proven useful in inducing anesthesia in hemodynamically unstable patients is the phencyclidine-class drug ketamine (Fig. 14–16). Ketamine can be given intravenously or intramuscularly to induce a dissociative state that permits endotracheal intubation or minor surgical procedures (eg, dressing changes in a burn patient). Ketamine also produces myocardial depression, but blood pressure is usually maintained because ketamine produces a centrally mediated increase in heart rate. In addition, ketamine produces copious secretions and should be given with an

Text continued on page 146

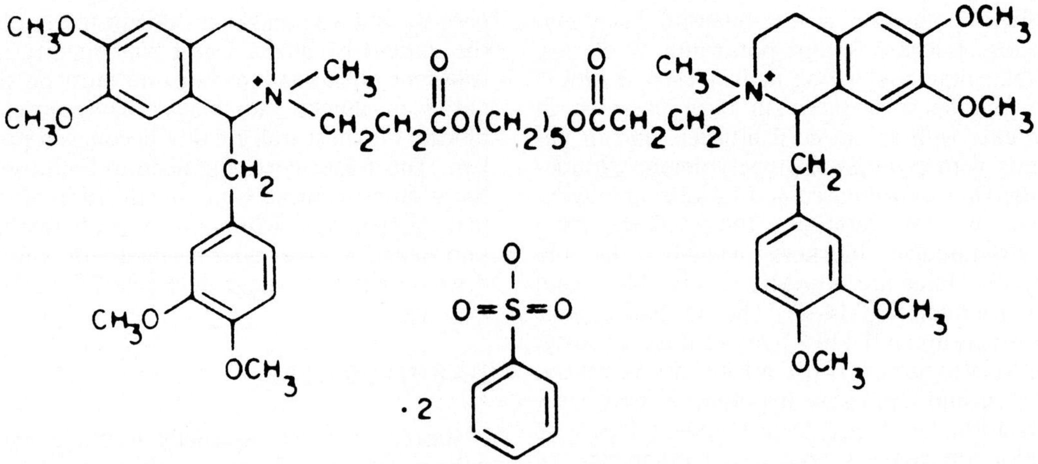

Figure 14–2. Atracurium.

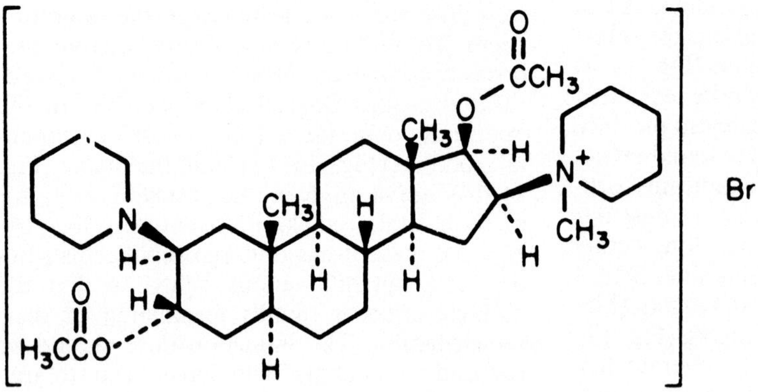

Figure 14–3. Vecuronium.

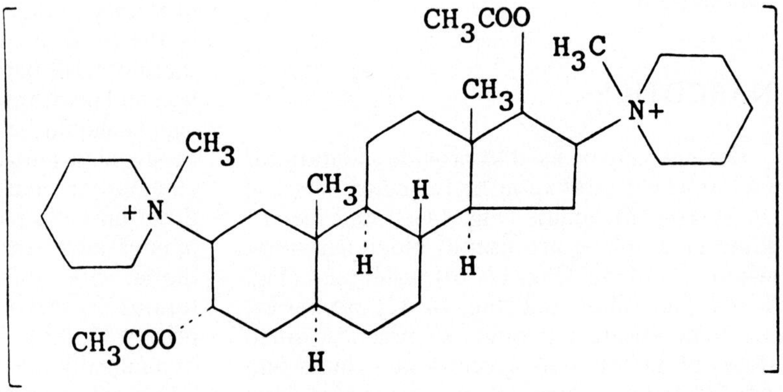

Figure 14–4. Pancuronium.

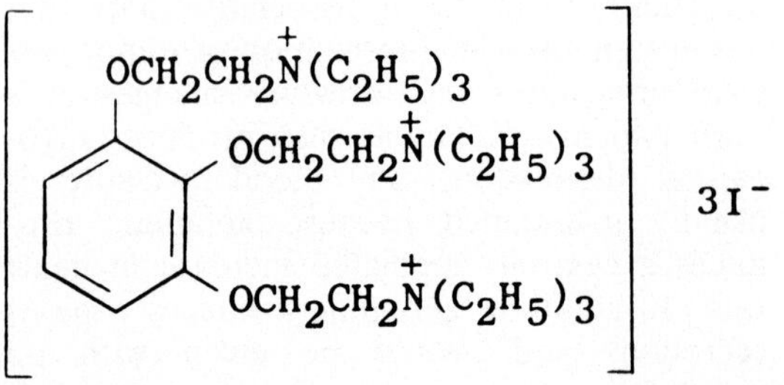

Figure 14–5. Gallamine.

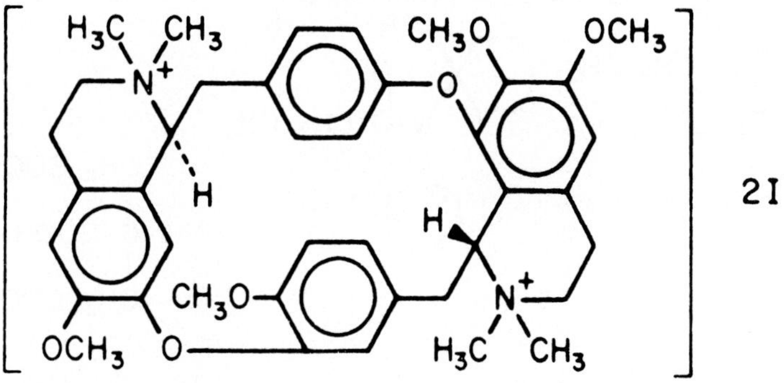

Figure 14–6. Metocurine.

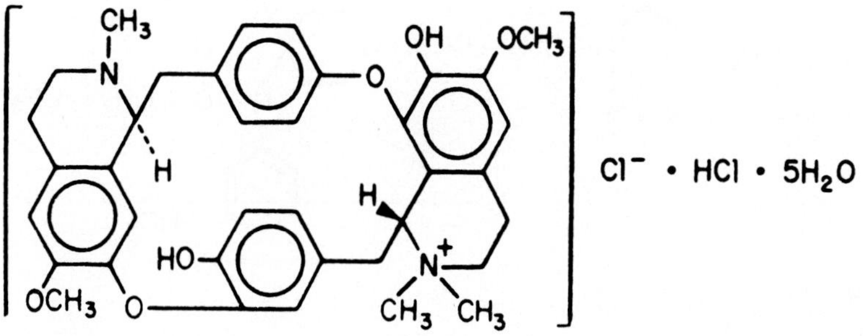

$2I^-$

$Cl^- \cdot HCl \cdot 5H_2O$ **Figure 14–7.** d-Tubocurarine.

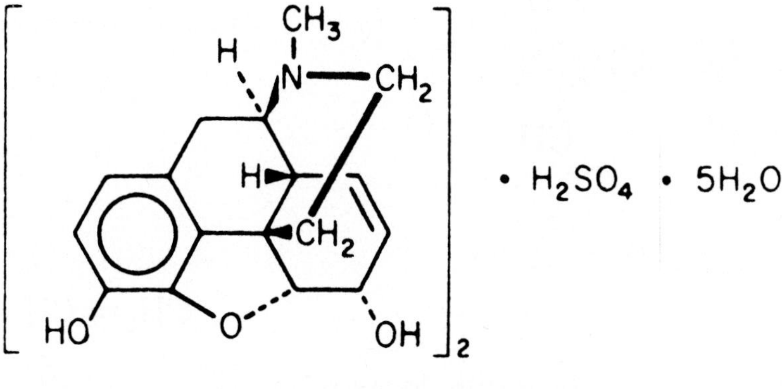

Figure 14–8. Morphine sulfate.

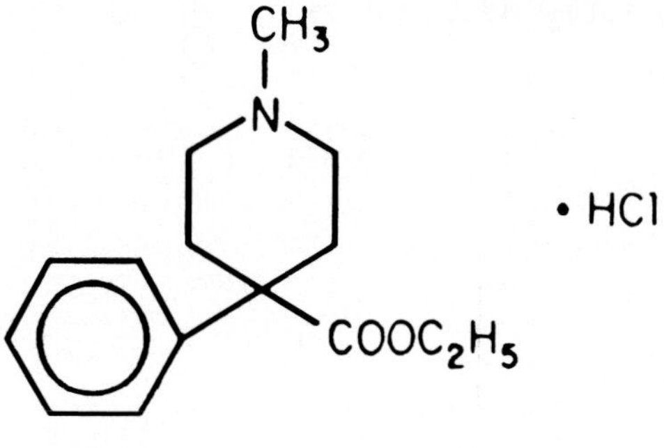

$\cdot H_2SO_4 \cdot 5H_2O$

$\cdot HCl$ **Figure 14–9.** Meperidine.

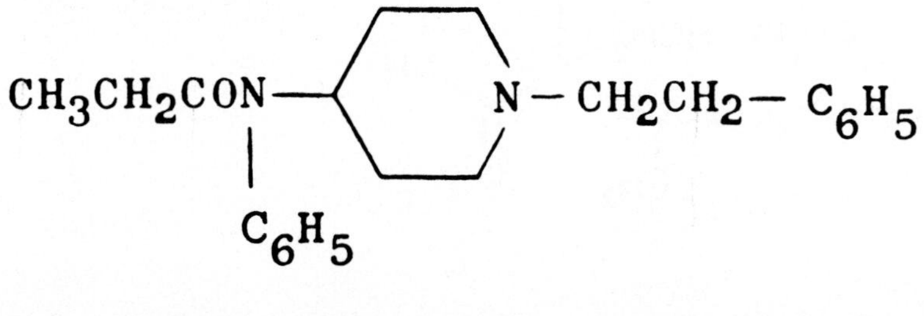

Figure 14–10. Fentanyl.

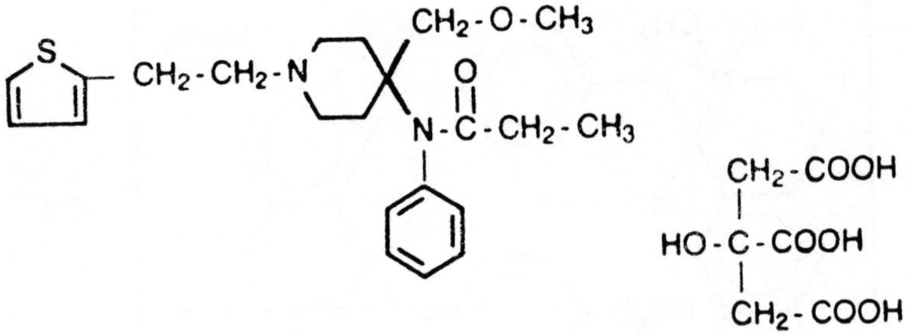

Figure 14–11. Sufentanil.

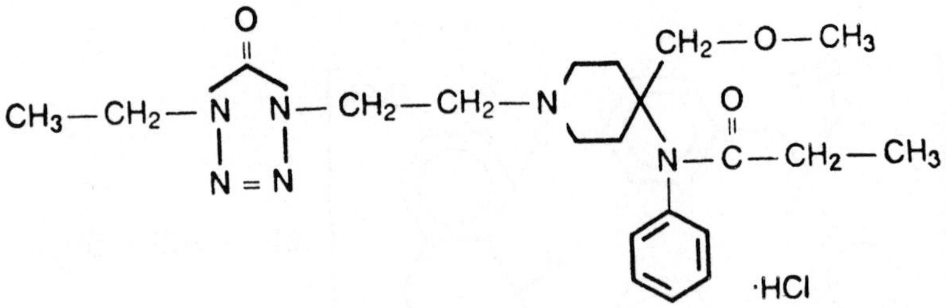

Figure 14–12. Alfentanil.

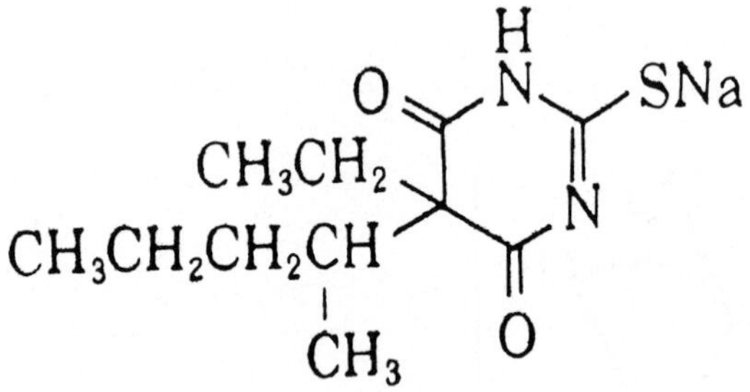

Figure 14–13. Thiopental sodium.

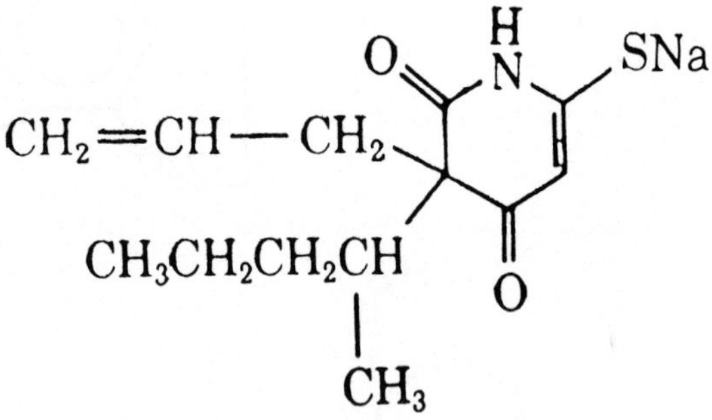

Figure 14–14. Thiamylal sodium.

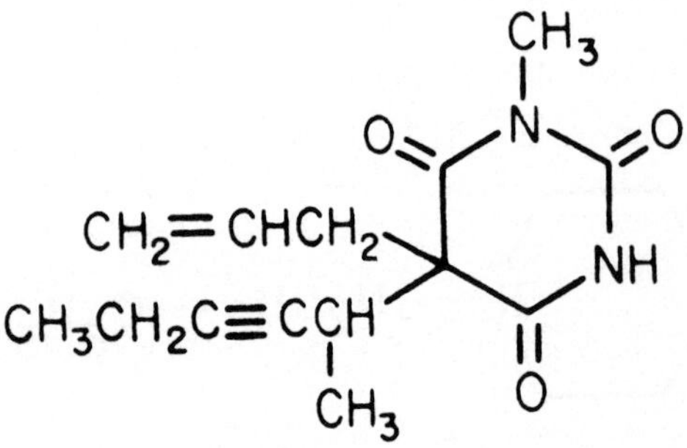

Figure 14–15. Methohexital.

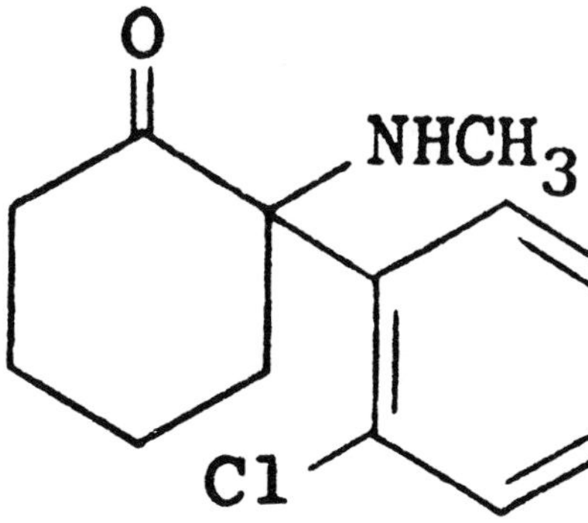

Figure 14–16. Ketamine.

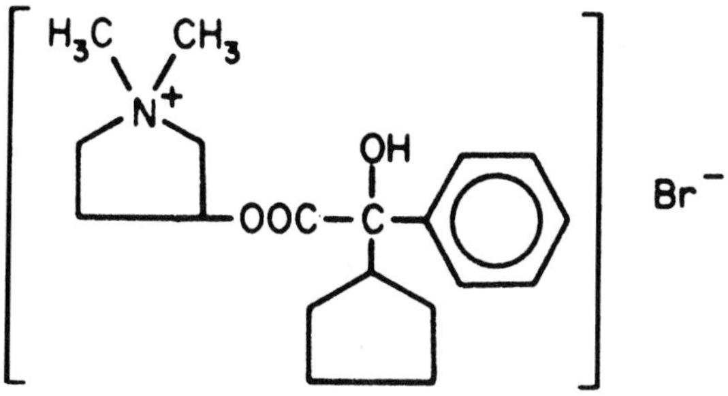

Figure 14–17. Glycopyrrolate.

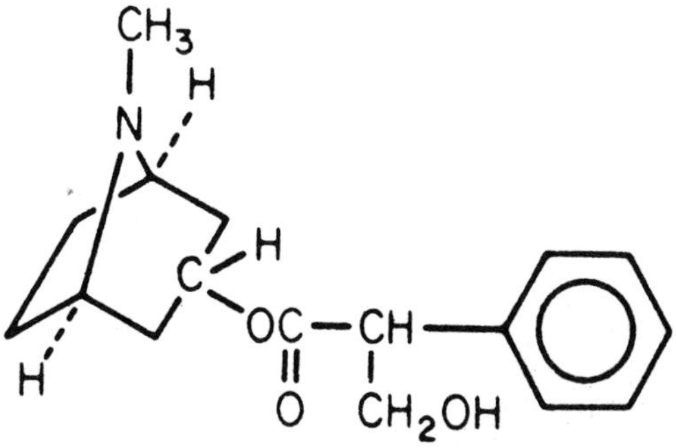

Figure 14–18. Atropine.

Figure 14–19. Propofol.

$C_{12}H_{18}O$

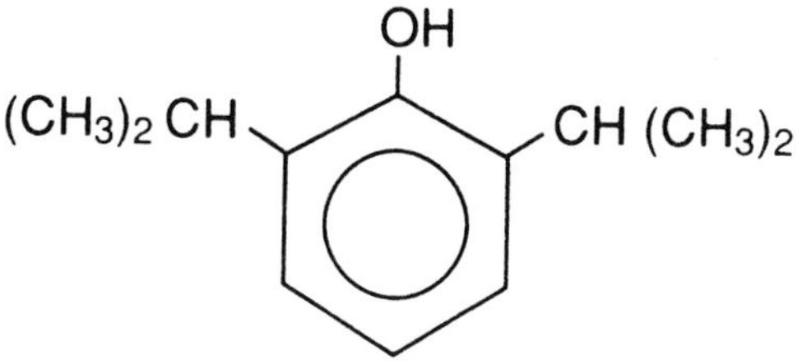

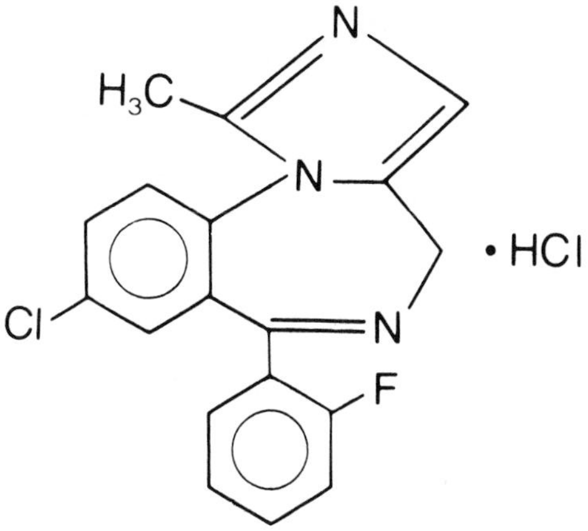

Figure 14–20. Midazolam.

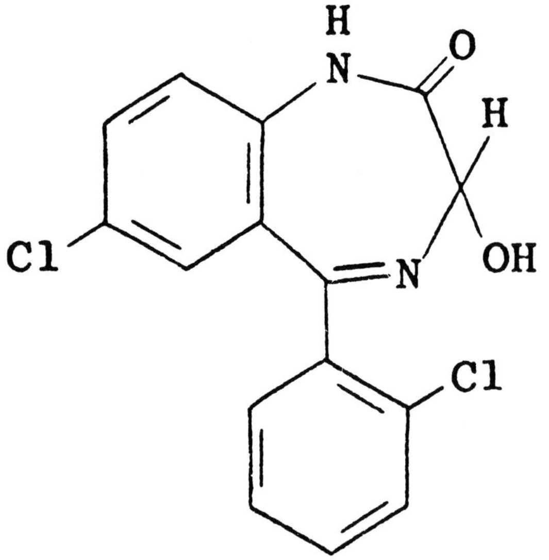

Figure 14–21. Lorazepam.

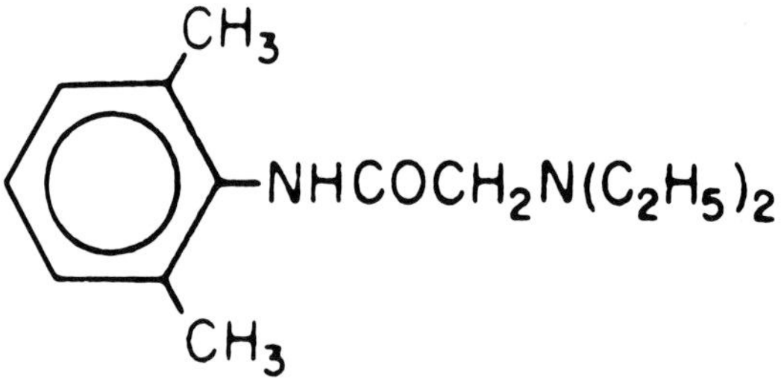

Figure 14–23. Lidocaine.

This emulsion can cause an unpleasant burning sensation at the site of administration. The more peripheral the site of injection, the greater the discomfort.

BENZODIAZEPINES

Benzodiazepines are useful agents for sedating patients for intubation. They are commonly used in the emergency room or intensive care unit for sedation of patients for emergency intubation. Benzodiazepines work rapidly after intravenous administration to produce sedation without analgesia. Benzodiazepines can also produce profound respiratory depression, so it is best to start with small, incremental doses that can be titrated to the desired effect. Midazolam (Fig. 14–20) is a relatively short-acting benzodiazepine that is particularly useful in these settings. Lorazepam (Fig. 14–21) and diazepam (Fig. 14–22) are also commonly used. Doses required for sedation vary widely from patient to patient and depend on such factors as patient age, presence of chronic benzodiazepine use, presence of ethanol abuse, and general overall health.

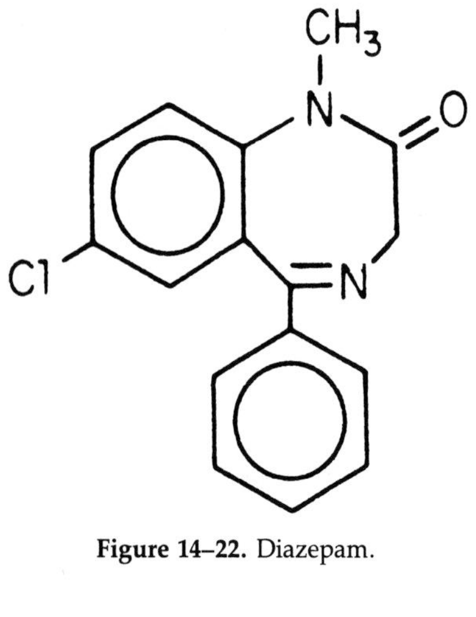

antisialagogue like glycopyrrolate (Fig. 14–17) or atropine (Fig. 14–18).

Propofol (Fig. 14–19) is another drug that can be used for intravenous sedation for intubation or for induction of general anesthesia. It is given intravenously at doses of 2 mg/kg for induction of anesthesia. It rapidly produces anesthesia, but has a short duration of action after a single bolus due to redistribution of the drug. Like the barbiturates, propofol causes vasodilatation and myocardial depression and should be used with caution in patients unlikely to tolerate these effects. An additional problem with propofol is that it is insoluble in aqueous solution; the drug is prepared in a lipid emulsion for intravenous administration.

LOCAL ANESTHETICS

Local anesthetics are commonly used to anesthetize airway structures when an awake intubation is anticipated. Indications for awake intubation and the techniques are discussed in Chapter 15. A variety of sprays, gels, and ointments that contain local anesthetics are available. These agents markedly reduce the requirement for intravenous sedation during intubation and can be quite helpful in reducing patient discomfort in the intensive care unit, as well as in the emergency and operating rooms. Lidocaine (Fig. 14–23) is probably the most widely used agent.

Figure 14–22. Diazepam.

CHAPTER 15

The Basics of Awake Intubation

Allan P. Reed, M.D., and Don G. Han, M.D.

Awake intubation is the partial realization of patients' worst perioperative fears and the antithesis of their most profound perioperative desires. Among the concerns they experience preoperatively is the apprehension of perioperative pain.[1] Patients usually prefer general anesthesia,[1] which they anticipate will protect them from physical and emotional suffering. Each patient must comprehend the extraordinary circumstances that require awake intubation and he or she must be assured of the increased margin of safety offered by its use. Patients and physicians profit from an in-depth discussion of the specific indications for awake intubation in a particular case, as well as the possible adverse sequelae. Those at increased risk for airway obstruction, hypoxemia, upper airway trauma, cervical spinal cord damage, or dental damage generally comprehend the need for awake intubation and grant permission,[2, 3] despite understandable reservations. Those motivated by an appreciation of the dangers associated with intubation under general anesthesia tend to cooperate better during the procedure and harbor less ill will afterward. The common indications for awake intubation are summarized in Table 15–1 and are detailed in previous chapters.

PREMEDICATION

Modern patients are familiar with medical calamities of all kinds. Such knowledge evokes fears, some of which are valid and some of which are without foundation. As patients advance toward the operating room, anxiety sometimes degenerates into terror. Prior administration of sedatives is a benevolent attempt to mitigate the horrors experienced prior to surgery. Despite outward calm following premedication, extreme internal emotional distress may coexist. The goal is to achieve anxiolysis.[4] Fostering a good doctor–patient relationship is the best method of preventing preoperative terrors.[5] Patients who develop trust in their physician's expertise and caring personality tend to be more relaxed. Therefore, the preanesthetic interview provides an opportunity not only to comprehend the patient's physiologic requirements, but also to establish the personal chemistry that will flourish into a strong doctor–patient relationship. Conduct the interview in a sincere and unhurried manner. Although the anesthesiologist has experienced many similar scenarios, the patient has not. Matters that are routine to the physician are unique and overwhelming to the average patient. The investment of time into a professional relationship pays premiums in patient acceptance and cooperation later on.[6]

Although the emotional preparation of the patient depends on personal interactions, the physiologic preparation requires judicious use of medications. Although numerous drugs might be used, one inviolate concept exists:

Table 15–1 FREQUENTLY ENCOUNTERED INDICATIONS FOR AWAKE LARYNGOSCOPY AND INTUBATION

History of difficult intubation

    Large tongue (Mallampati/Samsoon class IV)[58, 59]
    Micrognatha
    Short muscular or obese neck
    Protruding maxillary incisors
    Decreased temporomandibular joint range of motion
    Combinations of the above[60]
    Decreased range of motion of cervical vertebrae
    Microsomia
    Prominent maxilla
    Laryngeal tilt
    Hoarseness and rheumatoid arthritis
    Thyromandibular distance

Trismus due to mechanical problems

Unstable cervical vertebrae

Trauma of the
    Face
        Small mouth opening
        Hematomas
        Lacerations
    Upper airway
        Hematomas
        Lacerations
    Cervical spine
        Instability

Congenital airway abnormalities
    Large fixed tongue
    Clefts
    High-arched palate

Upper airway tumors
    Cysts
    Hygromas
    Cancers
    Abscesses

dry the airway.[7] Abundant airway secretions represent a two-fold problem. Secretions further obscure an already limited view through the fiberscope. Although various suctioning maneuvers usually restore the view, elimination or reduction of this impediment facilitates intubation. Furthermore, awake intubation requires use of topical local anesthetics. In order for these agents to work effectively, they must actually contact the mucosa. An intervening layer of secretions prevents local anesthetics from reaching the intended areas, resulting in failed sensory blockade.[8] Moreover, copious secretions could wash local anesthetics away from a particular site, thereby severely limiting their duration of action. Topical local anesthetics applied to the airway are of varying benefit when antisialogogue premedication is withheld.[9]

The antisialogogues commonly employed in clinical practice are atropine, glycopyrrolate, and scopolamine. Their pharmacologic profiles are summarized in Table 15–2. Antisialogogues prevent additional discharge of secretions, but they do not eradicate secretions that have already collected. Therefore, even a rapid-acting medication such as atropine must be administered sufficiently far in advance in order to hinder further collections and to provide for elimination of previous collections. Antisialogogues are typically administered parenterally and are optimally received approximately 1 ½ hours prior to application of topical local anesthetics.[10] One of the most important side effects of antisialogogue use is arrhythmias. Because arrhythmias are more likely to occur after intravenous administration, it is advisable to give them intramuscularly, subcutaneously, or by mouth. Although scopolamine offers the additional benefits of added amnesia and sedation, its use is limited by a predilection toward delirium. Additional premedicants usually include benzodiazepines, butyrophenones, or narcotics. Patients with significant airway compromise often require conscious muscle tone to maintain airway patency. Sedating such patients in the nursing unit may seriously jeopardize their ability to oxygenate and ventilate. Airway collapse may occur when they are unmonitored and alone in their rooms or in an elevator while attended by unskilled paramedical personnel. Under such conditions, institution of prompt, life-saving treatment is unlikely. Consequently, patients with such severe airway diseases should receive only atropine or glycopyrrolate premedication. Additional medications can be administered judiciously under close supervision in the operating room.

SEDATION

In the operating room, monitoring devices and venous access are secured. Baseline monitoring generally consists of blood pressure measurement, pulse and respiratory rates, and observation of cardiac rhythm on an electrocardiogram (ECG) display and oxygen saturation on a pulse oximeter. Procedures that depend on patient cooperation, such as gargling with 4% lidocaine, are accomplished before the administration of intravenous sedatives. The partially sedated patient may be unable to comply with instructions to gargle and expectorate. Even worse, the sedated patient might aspirate. The primary goals for sedation during awake intubation are mainte-

Table 15–2. ANTISIALAGOGUES EMPLOYED IN COMMON CLINICAL PRACTICE

	Antisialogogue (dose in mg)	Onset	Duration	Side effects
Atropine	0.4–0.8 IV, IM, SQ, PO	IV = rapid IM, SQ, PO = 1–2 h	IM, SQ, PO = 4 h	Tachyarrhythmias, PVCs Urinary retention Decreases GI motility Hyperthermia Delirium
Glycopyrrolate	0.1–0.2 IV, IM, SQ 1–2 PO	IV = 1–4 min IM, SQ = 20–40 min PO = 6 h	IV = 2–4 h IM, SQ, = 4–6 h PO = 6 h	Tachyarrhythmias, PVCs Urinary retention Decreases GI motility
Scopolamine	0.3–0.6 IV, IM, SQ	IV = 1 min		Delirium or excitement Tachyarrhythmias Hyperthermia Amnesia Sedation

GI, gastrointestinal; IM, intramuscular; IV, intravenous; PO, *per os* (orally); PVCs, premature ventricular contractions; SQ, subcutaneous.

From Reed AP, Han DG. Preparation of the patient for awake intubation. Anesth Clin North Amer 9:71, 1991; with permission.

nance of spontaneous respiration, adequate oxygenation, and sufficient ventilation. The patient's ability to inspire deeply on command facilitates ventilation and oxygenation. Deep breaths also help to align the vocal cords, larynx, and fiberscope. Secondary goals include amnesia and the ability to cooperate with instructions to take deep breaths. Amnesia of potentially uncomfortable procedures is desirable for the patient's psychologic outlook toward repeated awake intubations and other medical care. Lingering negative recall of previous medically related experiences can create sufficient anxiety over upcoming events to dissuade patients from accepting further medical care. Induction of amnesia under these circumstances represents a humane attempt to prevent overwhelming anxiety from entering into further decision-making processes. It is not an attempt to hide information from the patient.

Narcotics, benzodiazepines, and butyrophenones are most commonly used to achieve these goals. Ketamine is rarely employed for this purpose; its associated copious secretions and postoperative hallucinations contraindicate ketamine for this use. The benzodiazepines' rapid onset of sedation and anterograde amnesia make them a desirable option for awake intubations.[11, 12] The popular benzodiazepines are midazolam, diazepam, and lorazepam. Although lorazepam provides the most profound sedating and amnestic properties, it is difficult to use because of its relatively long onset time, 5 to 20 minutes (Table 15–3). Midazolam and diazepam, with onset times of 3 minutes or less, are both easier to use than lorazepam. Regardless of the specific drug selected, small incremental doses are administered until achieving a sedated but cooperative state. The interval between successive doses should be at least equivalent to the drug's maximal onset time. Otherwise, the patient soon becomes oversedated, uncooperative, and apneic. Midazolam is supplied as a watersoluble compound, but diazepam is prepared in a propylene glycol[13] and benzoic acid formulation that frequently produces a burning sensation on injection and causes irritation of endothelial linings, which predisposes to thrombosis. The burning sensation can be prevented by mixing lidocaine with diazepam before injection.

Although not pharmacologically equivalent, benzodiazepines are sometimes replaced by butyrophenones. Droperidol is classically selected for this purpose. It provides unusual effects: droperidol permits the patient to tolerate painful procedures without recoiling from noxious stimuli. Contrary to some reports, droperidol is not a good amnestic.[14] Patients exposed to painful stimuli while receiving droperidol recall the events clearly. Its onset of peak action may require 20 minutes, predisposing to cases of overdose whenever incremental administration proceeds too rapidly. Side effects include anxiety, restlessness, unusual physical sensations, extrapyramidal signs, and hypotension.[15] The onset of extrapyramidal effects may be delayed for 6 to 12 hours, thereby manifesting postoperatively.[16] Another beneficial property of droperidol is that of antiemesis.

Narcotics provide additional sedation, anal-

Table 15–3. CHARACTERISTICS OF SEDATIVES COMMONLY EMPLOYED FOR AWAKE
LARYNGOSCOPY AND INTUBATION*

Sedatives	Pharmacologic actions	Dose	Onset time	Duration	Side effects
Benzodiazepines	Sedation Anterograde Amnesia Antiepileptic				
Midazolam		IV, IM = 5–7 mg (0.075 mg/kg)	IV = 1–3 min[12] IM = 15–30 min	IV, IM = 2 h	Respiratory impairment in high doses
Diazepam		IV = 2–7 mg (0.03–0.1 mg/kg) IM = not recommended PO = 3–11 mg (0.05–0.15 mg/kg)	IV = <3 min IM = 15–30 min PO = 30–60 min	IV = min–h[11, 13]	Respiratory impairment in high doses IV and IM injections are painful Thrombophlebitis
Lorazepam		IV, IM, PO = 1–4 mg	IV = 5–20 min IM = 30–120 min PO = 60–120 min	IV = 4–6 h IM, PO = 8 h	Respiratory impairment in high doses
Butyrophenones	Sedation Antiemetic[61] Indifference				
Droperidol		IV, IM = 0.625–10.0 mg	IV, IM = 5–20 min	IV, IM = 6–12 h[18]	Dysphoria[62] Extrapyramidal symptoms[63] Mild alpha-adrenergic antagonist Prolongs emergence from anesthesia
Narcotics	Analgesia Sedation				
Morphine		IV, IM, SQ = 2–10 mg	IV = 5–10 min IM = 30–60 min SQ = 30–90 min	1–6 h	Respiratory depression Bronchospasm Chest wall rigid Bradycardia Vomiting Hypotension Biliary spasm
Fentanyl		IV, IM = 50–100 μg	IV = 2 min IM = 10–15 min	IV, IM = 30–45 min	Similar to morphine Bronchospasm, hypotension, and biliary spasm are less common

*Dosages and times quoted represent broad generalities. They may be highly variable for any one patient. Consequently, slow careful titration is required in each case.
IM, intramuscular; IV, intravenous; PO, *per os* (orally); SQ, subcutaneous.
From Reed AP, Han DG. Preparation of the patient for awake intubation. Anesth Clin North Am 9:73, 1991; with permission.

gesia, and euphoria. They also depress laryngeal reflexes.[17] Although all narcotics share these properties, morphine and fentanyl have been used most often. The onset of action of intravenous morphine is approximately 10 minutes. Fentanyl's onset of action is only 2 minutes. In order to hasten an already time-consuming procedure, agents with shorter onset times are desirable. Narcotics generally produce respiratory depression and often result in bradycardia.

Adding narcotics to droperidol creates neuroleptanalgesia. Neuroleptanalgesia offers moderate degrees of analgesia, sedation, and cardiovascular stability. It requires close observation to protect from recall, hypoxia, hypercarbia, tachycardia, and hypertension. Achievement of the desired goals requires mul-

tiple incremental doses, allowing for the clinical effect of each dose prior to administering more. A combined preparation of fentanyl and droperidol (Innovar Janssen Pharmaceutica, Piscataway, NJ) is commercially available. Its exclusive use is ill advised. Multiple repeat doses of Innovar provide excessive and cumulative amounts of droperidol that may last for 6 to 12 hours or more.[18] Fentanyl's actions usually last only 1 to 2 hours, depending on multiple factors. Consequently, postoperative patients tend to experience prolonged emergence, dysphoria, and pain following large doses of Innovar. Once an appropriate dose of droperidol is attained, subsequent episodes of pain are best treated solely with narcotics.

When administered individually, neither narcotics nor benzodiazepines produce signifi-

Table 15–4. SENSORY INNERVATION OF UPPER AIRWAY SEGMENTS

Structure		Innervation
Nose		Trigeminal N (V)
Tongue	Anterior	Lingual N (V)
	Posterior	Glossopharyngeal N (IX)
Pharynx		Glossopharyngeal N (IX)
		Vagus N (X)
Upper larynx		Superior laryngeal N (X)
Vocal cords		Recurrent laryngeal N (X)
Lower larynx		Recurrent laryngeal N (X)
Trachea		Vagus N (X)

N, nerve.
From Reed AP, Han DG. Preparation of the patient for awake intubation. Anesth Clin North Am 9:75, 1991; with permission.

cant cardiovascular impairment. However, combinations of diazepam and high doses of fentanyl have been shown to produce decreases in myocardial contractility, systemic vascular resistance, heart rate, and cardiac output and hypotension.[19–21] Even at moderate and low doses of midazolam and fentanyl, a synergism exists that potentiates the effects of both drugs.[22] Analgesia for awake intubation is provided with local anesthetics. Consequently, it is unlikely that sufficiently high doses of fentanyl will be required in order to interact adversely with the cardiovascular system, even in combination with diazepam.

Midazolam was originally thought to have been relatively innocuous. However, it has been implicated in over 80 deaths. Its use in these cases had been for sedation during diagnostic or therapeutic procedures; opioids had been used concurrently in many of these cases. Morbidity was associated mostly with spontaneous ventilation in the absence of supplemental oxygen administration. Subsequently, midazolam's respiratory safety has been confirmed at doses of 0.05 mg/kg^{-1}. Fentanyl 2.0 mg/kg^{-1} resulted in hypoxemia in half of all patients tested and in depression of the CO_2 response curve, but in no incidences of apnea. The combination of these two drugs produced hypoxemia in almost all patients and apnea in half of the patients tested without depressing the CO_2 response curve more than that seen with fentanyl alone.

AIRWAY ANESTHESIA

Awake intubation entails manipulations that generally produce convulsant withdrawal, projectile vomiting, or ferocious coughing. Indi-

vidually, any of these reactions will prevent laryngoscopy and intubation. Therefore, a plan for blocking sensory input from the airway must be devised. Accomplishing this task in a logical manner requires an understanding of the sensory innervation to the upper airway.

The upper airway begins simultaneously at both the nose and mouth (Table 15–4). Afferent input from the nose is carried by the trigeminal nerve (V). Sensation from the tongue is divided between two nerves. The lingual nerve (V) supplies the anterior tongue, and the glossopharyngeal nerve (IX) supplies the posterior tongue. The pharynx receives sensory input from the glossopharyngeal nerve (IX) and the vagus nerve (X). The upper larynx is supplied by the superior laryngeal nerve (X). Both the vocal cords and lower larynx receive afferents from the recurrent laryngeal nerve (X). Lastly, the trachea is supplied by the vagus nerve (X). The superior laryngeal nerve actually divides into internal and external branches. The internal branch of the superior laryngeal nerve supplies sensory innervation from the inferior aspect of the epiglottis down to (but excluding) the vocal cords.[23] This segment is called the upper larynx. It also sends afferent fibers to the most proximal portions of the hypopharynx.[24] The external branch of the superior laryngeal nerve supplies only motor innervation and does so to only one muscle, the cricothyroid muscle.[25, 26] The recurrent laryngeal nerve carries both sensory and motor fibers. The sensory portion of this nerve is distributed to the vocal cords, lower larynx, and trachea. Its motor contributions go to all the laryngeal muscles except the cricothyroid muscle[27] (Table 15–5).

Table 15–5. INNERVATION OF THE LARYNX

Nerve	Function
Internal branch of the superior laryngeal (vagus N)	Sensory from the inferior aspect of the epiglottis to (but excluding) the vocal cords (upper larynx)
External branch of the superior laryngeal (vagus N)	Motor to the cricothyroid muscle
Recurrent laryngeal (vagus N)	Sensory from the vocal cords to lower larynx and trachea
	Motor to all laryngeal muscles except the cricothyroid muscle

From Reed AP, Han DG. Preparation of the patient for awake intubation. Anesth Clin North Am 9:75, 1991; with permission.

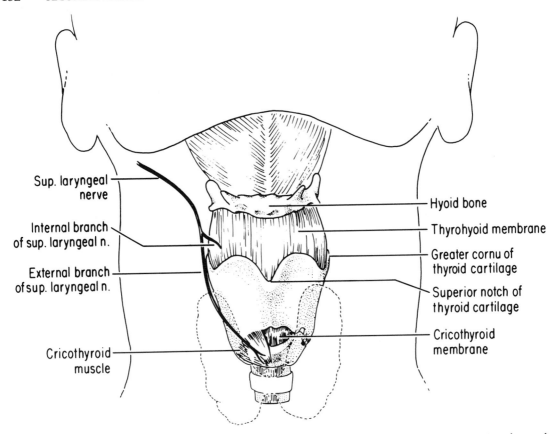

Figure 15–1. Anatomy of the anterior neck. (Adapted from Reed AP, Han DG. Preparation of the patient for awake fiberoptic intubation. Anesth Clin North Am 9:76, 1991; with permission.)

Sensory innervation of the upper airway is mediated by cranial nerves and their branches. Unlike major conduction anesthesia or perivascular anesthesia, upper airway anesthesia cannot be accomplished from any one central needle location. In fact, the cranial nerves that supply the airway are extremely difficult to anesthetize individually.

Numerous safe techniques of upper airway anesthesia exist and are divided into four major categories. In order of discussion, they are superior laryngeal nerve blocks, topical vasoconstrictors, topical local anesthetics, and transtracheal blocks.

Blockade of the Superior Laryngeal Nerve

The superior laryngeal nerve is a division of the vagus nerve (X). It courses inferiorly in the neck, running medial to the carotid artery. At the level of the hyoid bone, the superior laryngeal nerve dives deep to pierce the thyrohyoid membrane, which stretches from the hyoid bone to the thyroid cartilage. At about this point, the superior laryngeal nerve divides to produce an internal and an external branch.[28] The internal branch of the superior laryngeal nerve provides sensory innervation to the upper larynx, and the external branch of the superior laryngeal nerve gives off motor fibers to the cricothyroid muscle[25] (Fig. 15–1).

Sensory interruption of the superior laryngeal nerve is achieved at the level of the thyrohyoid membrane. The patient lies supine with the head extended. Labat's initial description of this nerve block used the hyoid bone as the primary landmark.[29] Unfortunately, the hyoid bone is difficult or impossible to feel in many patients. Also, it frequently requires deep palpation, which is uncomfortable for most individuals. Consequently, we prefer to employ the thyroid cartilage as the major landmark.[30, 31] The thyroid cartilage is located more superficially and is more readily identifiable.

The superior notch of the thyroid cartilage is commonly known as the Adam's apple. It is the most superficial aspect of the thyroid cartilage and is located in the midline. The superior notch of the thyroid cartilage is palpated and the operator's fingers are moved laterally across the neck until the end of the thyroid cartilage is identified. Prepare the skin over the greater cornu of the thyroid cartilage with isopropyl alcohol. Displace the thyroid cartilage laterally from the opposite side. Take a 3-mL syringe filled with 2 mL of 2% lidocaine and a 25-gauge needle and place the needle through the skin just above the greater cornu of the thyroid cartilage. Once there is resistance to passage of the needle, it lies at the greater cornu of the thyroid cartilage. "Walk" the needle off the greater cornu, in a superior direction. This places the needle between the greater cornu of the thyroid cartilage and the hyoid bone, the area through which the superior laryngeal nerve courses (Fig. 15–2). If an aspiration test does not yield blood or air, inject 2 mL of 2% lidocaine without epinephrine. Repeat this procedure on the opposite side. Depending on the relative positions of nerve and needle, the superior laryngeal nerve block may require 5 to 10 minutes for onset. In order to conserve time, perform this block first and attend to other matters while it is setting up. Its duration of action appears to be 4 to 6 hours when using 2% lidocaine.[30]

Another option is to perform superior laryngeal nerve blocks from the internal approach. A gauze sponge is soaked in 4% lidocaine and

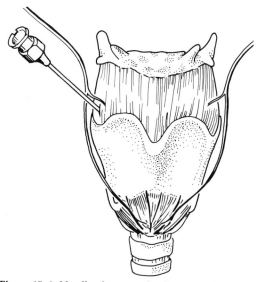

Figure 15–2. Needle placement for the external approach to the superior laryngeal nerve. (Adapted from Reed AP, Han DG. Preparation of the patient for awake fiberoptic intubation. Anesth Clin North Am 9:76, 1991; with permission.)

held with a Krause forceps. Have the patient open his or her mouth as wide as possible. Place the lidocaine-soaked sponge into the piriform fossa and hold it there for 5 minutes by the clock. This must be performed on both sides. The internal approach requires a minimum of 10 minutes and is only applicable to those patients who can open their mouths sufficiently wide.

Although originally designed as a treatment for painful laryngeal problems,[32] the superior laryngeal nerve block has found application providing analgesia for awake instrumentation of the airway during bronchoscopy, esophagoscopy, tracheal suctioning, and tracheal intubation.[24, 31–33] Most recently, superior laryngeal nerve block has been employed to facilitate passage of a transesophageal echocardiography probe in the awake patient.[32, 34] Whenever topical anesthesia to the upper larynx is inadequate, superior laryngeal nerve block improves patient comfort, reduces the total dose of topical local anesthetic required, and reduces the time required to successfully manipulate the upper larynx.[24]

Side effects of superior laryngeal nerve blocks are few. The most important potential complication is that of hematoma formation, which may arise from needle trauma to the superior laryngeal artery. The superior laryngeal artery courses with the internal branch of the superior laryngeal nerves as it pierces the thyrohyoid membrane. The bleeding, when it occurs, may be readily controlled with manual pressure over the site in question.[30] The close proximity of the superior laryngeal nerve and artery underscores the importance of careful aspiration prior to injecting local anesthetic.[25, 35] Other potential complications include needle penetration of the pharynx and needle plugging by cartilage.[31] Local infection or tumor are the only contraindications to this block.[35]

The external branch of the superior laryngeal nerve serves to tense the vocal cords. Simultaneous blockade of the external branch of the superior laryngeal nerve could theoretically result in difficulty in speaking.[25]

Vasoconstriction of the Nasal Mucosa

Instrumentation of the nose risks epistaxis. This includes passage of an endotracheal tube, fiberscope, or suction catheter. Even oral intubation risks epistaxis if laryngeal secretions must be suctioned through the nose. Once epistaxis occurs, visualization becomes impaired. Consequently, vasoconstriction of the nose should be considered, regardless of the intubation route intended.

Vasoconstriction of the nose is generally achieved with either cocaine or phenylephrine. For this purpose, cocaine has traditionally been used in concentrations as low as 4% and as high as 10%. Recent evidence suggests that 10% cocaine is associated with coronary artery vasoconstriction, diminished coronary blood flow, and an increase in myocardial oxygen demand.[36, 37] Because the potential risk of side effects is related to plasma levels, substitution of 4% cocaine for 10% cocaine should diminish the incidence of untoward reactions. Nevertheless, a small segment of the population is especially susceptible to cocaine toxicity because of impaired ability to hydrolyze the drug. Cocaine is degraded by serum cholinesterase, and the breakdown products are excreted in the urine. Quantitative or qualitative cholinesterase problems can impair cocaine metabolism, thereby effectively increasing plasma levels.[38] Although cocaine can be sprayed into the nose, application by cotton pledgets probably prevents excess absorption by limiting the amount that actually reaches alveoli.[39] Nevertheless, direct absorption from the nasal mucosa remains a theoretic possibility.[40] Cocaine-soaked cotton pledgets are introduced into both nares and then advanced slowly into the nasopharynx. Best results are obtained when pledgets remain in place for 10 minutes.

Phenylephrine is another commonly employed vasoconstrictor. It can be applied in concentrations ranging from 0.25% to 0.5%.[41] Although generally not commercially available, 0.5% phenylephrine solutions are readily formulated in any hospital. Phenylephrine is frequently supplied as a 1.0% solution. Simply add 1 mL of 1.0% phenylephrine to 1 mL of 4% lidocaine to manufacture the proper concentration of phenylephrine. Soak cotton pledgets in this solution and introduce them into both nares and advance into the nasopharynx as described for the cocaine solutions.

Alternatively, oxymetazoline can be substituted to help prevent epistaxis. Oxymetazoline is a pure alpha-adrenergic agonist that produces vasoconstriction of the nasal mucosa. It is not a controlled substance and therefore does not require the strict record keeping that is associated with employing cocaine. Oxymetazoline does not reduce catecholamine reuptake and therefore is devoid of euphoric effects, as well as of arrhythmogenic properties. Oxymetazoline is more effective than 4% lidocaine with 1:100,000 epinephrine or 10% cocaine for preventing epistaxis.[42] Therefore, oxymetazoline seems to represent a superior topical vasoconstrictor that eliminates the theoretic disadvantages of cocaine use. In actuality, side effects related to cotton pledget application of 4% cocaine to the nose seem to be minimal. The disadvantage of oxymetazoline is its lack of local anesthetic properties. When applied topically for vasoconstriction of the nares, oxymetazoline is used in a 0.05% concentration.

Topical Local Anesthetics

Topical local anesthetics are administered to either all or part of the airway. Nebulized 4% lidocaine easily and successfully anesthetizes the entire airway. Simply place 4 to 10 mL of 4% lidocaine into a nebulizer, flow oxygen through the nebulizer, and channel the nebulized lidocaine through a face mask. Instruct the patient to take deep breaths of the solution flowing through the oxygen mask. The nebulized lidocaine method is sufficiently effective to reduce the increases in heart rate and blood pressure that result from endotracheal intubation.[43, 44] Furthermore, this method prevents increases in intraocular pressure after laryngoscopy and intubation.[45] Although capable of producing profound anesthesia of the airway, inhalation of nebulized lidocaine usually requires 20 minutes or more to properly prepare the patient.

Alternatively, the anterior tongue, posterior tongue, and pharynx are anesthetized with 4% lidocaine administered by atomizer. Atomized lidocaine can be introduced deeper into the airway by administering each puff during a vital capacity inspiration. In fact, it is possible to anesthetize the entire airway using atomized 4% lidocaine or a similar agent.

Healthy children, especially those between 6 and 7 years of age, react adversely to local anesthetic sprayed into the larynx. Children are prone to severe bradycardia following this maneuver. Although preoperative intramuscular vagolytics do not protect against bradycardia, intravenous atropine or glycopyrrolate successfully block heart rate decreases under such circumstances.[46]

Topical local anesthetics necessitate employing high concentrations, which frequently travel to alveoli, where absorption is rapid.[47] Despite rapid absorption from alveoli, aerosolized lidocaine 4 mg kg^{-1} does not even produce therapeutic blood level (1 to 5 mg/mL).[48] Consequently, the likelihood of producing lidocaine toxicity from nebulized lidocaine 160 mg seems to be very low.

Anesthetic effects of topical lidocaine may last up to 1 hour in duration.[49] Onset time is between 1 and 5 minutes.[50, 51]

Alternatives to topical lidocaine include tetracaine, prilocaine, and benzocaine. Topical tetracaine is no longer recommended for total airway anesthesia because of its narrow margin of safety. The relatively large amounts of topical tetracaine required for total airway anesthesia are associated with toxic reactions. Topical prilocaine and benzocaine provide rapid onset and profound anesthesia. Unfortunately, they also produce significant methemoglobinemia. Pulse oximeters, which are used to guard against hypoxemia, overestimate oxygen saturation (SaO_2) in the face of methemoglobinemia.[52] Prilocaine and benzocaine are not only dangerous at the time of administration, but they continue to produce escalating levels of methemoglobinemia for up to 6 hours.[52]

Transtracheal Blocks

Transtracheal blocks furnish anesthesia of the vocal cords and trachea. Although rarely required, this method has enjoyed widespread use and is easily performed.

Permit the patient to lie supine with the head extended. Locate the Adam's apple, the midline superficial aspect of the thyroid cartilage, and run a finger inferiorly until a depression and another firm structure are appreciated. This depression is the cricothyroid groove, and the firm substance is the cricoid cartilage. A membrane runs from the cricoid cartilage across the groove to the thyroid cartilage and is called the cricothyroid membrane (see Fig. 15–1). Identify the cricothyroid groove and prepare the skin overlying it with isopropyl alcohol. Use a 3-mL syringe with 2 mL of 2% lidocaine and a 22-gauge needle. Insert the needle through the skin overlying the cricothyroid membrane and direct it posteriorly, until piercing the cricothyroid membrane. At this point, the needle bevel should reside within the trachea (Fig. 15–3). To confirm its proper location, simply aspirate air through the syringe. Warn the patient to expect vigorous coughing, and then rapidly inject the 2 mL of 2% lidocaine. Remove the needle immediately following injection. Coughing helps to spread the local anesthetic along the

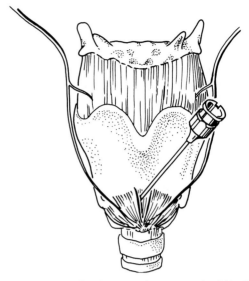

Figure 15–3. Needle placement for transtracheal block. (Adapted from Reed AP, Han DG. Preparation of the patient for awake fiberoptic intubation. Anesth Clin North Am 9:76, 1991; with permission.)

trachea and up against the inferior aspect of the vocal cords, thereby providing topical anesthesia to all these structures.[2] Significant amounts of local anesthetic also reach the alveoli, where it is rapidly absorbed. Successful transtracheal block is probably due to both topical anesthesia and, in some part, to local systemic absorption. Patients with good myocardial reserves and who are at increased risk for aspiration should not receive transtracheal blockade. Successful transtracheal block prevents coughing and expulsion of aspirated materials.[53]

The transtracheal block is minimally invasive and is associated with certain complications. Choking or gagging accompanies virtually all transtracheal blocks and is an anticipated side effect, not a complication of the procedure. Approximately 4% of blocks fail to produce adequate vocal cord anesthesia.[54] To improve sensory blockade, simply spray additional 4% lidocaine onto the vocal cords under direct vision.

If using a traditional, hand-held, retraction-blade laryngoscope, lidocaine is administered with an atomizer or syringe. If employing a fiberscope, then simply inject 1 to 2 mL of 4% lidocaine through the suction port. Allow several minutes for the lidocaine to take effect and instruct the patient to inspire deeply. As this is accomplished, the anesthetized vocal cords will abduct, allowing passage of the fiberscope or endotracheal tube.

Injection of local anesthetic into the trachea allows much of the solution to flow into the lungs, where alveolar absorption is rapid. High blood levels are achieved quickly, placing patients at risk for local anesthetic toxicity. Mechanical problems from needle placement are uncommon.[54] Although needles may break in the neck,[55] we have never seen this problem using 22-gauge needles. Puncture of the esophagus or other soft tissues has not led to problems. Hematoma formation from laceration of an aberrant artery that occasionally traverses the cricothyroid membrane is rare. Tracheocutaneous fistula formation is also extremely rare.[54]

Reflexes produce violent responses to foreign body invasion of the airway. Airway manipulations evoke coughing, vocal cord closure, withdrawal, and vomiting. Each one of these responses can hinder laryngoscopy and intubation. Traditional rigid laryngoscopy results in hypertension and tachycardia, and a correctly placed endotracheal tube predisposes to bronchoconstriction.[56] In the absence of deep general anesthesia, no amount of sedation can prevent these reactions to airway stimulation. Only profound sensory blockade offers conditions that are conducive to awake laryngoscopy and intubation. Awake intubation executed under successful airway anesthesia induces an average mean arterial pressure and heart rate increase of 10 mm Hg and 14 beats/min, respectively.[57]

References

1. Shevde K, Paoagopoulos G. A survey of 800 patients' knowledge, attitudes, and concerns regarding anesthesia. Anesth Analg 73:190–198, 1991.
2. Gold MI, Buechel DR: A method of blind nasal intubation of the conscious patient. Anesth Analg 39:257–263, 1960.
3. Ovassapian A, Dykes MHM. The role of fiberoptic endoscopy in airway management. Semin Anesth 6:93–104, 1987.
4. Norris W. The quantitative assessment of premedication. Br J Anaesth 41:778–784, 1969.
5. Egbert LD, Battit GL, Turndorf, Beecher HK. The value of the preoperative visit by an anesthetist. JAMA 185:553–555, 1963.
6. Leigh J, Walker J, Janaganathan P. Effect of preoperative anesthetic visit on anxiety. Br Med J 2:987–989, 1977.
7. Seward JB, Khandheria BK, Oh JK, Abel MD, Hughes BW, Edwards WD, Nichols BA, Freeman WK, Tajik AJ. Transesophageal echocardiography: Technique, anatomic correlations, implementation, and clinical applications. Mayo Clin Proc 63:649–680, 1988.
8. Geffin B. Anesthesia and the "problem upper airway." Int Anesthesiol Clin 28:106–114, 1990.
9. Laurito CE, Baughman VL, Becker GL, Polek WV, Riegler FX, Vade Boncouer TR. Effects of aerosolized and/or intravenous lidocaine on hemodynamic responses to laryngoscopy and intubation in outpatients. Anesth Analg 67:389–392, 1988.
10. Fassoulaki A, Kaniaris P. Does atropine premedication affect the cardiovascular response to laryngoscopy and intubation? Br J Anaesth 54:1065–1068, 1982.
11. Kortilla K, Lennoila M. Recovery and skills related to driving after intravenous sedation: Dose–response relationship with diazepam. Br J Anaesth 47:457–463, 1975.
12. Whitman JG, Al-Khudhain D, McCloy RF. Comparison of midazolam and diazepam in doses of comparable potency during gastroscopy. Br J Anaesth 55:773–777, 1983.
13. Greenblatt DJ, Koch-Wesen J. Intravascular injection of drugs. N Engl J Med 295:542–546, 1976.
14. Wolfson B, Skier ES, Wible LE, Dubnansky. Pneumonencephalography and neuroleptanalgesia. Anesth Analg 47:14–17, 1968.
15. Melnick B, Sawyer R, Karambelkar D, Phitayakorn P, Lim Uy NT, Patel R. Delayed side effects of droperidol after ambulatory general anesthesia. Anesth Analg. 69:748–751, 1989.
16. Patil VU, Stehling LC, Zauder HL. Fiberoptic Endoscopy in Anesthesia. Chicago: Year Book Medical Publishers, 1983; pp. 37–41.
17. Fry WA. Techniques of topical anesthesia for bronchoscopy. Chest 73:694–696, 1978.
18. Edmonds-Seal J, Prys-Roberts C. Pharmacology of drugs used in neuroleptanalgesia. Br J Anaesth 42:207–217, 1970.
19. Stanley THE, Webster LR. Anesthetic requirements and cardiovascular effects of fentanyl and fentanyl-diazepam-oxygen anesthesia in man. Anesth Analg 57:411–416, 1978.
20. Bailey PL, Willbrink J, Zwanikken P, Pace NL, Stanley TH. Anesthetic induction with fentanyl. Anesth Analg 64:48–53, 1985.
21. Tomichek RC, Rosow CE, Schenider RC, Moss J, Philbin DM. Cardiovascular effects of diazepam-fentanyl anesthesia in patients with coronary artery disease. Anesth Analg 61:217–218, 1982.
22. Ben-Shlomo I, Abdo-El-Khalim H, Ezry J, Zohan S, Tverskoy M. Midazolam acts synergistically with fentanyl for induction of anesthesia. Br J Anaesth 64:45–47, 1990.
23. Roberts JT. Fundamentals of Tracheal Intubation. New York: Grune & Stratton, 1983; pp. 23–26.
24. Gaskill JR, Gilles DR. Local anesthesia for peroral endoscopy using superior laryngeal nerve block with topical application. Arch Otolaryngol 84:654–657, 1966.
25. Durham CF, Harrison TS. The surgical anatomy of the superior laryngeal nerve. Surg Gynecol Obstet 118:38–44, 1964.
26. Roberts JT. Functional anatomy of the larynx. Int Anesthesiol Clin 28:101–105, 1990.
27. Ellis H, Feldman S. Anatomy for Anesthetists, 5th ed. Boston: Blackwell Scientific Publications, 1988; pp. 3–45.
28. Katz J. Atlas of Regional Anesthesia. Norwalk, CT: Appleton-Century-Crofts, 1985; p. 59.
29. Adriani J. Blocking of cranial nerves. In Labat's Regional Anesthesia: Techniques and Clinical Applications, 4th ed. St. Louis: Warren H. Green, 1985, pp. 187–191.
30. Gotta AW, Sullivan CA. Anaesthesia of the upper airway using topical anesthetic and superior laryngeal nerve block. Br J Anaesth 53:1055–1058, 1981.

31. Wycoff CC. Aspiration during induction of anesthesia: Its prevention. Anesth Analg 38:5–13, 1959.

32. Risk C, Fine R, D'Ambra MN, O'Shea JP. A new application for superior laryngeal nerve block: Transesophageal echocardiography. Anesthesiology 72:746–747, 1990.

33. DeMeester TR, Skinner DB, Evan RH, Benson DW. Local nerve block anesthesia for peroral endoscopy. Ann Thorac Surg 24:278–283, 1977.

34. Reed AP. Successful transesophageal echocardiography in an unsedated critically ill patient with superior laryngeal nerve blocks. Am Heart J 122:1472–1474, 1991.

35. Gotta AW, Sullivan CA. Superior laryngeal nerve block: An aid to intubating the patient with fractured mandible. J Trauma 24:83–85, 1984.

36. Lange RA, Cigarro RG, Yancy CW, Willard JE, Popma JJ, Sills MN, et al. Cocaine-induced coronary-artery vasoconstriction. 321:1557–1562, 1989.

37. Isner JM, Chokski SK. Cocaine and vasospasm. N Engl J Med, 321:1604–1606, 1989.

38. Verlander JM, Johns ME. The clinical use of cocaine. Otolaryngol Clin North Am 14:521–531, 1981.

39. Chiu YC, Brecht K, Das Gupta DS, Mhoon E. Myocardial infarction with topical cocaine anesthesia for nasal surgery. Arch Otolaryngol Head Neck Surg 112:988–990, 1986.

40. Pontiroli AE, Calderara A, Pozza G. Intranasal drug delivery—potential advantages and limitations from a clinical pharmacokinetic perspective. Clin Pharmacokinet 17:299–307, 1989.

41. Gross JB, Hartigan ML, Schaffer DW. A suitable substitute for 4% cocaine before blind nasotracheal intubation, 3% lidocaine–0.5% phenylephrine nasal spray. Anesth Analg 63:915–918, 1984.

42. Katz RI, Hovagim AR, Finkelstein HS, Grinberg Y, Boccio RV, Poppers PJ. A comparison of cocaine, lidocaine with epinephrine and oxymetazoline for prevention of epistaxis on nasotracheal intubation. J Clin Anesth 2:16–20, 1990.

43. Venus B, Polassani V, Pham CG. Effects of aerosolized lidocaine on circulatory responses to laryngoscopy and tracheal intubation. Crit Care Med 4:391–394, 1984.

44. Abou-Madi M, Keszler H, Yacoub O: A method for prevention of cardiovascular reactions to laryngoscopy and intubation. Can Anaesth Soc J 22:316–329, 1975.

45. Mostafa SM, Wiles JR, Dowd T, Bates R, Bricker S. Effects of nebulized lignocaine on the intraocular pressure responses to tracheal intubation. Br J Anaesth 64:515–517, 1990.

46. Ng WS. Pathophysiologic effects of tracheal intubation. In Latto IP, Rosen M (eds). Difficulties in Tracheal Intubation. Philadelphia: Bailliere Tindall, 1985; pp. 12–35.

47. Campbell D, Adriani J. Absorption of local anesthetics. JAMA 168:871–877, 1958.

48. Baughman VL, Laurito CE, Polek WV. Lidocaine blood levels following aerosolization and intravenous administration. J Clin Anesth 4:325–327, 1992.

49. Cohen MR, Levinsky WJ. Topical anesthesia and swallowing [letter]. JAMA 236:562, 1976.

50. Hamill JF, Bedford RF, Weaver DC, Colohan AR. Lidocaine before endotracheal intubation: Intravenous or laryngotracheal? Anesthesiology 55:578–581, 1981.

51. Delinger JK, Ellison N, Ominsky AJ. Effects of intratracheal lidocaine on circulatory responses to tracheal intubation. Anesthesiology 41:409–412, 1974.

52. Barker SJ, Tremper KK, Hyatt J. Effects of methemoglobinemia on pulse oximetry and mixed venous oximetry. Anesthesiology 70:112–117, 1989.

53. D'Hollander AA, Monteny E, Dewachter B, Sanders M, Dubois-Primo J. Intubation under topical supraglottic analgesia in unpremedicated and non-fasting patients: Amnesic effects of sub-hypnotic doses of diazepam and innovar. Can Anaesth Soc J 21:467–474, 1974.

54. Moore DC. Regional Block. A Handbook for Use in the Clinical Practice of Medicine and Surgery, 4th ed. Springfield: Charles C Thomas, 1981; pp. 321–324.

55. Adriani J. Labat's Regional Anesthesia Techniques and Clinical Applications, 4th ed. St. Louis: Warren H. Green, 1985, pp. 499–501.

56. Gal TJ, Suratt PM. Resistance to breathing in healthy subjects following endotracheal intubation under topical anesthesia. Anesth Analg 59:270–274, 1980.

57. Ovassapian A, Yelick SJ, Dykes MHM, Brunner EE. Blood pressure and heart rate changes during awake fiberoptic nasotracheal intubation. Anesth Analg 62:951–954, 1983.

58. Mallampati SR, Gatt SP, Gugino LD, Sesai SP, Waraksa B, Freiberger D, Liu PL. A clinical sign to predict difficult tracheal intubation: A prospective study. Can Anaesth Soc J 32:429–434, 1985.

59. Samsoon GLT, Young JRB. Difficult tracheal intubation: A retrospective study. Anaesthesia 42:487–490, 1987.

60. Rocke DA, Murray WB, Rout CC, Gouws E. Relative risk analysis of factors associated with difficult intubation in obstetric anesthesia. Anesthesiology 77:67–73, 1992.

61. Korttilla K, Kauste A, Auvinen J. Comparison of domperidone, droperidol, and metoclopramide in the prevention and treatment of nausea and vomiting after balanced general anesthesia. Anesth Analg 58:396–400, 1979.

62. Lee CM, Yeakel AE. Patient refusal of surgery following innovar premedication. Anesth Analg 54:224–226, 1975.

63. Patton CM. Rapid induction of acute dyskinesia by droperidol. Anesthesiology 43:126–127, 1975.

CHAPTER 16

Oral Intubation Techniques

James T. Roberts, M.D., M.A.

ROUTINE ORAL INTUBATION OF THE PATIENT WITH NORMAL ANATOMY

Preparation of the Patient

Foresight, provision, and training are the foundations for adroit intubation management. Cooperation, implying agreement and interaction, supports informed consent. Give patients as detailed a description as they desire of the benefits, risks, and complications of intubation. As physicians, we wish to free the patient from anxiety and discomfort, and not enhance such conditions. Even when patients desire an elaborate and extensive explanation of risks, we can still comfort them by informing them that we are prepared to avoid or to treat the existing risks.

Premedication, which is almost universally prescribed, is no substitute for dialogue with the patient. Drugs do help to calm a patient in a naturally anxiety-producing situation. Reassure patients. Do not deny a patient's anxiety by saying "now, don't be worried." Denial manages anxiety poorly. Recognize anxiety as a normal, legitimate response to a threatening situation. Tell the patient that there will be no surprises. Inform patients of what you intend to do before you do it. Premedicate with narcotics if the patient has pain or when you plan to do something painful to the patient.

Tranquilizers and sedatives are discussed in Chapter 14. Although often overlooked and underrated, positioning the patient promotes successful intubation. Proper positioning involves understanding the alignment of oral, pharyngeal, and tracheal axes. This changes with the head in the neutral position (Fig. 16-1), the head neutral with a pillow under the head (Fig. 16-2), and the head extended with a pillow under the head (Fig. 16-3). A pillow or blanket under the head aligns pharyngeal and laryngeal axes. Extension of the head aligns the oral axis with the pharyngeal-laryngeal axis to allow direct visualization of the laryngeal entrance.

Although usually supine, the patient may also be sitting, lateral, or prone. You may be unable to move the anesthetized patient to a supine position when he or she is inadvertently extubated during a surgical procedure.

General anesthesia, local anesthesia, and no anesthesia each has advantages and disadvantages for oral intubation. General anesthesia ensures patient cooperation; language barriers disappear, muscle relaxation improves with muscle relaxants, and amnesia results. Disadvantages include loss of reflex airway protection, rare reactions to the anesthetic or neuromuscular blocking agents, and perhaps even loss of an airway. Local anesthesia allows awake intubation, with the benefits of airway maintenance; positioning the patient awake;

158

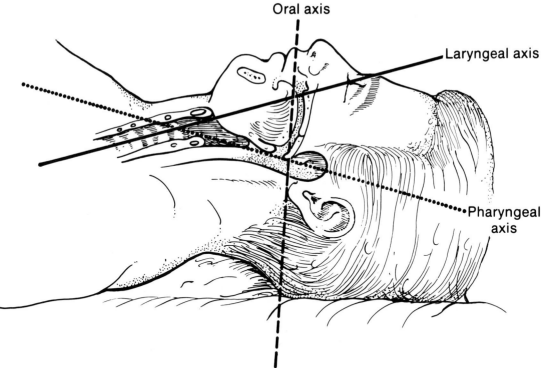

Figure 16–1. Head in neutral position. Oral, pharyngeal, and laryngeal axes are not aligned.

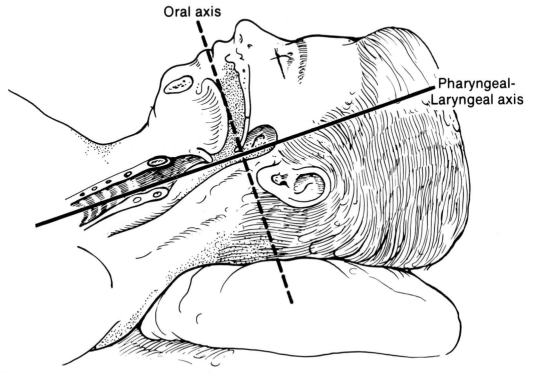

Figure 16–2. Head on a pillow in the neutral position; this gives cervical flexion, which aligns the pharyngeal and laryngeal axes.

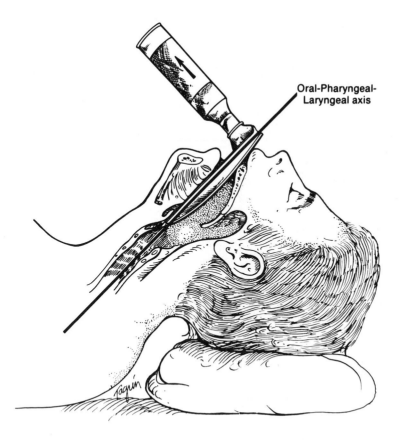

Oral-Pharyngeal-
Laryngeal axis

Figure 16–3. Placing the patient's head on a pillow with atlanto-occipital extension aligns the oral, pharyngeal, and laryngeal axes.

and avoidance of respiratory, cardiovascular, or central nervous system depression. Awake intubation is most difficult, however, without patient cooperation. Intubation without anesthesia may be appropriate in comatose patients, but remember that intubation may aggravate the cause of coma and that laryngospasm occurs more frequently without anesthesia. Patient preparation implies protection of the patient, our primary goal.

Access to the Airway: Laryngoscopy

Imagine intubating a patient using the equipment shown in Figure 16–4. The "endotracheal tube" was rigid and inserted into the larynx with no portion protruding from the mouth. Morbidity, mortality, and anxiety were high, but it was a beginning.

Examine the larynx directly. Laryngoscopes available for direct laryngoscopy are reviewed in Chapter 13. For routine oral intubation, master the use of two blades: the curved (MacIntosh) and the straight (Miller). Position the patient, as described, in the sniffing posi-

tion, with the head on a folded blanket, for the curved blade. Open the mouth with your fingers or extend the head. Avoid extending the head if you suspect a cervical spine injury. Hold the laryngoscope in your left hand, insert the blade in the right corner of the mouth, and visualize the right tonsillar fossa. Sweep the tongue to the left as you advance the blade to the midline, place the blade tip in the vallecula, and lift the laryngoscope up and away from you. Again, do not use this technique if you suspect cervical spine injury. This maneuver involves use of the triceps, rather than the stronger biceps muscle. If you fail to concentrate on producing the correct force vector, you naturally will use the upper teeth as a fulcrum for the laryngoscope. The prospect of inserting an endotracheal tube concentrates the mind on the laryngeal entrance. This, in combination with the natural propensity to use the biceps because of its greater strength, causes the careless clinician to produce force vector C in Figure 16–5. Practice and concentration help to overcome this natural tendency.

Apply a similar force vector to a laryngoscope with a straight blade. The tip of the straight blade, however, lifts the epiglottis

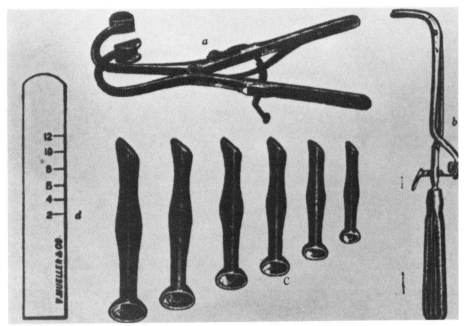

Figure 16–4. Equipment used for early endotracheal intubation.

from its posterior or dorsal side, rather than anteriorly, as described for the curved blade.

At times you may be unable to directly visualize the laryngeal opening. You may see only the tip of the epiglottis or the corniculate cartilages. In such cases, you must understand laryngeal anatomy to properly place an endotracheal tube (refer to Chap. 1). Should direct laryngoscopy fail, select another technique.

SPECIAL TECHNIQUES FOR ORAL INTUBATION

Useful Accessories

Learn to use several accessories for standard laryngoscope blades. The Huffman prism (see Fig. 11–4) clips to a #3 or #4 Macintosh blade and refracts light rays. It produces an upright

Figure 16–5. Optimal and sub-optimal force vectors for laryngoscopy.

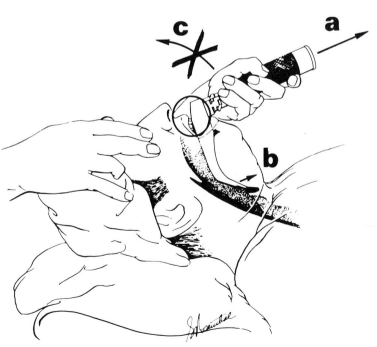

image of the tip of the blade, which is perhaps otherwise hidden from view with limited mouth opening or an anterior larynx. Placing the prism in warm water for 30 seconds or applying an antifog solution to it prevents fogging.

A Howland adapter (see Fig. 13–6) changes the force vector applied with the handle of a laryngoscope. Using the upper teeth as a fulcrum becomes more difficult; a "natural" motion is guided toward the correct force vector (vector A in Fig. 16–5). Both the blade and the handle hinge on the adapter. The adapter makes insertion of the blade into the mouth slightly more difficult, because the handle may now impinge on the chest wall.

Special Blades for Laryngoscopes

Special blades are described fully in Chapter 13. Insert these blades with force vectors similar to "standard" blades. With the Bizarri-Guiffrida blade (see Fig. 13–5), the absence of a ridge lessens the chance of injuring the upper teeth. Sometimes it appears that there are almost as many favorite varieties of blades as there are anesthetists.

Rigid Fiberoptic Laryngoscopes

The rigid fiberoptic stylette (see Fig. 16–6) has superb optics and a narrow diameter. Place an endotracheal tube over the stylette and guide it into the trachea. A standard laryngoscope facilitates introduction into the oral cavity. Gently pulling the tongue anteriorly also helps insertion. Although intended for difficult intubations, the instrument should not be used on patients suspected of having a neck injury, because extension of the neck may be required for its use.

Malleable Fiberoptic Stylette

The malleable fiberoptic stylette helps in oral intubation of the patient with a fractured cervical vertebra. Mold the curve of this stylette to the shape of the patient's oropharynx. Do not extend or flex the neck, but simply guide the stylette to the laryngeal opening. Prevent fogging of the lens by dipping the tip in warm water for 30 seconds immediately prior to use. Lubricate the stylette with an ointment or water-based lubricant. The malleable stylette does not contain a channel for suctioning secretions and administering oxygen or local anesthetics, as does the flexible fiberoptic laryngoscope.

Flexible Fiberoptic Laryngoscope

See Chapters 21, 22, and 23 for a full discussion of the use of the flexible fiberoptic laryngoscope.

Tracheal Guides

I formerly believed that the development of the flexible fiberoptic laryngoscope and malleable fiberoptic stylette made the use of a percutaneous retroguided tracheal guide wire passé. A skilled laryngoscopist, however, should have multiple methods at his or her disposal. A retrograde intubation may be particularly useful when blood fills the oral cavity and makes the use of a flexible fiberoptic instrument extremely difficult.

Digital Method

You may wish to direct an endotracheal tube into the larynx by palpation—the oldest method of introducing an endotracheal tube. Insert your middle finger and forefinger to palpate the posterior pharynx, perhaps the epiglottis. Guide the endotracheal tube between and along your fingers. Use the digital technique to intubate patients in abnormal positions.

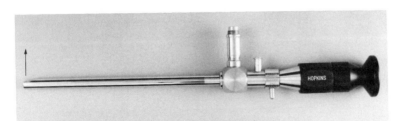

Figure 16–6. Rigid fiberoptic stylet.

Table 16–1. FOREWARNINGS OF A DIFFICULT
INTUBATION

Short muscular neck with full set of teeth
Receding lower jaw with obtuse mandibular angles
Protruding upper incisor teeth associated with relative
  overgrowth of premaxilla
Poor mobility of mandible
Long high-arched palate associated with long narrow
  mouth
Increased alveolar-mental distance necessitating wide
  opening of mandible
Small glottic opening
History of tracheal stenosis
Poor mobility of cervical vertebrae
Excessive anterior laryngeal tilt

Modified from Cass N, James N, Lines V. Difficult direct
laryngoscopy complicating intubation for anesthesia. Br Med J
1:488, 1956.

Abnormal Positions for Intubation

Reintubation with the patient in an abnormal position may be required when the patient is inadvertently extubated in the prone, lateral, or sitting position during general anesthesia. The emergency medical technician may be faced with the need to intubate a patient who cannot be removed from a motor vehicle involved in an accident.

No matter what the patient's position, direct your initial efforts toward ventilating the patient by mask; then work toward intubation. If the patient cannot be quickly and easily ventilated, intubated, or reintubated (in the prone position, for instance), stop surgery, turn the patient immediately to the supine position, then intubate (better to treat an infection with antibiotics than to explain an asphyxiation death to the patient's family). Reintubation is easier in the lateral than in the prone position, and easier in the left lateral than right lateral position; the tongue falls by gravity in the left lateral position, and laryngoscopes are designed to be held in the left hand. In the left lateral position, the endotracheal tube enters from the upper rather than the lower side, as would be the case in the right lateral position. A malleable stylette may be more useful than the standard laryngoscope for patients in the right lateral position. In the sitting position (for neurosurgical procedures), try the flexible fiberoptic laryngoscope for reintubation. You should, in any event, consider in advance how you would reintubate an inadvertently extubated patient in various positions.

SELECTION OF TECHNIQUE

The selection of the technique to be used is dictated by the clinical situation.

Predicting Difficult Intubation

Certain variations in normal anatomy predispose to difficult oral intubation. Cass and colleagues[1] listed six of these, and I have added four in Table 16–1.

Conditions Requiring Rapid-Sequence Induction of Anesthesia and Intubation

Intestinal obstruction, hematemesis, hiatal hernia (symptomatic), a full stomach, and preoperative vomiting all increase the likelihood of vomiting and aspirating gastric or esophageal contents. Empty the stomach with a nasogastric or Ewald tube prior to induction. This raises the question of intubation in the presence of a nasogastric tube. The advantages and disadvantages of leaving the nasogastric tube in place during rapid-sequence induction and intubation are listed in Table 16–2. The evidence strongly favors removal of the nasogastric tube under suction, immediately prior to intubation. You may, of course, intubate the awake patient using topical anesthesia prior to induction of general anesthesia. Use the Curry-Sellick maneuver to prevent regurgitation during rapid-sequence intubation attempts.

Removing a Sengstaken tube prior to intubation may flood the oral cavity with blood and make laryngoscopy impossible. Do an awake intubation in these cases.

Table 16–2. INTUBATION IN THE PRESENCE
OF A NASOGASTRIC TUBE FOR GENERAL
ANESTHESIA

Indications for Removal of Tube
It interferes with rapid sequence intubation
It breaks integrity of esophageal cardiac sphincter
It provides tract for vomitus to follow
Removal immediately before induction of anesthesia
  allows suctioning of stomach, esophagus, and
  pharynx as it is withdrawn
Ventilation by mask may be more difficult

Indications for Leaving Tube in Place
It decompresses stomach during intubation

Clinical Situations Making Oral Intubation Difficult

Facial Trauma

See Chapter 37 for a full discussion of facial trauma. Facial trauma may preclude the use of fiberoptic instruments. Blood obliterates the view through the laryngoscope. Avoid nasal intubation in cases of maxillary fracture. For awake patients with possible neck injury or facial trauma, use oral intubation. If the possibility of neck injury exists, avoid extending, flexing, or rotating the neck. Awake intubation allows the patient to tell you if you pinch the cervical cord (ie, cause pain). Intubate patients with mandibular fractures by a nasal route.

Tracheal Stenosis

See Chapter 29 for a full discussion of tracheal stenosis. In cases of tracheal stenosis requiring general anesthesia, induce anesthesia with a volatile agent and preserve spontaneous ventilation (Fig. 16–7). If intentionally paralyzed, such a patient may develop total airway obstruction.

Tomograms and magnetic resonance imaging (MRI) give some estimate of airway diameter and serve as a guide for selection of an appropriately sized endotracheal tube. In any event, have a complete array of tube sizes immediately available. Cricothyrotomy cannot be used to reestablish airway patency, because the obstruction to ventilation lies in the trachea, beyond this site. Agitation increases ventilation and negative inspiratory pressure, and tends to further collapse the tracheal wall and cut off the airway. *Calm the patient.* A similar situation exists in cases of epiglottitis. Calm agitated patients with airway obstruction.

Epiglottitis

In cases of epiglottitis, agitation causes further airway obstruction from increased negative pressure during inspiration. Calm, do not frighten, the child. If possible, have the mother hold the child. If you try to intubate an awake patient, you may completely lose the airway. Anesthesia and intubation should be performed by the most experienced anesthetist available.

Induce anesthesia gently and quietly, then intubate under direct vision. Remember, induction proceeds slowly because of reduced flow in the obstructed airway segment. Pre-

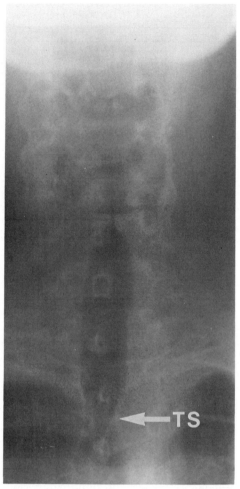

Figure 16–7. Frontal-sagittal section illustrating post-tracheostomy tracheal stenosis (TS) in a 55-year-old woman. (Courtesy of Jo-Anne O. Shepard M.D.)

mature attempts at laryngoscopy may precipitate laryngospasm.

Tumors of the Airway

Maintain spontaneous ventilation in patients with tumors of the airway. If you paralyze and control the patient's ventilation, the tumor may obstruct the airway completely. Tumor type and position dictate whether you intubate the patient awake or anesthetized.

Laryngeal Edema

Laryngeal edema may occur following extubation or after an airway burn. In cases of a burned airway, intubate early in the course of hospitalization or risk not being able to find the laryngeal opening (Fig. 16–8).

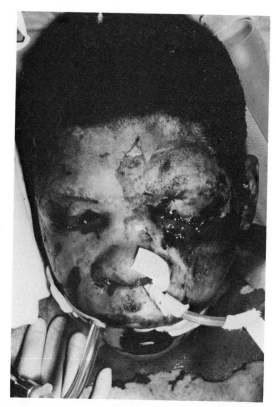

Figure 16–8. Post-burn with facial as well as laryngeal edema. It is key to intubate such a patient as early as possible. (Courtesy of Dr. Charles Coté.)

to the fistulous tract. Positioning the cuff proximal to the opening, if you control ventilation, will inflate the stomach and force the stomach contents into the trachea. Do not paralyze the patient until a cuffed endotracheal tube secures the airway beyond the fistula.

Pneumothorax

Pneumothorax deviates the trachea and lowers the larynx in the chest cavity (the trachea deviates toward the side of the pneumothorax). Beware—controlled ventilation after intubation may convert the pneumothorax into a tension pneumothorax.

Thoracic Aortic Aneurysm

A thoracic aortic aneurysm may compress the tracheal wall and make a smaller size endotracheal tube necessary (Fig. 16–10). Minimize blood pressure rise during intubation. The rise in blood pressure after intubation under deep thiopental (Pentothal) anesthesia is shown in Figure 16–11. Prevent reflex hypertension by topically anesthetizing the upper airway, by intravenous injection of lidocaine or esmolol, or by the use of a peripheral vasodilator. Monitor intra-arterial pressure closely.

Cervical Arthritis

Cervical arthritis may accompany temporomandibular arthritis. Inability to manipulate the neck makes the use of a standard laryngoscope difficult. The flexible fiberoptic laryngoscope neatly overcomes the problem.

Undersized Trachea

It is difficult to predict an undersized trachea except from past history or fortuitous radiographic diagnosis. Cadaver studies have shown tracheal size is unrelated to body size or habitat. Intubation was attempted in the patient in Figure 16–9, and the endotracheal tube just would not pass. The tube would not traverse the glottis until a smaller size (#6) was used.

Tracheo-Esophageal Fistula in Adults

In cases of adult tracheo-esophageal fistula, position the cuff of the endotracheal tube distal

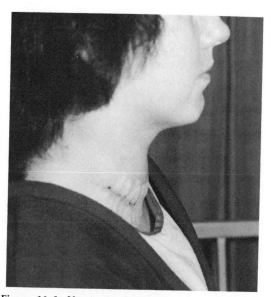

Figure 16–9. Unsuspected difficult intubation. Young patient for parathyroid surgery would accept no larger than a 6.0-mm endotracheal tube.

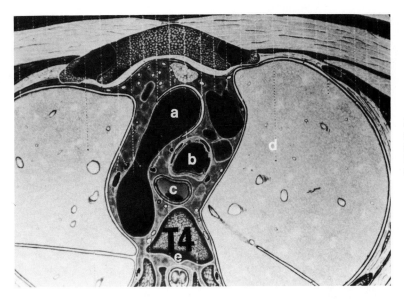

Figure 16–10. Note the proximity of the aortic arch to the trachea at the T4 level. Enlargement of the aorta at this level can easily compress the tracheal lumen.

Thyroid Enlargement

Unilateral thyroid enlargement causes contralateral deviation of the larynx. Following thyroid surgery, check for damage to the recurrent laryngeal nerves (Fig. 16–12). Damage to one nerve causes hoarseness; damage to both causes airway obstruction from unopposed action of the cricothyroideus muscles innervated by the superior laryngeal nerves. Beware of thyroid storm initiated by intubation of seriously hyperthyroid patients.

Cystic Hygroma

A patient with cystic hygroma is shown in Figure 16–13. As it turned out, this was not a terribly difficult intubation. Looking at the size of the mass, one would have expected otherwise.

Loose Teeth

The design of most rigid laryngoscopes leads the unskilled to use the upper teeth as a fulcrum. Check teeth before, as well as immediately after, intubation. Document their condition in the chart. Immediately retrieve a chipped or lost tooth during laryngoscopy, rather than force the patient to undergo a second anesthetic for this purpose.

Enlarged Tonsils

You may easily lacerate enlarged tonsils with the tip of the laryngoscope blade, or avulse an enlarged adenoid during nasal intubation. Hemorrhage may be excessive, and reintubation for control of bleeding after tonsillectomy may be hazardous. Consider awake oral intubation for these patients.

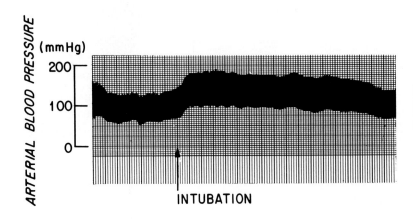

Figure 16–11. Typical rise in blood pressure after endotracheal intubation under general anesthesia.

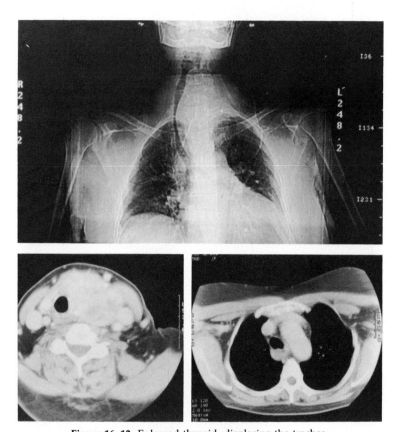

Figure 16–12. Enlarged thyroid, displacing the trachea.

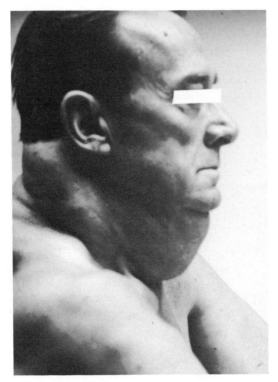

Figure 16–13. Cystic hygroma patient.

BEFORE   AFTER

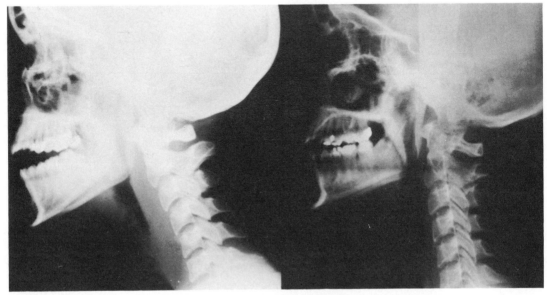

Figure 16–14. Ludwig's angina.

Pharyngeal Abscess

A case of Ludwig's angina is shown in Figure 16–14. Radiographs demonstrate anterior displacement of the larynx. Blind nasal intubation may rupture the abscess and spread the contents to the lungs. Gentle laryngoscopy and intubation under direct vision minimizes the risk of rupturing an abscess.

POSITIONING ORAL ENDOTRACHEAL TUBES

Single-Lumen Endotracheal Tubes

Preliminary placement of a single-lumen endotracheal tube should be done under direct vision. The tip of a standard tube should be placed in the middle third of the trachea.[2] Inflate the cuff. If an air leak exists despite a large amount of air in the cuff, reposition the cuff, probably further through the vocal cords. Deflate the cuff, advance the endotracheal tube slightly, then reinflate the cuff. A smaller amount of air should now prevent air leak. With the tube in position, be wary of encouraging an associate to "not let the tube come out." This encourages the person holding the tube in place to advance the tube so as not to let it come out. After taping the tube in place, auscultate both lungs, as well as the area over the stomach. Use only enough air in the cuff to prevent a leak. Cuff pressures in excess of 30 cm H_2O may compromise blood flow to tracheal mucosa.

Double-Lumen Endotracheal Tubes

Double-lumen tubes, designed for insertion into either the right or left mainstem bronchi, improve surgical access to the operative field by letting one lung collapse. These tubes use a tracheal as well as a bronchial cuff. Both the Carlens tube and the White tube hook onto the carina to guide positioning.

Use the following guidelines for placement of double-lumen tubes:

1. Place a stylet into the tracheal lumen.
2. Insert the tube into the mouth concave side up.
3. Rotate the endotracheal tube 180 degrees to facilitate passage of the tip through the glottic opening.
4. Rotate the tube 90 degrees as you advance the bronchial tube into the appropriate bronchus.
5. Position the contralateral bronchial orifice between the tracheal and bronchial cuffs.
6. Inflate the tracheal cuff and ventilate both lungs.
7. Clamp the Cobb extension with a hemostat, have the port open to the air, and ventilate the lung. Inflate the bronchial cuff to the point of no air leak through the open port.
8. Clamp the Cobb extension to the bronchial portion, then open the corresponding port to air.
9. Control ventilation to the other lung without a leak through the open port.
10. Remove the clamp and ventilate both lungs until it is appropriate to collapse one of the lungs, preferably not the one whose bronchus has been intubated. Open the bronchial Cobb extension to air to allow passive collapse of the nonintubated lung.

Whether a right-sided or left-sided tube is chosen is usually not important for a lobectomy. Do not, however, insert the bronchial tube into the side of the operation for a pneumonectomy.

For practice detecting malpositions of double-lumen tubes, match the descriptions of ventilation defects listed in Table 16–3 with the appropriate malposition schematic in Figure 16–15.[3] See Table 16–4 for correct answers.

Table 16–3. MALPOSITIONS OF DOUBLE-LUMEN ENDOTRACHEAL TUBES

Match the findings to the proper panels in Figure 16–15

Case 1
Left-sided tube (Answer _____)
 Bronchial lumen clamped—left side ventilates; right
  side no flow.
 Tracheal lumen clamped—right side ventilates; left
  side no flow.

Case 2
Left-sided tube (Answer _____)
 Bronchial lumen clamped—restricted flow both
  sides.
 Tracheal lumen clamped—both sides ventilate
  equally.

Case 3
Left sided tube (Answer _____)
 Bronchial lumen clamped—air into both sides; no air
  out.
 Tracheal lumen clamped—left side ventilates, right
  side slight ventilation.

Case 4
Left-sided tube (Answer _____)
 Bronchial lumen clamped—equal restricted flow to
  both sides.
 Tracheal lumen clamped—equal restricted flow to
  both sides.

Case 5
Right-sided tube (Answer _____)
 Bronchial lumen clamped—left side ventilates, right
  side traps air.
 Tracheal lumen clamped—right lung ventilates.

Case 6
Left-sided tube (Answer _____)
 Bronchial lumen clamped—right side restricted
  ventilation.
 Tracheal lumen clamped—left side ventilates.

Case 7
Left-sided tube (Answer _____)
 Bronchial side clamped—right side ventilates, left
  side ventilates poorly.
 Tracheal lumen clamped—both sides ventilate, right
  much more than left.

Case 8
Left-sided tube (Answer _____)
 Bronchial lumen clamped—flow to both sides
  blocked.
 Tracheal lumen clamped—both lungs ventilate
  equally.

Case 9
Left-sided tube (Answer _____)
 Bronchial lumen clamped—completely obstructed
  flow to both sides.
 Tracheal lumen clamped—right side ventilates.

Case 10
Left-sided tube (Answer _____)
 Bronchial lumen clamped—equal restricted flow to
  both sides.
 Tracheal lumen clamped—completely obstructed
  flow.

Case 11
Left-sided tube (Answer _____)
 Bronchial lumen clamped—right side ventilates.
 Tracheal lumen clamped—left side ventilates, gas
  trapping on right side.

Modified from Black A, Harrison G. Difficulties with positioning Robertshaw double lumen tubes. Anaesth Intensive Care 3:299, 1975.
The answer key is found in Table 16–4.

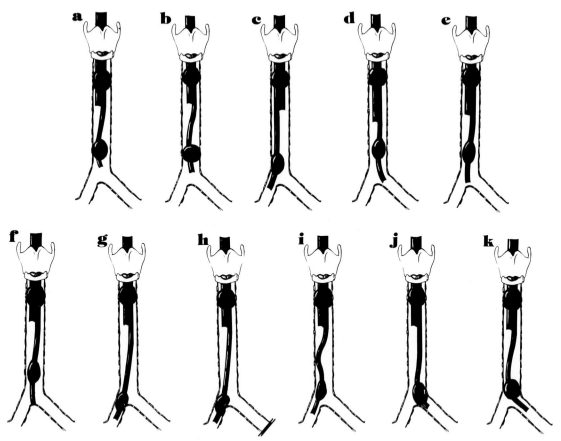

Figure 16–15. Schematic showing relative double-lumen endotracheal tube malpositions. Match the appropriate description of ventilation defects in Table 16–3 with the appropriate answer in Figure 16–15.

Table 16–4. ANSWERS: MALPOSITIONS OF DOUBLE-LUMEN ENDOTRACHEAL TUBES

The case descriptions in Table 16–3 match the pictures in Figure 16–15 as follows:

Case 1: G
Case 2: A
Case 3: K
Case 4: E
Case 5: C
Case 6: J
Case 7: I
Case 8: B
Case 9: H
Case 10: F
Case 11: D

For further discussion refer to Black A, Harrison G. Difficulties with positioning Robertshaw double lumen tubes. Anaesth Intensive Care 3:299–311, 1975.

References

1. Cass N, James N, Lines V. Difficult direct laryngoscopy complicating intubation for anesthesia. Br Med J 1:488, 1956.
2. Conrardy P, Goodman L, Lainge F, et al. Alteration of endotracheal tube position (flexion and extension of the neck). Crit Care Med 4:8–12, 1976.
3. Black A, Harrison G. Difficulties with positioning Robertshaw double lumen tubes. Anaesth Intensive Care 3:299–311, 1975.

CHAPTER 17

The Nasal Approach to Intubation

Takahisa Goto, M.D., and James T. Roberts, M.D., M.A.

Oral intubation is by far the most common technique of airway management. Nasal intubation is needed when the oral approach is either impractical or impossible, which often means that the airway is compromised and difficult. Many patients in the critical care setting are nasally intubated for prolonged ventilatory support, and this poses peculiar problems, such as paranasal sinusitis. In this chapter, basic as well as practical aspects of nasal intubation are discussed.

ADVANTAGES AND DISADVANTAGES OF NASAL INTUBATION

Before discussing the indications for nasal intubation, it is helpful to know its advantages and disadvantages, especially in comparison with oral intubation.

Advantages

The endotracheal tube is more easily secured, and the nasal passage itself helps keep the tube in place. Also, there is less risk of kinking. Nasal intubation is usually tolerated better by the awake patient. Nursing care is also easier. An orally placed tube is very irritating and increases the secretions in the mouth; it also disturbs the movement of the lips and makes communication more difficult. Nasal intubation eliminates the possibility of occlusion of the tube. Blind placement can be performed in a neutral head and neck position without general anesthesia or muscle paralysis, and can be performed in the uncooperative patient.

Disadvantages

Nasal intubation is more time-consuming than the oral approach. This is a serious disadvantage when the patient is in life-threatening respiratory failure or at a very high risk of aspiration. Aspiration can occur in less than 5 seconds, whereas nasal intubation takes longer. Oral intubation is the first choice if immediate establishment of the airway is necessary (for example, during cardiopulmonary resuscitation [CPR]) or if aspiration is a serious concern.

The nasal tube is smaller and longer than the oral tube and has higher resistance to air flow because the tube diameter is limited by choanal size. This causes a significant increase in breathing work, which may not be tolerated by critically ill patients and hence may reduce the probability of successful weaning from mechanical ventilation. Bolder and colleagues[1] reported that a 1 mm decrease in tube size resulted in an increase in breathing work of 34% to 150%.

There are some complications that are associated only with nasal intubation, such as paranasal sinusitis and nasal bleeding. These complications are discussed later in this chapter.

INDICATIONS

Inability to Open the Mouth

There are two main reasons for inability to open the mouth: pain or anatomic abnormalities. Pain is not a real indication for nasal intubation. You can anesthetize the patient first, then open the mouth and perform oral intubation.

If anatomic abnormalities such as perioral contracture scar or temporomandibular ankylosis make the mouth opening inadequate, nasal intubation is mandatory. If the patient does *not* have a full stomach, you can anesthetize the patient by either volatile or intravenous anesthetic, secure the airway by mask, then try either blind nasal or fiberoptic intubation. Awake intubation is necessary if the patient has a full stomach, or the airway will be compromised further by anesthetizing the patient.

Oral and Mandibular Surgery

Nasal intubation is beneficial, especially when the oral tube obstructs the view of the surgical field. If the mouth is to be wired or banded shut after surgery, a nasal tube must be used. The patient should be wide awake with full airway reflex before extubation. Scissors should be always at the patient's bedside to cut arch bar rubber bands in an emergency.

Anticipated Prolonged Intubation

As has been discussed in the section on the advantages of nasal intubation, better tube fixation, lower risk of kinking, greater comfort to the awake patient, and easier nursing care all make nasal intubation a preferable choice for prolonged intubation. When long-term postoperative ventilatory support is planned, the oral tube can be changed to the nasal tube at the end of the operation.

Laryngeal injury (vocal cord ulceration and crating) following extubation of the trachea has been reported to be less frequent and severe after nasal than oral tracheal intubation.[2] This may be due to the use of smaller tracheal tubes for nasal intubation and better stability, so that nasal tube movement is less likely with changes in head position.

Intubation Without Direct Laryngoscopy

In unstable patients, it may be preferable to avoid the stimulus of direct laryngoscopy or the cardiovascular and respiratory depressive effects of sedatives used to cover that stimulation (for example, when the patient in the emergency room with full stomach and unstable circulation needs semi-emergency intubation). Fiberoptic (nasal or oral) and blind nasal intubation are good techniques in these situations. Blind nasal intubation is also a good choice for the patient with oral trauma and bleeding that make visualization of the cords by laryngoscopy difficult.

CONTRAINDICATIONS

Skull Base Fracture or Cerebrospinal Fluid Leakage

Skull base fracture and cerebrospinal fluid (CSF) leakage are associated with higher risk of meningitis after nasal intubation. Migration of the endotracheal tube into the brain has also been reported.

Coagulopathy

Nasal intubation is often complicated with nasal bleeding, which is very difficult to stop if coagulopathy exists.

Other Contraindications

Severe nasal pathology and immunocompromise are other contraindications to nasal intubation. Prolonged intubation is associated with a high rate of paranasal sinusitis, which is sometimes very difficult to diagnose and can be a hidden source of sepsis or meningitis. Use of corticosteroids is also known to enhance the risk of sinusitis.

Table 17–1. COMPLICATIONS PECULIAR TO NASAL INTUBATION

Paranasal sinusitis
Nasal bleeding
Dissection of posterior pharyngeal wall mucosa
Dislodgement of pharyngeal tonsils (adenoids)
Pressure necrosis of external naris
Otitis due to auditory tube obstruction
Bacteremia

COMPLICATIONS

The complications of endotracheal intubation are discussed in detail in Chapter 41. In this section, complications peculiar to nasotracheal intubation are discussed (Table 17–1).

Paranasal Sinusitis

Recently, sinusitis has been recognized more frequently as a significant complication of nasal intubation. O'Really and associates[3] reported a 27% incidence of sinusitis after nasal intubation of more than 5 days. Prolonged nasotracheal intubation causes edema and occlusion of sinus drainage pathways, either by irritation of nasal mucosa or by direct mechanical obstruction by the tube. The normal flora of the sinuses become pathogenic when trapped in a closed space.[4]

Prompt diagnosis and treatment is paramount in managing sinusitis. If properly treated, most patients take a benign course and improve in a few days. Delay in diagnosis, however, can result in life-threatening sequellae such as meningitis, systemic sepsis, and pneumonia by the seeding of bacteria from sinuses.[5]

Diagnosis requires a high index of suspicion.[6] Sinusitis should be suspected whenever the nasally intubated patient is in a clinically septic course (ie, fever, leukocytosis, persistent hypermetabolism) and has no demonstrable source of infection. Purulent nasal drainage is a reliable clue, but is present in only 30% of the patients with sinusitis.[4] Facial tenderness, pain, and headache are very common complaints of outpatient sinusitis,[7] but often are very difficult to assess in nasally intubated patients because of the altered consciousness level and inability to talk.[8]

Diagnostic tests include sinus radiograph, computed tomography (CT) scan, and aspiration of sinus fluids. Signs on sinus radiograph and CT scan are mucosal thickening, sinus opacification, and the air–fluid level within the sinus (Fig. 17–1). To get the maximum diagnostic accuracy by sinus radiograph, Waters's view should be added to the standard four-view sinus series; this increases the confidence level from 24% to 88%.[7–9] A sinus radiograph can be obtained as a portable study in the critical care setting, without transporting the patient to the radiology area.

Involvement of the sphenoid or ethmoid

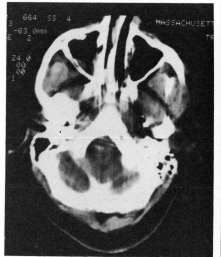
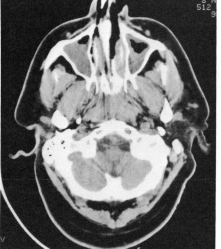

Figure 17–1. Computed tomography (CT) scan illustrating sinusitis. This head CT scan (*left*) of a motor vehicle accident victim shows clear maxillary sinuses on both sides. After nine (9) days of nasal endotracheal intubation and nasogastric tube placement, this patient (*right*) developed sinusitis as evidenced by opacification and air/fluid level in bilateral maxillary sinuses.

sinus is better evaluated by CT scan.[10–12] A sinus CT scan can be obtained simultaneously with scans of the chest or abdomen during a sepsis evaluation, or with head CT when the neurologic status of the patient warrants it.

The immediate and the most important treatment is to remove the nasotracheal and nasogastric tube and to switch to oral tube or trachostomy. Nasal decongestants may also be beneficial.

Antibiotics should be best administered according to the sensitivity of the organisms isolated from the sinus. Hospital-acquired organisms in the compromised patient, who usually is receiving broad-spectrum antibiotics, may be highly resistant to anti-microbial therapy. *Staphylococcus aureus,* Enterobacter, *Pseudomonas aeruginosa,* and other Gram-negative organisms are common,[13] and the infection is often polymicrobial. *Streptococcus pneumoniae* and *Haemophilus influenzae,* which are the main causative bacteria in outpatient acute sinusitis,[7] are rather rare. The isolated organisms from the sinus are different from those from lower respiratory tract secretions in more than half of the cases, and the cultures of tracheal secretions are of limited help.

Surgical drainage of the involved sinuses may be necessary in refractory cases.

Nasal Bleeding

To minimize the risk of nasal bleeding, use of vasoconstrictor (4% cocaine, 3% lidocaine–0.25% phenylephrine, or 2% lidocaine with 1:200,000 epinephrine) is highly recommended. Lubrication of the endotracheal tube also minimizes nasal bleeding.

If nasal bleeding occurs, it is probably wise to leave the tube in place to act as a tampon. In some instances, the tube may be withdrawn so that only the cuff remains in the naris; subsequent cuff inflation then tamponades the bleeding site. If the tube is removed, severe bleeding may occur and impair the visualization of the cords at the subsequent intubation attempt, or even jeopardize the ventilation.

Dislodgment of Pharyngeal Tonsils

Pharyngeal tonsils (adenoids) may be prominent, especially in children, and produce resistance to passage through the nasopharynx or bleeding if they are traumatized. If the adenoids are too large, nasotracheal intubation should be done under direct vision to prevent carrying a dislodged piece of tonsil into the trachea with the tube.

Bacteremia

The incidence of bacteremia after nasal intubation is reported to be between 5.5% and 17%.[5, 14, 15] Normal upper airway flora may enter into the circulation via traumatized nasal mucosa or may be transported by the tube from nose to trachea and enter into the circulation via vascular tracheal mucosa. If nasal intubation is planned for the patient with heart disease or a prosthetic valve who is at an increased risk of bacterial endocarditis, prophylactic antibiotics may be needed.

TECHNIQUE

Because most instructions for oral intubation apply equally to nasal intubation, they are not repeated in their entirety here. Positioning the patient, preoxygenation, laryngoscopy technique, correct depth of tube insertion, and marking and securing the tube are the same for either method.

Preparation of the Patient

First, the patient should be asked to judge which nasal passage is larger by alternately occluding each nostril and determining the ease of breathing through the open one. If awake intubation is planned, explain the procedures thoroughly to the patient so that good cooperation can be obtained.

Anesthesia is provided to both nares with 4% cocaine, 0.25% phenylephrine containing 3% lidocaine, or even 2% lidocaine with 1:200,000 epinephrine (which is most readily available). These local anesthetics also have vasoconstricting properties, which make the nasal passage larger by causing shrinkage of nasal mucosa and thereby help the passage of endotracheal tube and minimize the risk of bleeding. Using 3% lidocaine with 0.25% phenylephrine has been shown to be as effective as 4% cocaine in preventing epistaxis and hemodynamic responses associated with nasal intubation.[16] Because of the potential problems of systemic toxicity and illicit use of cocaine, lidocaine with phenylephrine is now used at the Massachusetts General Hospital. This nasal preparation should be done to both nares in case the endotracheal tube cannot be passed through the selected nostril or in case a nasogastric tube needs to be placed through the other side.

Topical spray of a local anesthetic to pharynx, superior laryngeal nerve block, and transtracheal block may also be performed to provide comfort to the awake patient and to minimize coughing and gagging. Adequate intravenous sedation may be given. Remember that intravenous sedation is *not* a substitute for good topical anesthesia. Intravenous sedation should be minimized in patients with a full stomach or a compromised airway. Superior laryngeal nerve block and transtracheal block are contraindicated in the full-stomach patient.

A soft, well-lubricated nasal airway may be inserted into the selected nare before the endotracheal tube is placed in order to dilate the nasal pathway even more and to evaluate the appropriate size of the endotracheal tube.

Topical anesthesia of the nose and vasoconstriction should also be used for nasal intubation under general anesthesia. Preoxygenation is even more important than in oral intubation, because nasal intubation usually takes longer.

Tube Selection

Select a tube 0.5 to 1.0 mm smaller in inner diameter than that for oral intubation. In an adult, a 7.0- to 7.5-mm inner diameter tracheal tube is usually adequate. For detailed discussion about the design of endotracheal tubes, see Chapter 12.

Technique

Three approaches to nasotracheal intubation are commonly used. Blind nasal intubation was the technique of choice prior to the development of useful laryngoscopes. This was followed by direct laryngoscopy, and only recently by flexible fiberoptic laryngoscopy. In this section, the first two are discussed. For detailed discussion of flexible fiberoptic laryngoscopy, see Chapters 21 through 23.

Direct Laryngoscopy

Pass the endotracheal tube through the larger nostril. The right side is preferred if both sides are about the same in size, because (1) a left nasotracheal tube is clumsy to manipulate with the intubationist's left hand holding the laryngoscope, and (2) when passed through the right nostril, the bevel of most endotracheal tubes faces the flat nasal septum, possibly reducing damage to the large inferior turbinate and Kiesselbach's plexus.

Direct the tube *not* partially cephalad, which is a common mistake of beginners, but in the plane that is roughly perpendicular to the face. As the tube passes through the nose into the nasopharynx, it must turn downward to pass through to the oropharynx. While making this turn, it may impact against the posterior nasopharyngeal wall and resist any attempt to push it further. The tube should be pulled back a short distance, and the patient's head should be extended further to facilitate attempts to pass this point smoothly and atraumatically. If this is not done and the tube is forced, the mucosal covering of the posterior nasopharyngeal wall may be torn open, and the tube may be passed into the submucosal tissues and create false passage. If the tube cannot be passed, you should try the other nostril, use a smaller tube, or resort to oral intubation.

After the tube has entered the oropharynx, visualize the glottic opening with the direct laryngoscopy. The tube may be guided into the larynx under direct vision by manually advancing at the nasal end. More commonly, the tube is grasped in the oropharynx with Magill forceps, directed toward the larynx, and then advanced by the assistant (Fig. 17–2). There are two important points in using Magill forceps. (1) Never grasp the cuff of the endotracheal tube with Magill forceps. The cuff is extremely vulnerable to damage by the forceps. Grasp the tube proximal to the cuff (ie, cephalad in the pharynx). The soft palate may have to be pushed up with Magill forceps to do so. If the tip of the tube is grasped, the forceps may hinder visualization of the larynx as the tube is advanced, and the tube may have to be released before it is securely placed between the cords. (2) Never advance the tube with Magill forceps. Always ask your assistant to advance the tube. Use forceps only to direct the tube to the glottic opening. Otherwise, forceps may traumatize the cuff.

Blind Nasal Intubation

Blind nasal intubation offers a practical solution to the problem of the alert, agitated patient with a full stomach who requires intu-

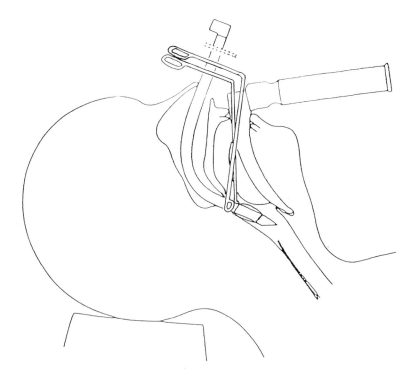

Figure 17–2. Magill forceps used to direct an endotracheal tube to the glottic opening. The tube is grasped not by the tip or the cuff, but more proximally.

bation in the emergency room or ICU.[17] In 1902, Kuhn[18] first reported blind nasal intubation. In 1920, Rowbotham[19] recognized that blind nasal catheters frequently entered the trachea, but it was not until 10 years later that Magill's article in the *British Medical Journal*[20] led to the expanded use of this technique. Although largely replaced by oral intubation or nasal intubation using the fiberoptic laryngoscope, it still has a place in today's practice of medicine.

Pass the tube to the oropharynx as described in the previous section. For this technique to be most successful, the patient must ventilate spontaneously, although apneic patients have been successfully intubated by blind nasal technique.[21, 22] Listen carefully to the exhaled air passing from the proximal end of the tube. Advance the tube as long as breath sounds are maximal. If they decrease, pull back the tube until maximal breath sounds can be heard again, redirect it, then advance it again. The intubationist must keep an ear close to the tube connector to readily detect changes in breath sounds. The tube is then inserted into the glottis during inspiration, because this is the time when vocal cords are separated most widely. As soon as the tube enters the trachea, the patient usually coughs, and condensation of water vapor is seen in the tube lumen.

Proper positioning of the tube should be confirmed immediately by the same way as in oral intubation; ie, equal bilateral breath sounds, symmetrical chest wall movement, and absence of breath sounds over the epigastrium. Because entry into the glottis is not seen directly, it is helpful to have capnography or a bronchoscope to confirm the endotracheal placement, because the indirect signs of intubation listed above are sometimes misleading.[23] The American Society of Anesthesiologists Standards for Basic Intraoperative Monitoring now requires that the proper placement of the endotracheal tube be verified by identifying carbon dioxide in the expired gas.[24]

If the tube does not enter the trachea, it has only four places to go: off the midline (the pyriform recess), too anteriorly (the vallecula), too posteriorly (the esophagus), or it is hung up at the entrance to the larynx. The tip of the tube should be aligned to the midline of the pharynx, because the glottic opening and trachea are also on the midline. Unfortunately, a nasally inserted tube is usually offset toward the side of the naris it passes through, so you may have to rotate the tube to guide its tip onto the center or manually move the larynx to the side of the tube; for example, the tube inserted through the right naris usually appears on the right side in the pharynx, and counter-

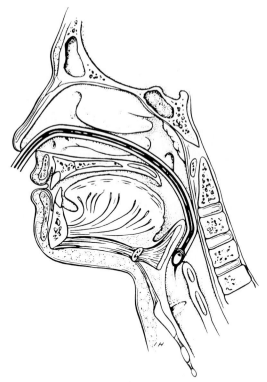

Figure 17-3. A malleable stylet used as an aid for blind nasal intubation. (From Berry FA. The use of a stylet in blind nasotracheal intubation. Anesthesiology 61:470, 1984; with permission.)

clockwise rotation of the tube brings the tip to the midline and facilitates endotracheal placement of the tube.

If the tube is felt anteriorly or bulging of the neck is observed, flexion of the head may help.

Most of the time, the tube enters the esophagus and extension of the head helps. Cricoid pressure may also be useful to bring the larynx posteriorly. Posterior direction can also be corrected by using a ring tube (Endotrol; Mallinckrodt, Inc., Glens Falls, NY 12801). A ring has a cord that runs from the anterior surface of the tip of the tube up the length of the tube to a ring on the proximal end of the tube. Pulling on the ring causes anterior bending of the tip of the tube. A malleable stylet or suction catheter has also been shown to be an effective aid in blind nasal intubation[25-27] (Fig. 17-3).

For better understanding of how the change of a patient's head position with respect to the torso affects the relative position of the tube and the larynx, two series of radiographs are presented. The first series shows the effect of extension and flexion of the neck (Fig. 17-4). In the neutral position (Fig. 17-4A), the tip of the endotracheal tube lies just posterior to the epiglottis. The axis of the tube and the axis of the trachea are shown as white lines. Flexion (Fig. 17-4B) aligns the axis of the tube with the axis of the esophagus. Extension (Fig. 17-4C) aligns the axis of the tube with the opening of the larynx, thus bringing the tip of the tube more anteriorly.

Tilting and rotating the head with respect to the torso are illustrated in the second series of radiographs (Fig. 17-5). In the neutral position (Fig. 17-5A), the axis of the nasotracheal tube parallels the axis of the trachea, offset toward the side of the tube insertion (in this case, the left side). Rotation of the head (Fig. 17-5B) aligns the axis of the tube with soft tissues

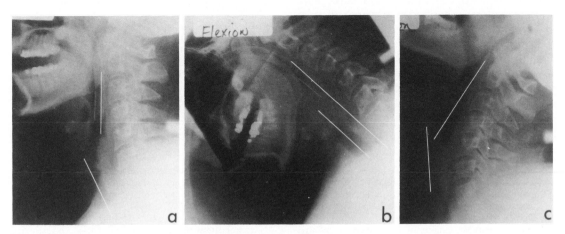

Figure 17-4. Effect of cervical flexion and extension. A, In the neutral position, the tip of the endotracheal tube lies just posterior to the epiglottis. B, Cervical flexion aligns the axis of the tube with the axis of the esophagus. C, Cervical extension aligns the axis of the tube with the opening of the larynx, thus bringing the tip of the tube more anteriorly. (From Roberts JT. Fundamentals of Tracheal Intubation, p. 101. Orlando: Grune & Stratton, 1983; with permission.)

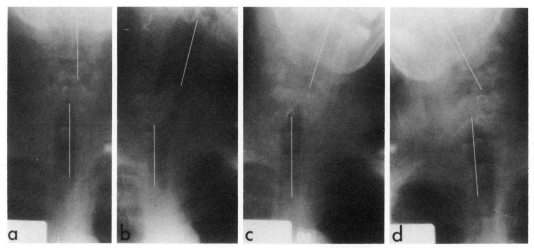

Figure 17–5. Tilting and rotating the head with respect to the torso. *A*, In the neutral position, the axis of the nasotracheal tube parallels the axis of the trachea, offset toward the side of the tube insertion (in this case, the left side). *B*, Rotation of the head aligns the axis of the tube with the soft tissue, rather than with the entrance of the larynx. *C*, Tilting the head to the side of the insertion (in this example, the left) guides the axis of the tube toward the axis of the trachea, making passage into the trachea more likely. *D*, Tilting the head toward the opposite side guides the tube toward the piriform recess, lateral to the opening of the larynx. (From Roberts JT. Fundamentals of Tracheal Intubation, p. 102. Orlando: Grune & Stratton, 1983; with permission.)

rather than with the entrance of the larynx. Tilting the head to the side of the tube insertion (in this example, to the left; Fig. 17–5*C*) guides the axis of the tube toward the axis of the trachea, making passage into the trachea more likely. Tilting the head toward the opposite side (Fig. 17–5*D*) guides the piriform recess, lateral to the opening of the larynx.

Finally, one of the major drawbacks of blind nasal intubation is a high failure rate. Failed attempts may trigger gagging and vomiting, or may further compromise the airway. Always observe the patient carefully and make sure you are not exacerbating the patient's distress by repeating intubation attempts. Also, in case this technique turns out to be impossible, you should always have in mind alternative plans to secure the airway; ie, direct laryngoscopy, fiberoptic laryngoscopy, retrograde intubation, oral intubation, or even cricothyroid puncture or tracheostomy.

References

1. Bolder P, Healy T, Bolder A, Beatty P, Kay B. The extra work of breathing through adult endotracheal tubes. Anesth Analg 65:853–859, 1986.
2. Dubick M, Wright B. Comparison of laryngeal pathology following long-term oral and nasal endotracheal intubations. Anesth Analg 57:663–668, 1978.
3. O'Really M, Reddick E, Black W, Carter P, Erhardt J, Fill W, Maughn D, Sado A, Klatt G. Sepsis from sinusitis in nasotracheally intubated patients: A diagnostic dilemma. Am J Surg 147:601–604, 1984.
4. Caplan E, Hoyt N. Nosocomial sinusitis. JAMA 247:639–641, 1982.
5. Berry F, Blankenbaker W, Ball C. A comparison between bacteremia occurring with nasotracheal and orotracheal intubation. Anesth Analg 52:873–877, 1973.
6. Deutschman C, Wilton P, Sinow J, Dibbell D Jr, Konstantinides F, Cerra F. Paranasal sinusitis associated with nasotracheal intubation: A frequently unrecognized and treatable source of sepsis. Crit Care Med 14:111–114, 1986.
7. Hamory B, Sande M, Sydnor A Jr, Seale D, Gwaltney J. Etiology and antimicrobial therapy of acute maxillary sinusitis. J Infect Dis 139:197–202, 1979.
8. Knodel A, Beekman J. Unexplained fevers in patients with nasotracheal intubation. JAMA 248:868–870, 1982.
9. Chidekel N, Jensen G, Axelsson A, Grebelius N. Diagnosis of fluid in the maxillary sinus. Acta Radiol 10:433–440, 1970.
10. Abramovich S, Smelg GJC. Acute sphenoiditis, alone and in concert. J Laryngol Otol 96:751–757, 1982.
11. Carter B, Bankoff M, Fisk M. Computed tomographic detection of sinusitis responsible for intracranial and extracranial infections. Radiology 147:739–742, 1983.
12. Lew D, Southwick F, Montgomery W, Weber A, Baker A. Sphenoid sinusitis. N Engl J Med 309:1149–1154, 1983.
13. Kronberg F, Goodwin W. Sinusitis in intensive care unit patients. Laryngoscope 95:936–938, 1985.
14. McShane A, Hone R. Prevention of bacterial endocarditis: Does nasal intubation warrant prophylaxis? Br Med J 292:26–27, 1986.
15. Dinner M, Tjeuw M, Artusio J. Bacteremia as a complication of nasotracheal intubation. Anesth Analg 66:460–462, 1987.
16. Gross J, Hartigan M, Schaffer D. A suitable substitute for 4% cocaine before blind nasotracheal intubation: 3% lidocaine–0.25% phenylephrine nasal spray. Anesth Analg 63:915–918, 1984.

17. Danzl D, Thomas D. Nasotracheal intubations in the emergency department. Crit Care Med 8:677–682, 1980.
18. Kuhn F. Die pernasale Tubage. Munch Med Wochenschr 49:1456, 1902.
19. Rowbotham S. Intratracheal anaesthesia by the nasal route for operations on the mouth and lips. Br Med J 2:590, 1920.
20. Magill I. Technique in endotracheal anaesthesia. Br Med J 2:817, 1930.
21. Maltby J, Cassidy M, Nanji G. Blind nasotracheal intubation using succinylcholine. Anesthesiology 69:946–948, 1988.
22. Williamson R. Blind nasal intubation of an apneic neonate. Anesthesiology 69:633–634, 1988.
23. Birmingham P, Cheney F, Ward R. Esophageal intubation: A review of detection techniques. Anesth Analg 65:886–891, 1986.
24. American Society of Anesthesiologists, Park Ridge, IL, 1990.
25. Berry F: The use of a stylet in blind nasotracheal intubation. Anesthesiology 61:469–471, 1984.
26. Reeves J. Blind nasal intubation. Anesth Intensive Care 17:115–116, 1989.
27. Meyer R. Suction catheter to facilitate blind nasal intubation. Anesth Analg 68:698, 1989.

CHAPTER 18

The Prediction of Difficult Intubation

James T. Roberts, M.D., M.A.
and George D. Shorten, M.D., F.F.A.R.C.S.(I.), F.C.Anaes.

Most life-threatening clinical problems that involve a difficult airway occur infrequently. A difficult intubation occurs in approximately one in 2000 patients in the general surgical population, but in one in 300 obstetric patients.[1] With newer fiberoptic techniques, once-difficult problems of intubation are now usually easily overcome. Although only a small population of patients present with a difficult endotracheal intubation, the absolute prevalence of the problem is high. It may be that there are 600 deaths annually in the developed world due to hypoxia during difficult intubation, failed endotracheal intubation, or Mendelson's syndrome. One closed-claim study estimated that 4% of the anesthetic mishaps examined (22 of 624) were related to difficult intubation.[2] Of these 22 patients, 9 died and 4 suffered brain damage.

Many devices, including flexible fiberoptic laryngoscopes, lightwands, retrograde wires, intubating stylets, and a multiplicity of rigid laryngoscope blades—some with a coherent fiberoptic bundle for visualizing the laryngeal opening—are now available to facilitate intubation. This is indicative of the widespread awareness of the problem. What has been published concerning identification of predictive features in patients that may indicate a difficult laryngoscopy or difficult intubation? In this chapter we refer specifically to either laryngoscopy or to intubation in an attempt to avoid the assumption that an inadequate view of the larynx necessarily implies a difficult intubation.

Investigators must address the problem of standardization of compared groups. They must quantitate the parameters studied and examine large numbers of patients to produce a satisfactory prospective study. Ideally, control and study groups in a clinical trial are well matched for all factors except those to be studied. When a particular intubation is found to be difficult, one must know many factors other than the anatomic features of the patient; these include the experience of the intubator, the laryngoscope handle and blade used, the relative position of the patient's head and neck, whether profound muscle relaxation was achieved with general anesthesia, and whether a trained assistant was present. Horton and colleagues have proposed a standard intubating position, based on the degree of lower neck flexion and extension of the plane of the face relative to the horizontal, which would serve as a research standard.[3]

Relevant anatomic features have not been easily quantitated. How high is a high arched palate? How anterior is an anterior larynx, and anterior to what? Structural images examined radiologically may be accurately measured and the influence of structural changes clearly demonstrated. Routine use of radiographs, however, for preanesthetic assessment is impractical and expensive. Mallampati has reported examining and classifying the oropharyngeal appearance of the sitting patient with the mouth wide open and the tongue protruded maximally.[4, 5] In a prospective trial, he clearly demonstrated that such appearances are predictive of the ease of laryngoscopy. This simple test may be performed easily at the bedside and appears to have gained widespread acceptance.[6-8] Recently, we described a device, the laryngeal indices caliper, designed to measure a number of upper airway variables relative to a predefined standard (the laryngeal indices line, joining the upper incisor to the external auditory canal in a lateral view of the subject).[9] A second device, the bubble inclinometer, may be used to measure the degree of anterior tilt of the thyroid cartilage relative to the horizontal.[10] Both of these instruments are easy to use, involve no patient discomfort, and the measurements obtained are reproducible and relevant to the prediction of difficult laryngoscopy. The range of atlanto-occipital extension may be accurately measured using a goniometer (a pair of articulated rulers calibrated to read the angle between them). Other measurements—eg, maximal incisor separation and chin to suprahyoid notch distance—are simply made with a ruler.

If one of each 2000 general surgical patients proves difficult to intubate, perhaps a single proposed factor may contribute to one fifth of such cases. Thus, 10,000 patients requiring intubation must be studied to encounter one in whom the proposed factor is responsible. To study such a factor prospectively, perhaps 10 such cases are required to achieve statistical significance. Therefore, a conclusion may be drawn only when 100,000 patients have been studied using a carefully standardized intubation technique. Although the actual figures mentioned previously represent guesswork, the numerical difficulties to be overcome may be appreciated.

The experienced anesthetist has long been alert to the difficulties of intubating patients with certain characteristics. In 1956, Cass and associates described anatomic features that cause difficult intubation.[11] Although five of these features had previously been recognized, these researchers supported their conclusion with a series of six brief case reports. In 1968, Brechner emphasized the importance of the mobility of the cervical vertebrae in proper positioning of the head and neck for intubation.[12] Measurements made using lateral, posteroanterior, and submental-vertical radiographs by White and Kander suggested that the reduction in the distance between the occiput and the spinous process of C1 and, to a lesser extent, the C1–C2 interspinous gap were important factors.[13] They concluded that the most significant determinant of ease of laryngoscopy is the posterior depth of the mandible, a finding that has not been confirmed in other studies. Bellhouse and Dore analyzed measurements made using lateral radiographs and concluded that reduced atlanto-occipital extension, reduced mandibular space, and increased anteroposterior thickness of the tongue were the three most reliable factors in distinguishing between difficult and straightforward intubation.[14] More importantly, they described a method of assessing these variables clinically. They recommended a combination of Mallampati-style inspection of the oropharynx with a grading of reduction of head extension (none, 1/3, 2/3, complete) and estimation of mandibular space. Nichol and Zuck explained the importance of a small atlanto-occipital gap by pointing out that, in such cases, attempts to extend the head result in anterior bowing of the cervical spine, thus displacing the larynx forward, out of the laryngoscopist's line of vision.[15]

Our recent work identifies one previously undocumented variable that influences ease of laryngoscopy; namely, the degree of anterior tilt of the larynx.[9, 10] This concept may be best understood if one envisions that when the longitudinal axis of the larynx forms a large angle with the line of vision achievable with a laryngoscope blade, direct laryngoscopy is more difficult. We measured a number of upper airway variables, using the laryngeal indices caliper for association with laryngoscopic appearance. Of these, only laryngeal tilt showed a strong positive association. Subsequently, we demonstrated that the laryngeal tilt, relative to the horizontal measured with a bubble inclinometer, was equally predictive of laryngoscopic appearance.

From published work in this field, three principles have clearly emerged. First, in order to gain widespread support, a predictive test must be amenable to simple, painless application at the bedside. Second, no single factor is predictive of difficult intubation or laryngoscopy in all cases.[16] Third, the predictive value of any factor depends on the accuracy with which it can be measured. A number of attempts to combine a predictive index have been made.

The anesthetic literature contains a long and

growing list of clinical conditions said to be associated with difficult intubation. These, for the most part, pose less of a problem of prediction than of awareness that an airway problem may exist. If this possibility is considered, one need not resort to clinical tests or radiographic measurements to detect the gross anatomic abnormalities present. Trauma, burns, and radiation are common conditions encountered in anesthesia practice. A detailed review is given by Jones and Pelton.[17]

Endotracheal intubation is now an essential part of the practice of medicine. The risks of a failed intubation attempt are great. Therefore, assessment of the patient's upper airway must be a part of any preintubation visit. There are two objectives in this assessment. First, one should identify those patients in whom intubation is likely to be difficult and try to assess the anatomic basis for such a prediction; second, one must make a decision as to how the patient's airway may be safely secured.

McIntyre suggests a systematic approach to meet these objectives.[18] He emphasizes the importance of a complete history at the preintubation visit, "as diseases or syndromes primarily affecting other parts of the body may have a component that makes intubation difficult."[18] His comprehensive plan for clinical examination includes six steps: (1) viewing the patient from the lateral and anterolateral position; (2) viewing and palpating the neck anteriorly and laterally; (3) extending the neck maximally; (4) flexing the neck maximally; (5) examining the mouth opening, teeth, and oral cavity; and (6) determining the patency of the nostrils.

We recommend an approach to examination that differs in emphasis from that of McIntyre. We concentrate on the line of vision (LOV) that the laryngoscopist hopes to achieve; in so doing, we assess all those factors shown to influence ease of laryngoscopy. The LOV is potentially created when the axes of the buccal cavity, oropharynx, and larynx are brought into line. Lower neck flexion and atlanto-occipital extension are assessed by placing the awake supine patient in the standard intubating position. Ask the patient to sit, open his or her mouth, and protrude his or her tongue maximally (as suggested by Mallampati). Potential obstacles to the proximal LOV may then be assessed (ie, limited mouth opening, prominent incisors, macroglossia, oropharyngeal structures).

The distal LOV depends primarily on laryngeal position (the "high, anterior larynx") or

tilt. When the distance from chin to thyroid prominence is less than 6 cm, laryngoscopy may well be impossible. The laryngeal opening is difficult to visualize when the tilt of the anterior surface of the thyroid cartilage is greater then 40 degrees as measured by the bubble inclinometer.

These four steps may easily be performed in less than 1 minute and will predict most difficult intubations. The posterior mandibular depth deliberately has been ignored because its significance is doubtful. Other factors, such as obesity and sternal prominence, are obvious on general inspection of the patient. The use of an objective grading system or actual measurement reduces the extent to which an assessment is based on the observer's experience.

The information thus obtained will be useful in selecting the safest intubation technique in a specific patient (the second objective of the preintubation assessment). Although elective tracheostomy using local anesthesia remains an option, awake fiberoptic intubation will overcome many of the anatomic obstacles. However, neither a fiberoptic laryngoscope nor personnel trained in its use are available in every center. Adequate topicalization is essential, because a flexible fiberscope may precipitate laryngospasm.

McIntyre has cleverly matched rigid laryngoscope characteristics with some of the commonly encountered problems.[19] For instance, the protruding sternal region that makes introduction of the blade into the mouth impossible is best managed by increasing the angle between the blade and the handle, by offsetting the blade from the handle, or by shortening the length of the laryngoscope handle. For a reduced intraoral cavity, he recommends a blade with a substantial flange such as the Wisconsin, Flagg, or Guedel laryngoscopes. A straight blade with a distal curve or beak directed anteriorly may be useful in obtaining a view of the anterior larynx.

In summary, we emphasize the importance of anticipating specific causes of difficult laryngoscopy and intubation. We pointed out some of the hazards to be overcome in any scientific appraisal of the problem. Factors proven to be useful predictors of difficult intubation were enumerated and discussed. Alternative techniques of airway assessment suitable for routine clinical use during the preintubation visit are described. The best intubation plan is chosen with the aid of such an assessment.

References

1. Samsoon GLT, Young JRB. Difficult tracheal intubation: A retrospective study. Anaesthesia 42:487–490, 1987.
2. ASA preliminary data. Closed claims study in safety and cost containment. In Gravenstein JS, Holzer JF (eds). Anesthesia. London: Butterworth, 1988; p. 16.
3. Horton WA, Fahy L, Charteus P. Defining a standard intubation position using 'angle finder.' Br J Anaesth 62:6–12, 1989.
4. Mallampati SR. Clinical sign to predict difficult tracheal intubation (hypothesis) [letter]. Can Anaesth Soc J 30:316–317, 1983.
5. Mallampati SR, Gatt SP, Gugino LD. A clinical sign to predict difficult tracheal intubation: a prospective study. Can Anaesth Soc J 32:429–434, 1985.
6. Charters P, Perera, Horton WA. Visibility of the pharyngeal structures as a predictor of difficult intubation. Anaesthesia 42:1115, 1987.
7. Cohen SM, Laurito CE, Segil LS. Oral exam to predict difficult intubations: A larger prospective study. Anesthesiology 71:A937, 1989.
8. Wilson ME, John R. Problems with the Mallampati sign. Anaesthesia 45:486–502, 1990.
9. Roberts JT, Ali HH, Shorten GD. Using the laryngeal indices caliper to predict difficulty of intubation with a Macintosh #3 laryngoscope. J Clin Anesth 5:302–305, 1993.
10. Roberts JT, Ali HH, Shorten GD. Using the bubble inclinometer to measure laryngeal tilt and predict difficulty of laryngoscopy. J Clin Anesth 5:306–309, 1993.
11. Cass NM, James NR, Lines V. Difficult direct laryngoscopy complicating intubation for anaesthesia. Br Med J 1:488–489, 1956.
12. Brechner VL. Unusual problems in the management of airways. I: Flexion-extension mobility of the cervical vertebrae. Anesth Analg 47:362–373, 1968.
13. White A, Kander PL. Anatomical factors in difficult direct laryngoscopy. Br J Anaesth 47:468–473, 1975.
14. Bellhouse CP, Dore C. Criteria for estimating likelihood of difficulty of endotracheal intubation with the Macintosh laryngoscope. Anaesth Intensive Care 16:329–337, 1986.
15. Nichol HC, Zuck D. Difficult laryngoscopy—the anterior larynx and the atlanto-occipital gap. Br J Anaesth 55:141–144, 1983.
16. Wilson ME, Spiegelhalter D, Robertson JA, Lesser P. Predicting difficult intubation. Br J Anaesth 61:211–216, 1988.
17. Jones AEP, Pelton DA. An index of syndromes and their anaesthetic implications. Can Anaesth Soc J 23:207–226, 1976.
18. McIntyre JWR. The difficult tracheal intubation. Can J Anaesth 34:204–213, 1987.
19. McIntyre JWR. Laryngoscope design and the difficult adult tracheal intubation. Can J Anaesth 36:94–98, 1989.

CHAPTER 19

The Failed Intubation: Maximizing Successful Management of the Patient with a Compromised or Potentially Compromised Airway

James T. Roberts, M.D., M.A., Amr E. Abouleish, M.D., Frederick J. Curlin IV, M.D., and Andrew Patterson, M.D.

Of the menacing events possible in medical practice, few surpass in jeopardy the unprotected airway following a failed intubation attempt. This chapter attempts to develop an awareness of the variety of *causes* of impaired airway function that may lead to failed intubation; to understand how the *sequelae* of an obstructed airway may affect further efforts at

Table 19–1. CHAPTER GOALS

1. To understand how causes of an impaired airway may lead to failed intubation
2. To review how sequelae of an obstructed airway may impact on continued attempts at intubation
3. To establish a game plan for a patient with a known prior difficult or failed intubation (prior may mean 5 minutes ago or 5 years ago)

intubation; and to develop a game plan to *secure oxygenation and ventilation,* taking the first two goals into account after an unsuccessful intubation attempt (Table 19–1).

AIRWAY IMPAIRMENTS THAT MAY LEAD TO FAILED INTUBATION

Over 900 articles have been published on impaired airway function since 1986. Many cited abnormal anatomic causes, including abnormal head size, congenital syndromes, limited neck mobility, limited mouth opening, loose teeth, enlarged tongue, enlarged tonsils, thyroglossal duct cyst, abnormal epiglottis, limited laryngeal opening, obesity, trauma, hiatal hernia, infections, an abnormal trachea or esophagus, tumors, and radiation effects. Other articles cited causes with normal anatomy but with extenuating circumstances, such as functional abnormalities, foreign bodies, chronic smoking, alcohol ingestion, and acute or chronic drug use, as well as iatrogenic causes.

Abnormal Anatomy

Table 19–2 lists abnormal anatomy leading to difficult or failed intubation.

Head Size. Patients with hydrocephalus or craniosynostosis should be evaluated for potential airway difficulties.

Congenital Syndromes. Syndromes cited as causes of airway obstruction include Hurler's,[1] Goltz,[2] Pierre-Robin,[3–5] and Sjögren's.[6] Refer to Chapter 35 for a discussion of these congenital pediatric problems. The infant with the encephalocele in Figure 19–1 shows the difficulty in placing the infant in the supine position. In this case, the infant was successfully intubated in the lateral position using a standard rigid laryngoscope.

Neck Mobility. Neck mobility is of particular importance in rheumatoid arthritis,[7–13] anky-

losing spondylitis,[14–20] and in the patient with an unstable neck.[21]

Limited Mouth Opening. Ability to open the mouth must be considered in Whistler's syndrome, temporomandibular joint (TMJ) disorders,[22–25] hemifacial patients,[26, 27] and patients who have had cancer and reconstructive surgery (Fig. 19–2).

Loose Teeth. The design of most rigid laryngoscope blades leads the unskilled to use the upper teeth as a fulcrum. Check teeth before as well as immediately after intubation; document their condition in the chart. Immediately retrieve a chipped or lost tooth during laryngoscopy, rather than anesthetize the patient a second time for this purpose.

Enlarged Tongue. The patient in Figure 19–3 has a markedly enlarged tongue due to a venous malformation. She was anesthetized and intubated for sclerotherapy (ethanol injection) to shrink the malformation. A flexible fiberoptic laryngoscope was used for an oral intubation. Rigid laryngoscopy would have proved difficult in this case. Following sclerotherapy, the tongue was quite edematous, and the patient was allowed to fully awaken prior to extubation. In this case, emergence from enflurane anesthesia was prolonged (1 h) by the high blood alcohol level.

Enlarged Tonsils. It is possible to lacerate enlarged tonsils with the tip of a rigid laryngoscope blade or to avulse an enlarged adenoid during nasal intubation. Hemorrhage may be

Table 19–2. ABNORMAL ANATOMY LEADING TO DIFFICULT OR FAILED INTUBATION

1. Head size
2. Congenital syndromes
3. Neck mobility
4. Limited mouth opening
5. Loose teeth
6. Enlarged tongue
7. Enlarged tonsils
8. Thyroglossal duct cyst
9. Epiglottitis
10. Limited laryngeal opening
11. Laryngeal polyposis
12. Trauma
13. Laryngeal edema
14. Infections
15. Burn patients
16. Small or narrowed trachea
17. Tracheoesophageal fistula
18. Esophageal achalasia
19. Goiter
20. Tension pneumothorax
21. Hiatal hernia
22. Tumors
23. Radiation effects

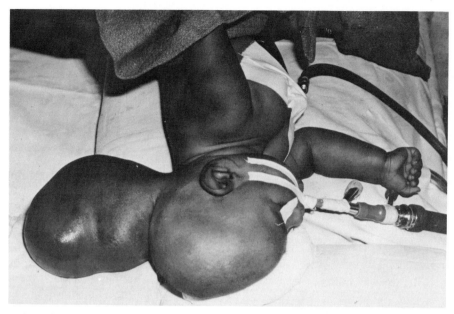

Figure 19–1. This infant was positioned for intubation with some difficulty. The lateral position was chosen, and a rigid laryngoscope was used.

excessive, and reintubation for control of bleeding after tonsillectomy may be hazardous. Awake oral intubation should be considered for these patients.[28]

Thyroglossal Duct Cyst. Figure 19–4 illustrates a thyroglossal duct cyst in the vallecula directly above the juvenile epiglottis. A differential diagnosis should include thyroid carcinoma, adenoma, thyroiditis, thyrotoxicosis, inflammation, and infection. Obstructive symp-

toms occur primarily in children and infants and rarely in the adult. Several reviews that include diagnostic errors and causes of recurrence have appeared in the literature.[29–32] Horisawa and colleagues presented an anatomic reconstruction of the thyroglossal duct.[33] Diagnosis by ultrasonography and computed tomography (CT) scan of seven cases was reported by Mozen and associates.[34] Issa and deVries reported a case of familial thyroglossal

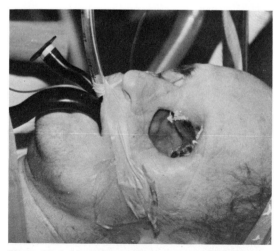

Figure 19–2. Limited mandibular opening secondary to radiation scarring. The patient was intubated orally while asleep with a flexible fiberoptic laryngoscope (he absolutely refused an awake intubation). Spontaneous ventilation was continuously maintained.

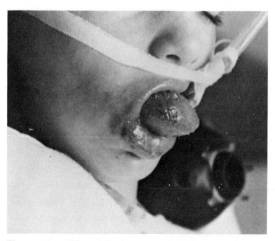

Figure 19–3. This child has an enlarged tongue from a venous malformation. She was anesthetized, then intubated orally using a flexible fiberoptic laryngoscope. Following ethanol sclerotherapy of the venous malformation, the child was fully awakened prior to extubation.

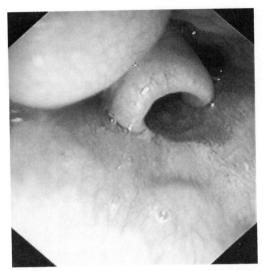

Figure 19–4. Young man with a thyroglossal duct cyst.

duct cyst and cited two other reports of familial thyroglossal duct cyst in the literature.[35] Management of 79 cases of thyroglossal duct cyst was reported by Katz and Hachigian, who recommend the Sistrunk procedure as the operation of choice.[36]

Epiglottitis. Although usually found in the pediatric age group, epiglottitis may also occasionally occur in the adult. Intubation of the patient with epiglottitis requires special skills.[37] The most skilled anesthetist available should be present. The child must be kept calm; agitation may cause further airway obstruction from an increased negative pressure during inspiration. A parent should hold the child while general anesthesia is slowly and gently induced with spontaneous ventilation, and intubation should be performed under direct visualization. Muscle relaxants are contraindicated. A premature or awake intubation attempt may well precipitate laryngospasm and complete obstruction. Remember, induction proceeds slowly because of reduced flow in the obstructed airway.

Limited Laryngeal Opening. Figure 19–5 highlights a mass at the laryngeal opening that limits access to the laryngeal cavity and trachea.

Laryngeal Polyposis. Hill and Cardig reported 10 patients with laryngeal polyposis.[38] They found that narrow-based polyps splinted the glottis open during phonation, which increased mean air flow rates, whereas large, broad-based polyps tended to obstruct the glottis and reduce airflow.

Obesity. Figure 19–6 shows an obese patient having an awake flexible fiberoptic intubation. Refer to Chapter 15 for details on awake intubation. Due to their reduced functional residual capacity (FRC), obese patients do not tolerate prolonged apnea or diminished ventilation. Leech and coworkers[39] studied 27 patients with occlusive sleep apnea syndrome, and found that six of 13 of these patients with airflow obstruction could not hyperventilate to eucapnia, suggesting mechanical impairment in obesity hypoventilation. The sitting or semi-sitting position may be preferred for intubation.

Fat may be layered immediately outside or may surround the laryngeal inlet, as illustrated in Figure 19–7. Adequate topicalization with local anesthetics is more difficult, because the local anesthetic may not reach the nerve endings of the laryngeal mucosa.

Misdiagnosis of mediastinal tumor with trachea compression, "sabre sheath" trachea, is also possible with mediastinal lipomatosis, which is a benign condition.[40]

Trauma. Kattan and Snyder[41] reported a case of lingual artery hematoma and airway obstruction after suturing the lingual artery following a puncture wound of the tongue. Another patient (Fig. 19–8) had surgery earlier in the day and postoperatively developed swelling and bleeding at the base of the tongue. Awake flexible fiberoptic intubation was performed nasally. The patient remained intu-

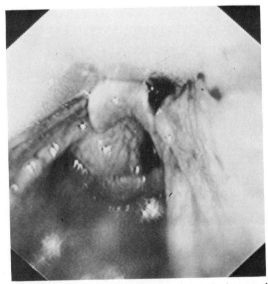

Figure 19–5. Tumor mass limiting access to the laryngeal opening.

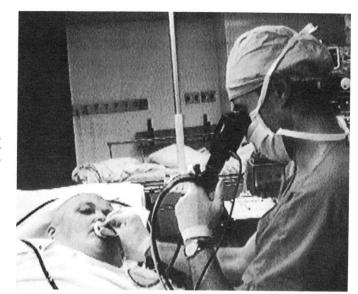

Figure 19–6. Obese patient having an awake flexible fiberoptic intubation. The patient is in a semi-sitting position to help her ventilate, with the operator facing her.

bated postoperatively until the swelling subsided.

Wells[42] reviewed the importance of airway management of the patient with a cervical spine injury from blunt trauma. Kellman[43] reviewed the implications of cervical spine injury associated with maxillofacial trauma. Radio-logic diagnosis of upper airway obstruction in maxillofacial trauma was reviewed by Teich-graeber and colleagues.[44]

Woo and associates[45] followed 50 head-injured patients who underwent a tracheostomy

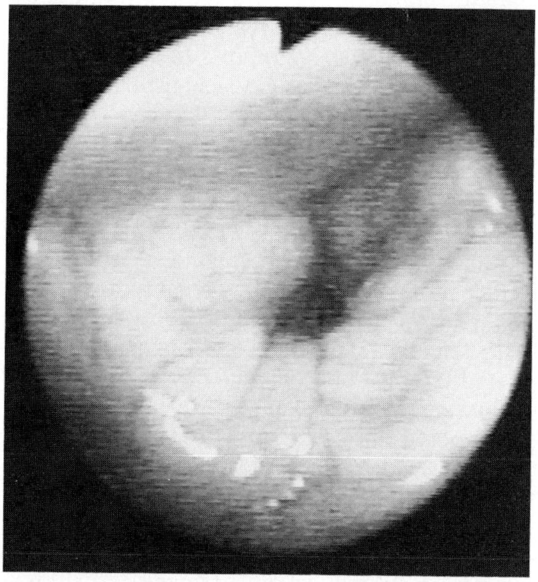

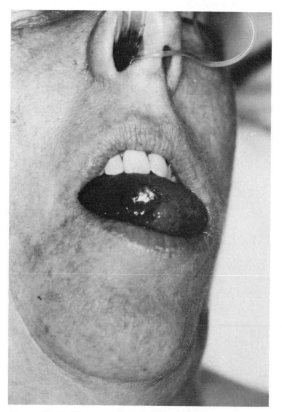

Figure 19–7. Fiberoptic view of another obese patient, illustrating adipose tissue surrounding the entrance to the larynx. It is doubtful whether the topical local anesthetic that was applied penetrated through the fat to the underlying mucosa. Her glottic opening remained very active during the awake intubation, despite copious amounts of local anesthetic applied both topically by direct intraoral spray and through the channel of the flexible fiberoptic laryngoscope.

Figure 19–8. Postoperative swelling of the tongue. The patient was reintubated nasally with an awake intubation.

with video laryngoscopy. Significant airway obstruction was seen in both laryngeal and tracheal sites. Even when there was proper surgical anatomic repair, neurologic injury could disrupt postdecannulation function, resulting in central laryngeal muscle movement disorder.

An isolated hyoid fracture that caused severe and sudden upper airway obstruction was reported by Szeremeta and Morovati.[46] Fortunately, isolated hyoid fractures are rare and have few complications. Nakayama and coworkers,[47] reviewed 605 pediatric trauma cases that required endotracheal intubation. Maxillofacial trauma is fully discussed in Chapter 37.

Laryngeal Edema. Congestive heart failure has been associated with peripheral and/or pulmonary edema. Our recent video examination of a patient's oropharynx and laryngeal entrance documented significant laryngeal edema associated with congestive heart failure (Fig. 19–9). Laryngeal edema also may present following multiple attempts at laryngoscopy with a rigid laryngoscope blade and has been reported to be associated with complications of thyroid surgery,[48, 49] systemic lupus erythematosus,[50] angiotensin-converting enzyme (ACE) inhibitors,[51, 52] pregnancy,[5, 54–56] antimony therapy for mucosal leishmaniasis,[57] hereditary angioedema,[58–62] respiratory burns,[63] regional enteritis,[64] and with multiple attempts at awake intubation.[65] Corren and Schocket have reviewed management of laryngeal edema as a complication of anaphylaxis.[66]

Infections. Welsh and associates[67] reviewed cases and management of massive orofacial abscesses of dental origin. Ekberg and Feinberg cited Ludwig's angina, retropharyngeal infection, acute epiglottitis, diphtheria, tetanus, and peritonsillar abscess as infectious processes leading to airway obstruction.[68] Infections of the airway are discussed in Chapter 32.

Burn Patients. Burn patients are discussed in Chapter 38.

Small or Narrowed Trachea. Tumors are a prominent cause of tracheal narrowing. Tracheal narrowing may also result from displacement by a goiter, be caused by scarring from prolonged intubation, or may result from an old tracheostomy site. In the former case, an endotracheal tube usually passes easily past the narrowed area. Scarring may dramatically limit the size of the endotracheal tube that will pass the stenosis.

Tracheoesophageal Fistula. In cases of adult tracheoesophageal fistula, the endotracheal tube cuff should be positioned distal to the fistulous tract. If it is proximal, positive pressure ventilation will inflate the stomach, forcing stomach contents into the trachea. The patient should not be paralyzed until a cuffed endotracheal tube secures the airway beyond the fistula. Numerous reports of surgical management of tracheal esophageal fistula are present in the literature.[69–76]

Esophageal Achalasia. Westbrook[77] reported a case of massive esophageal achalasia successfully treated with sublingual nitroglycerine; presumably, this worked by relieving spasm of the lower esophageal sphincter. Other individual cases have been reported.[78–81] Figure 19–10 shows a radiograph of a patient with significant esophageal achalasia. Distorted tracheal anatomy as well as esophageal reflux are constant dangers during intubation attempts in these patients.

Goiter. Figure 19–11 shows tracheal displacement by a large goiter. Articles involving airway obstruction secondary to thyroid enlargement have originated from around the world, including several reviews.[82–86] Flow–volume loops have been reported to be helpful in diagnosing tracheal stenosis caused by goiter.[87] A report of a lingual thyroid in a pediatric patient[88] and of goiters resulting in airway obstruction in older patients[89] have also appeared in the literature.

Tension Pneumothorax. A tension pneu-

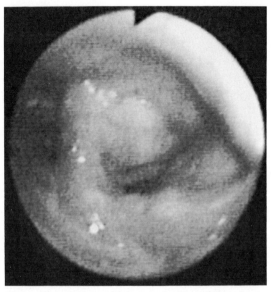

Figure 19–9. Patient with congestive heart failure manifesting by edema of the pharynx. This video photograph was taken under mask general anesthesia.

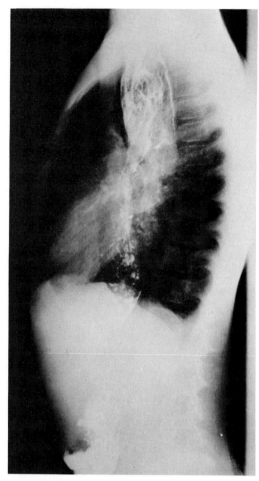

Figure 19–10. Radiograph of a patient with esophageal achalasia. (Courtesy of Jo-Anne O. Shepard, M.D.)

mothorax arises from air movement into the pleural space after lung puncture, and progresses from collapse of the lung, development of tension in the pleural cavity, to shift of the mediastinum toward the contralateral lung with contralateral lung compression and decreased venous return to the heart. This relatively rare event is pictured in Figure 19–12, which illustrates marked deviation of the trachea. Treatment involves immediate thoracentesis with a syringe and needle to release air from the pleural space. Intubation may be difficult due to tracheal deviation. Remember, positive pressure ventilation after successful intubation may worsen the pneumothorax by increasing the leakage of air from the affected lung into the pleural space.[90–92]

Hiatal Hernia. Acid reflux and delayed gastric emptying are normally associated with hiatal hernia.[93] Hiatal hernia markedly increases the risk of aspiration of stomach contents during attempted tracheal intubation. Posterior pressure applied to the cricoid ring minimizes this risk by interrupting the exit of stomach contents from the esophagus. Figure 19–13 shows a massive hiatal hernia. In the face of such a large hernia, the stomach should be emptied with an Ewald or a nasogastric tube prior to induction of anesthesia.

Tumors. Tumors of the upper airway are discussed in Chapter 2. An example of a vascular tumor (venous malformation) obstructing the entrance to the larynx is presented in Figure 19–14. An elective tracheostomy by-

Figure 19–11. Computed tomography (CT) scan of a patient with a goiter that displaces the trachea.

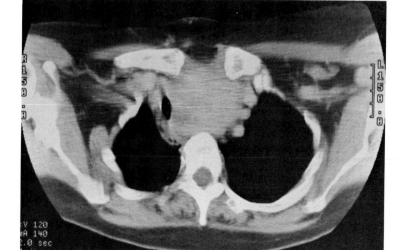

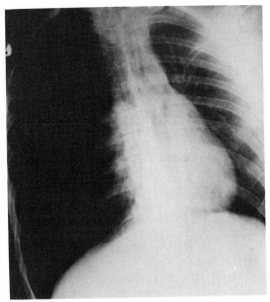

Figure 19–12. Radiograph of a patient with a tension pneumothorax. (Courtesy of Jo-Anne O. Shepard, M.D.)

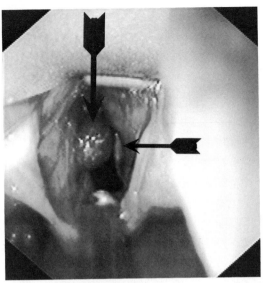

Figure 19–14. A patient with a tumor obstructing the laryngeal entrance. The *vertical arrow* indicates the venous malformation; the *horizontal arrow* indicates the vocal fold.

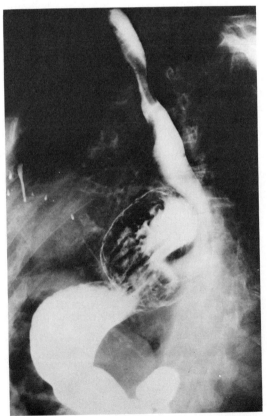

Figure 19–13. Radiograph of a patient with a hiatal hernia that penetrates the diaphragm into the chest. (Courtesy of Jo-Anne O. Shepard, M.D.)

passed the problem, whereas laser surgery fixed it.

Radiation Effects. Radiation may be used to shrink airway tumors[94, 95] and to relieve airway obstruction, or it may cause radiation fibrosis that secondarily induces significant airway obstruction.[96]

Normal Anatomy With Aggravating Circumstances

Table 19–3 lists extenuating circumstances that may lead to difficult or failed intubation in the patient with normal anatomy.

Drug Induced. Chronic ethanol ingestion has many effects.[97–110] It induces airway problems by modifying the action or inactivation of drugs administered for anesthesia, and it increases the likelihood of emesis. Acute alcohol ingestion may also increase the combat-

Table 19–3. HOW EXTENUATING CIRCUMSTANCES IN THE PATIENT WITH NORMAL ANATOMY MAY LEAD TO DIFFICULT OR FAILED INTUBATION

1. Drug induced
2. Cardiovascular causes
3. Reflex closure of the laryngeal entrance
4. Emesis, hematemesis, and secretions
5. Laryngeal dysfunction
6. Foreign body in the airway
7. Iatrogenic causes

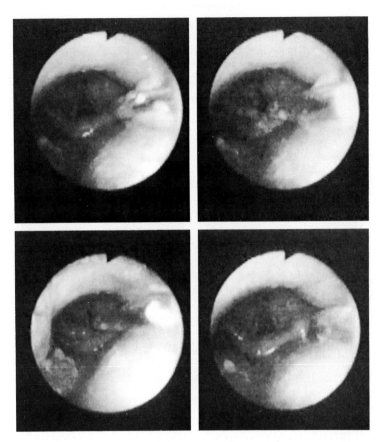

Figure 19–15. Video photographs illustrating a very sensitive reflex closure of the laryngeal opening in response to a suction catheter. When the catheter was removed, the glottic opening relaxed. The patient was ventilating spontaneously under general anesthesia and not responding to the pain of concurrent fulguration of his bladder.

ive nature of the patient during an awake intubation attempt.

Cardiovascular Causes. Pulmonary edema resulting from congestive heart failure may flood the airway with secretions, making it impossible to visualize landmarks during an intubation attempt. Wright and Alexander[111] report an interesting case where a tortuous aorta impinged on the anterior tracheal wall, causing airway obstruction. The tracheal obstruction was relieved by general anesthesia, presumably by lowering the patient's blood pressure.[111]

Reflex Closure of the Laryngeal Entrance. Figure 19–15 illustrates the sequential opening and closing of the supraglottic structures in response to stimulation by a suction catheter. The patient was under general anesthesia and not responding to fulguration of his bladder cancer.

Emesis, Hematemesis, and Secretions. The presence of emesis, hematemesis,[112] or secretions in the oral cavity represents a threat of aspiration, as well as the threat of blocking the visual pathway for intubation by both direct and indirect (flexible fiberoptic) laryngoscopy.

The immediate need is to clear the obstructing material by suctioning, prevent reappearance of the material by cricoid pressure, implement optimal patient positioning for intubation, and prevent further accumulation.

Laryngeal Dysfunction. George and associates[113] reported two cases of stridor due to paradoxic vocal cord motion that caused functional airway obstruction. Only 12 cases have been reported in the literature in the past 15 years.

Foreign Body in the Airway. Many foreign bodies have been reported in the airway.[114–124] Choking on food probably represents the most common foreign body that causes airway difficulty. Either the Heimlich maneuver or a slap on the back is the immediate therapeutic step to be taken.

Iatrogenic. Iatrogenic causes of a difficult airway may precede or follow an unsuccessful intubation attempt. These include edema from excessive fluid administration, inappropriate selection of an oral airway, unsuitable selection of a laryngoscope blade, improper positioning of the patient, and inadequate management of the patient's airway reflexes.[125–127]

Table 19–4. HOW SEQUELAE OF AN OBSTRUCTED AIRWAY MAY IMPACT ON CONTINUED ATTEMPTS AT INTUBATION

1. Hypoxia
2. Hypercarbia
3. Alteration of drug distribution, action, and metabolism

SEQUELAE OF AN OBSTRUCTED AIRWAY AND THEIR EFFECT ON CONTINUED ATTEMPTS AT INTUBATION

Sequelae of an obstructed airway include (1) hypoxia; (2) hypercapnia; (3) alteration of drug distribution, action, or metabolism; and (4) miscellaneous effects such as respiratory efforts against a closed glottis, agitation, restlessness, modified action of laryngeal muscles, and an increased possibility of esophageal placement when intubating during laryngospasm. Table 19–4 lists how sequelae of an obstructed airway may impact on continued attempts at intubation.

Hypoxia

Hypoxia is the end point of an obstructed airway. Adult residual capacity is approximately 3500 mL, assuming 20% O_2 and VO_2 of 250 mL/min. This gives roughly 3 minutes' oxygen reserve following cessation of ventilation. With removal of nitrogen by preoxygenation, reserve oxygen lasts 10 to 12 minutes in the ideal case (allowing for water vapor and dead space), less in the presence of lung disease or a decreased FRC (pregnancy or obesity). Aerobic metabolism is reduced when Pa_{O_2} within the mitochondria falls below 36 mm Hg. With a further reduction in Pa_{O_2} to 20 mm Hg (corresponding to 32% saturation of hemoglobin or an oxygen content of 4 to 5 mL/100 mL blood), neurons cease to function and consciousness is lost.

Means of assessing oxygenation include blood gases, oximetry, and, to some extent, direct examination of the patient's color. Blood gas determination is precise, but it requires taking an invasive sample and results may be significantly delayed. Pulse oximetry is continuous and real time but difficult to perform in cold or hypotensive patients. Assessment of a patient's color is quick but imprecise. Factors that influence the rate of onset of hypoxia include the supply of oxygen, the volume of oxygen stored in the body, and the rate of use of these stores.

Supply of Oxygen

The supply of oxygen may be supplemented simply by increasing the inspired oxygen concentration or by increasing the barometric pressure (as in a hyperbaric chamber).

Volume of Stored Oxygen

The primary storage site for supplemental oxygen at atmospheric pressure is the lungs. The volume of pulmonary oxygen depends on the functional residual capacity of the lungs; ie, the lung volume at the end of a normal expiration—approximately 3500 mL. Oxygen storage in the blood, myoglobin, and tissues remains relatively constant despite increased inspired concentration.

Blood carries oxygen in two forms: bound to hemoglobin and dissolved in plasma. Most of the oxygen (19.5 mL/100 mL blood) binds to hemoglobin; only 0.3 mL oxygen dissolves in solution, assuming a hemoglobin concentration of 14 to 15 g/100 mL and a Pa_{O_2} of 100 mm Hg. Cooperativity of hemoglobin subunits produces a nonlinear (sigmoidal) relationship between the percentage of oxygen saturation and Pa_{O_2}; ie, hemoglobin binds oxygen more tightly at a high Pa_{O_2} (in the lung) and gives up oxygen more readily at a low Pa_{O_2} (in the tissues).

Preoxygenation is important for several reasons. First, it maximizes oxygen reserve in the lungs of an apneic patient by replacing nitrogen with oxygen. Second, it maximizes oxygen reserves in the blood and tissues, although this is considerably less than the oxygen stores in the lungs. Patients with smaller FRCs (seen in pregnancy and obesity) require less time to denitrogenate, but also desaturate more quickly. These patients should be preoxygenated for a longer, rather than a shorter, period of time.

Rate of Use of Oxygen Stores

Factors influencing the rate of oxygen use include MV_{O_2}, and physiologic functions such as pH, concentration, and type of hemoglobin; temperature; available 2,3-diphosphoglycerate (2,3-DPG); poisons such as carbon monoxide or cyanide; and functional abnormalities of the pulmonary alveolar membrane.

MV_{O_2}. Differences in the rate of oxygen consumption (MV_{O_2}) and recognition of increased MV_{O_2} states, such as in children (twice that of adults), pregnancy, anxiety, sepsis or fever, shivering, and thyroid storm are important to keep in mind.

Bohr Effect. Increased P_{CO_2} causes a shift to the right of the Hgb–O_2 curve.

pH. Acidosis increases the availability of oxygen at the tissue level by shifting the oxyhemoglobin dissociation curve to the right. Acidosis in the lungs produces a similar shift, making uptake of oxygen more difficult. Does one effect negate the other? Due to cooperativity (sigmoidal shape of the oxyhemoglobin dissociation curve), acidosis produces a greater effect at low Pa_{O_2} values (found at the tissues) than near saturation levels (as found in the lung capillaries). Tissue oxygenation increases during acidosis, even though binding of oxygen to hemoglobin may be somewhat decreased in the lungs.

Concentration of Hemoglobin. One gram of hemoglobin binds 1.34 mL oxygen. Oxygen capacity therefore varies directly with hemoglobin concentration. Increased cardiac output may compensate for a low hemoglobin concentration.

Type of Hemoglobin. Abnormal hemoglobin species exist that may either increase or decrease the ability of hemoglobin to bind oxygen. Those that tend to increase affinity for oxygen cause a polycythemia, whereas those that decrease affinity cause anemia. Examples of those that increase affinity for oxygen include hemoglobins S, C, D, E, and H; examples of those that decrease affinity include hemoglobins J, Chesapeake, and Hiroshima.

Temperature. Increased temperature releases oxygen from hemoglobin, similar to pH, by shifting the oxyhemoglobin dissociation curve to the right. This facilitates oxygen delivery to areas of higher metabolism. An endogenous increase in body temperature accelerates oxygen consumption, as described by the Q10 law; ie, for every 10°C rise in temperature, the metabolic rate doubles. An exogenous increase in body temperature (ie, increasing environmental temperature) does not affect basal metabolic rate. Pa_{O_2} readings should be corrected for body temperature.

2,3-DPG. The major organic phosphate in erythrocytes in humans, 2,3-DPG, decreases the affinity of oxygen for hemoglobin. Mutually interdependent with carbon dioxide and hydrogen ion, 2,3-DPG levels increase when erythrocytes are exposed to low oxygen ten-

sions.[128] This augments distal oxygen delivery by forcing the dissociated hemoglobin state.

Carbon Monoxide. Carbon monoxide produces its toxic effect by competing with oxygen for the hemoglobin iron (II) ion with much higher affinity. Decreasing the oxygen content of the blood may not significantly affect the measured Pa_{O_2} of blood; thus, arterial blood gases give an inadequate indication of the degree of poisoning with carbon monoxide. Diagnose carbon monoxide poisoning first by suspicion (smoke exposure, soot or carbon in the upper airway), then by measuring arterial carbon monoxide hemoglobin saturation. Carbon monoxide-poisoned blood is cherry red, making oxygen saturation measurements unreliable.

Cyanide. This is a cytotoxic agent and does not affect oxygen binding to hemoglobin or transport. Oxygen content and Pa_{O_2} are thus normal and useless for diagnosis.

Hypercapnia

Normal P_{CO_2} ranges between 36 and 44 mm Hg. With complete cessation of ventilation, under basal metabolic conditions, P_{CO_2} increases at a rate of 3 to 6 mm Hg/min, causing both direct and indirect effects.[129, 130]

Direct effects include a decrease in myocardial contractility, negative chronotropic effect, hypotension in the presence of ganglionic blockade, increased myocardial perfusion, decreased skeletal muscle perfusion, potassium release into the serum from the liver, increased excitability of peripheral nerves, cerebral vasodilatation, epinephrine and norepinephrine release, and depressed activity of acetylcholine.

Hypercapnia also causes the following indirect effects: it increases cardiac output (with an intact sympathetic nervous system), increases heart rate via the autonomic nervous system, increases blood pressure with an intact autonomic nervous system, increases myocardial oxygen use, causes anuria secondary to constriction of afferent glomerular arterioles, and increases parasympathetic activity, but it produces no change in potassium in hepatectomized animals.

Alteration of Drug Distribution, Action, and Metabolism

Drugs for intubation should be administered intravenously.[131] In the intravascular space, they distribute to (1) receptor sites, initiating the characteristic action of the drug; as well as to (2) plasma and tissue proteins for distribution and storage. The pH, anoxia, concurrent administration of other drugs, the state of the circulation, preexisting malnutrition, and temperature influence drug action during obstructed ventilation.

pH. pH may be high from hyperventilation prior to intubation of a conscious patient, or it may reach extremely low levels with failed intubation attempts or cardiac arrest. pH changes secondary to metabolic acidosis are reflected to a lesser degree in the cerebrospinal fluid than are pH changes secondary to elevated P_{CO_2}, because carbon dioxide freely diffuses across cellular membranes. Elevated P_{CO_2} increases the migration of weak organic acids to the brain. In general, weak organic acids such as succinylcholine and d-tubocurarine diffuse to areas of higher pH, whereas organic bases diffuse to areas of lower pH.

Anoxia. Anoxia increases permeability and decreases selectivity of cell membranes, allowing greater penetration of drugs to intracellular space. The relative importance of anoxia and hypercapnia in humans was investigated by Frumin and colleagues.[132] They found tolerance to hypercapnia when not accompanied by hypoxia.

Altered Circulation. Patients with depressed circulation secondary to congestive heart failure in general require lower drug doses. Volatile anesthetics used to facilitate intubation reach anesthetizing partial pressures more rapidly because the drug is not as readily removed from the blood stream.

Malnutrition. Preexisting malnutrition, pregnancy, decreased liver function, starvation, or chronic alcoholism may result in diminished plasma cholinesterases. Plasma protein levels may also be lowered, reducing available inactive binding sites and, therefore, reducing the amount of succinylcholine needed to achieve relaxation. This may or may not prolong the action of succinylcholine and mivacurium, *but* the same dose is needed to achieve relaxation.

Miscellaneous Effects. Laryngospasm and simultaneous respiratory efforts against a closed glottis may hinder efforts at intubation, not only by closing the glottis but also by lowering the larynx in relation to the oral cavity, making visualization during laryngoscopy more difficult. Muscle relaxants reverse these effects: visualization becomes easier, the pathway is opened, and the larynx ceases to

be lowered. Agitation and restlessness may be signs of hypoxia; thus, attempts at reasoning with the patient are meaningless. Sedation of these patients may aggravate the agitation. You must oxygenate. In the alcoholic patient, agitation may reflect hypoglycemia as well as hypoxemia. Administering 50 mL of 50% glucose may be valuable. If initial efforts at intubation are unsuccessful, but you can ventilate the patient by mask, a judicious dose of a muscle relaxant may be useful.

Hypoxia and hypercarbia potentiate laryngospasm, hindering laryngoscopy and intubation; a muscle relaxant breaks this vicious cycle. Intubation attempts during laryngospasm may result in esophageal intubation, the path that offers the least resistance to the endotracheal tube. Pulmonary edema may also result from laryngospasm.

The rate of induction of anesthesia via inhalation agents is usually faster with a decreased cardiac output, in children, in obesity, and during pregnancy. A slower inhalation induction of anesthesia may be expected with an increase in cardiac output states (fever) or with airway obstruction.

SECURING OXYGENATION AND VENTILATION

General Assessment of the Patient

Prior to *any* intubation attempt, one should create a game plan specific for that patient. The process should begin with an assessment of the patient, including (1) an evaluation of the patient's history, (2) an examination of the patient and the airway, (3) measurement of the movement of critical airway structures, and (4) a determination of the influence of the patient's current status on the airway (Table 19–5).

Table 19–5. GENERAL ASSESSMENT OF THE PATIENT

1. Evaluate the patient's history
2. Examine the patient and the airway
3. Measure the movement of critical airway structures
   Mandible
   Cervical vertebrae
   Atlanto-occipital joint
   Tongue
   Teeth
4. Determine the influence of the patient's current status on the airway

Table 19–6. ESTABLISHING A GAME PLAN
FOR A PATIENT WITH A KNOWN PRIOR
DIFFICULT INTUBATION

1. Bypass the problem
2. Delay the case
3. Deal with the problem immediately

Table 19–7. AGENDA FOR SECURING
THE AIRWAY

1. Properly position the patient
2. Decide on how to approach the airway
3. Select appropriate instruments
4. Adequately suppress the patient's airway reflexes

Establishing a Game Plan for a Patient With a Known Prior Difficult Intubation

Table 19–6 summarizes options for a patient with a known prior difficult intubation.

Bypass the Airway Problem. In the past, an absolute contraindication to a regional anesthetic technique was the patient with a potentially difficult airway to control in an emergency. More recently, as anesthesiologists have become more confident in their ability to perform a safe and controlled regional anesthetic, this dogma has become a relative, rather than an absolute, contraindication. That is, an anesthesiologist may choose a judicious regional technique rather than opting for not needing to manage a difficult airway. The anesthesiologist must weigh the risks needed to control the airway intraoperatively.

Three situations may lead to emergent airway management: inadvertent total spinal (while performing an epidural, or interscalene block, etc); inadvertent intravascular injection; and the need for anesthesia of longer duration than the regional technique can offer. Judicious techniques to avoid these situations include incremental dosing with epinephrine or regional technique in order to recognize inadvertent intrathecal or intravascular injections; and avoidance of single-shot spinal anesthesia and the use of epidurally or intrathecally placed catheters. This allows a controlled level and duration of anesthesia.

Delay the Case. When the patient with a potentially difficult airway has a full stomach, the surgery may be delayed until stomach emptying occurs if the surgery is not of an emergent nature.

Deal With the Airway Problem Immediately. With the decision to secure the airway, four challenges must be met: (1) the patient should be ideally positioned, (2) an approach to the airway must be determined, (3) appropriate instruments must be selected, and (4) adequate suppression of the patient's airway reflexes must be achieved (Table 19–7).

Positioning the Patient. Table 19–8 offers options in positioning the patient.

Choices for head positioning involve changes in the curvature of the cervical vertebrae and flexion or extension of the atlanto-occipital joint or, infrequently, rotation of the head (Table 19–9). Classically, to optimize positioning for laryngoscopy with a Macintosh blade, the patient is placed in cervical flexion by placing a blanket under the patient's head, and the atlanto-occipital joint is extended to align the oral–pharyngeal and tracheal axes (see Figs. 16–1, 16–2, and 16–3).

Roberts and associates[133] examined the relationship between flexion–extension of the cervical vertebrae and flexion–extension of the atlanto-occipital joint on the position of the larynx relative to the laryngeal indices line, a line connecting the upper teeth to the external auditory canal. The relative position was determined with a laryngeal indices caliper (Fig. 19–16) and plotted on a representative graph (Fig. 19–17), with the laryngeal indices line being the X axis and a perpendicular line through the upper being the Y axis. Figure 19–18 illustrates the relative changes in position of the larynx with changes in cervical flexion–extension. Cervical flexion (a pillow under the occiput) moves the larynx posteriorly relative to the upper teeth (historically, it is the anterior larynx that proves difficult to intubate). Cervical extension moves the larynx anteriorly along the laryngeal indices line, thus theoretically making it more difficult to perform laryngoscopy with a Macintosh laryngoscope blade.

Changes in the position of the larynx relative to the laryngeal indices line with flexion–extension of the atlanto-occipital joint are illus-

Table 19–8. POSITIONING THE PATIENT

1. Positioning the patient's head
2. Positioning the patient's torso
3. Positioning the patient's larynx
4. Positioning the table

Table 19–9. POSITIONING THE PATIENT'S HEAD

1. Cervical flexion or extension
2. Atlanto-occipital flexion or extension

trated in Figure 19–19. Atlanto-occipital flexion moves the larynx anteriorly, whereas atlanto-occipital extension moves the larynx posteriorly along the same line.

Thus, both cervical flexion and atlanto-occipital extension move the larynx posteriorly along the laryngeal indices line, making it easier to visualize the laryngeal opening with the Macintosh laryngoscope. Although this produces an ideal patient position for direct laryngoscopy, it is not an ideal position for intubation with the flexible fiberoptic laryngoscope. The ideal patient position for flexible fiberscopy is cervical extension and atlanto-occipital extension; this position lifts the epiglottis from the posterior pharyngeal wall and opens a channel for the fiberscope bundle as it approaches the laryngeal entrance.

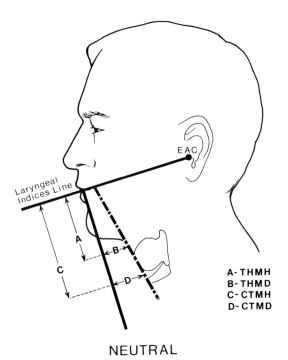

A - THMH
B - THMD
C - CTMH
D - CTMD

NEUTRAL

Figure 19–17. Graph generated by laryngeal indices caliper shown in Figure 19–16, showing the laryngeal indices line (LIL, X axis) passing through the upper teeth and the external auditory canal and a perpendicular line passing through the upper teeth representing the Y axis.

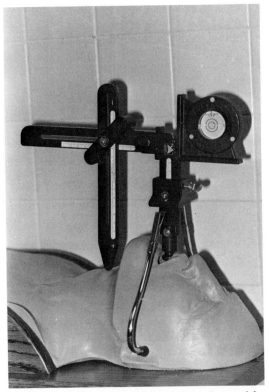

Figure 19–16. A laryngeal indices caliper designed by the author to take noninvasive measurements that indicate the relative position of the larynx in relation to the skull.

The patient's torso may be positioned supine with the operator at the patient's head or supine with the operator at the side. The patient may be sitting with the operator facing the patient. The patient may be positioned laterally with the operator at the patient's head for direct or for flexible fiberoptic laryngoscopy or at the patient's side for flexible fiberoptic laryngoscopy. A patient may also be positioned prone, as in Figure 19–20, with the

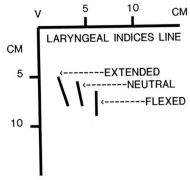

Figure 19–18. Changes in laryngeal position with changes in cervical flexion–extension.

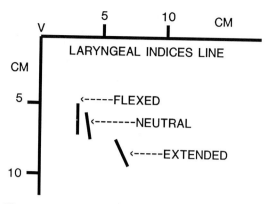

Figure 19–19. Changes in laryngeal position with changes in atlanto-occipital extension.

operator sitting at the patient's head. The prone position has the advantage that, if the patient vomits, there is less likelihood of pulmonary aspiration. It also has the advantage that the epiglottis falls forward by gravity, making flexible fiberoptic intubation easier (Fig. 19–21). The prone position has the disadvantage of making mask ventilation somewhat more difficult. Table 19–10 summarizes these positioning options.

Whereas the relative position of the larynx changes with changes in head position, the position of the larynx itself may be altered directly (Table 19–11). Once the importance

Table 19–10. POSITIONING THE PATIENT'S TORSO

1. Supine with the operator at the patient's head
2. Supine with the operator at the patient's side
3. Lateral with the operator at the patient's head
4. Lateral with the operator at the patient's side
5. Sitting with the operator facing the patient
6. Prone with the operator sitting, facing the patient, at the patient's head

of the tilt of the larynx was determined, a carpenter's level was modified (bubble inclinometer) so that the tilt of the larynx could be measured directly with the patient in the supine position (Fig. 19–22).[134] Figure 19–22 shows a patient with a normal tilt to the larynx. Figure 19–23 shows a patient with a difficult airway; ie, an anterior tilt greater than 40 degrees indicates a difficult direct laryngoscopy. Figure 19–24 illustrates what could be seen during direct laryngoscopy with a Macintosh #3 laryngoscope. The graph in Figure

Table 19–11. POSITIONING THE PATIENT'S LARYNX

1. Cricoid pressure
2. Thyrohyoid pressure
3. Combined thyrohyoid and cricoid pressure
4. Anterior traction on the larynx

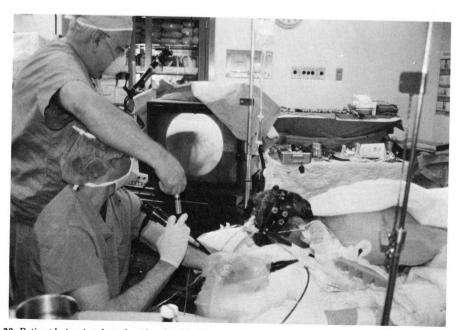

Figure 19–20. Patient being intubated with a flexible fiberoptic laryngoscope while in the prone position. The operator is sitting at the patient's head, viewing the larynx on a video monitor.

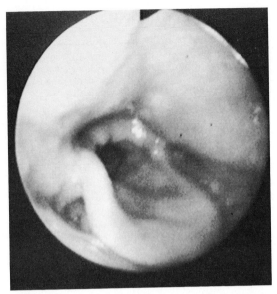

Figure 19–21. Video photograph taken with the patient in the prone position with the operator sitting at the patient's head. With gravity, the epiglottis falls anteriorly and opens the laryngeal entrance. The image is inverted 180 degrees from the view normally seen during direct laryngoscopy with the patient supine.

19–25 indicates that the greater the anterior tilt of the larynx, the more difficult it is to see the vocal cords on direct laryngoscopy with the Macintosh #3 laryngoscope.

Cricoid pressure (increasing the anterior tilt of the larynx) applied during rapid-sequence intubation may actually make direct laryngoscopy harder, whereas thyrohyoid pressure should decrease the anterior tilt, making direct laryngoscopy easier. It thus seems reasonable to apply thyrohyoid pressure in addition to cricoid pressure during rapid-sequence intubation. Lateral thyroid movement may facili-

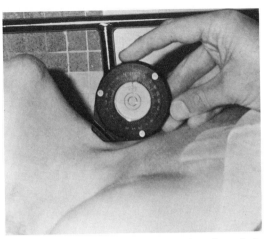

Figure 19–23. Bubble inclinometer against the anterior surface of the thyroid cartilage of a patient who had a very difficult intubation with a Macintosh #3 laryngoscope. Note the excessive anterior tilt of the thyroid cartilage, 40 degrees or greater.

tate visualization of the laryngeal opening when there is lateral displacement of the larynx by a neck mass. Anterior thyroid traction may facilitate passage of a nasogastric tube.

The operating room table or stretcher is usually elevated for direct laryngoscopy but should be lowered for flexible fiberoptic laryngoscopy (Table 19–12). The low level forces the operator to keep the flexible fiberoptic laryngoscope fully extended in order to ensure proper orientation of the tip of the fiberscope to the movement of the image in the eyepiece.

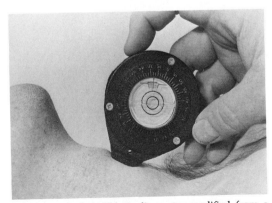

Figure 19–22. A bubble inclinometer modified from a carpenter's level by the author, placed against the anterior surface of the thyroid cartilage in a patient with a normal anterior tilt.

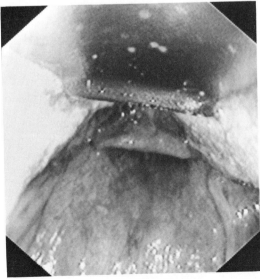

Figure 19–24. Video photograph illustrating visualization of the epiglottis, but not of the vocal cords, under direct laryngoscopy with a Macintosh #3 laryngoscope.

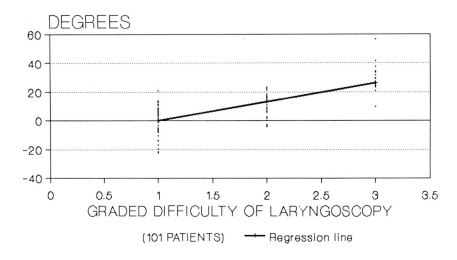

DEGREES

GRADED DIFFICULTY OF LARYNGOSCOPY

(101 PATIENTS)   —+— Regression line

1-ALL, 2-HALF, 3-NONE OF CORDS SEEN

Figure 19–25. Graph illustrating ability to see the laryngeal opening with a Macintosh #3 laryngoscope versus the tilt of the thyroid cartilage measured with a bubble inclinometer. Grade 1—all of the vocal cords could be seen; grade 2—some of the vocal cords could be seen; grade 3—none of the vocal cords could be seen.

The image in the eyepiece always moves from 6 to 12 o'clock, even when the tip is moving in a horizontal rather than a vertical direction.

Approaching the Airway. The oral approach is examined in Chapter 16, whereas the nasal approach is discussed in Chapter 17. Description of the techniques, as well as the advantages and disadvantages of tracheostomy and cricothyrotomy, are found in Chapter 10. In very selective conditions, a retrograde wire may be inserted percutaneously through the cricothyroid membrane, passed cephalad out the nose or mouth, and used as a guide for an endotracheal tube. Table 19–13 lists options for approaching the airway.

Instruments. Table 19–14 reviews the selection of appropriate instruments.

Mask ventilation: should an intubation attempt fail, immediate action depends on whether or not the airway is obstructed. With an adequate patent airway, controlled ventilation depends on a proper mask fit. Proper one- or two-handed face mask application is essential. Raise the mandible and face to meet the mask. Divide your relative effort in applying mask to face: 10% of your effort pushes the mask toward the face, and 90% brings the face (mandible) upward to meet the mask. With reverse percentages (the natural tendency), the result may well be obstruction of the airway from pressure of the tongue against the posterior pharyngeal wall. Inexperienced personnel who use this technique make maintenance of the airway difficult or even impossible. Oral or nasal airways may be of immense help during mask ventilation.

Maintain a mask fit with an edentulate patient by bringing the cheeks forward around the edges of the mask. This helps maintain a seal between mask and skin. A gauze pad in each of the buccal pouches may also help maintain a good mask fit, but great care must be exercised and these pads must be removed later on.

An Ambu bag or anesthesia machine should be available to deliver 100% oxygen with mask ventilation. Controlling ventilation with a mask may require the assistance of another individual (one individual maintaining a mask fit, the other individual ventilating the patient). Exercise extreme care in order to prevent forcing air into the esophagus and stomach. A dis-

Table 19–12. POSITIONING THE OPERATING ROOM TABLE OR STRETCHER

1. Elevating the table
2. Lowering the table
3. Changing the sitting position of the table
4. Trendelenburg
5. Reverse Trendelenburg

Table 19–13. APPROACHING THE AIRWAY

1. Oral techniques
2. Nasal techniques
3. Techniques that access the airway through the neck

Table 19–14. SELECTING APPROPRIATE
INSTRUMENTS

1. Mask ventilation
2. Laryngeal mask airway
3. Rigid laryngoscopes
4. Specialized rigid laryngoscopes
5. Flexible fiberoptic laryngoscopes
6. Combitube
7. Lightwand
8. Transtracheal jet ventilator
9. Retrograde guidewire
10. Specialized endotracheal tubes

tended stomach may embarrass ventilatory movements of the diaphragm or induce vomiting by build up of intragastric pressure. By placing a stethoscope over the stomach just below the xiphoid and listening for gurgling (air bubbles) during controlled inspiration, one may detect air being forced into the stomach. To prevent this, reduce inspiratory pressure and ventilate with a smooth motion, using smaller tidal volumes. When ventilating with an Ambu bag with 100% FiO_2, limit inspiratory pressures to 20 mm Hg in order to minimize gastric air.

The laryngeal mask airway (LMA) was recently introduced in the United States and approved for use by the Food and Drug Administration (FDA). Although the laryngeal mask airway is discussed in Chapter 20, its usefulness in critical airway situations cannot be overemphasized. The laryngeal mask airway is particularly useful in the morbidly obese patient when the patient does not need to be intubated with an endotracheal tube but does need to have oxygenation and ventilation established.

Flexible fiberoptic laryngoscopy has emerged as the premier technique for intubating the patient with a difficult airway. The flexible fiberoptic laryngoscope may also be used to check the position of endotracheal tubes. See Chapters 21, 22, and 23 for select discussions on the use of the flexible fiberoptic laryngoscope.

The Combitube is discussed in Chapter 26.

Standard rigid laryngoscope blades for oral intubations are covered in Chapter 13.

Specialized rigid laryngoscope blades, such as for the Bullard laryngoscope, may be useful if the operator is familiar with their use. These blades are designed only for oral intubations, whereas the flexible fiberoptic laryngoscope is designed for oral or nasal use, as well as to check the position of an endotracheal or tracheostomy tube.

A lightwand, shown in Figure 19–26, may be used as a stylet to semiblindly guide an endotracheal tube through the mouth to the patient's larynx. The light at the tip of the stylet is visualized through the skin of the anterior neck. A semidarkened room is of some value. It is our opinion that direct visualization of the laryngeal entrance is preferred.

Transtracheal oxygenation/ventilation: individuals may withstand high P_{CO_2} levels as long as they are not hypoxic; ie, as a temporary measure, it may not be necessary to ventilate and remove carbon dioxide as long as oxygen can be supplied to the lungs.[5] It is hypoxia that damages tissue in airway obstruction. Attia and colleagues[135] described pressures required to achieve adequate flows of oxygen through various sizes of catheters. The term *transtracheal ventilation* assumes exhalation through an open glottis; if the airway is totally obstructed, passive exhalation through a transtracheal catheter is inadequate to sustain ventilation. Negative pressure must be applied to the catheter in order to remove adequate

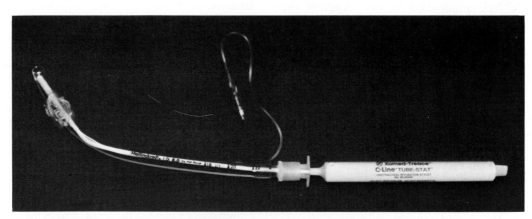

Figure 19–26. A lightwand inserted through an endotracheal tube.

amounts of inspired air to maintain a normal P_{CO_2}.[136–139] Equipment to produce this alternating positive and negative pressure sufficient to allow ventilation through a 14-gauge catheter with normal tidal volumes is not readily available.

In the last 10 years, a method of ventilation that uses significantly lower tidal volumes with much higher frequencies has appeared in the literature: high-frequency positive-pressure ventilation.[140–146] Although it is still under investigation in many centers, it holds promise for ventilation in emergency situations such as complete obstruction of the airway (as long as one can apply negative pressure to the catheter during exhalation). In the meantime, transtracheal ventilation should not be confused with transtracheal oxygenation. Transtracheal oxygenation creates a diffusion gradient along the pulmonary tree. Oxygen, supplied at the tracheal end, diffuses to the alveolar end. Oxygenating the patient by this method buys time in a critical situation, until more appropriate means of oxygenation can be instituted.

A retrograde guidewire technique has also been used to facilitate intubation when direct laryngoscopy has failed.[147] An arteriographer, S. I. Seldinger, originally described the guidewire technique to facilitate cannulation of arteries. For retrograde intubation, a cannula is used to percutaneously puncture the cricothyroid membrane. A guidewire is then passed through the cannula and out the mouth. The endotracheal tube is then passed over the guidewire, through the mouth, and through the laryngeal entrance. Once the tip of the endotracheal tube passes through the vocal cords, the wire is withdrawn and the endotracheal tube is advanced to optimal position.

A specialized endotracheal tube, the Endotrol tube (Mallinckrodt Co.), may be particularly useful when it becomes necessary to bend the tip of the endotracheal tube anteriorly. This is frequently the case with the patient with ankylosing spondylitis or the patient with an "anterior" larynx (see Chapter 12 and Fig. 12–13).

Reflex Responses. Autonomic reflexes are summarized in Table 19–15, with the stimulus, response, and possible treatment listed. Specific reflexes that need to be controlled to secure the airway include the gag reflex, the cough reflex, the vomiting reflex, reflex laryngeal closure, bronchospasm, cardiovascular reflexes, and secretory responses.

Gag reflex: the afferent limb of the gag reflex originates from the sensory branches of the

Table 19–15. DEALING WITH AIRWAY REFLEXES

1. Gag reflex
2. Cough reflex
3. Vomiting reflex
4. Reflex laryngeal closure
5. Bronchospasm
6. Cardiovascular reflexes
7. Secretory responses

glossopharyngeal nerve (IX). From there, impulses travel to the dorsal nucleus of the vagus, from which efferents emerge. The gag reflex has been reported to be diminished in various disease states, including stroke patients,[148, 149] patients with prolonged endotracheal intubation,[150] mentally retarded patients,[151] patients with a lateral medullary syndrome,[152] patients with a vagal neuropathy,[153] comatose head-injured patients,[154] and schizophrenic patients.[155, 156] Hyperactivity of the gag reflex is of great concern to dentists, as well as to physicians, and therefore there are a number of reports in the dental and medical literature on various management techniques.[157–169]

Commonly, the oropharyngeal distribution of the glossopharyngeal nerves may be anesthetized by a direct nerve block or by applying a topical anesthetic to the posterior pharyngeal wall. With the patient supine, 5% lidocaine ointment can be applied to an oral airway: as the ointment melts in the patient's mouth, it coats the posterior pharyngeal wall with its pleasing peppermint taste. The gag reflex may also be blocked with an aerosol or spray of lidocaine or with a general anesthetic (with or without a muscle relaxant).

Cough reflex: initially, the laryngeal entrance opens and air is insufflated into the lungs. This is followed by closure of both the vocal cords and the supraglottic structures. These structures then open and air is forcibly expelled. The effect is to clear the airway of the irritating foreign substances that initiate the reflex. The sensory branch of the superior laryngeal nerves innervates the vallecula, the epiglottis, and the piriform recesses down to the superior aspect of the vocal cords. The reflex arc travels to the spinal cord and hence to the motor portion of the superior laryngeal nerve to the cricothyroideus muscle, the only tensor of the vocal cords, and to the other muscles that close the glottis and are controlled by the efferent branches of the recurrent laryngeal nerves.

Tracheal stimulation is transmitted via afferent fibers from the recurrent laryngeal nerves to the nucleus of the tractus solitarius and to the dorsal motor nucleus of the vagus, and from there to the efferent fibers of the recurrent laryngeal nerves that innervate all of the other intrinsic muscles of the larynx (other than the cricothyroideus muscle). Mucus affects the sensory response to stimulation; ie, the greater the amount of mucus present, the lower the response to the stimulus. Viral infections of the lungs increase the reflex response on both the afferent and efferent sides of the reflex arc.

The cough reflex may be blocked to varying degrees, depending on the depth of general anesthesia, the presence of muscle relaxants, or the use of topical or intravenous local anesthetics.

Vomiting reflex: an obstetric patient undergoing anesthesia frequently does so with a full stomach. Vomiting may occur during any intubation attempt, whether the patient is awake or anesthetized. Stimuli to vomiting arise from a variety of sources, such as laryngoscopy or an oral airway. Intestinal obstruction, particularly duodenal, may induce regurgitation. Stimuli carried by either sympathetic or parasympathetic afferents to the vomiting center in the medulla oblongata initiate a series of muscular contractions and relaxations mediated by the phrenic, vagal, and sympathetic nerves. The sequence of events during vomiting is shown in Figures 19–27 and 19–28.

Topical anesthetics applied to the oral cavity may block oral or pharyngeal stimulation of the gag and subsequent vomiting reflexes but have no effect on the intestinal causes of vomiting. Oral or intravenous cimetidine or oral magnesium hydroxide/aluminum hydroxide (Maalox) helps to neutralize stomach acid. Emptying the stomach with an Ewald tube or nasogastric tube before induction of general anesthesia cannot be counted on to remove all of the stomach contents. Several techniques for anesthetizing a patient with a full stomach have been suggested.

Regional anesthesia bypasses the need for general anesthesia but does not guarantee against vomiting. It leaves the laryngeal reflexes intact to protect against aspiration if vomiting does occur. However, regional anesthesia is suitable for only a limited number of procedures. For rapid-sequence induction of general anesthesia, currently in common use, place the patient in either a head-up or a lateral head-down position. The lateral head-down position helps minimize aspiration, although regurgitation may actually be more likely with the head-down position; intubation is more difficult in this position, particularly for the inexperienced anesthetist. The intravenous route gains anesthesia and muscle relaxation for intubation. A drawback of rapid-sequence intubation and anesthesia occurs when the trachea cannot be intubated on the first attempt. The Curry maneuver minimizes

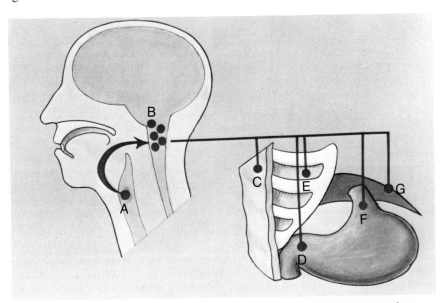

Figure 19–27. Reflex vomiting pathway. *A*, Stimulation of sensory receptors at the laryngeal entrance; *B*, dorsal nucleus of the vagus; *C*, abdominal muscles contract; *D*, gastroduodenal junction; *E*, intercostal muscles contract; *F*, esophagogastric relaxation; *G*, diaphragm contracts. (From Roberts JT. Fundamentals of tracheal intubation. Orlando: Grune & Stratton, 1983; with permission.)

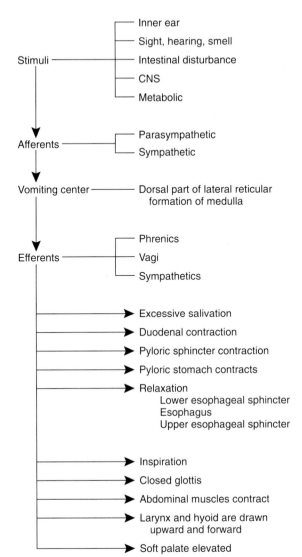

Figure 19–28. Sequence of events during reflex vomiting. (From Roberts JT. Fundamentals of tracheal intubation. Orlando: Grune & Stratton, 1983; with permission.)

the risk of forcing air into the stomach during controlled ventilation, and the Sellick maneuver minimizes the chance of regurgitation of stomach or esophageal contents. Both maneuvers apply cricoid pressure against the upper esophagus.

Use awake intubation as an alternative to prevent aspiration if vomiting or regurgitation is anticipated. Optimal areas to anesthetize with a local anesthetic for awake intubation of the patient with a full stomach are the base of the tongue, the vallecula, and the epiglottis. Avoid the piriform recess, the vocal folds, and the trachea. Although this leaves the laryngeal reflexes intact to protect the airway from as-

piration, it almost always ensures violent coughing with the introduction of the endotracheal tube into the trachea. Vomiting may accompany coughing. Inflating the cuff of an endotracheal tube does not absolutely guarantee against aspiration (although it undoubtedly helps). Various premedicant techniques have been advocated to prevent aspiration with awake intubation of the patient with a full stomach.

Reflex laryngeal closure: stimulation of the sensory area innervated by the superior laryngeal nerves initiates the afferent limb of the reflex path for laryngeal closure and possibly laryngospasm. Impulses travel to the central vagal nuclei, then out vagal efferents to one or more of the muscle groups protecting the laryngeal entrance—the cricothyroids tense the vocal cords (Fig. 19–29), the thyroarytenoids relax the vocal cords (Fig. 19–30A), the lateral cricoarytenoids adduct the arytenoids (Fig. 19–30B), the transverse arytenoids adduct the arytenoids (Fig. 19–31A), and the posterior cricoarytenoids abduct the vocal cords (Fig. 19–31B). Figure 19–32 shows the intrinsic muscles of the larynx as they would appear if the mucosal surface were peeled away and the structure was visualized from the oral cavity.

In addition to general anesthesia with or without a muscle relaxant, techniques to block reflex laryngeal closure include topical application, intraoral spray, inhaled vapor, or percutaneous transtracheal application of a local anesthetic.

Bronchospasm: the closely intertwined upper airway and digestive tract have developed complex reflexes to ensure appropriate conduction of food and air. Although normal pharyngeal and laryngeal reflexes serve protective functions against aspiration into the upper airway, abnormally exaggerated respiratory and cardiovascular responses may prove disastrous during the induction of anesthesia. Instrumentation of the upper airway, including fiberoptic bronchoscopy, has been associated with fatal acute bronchospasm and cardiopulmonary arrest.[170, 171]

Bronchospasm is primarily a vagally mediated increase in bronchial smooth muscle tone with expiratory airflow obstruction. Increased secretions and mucosal edema, seen as components of the inflammatory response, may potentiate obstruction, most notably in patients with reactive airway disease. This can lead to clinically significant changes in pulmonary mechanics, including increased functional

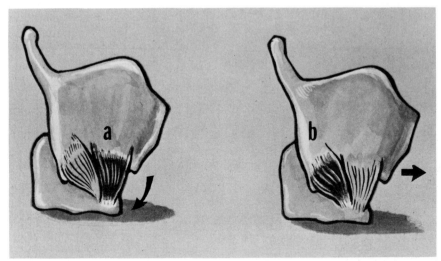

Figure 19–29. Thyroid and cricoid cartilages and the cricothyroid muscle. *A*, Pars anterior; *B*, Pars oblique. Contraction of these muscles tenses the vocal cords.

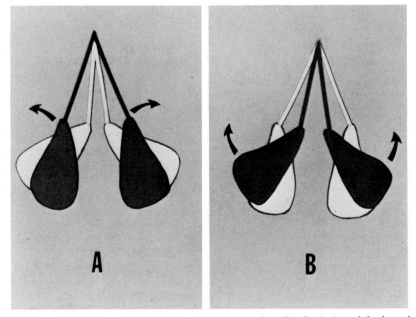

Figure 19–30. *A*, Action of the thyroarytenoid muscles (relax the vocal cords). *B*, Action of the lateral cricoarytenoid muscles (adducts arytenoids) Unshaded areas represent the position prior to the action of the muscle; shaded areas represent the position after the action of the muscle. (From Roberts JT. Fundamentals of tracheal intubation. Orlando: Grune & Stratton, 1983; with permission.)

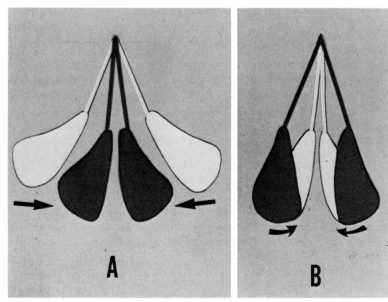

Figure 19–31. *A*, Action of the transverse arytenoid muscles (adduct arytenoids). *B*, Action of the posterior cricoarytenoid muscles (abducts the vocal cords). Unshaded areas indicate the position prior to the action of the muscle; shaded areas indicate the position after the action of the muscle. (From Roberts JT. Fundamentals of tracheal intubation. Orlando: Grune & Stratton, 1983; with permission.)

residual capacity (FRC), decreased arterial O_2 tension, vital capacity (Vc), and first-second expiratory volume flow (FEV$_1$).[172]

Many different stimuli can trigger a bronchospastic attack. Indirect, immune-mediated

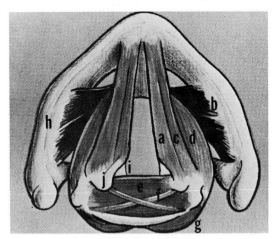

Figure 19–32. Intrinsic muscles of the larynx from above. a, Vocal cord; b, cricothyroids—tense the vocal cords; c, thyroarytenoids—relax the vocal cords (main function), lateral portion adducts arytenoids; d, lateral cricoarytenoids—close glottis; e, transverse arytenoids—close glottis; f, oblique arytenoids—close glottis; g, posterior cricoarytenoids—open glottis; h, thyroid cartilage; i, arytenoid cartilage; j, cuneiform cartilage. (From Roberts JT. Fundamentals of tracheal intubation. Orlando: Grune & Stratton, 1983; with permission.)

stimuli such as dust or pollen may trigger mast cell degranulation and begin the inflammatory cascade in susceptible individuals. Release of inflammatory mediators, including histamine and the leukotrienes, both directly stimulate smooth muscle contraction and sensitize rapidly adapting subendothelial irritant receptors in the tracheobronchial tree. Touch, mechanical pressure, cold air, smoke, water, and acid or alkaline fluids (pH <4.5 or >8.8) all elicit laryngeal and pharyngeal reflexes. Irritant and specialized mechanoreceptors are thought to represent the afferent limb. Stimuli then travel via the superior laryngeal nerves (for tissues above the vocal cords) and glossopharyngeal nerves (portions of the pharynx) to the nucleus of the tractus solitarius. Interneurons then project to vagal efferent motor nuclei in the ventrolateral medulla, to descend with the vagus nerve to the tracheobronchial tree. Receptors in the upper tracheobronchial tree travel via afferent fibers from the recurrent laryngeal nerves to the nucleus of the tractus solitarius. Interneurons then project from the tractus solitarius to efferent neurons in the ventrolateral medulla, which innervate bronchial smooth muscle and mucus-secreting cells by cholinergic synapses. Efferent vagal function may also modulate mast cell activity, although this has not been fully elucidated.

Both laryngeal and pharyngeal stimulation may provoke bronchospasm.

Prevention and treatment of bronchoconstriction may take place on several levels. Direct stimulation of mechanoreceptors may be blocked by topical anesthetics, including viscous lidocaine, benzocaine (Cetacaine) spray, or intratracheal lidocaine injection through the cricothyroid membrane. Aerosolized lidocaine has been used experimentally to demonstrate the differential sensitivity of the upper portion of the tracheobronchial tree to stimulation. Gentle handling of an endotracheal tube or other invasive devices minimizes mechanoreceptor activation. Decreases in vagal tone and secretions may be achieved with either nebulized or intravenous anticholinergics (atropine 0.4 mg IV or nebulized). Inhaled β_2 agonists counteract increased vagal tone. Finally, induction of general anesthesia decreases reflex autonomic outflow.

Cardiovascular reflexes: protective glottic and laryngeal reflexes elicit sympathetic discharge on intubation. Impulses from irritant upper airway receptors travel via cranial nerves to the brainstem. Hypothalamic, cortical, and brainstem centers integrate afferent information and supply efferents to mediate neuromuscular, cerebral, and cardiovascular responses. Mechanical stimulation of the trachea is an extremely noxious stimulus that can elicit strong cardiovascular reflex responses, including bradycardia, hypertension, and tachycardia. Increased heart rate and blood pressure raise myocardial oxygen demand, with the possibility of ischemia and infarction.[173] Reflex sympathetic discharge predisposes to cardiac arrhythmias, seen in up to 15% of patients during and after intubation.[174] Attenuation of these responses has been described with a variety of pharmacologic agents (Table 19–16). The most commonly used agent is an intravenous opioid premedication. Mechanoreceptors in the upper airway and trachea provide strong afferent stimuli during direct laryngoscopy. Supraglottic structures are innervated by the glossopharyngeal and superior laryngeal nerves, whereas infraglottic structures are innervated by the recurrent nerves. There is, however, some overlap of receptive fields. Vagal afferents have been important in animal models and, occasionally, in pediatric patients, as part of the bradycardiac response to intubation or endotracheal suctioning. These afferent impulses travel to the ventrolateral medulla, with projections to higher centers. Cortical, hypothalamic (medial preoptic and posterior), and brainstem centers are integrated to produce the cardiovascular response to intubation. This in part accounts for the extreme variability of responses.

Cholinergic efferents to the heart may produce bradycardia and hypotension during intubation. Vagal responses seem to be age related, occurring most prominently in the pediatric population, probably due to receptor

Table 19–16. ATTENUATION OF CARDIOVASCULAR REFLEXES

Modality	Advantages	Disadvantages
Local anesthetics	Lower systemic anesthetic levels	Reflexes may be triggered by spray; injection invasive
Recurrent laryngeal nerve block, topical spray		
Oral anesthetic rinse	Avoids laryngoscopy	No tracheal block
Intratracheal injection	Avoids laryngoscopy	No oropharyngeal block
Nebulized local anesthetic	Avoids laryngoscopy, includes tracheal block	Effective dose uncertain
Parenteral medications		
Opioids and anesthetics	BP, HR control	Potential for respiratory depression
Peripheral vasodilators	BP control	No protection against tachycardia
Ca^{++} channel blockers	BP control	No protection against tachycardia, negative inotropic effect
Central alpha-blockers	BP, HR control	Requires administration long before surgery; poorly reversible if patient develops hemodynamic instability
Peripheral alpha and beta blockade	BP, HR control	Beta alone inadequate; poorly reversible in the event of hemodynamic instability or bronchospasm

BP—blood pressure; HR—heart rate.
Adapted from Kaplan JD, Schuster DP. Physiologic consequences of tracheal intubation. Clin Chest Med 12:425–432, 1991; with permission.

field overlap in the nucleus of the tractus solitarius.[170] Asystole has been described; treatment with an anticholinergic is often effective.

Hypertension and tachycardia are more commonly seen in the adult population. Sympathetic responses to endotracheal intubation are mediated both directly via sympathetic nervous system efferents and indirectly by catecholamine release from the adrenal medulla. Efferents from the thoracolumbar ganglia travel to the heart (T1 to T5 branches), adrenal glands (T6 to T12), and directly to the vascular bed (the entire chain from T1 to L2). Within 5 seconds of epiglottic stimulation, Stoelting describes increases in systolic and diastolic blood pressure of 50 and 30 mm Hg, respectively, which peak at 45 seconds.[175] Intubation resulted in additional hypertension and tachycardia, with a mean heart rate increase. The principal determinants of the cardiac response to intubation appear to be epinephrine and norepinephrine released from the adrenal medulla, which produces a mixed alpha and beta response.[176] This response changes with patient age. Pediatric patients demonstrate a greater degree of cholinergic response to upper airway stimulation. With advancing age, the relative importance of β_1 effects diminishes, but an alpha hypertensive response continues.[177]

Studies of pharmacologic blockade of these responses have focused on every phase of the reflex arc. Adequate topical anesthesia decreases receptor activation, although this is difficult to achieve below the glottis on a routine basis. Alpha-blockers, either clonidine or phentolamine, have been tried. Nitroprusside has been used to blunt the hypertensive response to intubation, although with no effect on the tachycardia. Massive preinduction doses of opioids, such as fentanyl 50 μg/kg, have been shown to blunt the catecholamine surge for a stress-free induction for cardiac surgery; such large doses are not suitable, however, for routine surgery.

Secretory responses: secretory fibers to the sublingual, submaxillary, nasopalatine, and lacrimal glands originate in the superior salivatory and lacrimal nuclei located in the middle hindbrain. These nuclei give rise to two groups of secretory nerves: the nervus intermedius and the greater superficial petrosal nerve. The nervus intermedius travels with the facial nerve, passes the chorda tympani through the middle ear, then travels with the lingual nerve to synapse in the submaxillary ganglion. From there it innervates the sublingual, submaxillary, and nasopalatine glands. The greater superficial petrosal nerve synapses in the sphenopalatine ganglion and innervates the lacrimal glands.

The dorsal vagal nucleus, located in the floor of the fourth ventricle, gives rise to autonomic efferents; the ventral vagal nucleus gives rise to fibers that supply striated muscle. Secretory fibers to the mucous glands of the larynx, below the vocal folds, and to mucous glands in the trachea travel with the recurrent laryngeal branch of the vagus. The mucous cells constitute approximately one sixth of the cells lining the trachea. The other five sixths are ciliated epithelial cells that contain as many as 200 cilia per cell. These cells sweep the respiratory tract of mucus and dust particles.

Efferent autonomic fibers, accompanying the glossopharyngeal nerve and arising from the inferior salivatory nucleus in the reticular formation, innervate the parotid gland, oropharyngeal isthmus, tonsils, and meninges.

Electrical stimulation of the parasympathetic nerve supply to the salivary glands produces vasodilatation and a watery secretion proportional to the rate of stimulation. Stimulation of sympathetic nerves to the salivary glands produces vasoconstriction and a small secretory response. Respiratory tract secretions in humans approximate 0.09 g/m²/min.

SUMMARY

Failed intubation can be a devastating experience if it is not properly prepared for. Initial evaluation must include assessment of the patient's airway for factors that predict a difficult intubation. A structured approach must then be developed, considering anatomy and airway; superimposed conditions (trauma, aspiration, obesity); and patients with preexisting medical problems.

The operator has at his or her disposal: (1) patient positioning; (2) choice of approach to the airway; and (3) selected instruments. Any plan must also include measures to control potentially life-threatening reflexes, including cough, gag, vomiting, secretions, bronchospasm, and cardiovascular responses. These measures include ablating afferent impulses (topical anesthesia, nerve block), modulating autonomic reflexes (general anesthesia or sedation), and blocking completion of the reflex arc with alpha- and beta-blockers, opioids, and so forth.

Tables 19–17 through 19–27 offer guidelines (in terms of positioning, approach, instruments, and reflexes) to secure the difficult airway.

Table 19–17. GAME PLAN FOR A PATIENT WITH AN UNSTABLE NECK

Position
  Head—neutral
  Torso—supine or prone
  Larynx—no thyroid pressure
  Table—lowered when supine, elevated when prone
  Operator—at patient's head or side
Approach
  Awake, oral or nasal
Instruments
  Flexible fiberoptic
Reflexes
  Topical anesthesia—lidocaine
  Aerosol lidocaine
  Regional block (superior laryngeal nerves)
  Sedation

Table 19–18. GAME PLAN FOR THE PATIENT WITH BLOOD IN THE OROPHARYNX

Position
  Head—neutral
  Torso—supine or lateral
  Larynx—cricoid–thyrohyoid pressure
  Table—elevated
  Operator—at patient's head
Approach
  Awake—oral
Instruments
  Rigid laryngoscope—minimal blood
  Retrograde wire—gross blood
Reflexes
  Topical anesthesia
  Aerosol lidocaine
  Regional block with lidocaine (superior laryngeal nerves)

Table 19–19. GAME PLAN FOR THE PATIENT WITH GROSS ASCITES

Position
  Head—neutral
  Torso—lateral
  Larynx—cricoid + thyrohyoid pressure
  Table—elevated
  Operator—at patient's head or side
Approach
  Awake—oral
Instruments
  Flexible fiberoptic laryngoscope with operator at patient's side
  Rigid laryngoscope with operator at patient's head
Reflexes
  Topical anesthesia
  Aerosol lidocaine
  Regional block (superior laryngeal nerves)
  Sedation

Table 19–20. GAME PLAN FOR THE PATIENT WITH A LIMITED JAW OPENING

Position
  Head—neutral
  Torso—supine
  Larynx—neutral
  Table—lowered
  Operator—at patient's head
Approach
  Awake—nasal
Instruments
  Flexible fiberoptic laryngoscope
Reflexes
  Topical anesthesia
  Aerosal lidocaine
  Regional block (superior laryngeal nerves)
  Sedation

Table 19–21. GAME PLAN FOR THE PATIENT WITH A FULL STOMACH

Position
  Head—sniffing
  Torso—supine
  Larynx—cricoid and thyrohyoid pressure
  Table—elevated
  Operator—at patient's head
Approach
  Oral
Instruments
  Rigid standard laryngoscope
  Styletted endotracheal tube
Reflexes
  Topical anesthesia
  General anesthesia with rapid sequence induction

Table 19–22. GAME PLAN FOR THE PATIENT WITH COPIOUS ORAL SECRETIONS

Position
  Head—neutral
  Torso—supine or lateral
  Larynx—cricoid pressure if necessary
  Table—elevated
  Operator—at patient's head
Approach
  Oral or nasal
Instruments
  Rigid standard laryngoscope
  Flexible fiberoptic laryngoscope
Reflexes
  Antisialagogues
  Topical anesthesia
  Aerosol lidocaine
  Sedation

Table 19–23. GAME PLAN FOR THE PATIENT
WITH HEAD OR NECK TRAUMA

Position
  Head—neutral
  Torso—supine
  Larynx—cricoid + thyrohyoid pressure
  Table—elevated
  Operator—at patient's head
Approach
  Oral
  Nasal
  Through the neck
    Retrograde wire
    High-frequency jet ventilation
    Cricothyrotomy
    Surgeon standing by for surgical airway
Instruments
  Complete array of instruments available
Reflexes
  Topical anesthesia
  General anesthesia with rapid sequence induction

Table 19–24. GAME PLAN FOR THE PATIENT
WITH GROSS OBESITY

Position
  Head—sniffing for rigid standard laryngoscopy;
    extended for flexible fiberoptic laryngoscopy
  Torso—supine or sitting
  Larynx—no pressure
  Table—lowered
  Operator—standing at patient's head or facing
    patient who is in a sitting position
Approach
  Oral
Instruments
  Laryngeal mask airway
  Rigid standard laryngoscope
  Flexible fiberoptic laryngoscope
Reflexes
  Topical anesthesia with patient awake
  Aerosol lidocaine
  Regional block (superior laryngeal nerves)
  Sedation

Table 19–25. GAME PLAN FOR A PEDIATRIC
PATIENT WITH EPIGLOTTITIS

Position
  Head—neutral
  Torso—in parent's arms
  Larynx—undisturbed
  Table—elevated
  Operator—(most experienced operator available)
    stand beside parent and patient for an inhalation
    induction
Approach
  Oral
Instruments
  Rigid standard laryngoscope
Reflexes
  General anesthesia with gentle mask induction;
    maintain spontaneous ventilation
  No needles prior to general anesthesia
  Emergency/desperation maneuver: if the airway is
    lost, push on the chest and, under direct vision,
    intubate where air bubbles are seen to be
    emerging

Table 19–26. GAME PLAN FOR A PATIENT
WITH AN ASPIRATED PEANUT

Position
  Head—neutral
  Torso—supine
  Larynx—no pressure
  Table—elevated
  Operator—at patient's head
Approach
  Oral
Instruments
  Rigid bronchoscope
Reflexes
  General anesthesia with spontaneous ventilation
    induction and maintenance

Table 19–27. GAME PLAN FOR THE
AGITATED PATIENT

Position
  Head—neutral or sniffing
  Torso—supine
  Larynx—cricoid + thyrohyoid pressure
  Table—elevated
  Operator—standing at patient's head
Approach
  Oral
Instruments
  Rigid standard laryngoscopes
Reflexes
  Treat hypoxia
  Treat hypoglycemia
  Sedate appropriately
  General anesthesia
  Topical anesthesia

References

1. Myer CM III. Airway obstruction in Hurler's syndrome—radiographic features. Int J Pediatr Otorhinololaryngol 22:91–96, 1991.
2. Holzman RS. Airway involvement and anesthetic management in Goltz's syndrome. J Clin Anesth 3:422–425, 1991.
3. Lynch M, Underwood S. Pulmonary oedema following relief of upper airway obstruction in the Pierre-Robin syndrome: A consequence of early palatal repair? Br J Anaesth 66:391–393, 1991.
4. Scheller JG, Schulman SR. Fiber-optic bronchoscopic guidance for intubating a neonate with Pierre-Robin syndrome. J Clin Anesth 3:45–47, 1991.
5. Bull MJ, Givan DC, Sadove AM, Bixler D, Hearn D. Improved outcome in Pierre Robin sequence: Effect of multidisciplinary evaluation and management. Pediatrics 86:294–301, 1990.
6. Kelly CA, Griffiths ID. Major upper airways obstruction associated with Sjogren's syndrome: A case report and literature review. Br J Rheumatol 28:543–545, 1989.
7. Bollensen E, Schonle PW, Braun U, Prange HW. An unnoticed dislocation of the dens axis in a patient with primary chronic polyarthritis undergoing intensive therapy. Anaesthesist 40:294–297, 1991.
8. Yaszemski MJ, Shepler TR. Sudden death from cord compression associated with atlanto-axial instability in rheumatoid arthritis. Spine 15:338–341, 1990.
9. Crosby ET, Lui A. The adult cervical spine: Implications for airway management. Can J Anaesth 37:77–93, 1990.
10. Bamshad M, Rosa U, Padda G, Luce M. Acute upper airway obstruction in rheumatoid arthritis of the cricoarytenoid joints. South Med J 82:507–511, 1989.
11. Goldhagen J. Cricoarytenoiditis as a cause of acute airway obstruction in children. Ann Emerg Med 17:532–533, 1988.
12. Roelofse JA, Shipton EA. Difficult intubation in a patient with rheumatoid arthritis: A case report. S Afr Med J 64:679–680, 1983.
13. Messeter KH, Pettersson KI. Endotracheal intubation with the fibre-optic bronchoscope. Anaesthesia 35:294–298, 1980.
14. Fox MW, Onofrio BM, Kilgore JE. Neurological complications of ankylosing spondylitis. J Neurosurg 78:871–878, 1993.
15. Steib A, Beller JP, Lleu JC, Otteni JC. Difficult intubation managed by laryngeal mask and fibroscope. Ann Fr Anesth Reanim 11:601–603, 1992.
16. Hyman SA, Rogers WD, Bullington JC III. Cervical osteotomy and manipulation in ankylosing spondylitis: Successful general anesthesia after local anesthesia with sedation. J Spinal Disord 3:423–426, 1990.
17. Yamakage M, Yamazaki Y, Iwasaki H, Namiki A. Utility of Bullard intubating laryngoscope with a special stylet in two cases of difficult tracheal intubation. Masui 40:1404–1406, 1991.
18. Wittmann FW, Ring PA. Anaesthesia for hip replacement in ankylosing spondylitis. J IR Soc Med 79:457–459, 1986.
19. Sinclair JR, Mason RA. Ankylosing spondylitis: The case for awake intubation. Anaesthesia 39:3–11, 1984.
20. Edens ET, Sia RL. Flexible fiberoptic endoscopy in difficult intubations. Ann Otol Rhinol Laryngol 90(4 pt 1):307–309, 1981.
21. Daum RE, Jones DJ. Fiberoptic intubation in Klippel-Feil syndrome. Anaesthesia 43:18–21, 1988.
22. Roelofse JA, Morkel JA. Anesthesia for temporomandibular arthroplasty in a quadriplegic patient: A case report. Anesth Pain Control Dent 1:153–156, 1992.
23. Aiello G, Metcalf I. Anaesthetic implications of temporomandibular joint disease. Can J Anaesth 39:610–616, 1992.
24. Lipp M, Daublander M, Ellmauer ST, vonDomarus H, Stauber A, Dick W. Changes in temporomandibular joint functions in various general anesthesia procedures. Anaesthesist 37:366–373, 1988.
25. Lipp M, vonDomarus H, Daublander M, Leyser KH, Dick W. Effects of intubation anesthesia on the temporomandibular joint. Anaesthesist 36:442–445, 1987.
26. Krucylak CP, Schreiner MS. Orotracheal intubation of an infant with hemifacial microsomia using a modified lighted stylet. Anesthesiology 77:826–827, 1992.
27. Handler SD, Keon TP. Difficult laryngoscopy/intubation: The child with mandibular hypoplasia. Ann Otol Rhinol Laryngol 92(4 pt 1):401–404, 1983.
28. Licht JR, Smith WR, Glauser RL. Tonsillar hypertrophy in an adult with obesity-hypoventilation syndrome: The use of the flow-volume loop. Chest 70:672–674, 1976.
29. Anton-Pacheco J, Cano-Novillo I, Vilarino-Mosquere A, Herrero-Lopez E, Cuadros-Garcia J, Berchi-Garcia FJ. Cysts of the thyroglossal duct: Analysis of diagnostic errors and causes of recurrence. An Esp Pediatr 36:121–124, 1992.
30. Liu TP, Jeng KS, Yang TL, Wang TC, Hwang KF. Thyroglossal duct cyst: An analysis of 92 cases. Chung Hua I Hsueh Tsa Chih 49:72–75, 1992.
31. Girard M, DeLuca SA. Thyroglossal duct cyst. Am Fam Physician 42:665–668, 1990.
32. Topf P, Fried MP, Strome M. Vagaries of thyroglossal duct cysts. Laryngoscope 98:740–742, 1988.
33. Horisawa M, Ninomi N, Ito T. Anatomical reconstruction of the thyroglossal duct cyst. J Pediatr Surg 26:766–769, 1991.
34. Mozen Y, Watanabe T, Nakanishi K, Iwasaki K, Mori H, Aikawa H, Ashizawa A. Ultrasonography and CT of thyroglossal duct cysts: Nippon Igaku Hoshasen Gakkai Zasshi 51:400–405, 1991.
35. Issa MM, deVries P. Familial occurrence of thyroglossal duct cyst. J Pediatr Surg 26:30–31, 1991.
36. Katz AD, Hachigian M. Thyroglossal duct cysts: A thirty year experience with emphasis on occurrence in older patients. Am J Surg 155:741–744, 1988.
37. Benjamin B. Acute epiglottitis. Ann Acad Med Singapore 20:696–699, 1991.
38. Hill J, Cardig P. Mean airflow rates in laryngeal polyposis. Clin Otolarlyngol 18:121–124, 1993.
39. Leech H, Onal E, Aronson R, Lopata M. Voluntary hyperventilation in obesity hypoventilation. Chest 100:1334–1338, 1991.
40. Hoskins MC, Evans RA, King SJ, Gishen P. 'Sabre sheath' trachea with mediastinal lipomatosis mimicking a mediastinal tumour. Clin Radiol 44:417–418, 1991.
41. Kattan B, Snyder HS. Lingual artery hematoma resulting in upper airway obstruction. J Emerg Med 9:421–424, 1991.
42. Wells RM. Airway management in the blunt trauma patient: How important is the cervical spine? Can J Surg 35:27–30, 1992.
43. Kellman R. The cervical spine in maxillofacial

trauma: Assessment and airway management. Oto-laryngol Clin North Am 24:1–13, 1991.
44. Teichgraeber JF, Rappaport NH, Harris JH Jr. The radiology of upper airway obstruction in maxillofacial trauma. Ann Plast Surg 27:103–109, 1991.
45. Woo P, Kelly G, Kirshner P. Airway complications in the head injured. Laryngoscope 99(7 pt 1):725–731, 1989.
46. Szeremeta W, Morovati SS. Isolated hyoid bone fracture: a case report and review of the literature. J Trauma 31:268–271, 1991.
47. Nakayama DK, Gardner MJ, Rowe MI. Emergency endotracheal intubation in pediatric trauma. Ann Surg 211:218–223, 1990.
48. Lacoste L, Gineste D, Karayan J, Montaz N, Le-huede MS, Girault M, Bernit AF, Barbier J, Fusciardi J. Airway complications in thyroid surgery. Ann Otol Rhinol Laryngol 102:441–446, 1993.
49. Wade JS. Cecil Joll Lecture, 1979: Respiratory obstruction in thyroid surgery. Ann R Coll Surg Engl 62:15–24, 1980.
50. Teitel AD, MacKenzie CR, Stern R, Paget SA. Laryngeal involvement in systemic lupus erythematosus. Semin Arthritis Rheum 22:203–214, 1992.
51. Thompson T, Frable MA. Drug-induced, life-threatening angioedema revisited. Laryngoscope 103(1 pt 1):10–20, 1993.
52. Ulmer JL, Garvey MJ. Fatal angioedema associated with lisinopril. Ann Pharmacother 26:1245–1246, 1992.
53. Ebert RJ. Post partum airway obstruction after vaginal delivery. Anaesth Intensive Care 20:365–367, 1992.
54. Rocke DA, Scoones GP. Rapidly progressive laryngeal oedema associated with pregnancy-aggravated hypertension. Anaesthesia 47:141–143, 1992.
55. Laitinen K. Life-threatening laryngeal edema in a pregnant woman previously treated for thyroid carcinoma. Obstet Gynecol 78(5 pt 2):937–938, 1991.
56. Hardy F, Ngwingtin L, Bazin C, Babinet P. Hereditary angioneurotic edema and pregnancy. J Gynecol Obstet Biol Reprod (Paris) 19:65–68, 1990.
57. Costa JM, Netto EM, Marsden PD. Acute airway obstruction due to edema of the larynx following antimony therapy in mucosal leishmaniasis. Rev Soc Bras Med Trop 19:109, 1986.
58. Reimold WV. Pathogenesis of hereditary angioedema. Z Gastroenterol 25:316–324, 1987.
59. Poppers PJ. Anaesthetic implications of hereditary angioneurotic oedema. Can J Anaesth 34:76–78, 1987.
60. Correll RW, DeBoom GW, Jensen JL. Rapidly developing, edematous swelling of the upper lip. J Am Dent Assoc 113:69–70, 1986.
61. Schar B. Anesthesia in a patient with hereditary angioedema. Anaesthesist 33:140–141, 1984.
62. Delfino JJ, Sclaroff A, Giglio JA, Travis M. Management of a patient with hereditary angioneurotic edema. J Oral Surg 36:890–892, 1978.
63. Sataloff DM, Sataloff RT. CME program: Tracheotomy and inhalation injury. Head Neck Surg 6:1024–1031, 1984.
64. Kelly JH, Montgomery WW, Goodman ML, Mulvaney TJ. Upper airway obstruction associated with regional enteritis. Ann Otol Rhinol Laryngol 88(1 pt 1):95–99, 1979.
65. Benumof JL. Management of the difficult adult airway: With special emphasis on awake tracheal intubation. Anesthesiology 75:1087–1100, 1992.
66. Corren J, Schocket AL. Anaphylaxis: A preventable emergency. Postgrad Med 87:167–168, 171–178, 1990.
67. Welsh LW, Welsh JJ, Kelly JJ. Massive orofacial abscesses of dental origin. Ann Otol Rhinol Laryngol 100(9 pt 1):768–773, 1991.
68. Ekberg O, Feinberg M. Clinical and demographic data in 75 patients with near-fatal choking episodes. Dysphagia 7:205–208, 1992.
69. Filler RM, Messineo A, Vinograd I. Severe tracheomalacia associated with esophageal atresia: Results of surgical treatment. J Pediatr Surg 27:1136–1140, 1992.
70. Wiseman RS, Gravlee GP, Koufman JA, Kon ND. The perils of esophageal prosthesis placement in malignant tracheoesophageal fistula. J Clin Anesth 4:134–138, 1992.
71. Heiss K, Wesson D, Bohn D, Smith C, Wiseman N. Respiratory failure due to retained esophagus: A complication of esophageal replacement. J Pediatr Surg 26:1359–1361, 1991.
72. Griscom NT. Caldwell lecture: Respiratory problems of early life now allowing survival into adulthood: Concepts for radiologists. AJR 158:1–8, 1992.
73. Kao SC, Smith WL, Sato Y, Franken EA Jr, Kimura K, Soper RT. Ultrafast CT of laryngeal and tracheo-bronchial obstruction in symptomatic postoperative infants with esophageal atresia and tracheoesophageal fistula. AJR 154:345–350, 1990.
74. Biller JA, Allen JL, Schuster SR, Treves ST, Winter HS. Long-term evaluation of esophageal and pulmonary function in patients with repaired esophageal atresia and tracheoesophageal fistula. Dig Dis Sci 32:985–990, 1987.
75. Templeton JM Jr, Templeton JJ, Schnaufer L, Bishop HC, Ziegler MM, ONeill JA Jr. Management of esophageal atresia and tracheoesophageal fistula in the neonate with severe respiratory distress syndrome. J Pediatr Surg 20:394–397, 1985.
76. Oliver AM, Orlowski JP. A double-crossover study comparing conventional ventilation with high frequency ventilation in a patient with tracheoesophageal fistula. Resuscitation 12:225–231, 1985.
77. Westbrook JL. Oesophageal achalasia causing respiratory obstruction. Anaesthesia 47:38–40, 1992.
78. Becker DJ, Castell DO. Acute airway obstruction in achalasia: Possible role of defective belch reflex. Gastroenterology 97:1323–1326, 1989.
79. Zikk D, Rapoport Y, Halprin D, Papo J, Himelfarb MZ. Acute airway obstruction and achalasia of the esophagus. Ann Otol Rhinol Laryngol 98(8 pt 1):641–643, 1989.
80. Barr GD, MacDonald T. Management of achalasia and laryngo-tracheal compression. J Laryngol Otol 103:713–714, 1989.
81. Cousar JI Jr, Berman JS. Respiratory muscle fatigue from functional upper airway obstruction. Chest 96:689–690, 1989.
82. Brown NJ, Morgan HJ. Multinodular goiter causing airway obstruction. J Tenn Med Assoc 85:65–66, 1992.
83. Ayabe H, Kawahara K, Tagawa Y, Tomita M. Upper airway obstruction from a benign goiter. Surg Today 22:88–90, 1992.
84. Smallridge RC. Metabolic and anatomic thyroid emergencies: A review. Crit Care Med 20:276–291, 1992.
85. Shaha AR. Surgery for benign thyroid disease causing tracheoesophageal compression. Otolaryngol Clin North Am 23:391–401, 1990.

86. Shaha AR, Burnett C, Alfonso A, Jaffe BM. Goiters and airway problems. Am J Surg 158:378–380, 1989.
87. Geraghty JG, Coveney EC, Kierman M, OHiggins NJ. Flow volume loops in patients with goiters. Ann Surg 215:83–86, 1992.
88. Muckart DJ, Aitchison JM. Fatality from blind intubation of suspected tension pneumothorax. Injury 20:175–176, 1989.
89. Holcomb GW III, Templeton JM Jr. Iatrogenic perforation of the bronchus intermedius in a 1,100-g neonate. J Pediatr Surg 24:1132–1134, 1989.
90. Rollins RJ, Tocino I. Early radiographic signs of tracheal rupture. AJR 148:695–698, 1987.
91. Gold MI, Joseph SI. Bilateral tension pneumothorax following induction of anesthesia in two patients with chronic obstructive airway disease. Anesthesiology 38:93–96, 1973.
92. Newton NI, Adams AP. Excessive airway pressure during anaesthesia: Hazards, effects and prevention. Anaesthesia 33:689–699, 1978.
93. Ward PH, Zwitman D, Hanson D, Berci G. Contact ulcers and granulomas of the larynx: New insights into their etiology as a basis for more rational treatment. Otolaryngol Head Neck Surg 88:262–269, 1980.
94. Mehta M, Petereit D, Chosy L, Harmon M, Fowler J, Shahabi S. Sequential comparison of low dose rate and hyperfractionated high dose rate endobronchial radiation for malignant airway occlusion. Int J Radiat Oncol Biol Phys 23:133–139, 1992.
95. Mehta MP, Shahabi S, Jarjour NN, Kinsella TJ. Endobronchial irradiation for malignant airway obstruction. Int J Radiat Oncol Biol Phys 17:847–851, 1989.
96. Francfort JW, Smullens SN, Gallagher JF, Fairman RM. Airway compromise after carotid surgery in patients with cervical irradiation. J Cardiovasc Surg (Torino) 30:877–881, 1989.
97. Dawson A, Lehr PP, Bigby BG, Mitler MM. Effect of bedtime ethanol on total inspiratory resistance and respiratory drive in normal nonsnoring men. Alcohol Clin Exp Res 17:256–262, 1993.
98. Berry RB, Bonnet MH, Light RW. Effect of ethanol on the arousal response to airway occlusion during sleep in normal subjects. Am Rev Respir Dis 145(2 pt 1):445–452, 1992.
99. Jakkupi M, Dreshaj IA, Mandura I, Haxhiu MA. Effect of ethanol on tone of isolated smooth muscle of the pulmonary artery. Plucne Bolesti 43:16–20, 1991.
100. Greiff L, Erjefalt I, Wollmer P, Pipkorn U, Persson CG. Effects of histamine, ethanol, and a detergent on exudation and absorption across guinea pig airway mucosa in vivo. Thorax 46:700–705, 1991.
101. Morio H, Osegawa M, Matsucka Y, Yokota M, Kohno N, Mitsunaga S, Fujisawa T, Yasumi K, Mikata A. Effect of ethanol injection in tracheal large cell carcinoma—a case report. Nippon Kyobu Shikkan Gakkai Zasshi 28:623–627, 1990.
102. Richards IS, Kulkarni AP, Brooks SM. Ethanol-induced bronchodilatation in TEA-treated canine tracheal smooth muscle is mediated by a beta-adrenoceptor-dependent mechanism. Eur J Pharmacol 167:155–160, 1989.
103. Drummond WH, Gause GE, Polak MJ, Lyles D, Cassin S. Ethanol induces acute pulmonary vasoconstriction in salt-perfused rat lungs. Exp Lung Res 15:447–458, 1989.
104. Mitler MM, Dawson A, Henriksen SJ, Sobers M, Bloom FE. Bedtime ethanol increases resistance of upper airways and produces sleep apnea in asymptomatic snorers. Alcohol Clin Exp Res 12:801–805, 1988.
105. Fujisawa T, Hongo H, Yamaguchi Y, Shiba M, Kadoyama C, Kawano Y, Fukasawa T. Intratumoral ethanol injection for malignant thracheobronchial lesions: A new bronchofiberscopic procedure. Endoscopy 18:188–191, 1986.
106. Jakupi M, Djokic TD, Karahoda-Gjurgjeala N, Zuskin E, Haxhiu MA. Effect of ethanol on the isolated airway smooth muscle tone. Acta Med Iugosl 40:207–214, 1986.
107. Bonora M, Shields GI, Knuth SL, Bartlett D Jr, St-John WM. Selective depression by ethanol of upper airway respiratory motor activity in cats. Am Rev Respir Dis 130:156–161, 1984.
108. Hadfield JM, Stoner HB. Interactions between ethanol and the responses to injury. J Trauma 23:518–522, 1983.
109. Kruhoffer PW. Handling of inspired vaporized ethanol in the airways and lungs (with comments on forensic aspects). Forensic Sci Int 21:1–17, 1983.
110. Ayres J, Clark TJ. Alcohol in asthma and the bronchoconstrictor effect of chlorpropamide. Br J Dis Chest 76:79–87, 1982.
111. Wright PM, Alexander JP. Acute airway obstruction, hypertension and kyphoscoliosis. Anaesthesia 46:119–121, 1991.
112. Merchant FJ, Nichols RL, Bombeck CT. Unusual complication of nasogastric esophageal intubation-erosion into an aberrant right subclavian artery. J Cardiovasc Surg 18:147–150, 1977.
113. George MK, OConnell JE, Batch AJ. Paradoxical vocal cord motion: an unusual cause of stridor. J Laryngol Otol 105:312–314, 1991.
114. Tatsumi K, Furuyz H, Nagahata T, Hashimoto M, Sha K, Tanake O, Matsunaga T, Okuds T. Removal of a bronchial foreign body in a child using the laryngeal mask. Masui 42:441–444, 1993.
115. Todres ID. Pediatric airway control and ventilation. Ann Emerg Med 22(2 pt 2):440–444, 1993.
116. Travassos RR Jr, Barbas SV, Fernandes JM, Mendes MJ, Fiks IN, Ribeiro CS, Barbas-Filho JV. Foreign-body aspiration in adults. Rev Hosp Clin Fac Med Sao Paulo 46:193–195, 1991.
117. Nichol JW, Yardley MP, Parker AJ. Pharyngolaryngeal migration: A delayed complication of an impacted bullet in the neck. J Laryngol Otol 106:1091–1093, 1992.
118. Kimura M, Hara H, Matsushima T, Kobori M. A case of obstructive ventilatory disturbance caused by bronchial wall granulation due to a fish bone. Nippon Kyobu Shikkan Gakkai Zasshi 30:2013–2017, 1992.
119. Eyrich JE, Riopelle JM, Naraghi M. Elective transtracheal jet ventilation for bronchoscopic removal of tracheal foreign body. South Med J 85:1017–1019, 1992.
120. Anderson CE, Savignac AC. Nasoendotracheal tube obstruction secondary to inferior turbinate impaction. AANA J 59:538–540, 1991.
121. Roach JM, Ripple G, Dillard TA. Inadvertent loss of bronchoscopic instruments in the tracheobronchial tree. Chest 101:568–569, 1992.
122. Parsons DS, Kearns D. The two-headed stethoscope: Its use for ruling out airway foreign bodies. Int J Pediatr Otorhinolaryngol 22:181–185, 1991.

123. Haines DJ Jr. Wheezing as a sign of foreign-body aspiration in infants and children. Postgrad Med 90:153–154, 1991.

124. Conacher ID. Foreign body in a laryngeal mask airway [letter]. Anaesthesia 46:164, 1991.

125. Perper JA, Kuller LH, Shim YK. Detection of fatal therapeutic misadventures by an urban medico-legal system. J Forensic Sci 38:327–338, 1993.

126. Streitz JM Jr, Shapshay SM. Airway injury after tracheotomy and endotracheal intubation. Surg Clin North Am 71:1211–1230, 1991.

127. Todd DA, John E, Osborn RA. Tracheal damage following conventional and high-frequency ventilation at low and high humidity. Crit Care Med 19:1310–1316, 1991.

128. Woodson R. Physiological significance of oxygen dissociation curve shifts. Crit Care Med 7:368–373, 1979.

129. Hlastala M. Physiological significance of the interaction of oxygen and carbon dioxide in blood. Crit Care Med 7:374–379, 1979.

130. Tenny S, Lamb T. Physiological consequences of hypoventilation and hyperventilation. In Handbook of Physiology, vol. 1. Washington, DC: American Physiological Society, 1964; pp 979–1010.

131. Hug C. Pharmacokinetics of drugs administered intravenously. Anesth Analg 57:704–723, 1978.

132. Frumin M, Epstein R, Cohen G. Apneic oxygenation in man. Anesthesiology 20:789, 1959.

133. Roberts JT, Ali HH, Shorten GD. Using the laryngeal indices caliper to predict difficulty of laryngoscopy with a Macintosh #3 laryngoscope. J Clin Anesth 5:302–305, 1993.

134. Roberts JT, Ali HH, Shorten GD. Using the bubble inclinometer to measure laryngeal tilt and predict difficulty of laryngoscopy. J Clin Anesth 5:306–309, 1993.

135. Attia R, Battit G, Murphy J. Transtracheal ventilation. JAMA 234:1152, 1975.

136. Neff CC, Pfister RC, Van Sonnenberg E. Percutaneous transtracheal ventilation: Experimental and practical aspects. J Trauma 23:84–90, 1983.

137. Dunlap L, Oregon E. A modified, simple device for the emergency administration of percutaneous transtracheal ventilation. JACEP 7:42–46, 1978.

138. Spoerel W, Narayanan P, Singh N. Transtracheal ventilation. Br J Anaesth 43:932–939, 1971.

139. Jacobs H. Emergency percutaneous transtracheal catheter and ventilator. Trauma 12:50–55, 1972.

140. Jonzon A, Sedin G, Sjostrand U. High-frequency positive-pressure ventilation (HFPPV) applied for small lung ventilation and compared with spontaneous respiration and continuous positive airway pressure (CPAP). Acta Anaesthesiol Scand Suppl 53:23–36, 1973.

141. Heijman K, Heijman L, Jonzon A, et al. High frequency positive pressure ventilation during anesthesia and routine surgery in man. Acta Anaesthesiol Scand 16:176–187, 1972.

142. Jonzon A, Oberg, Sedin G, et al. High-frequency positive-pressure ventilation by endotracheal insufflation. Acta Anaesthesiol Belg Suppl 43:1–43, 1971.

143. Eriksson I, Nilsson LG, Nordstrom S, et al. High-frequency positive-pressure ventilation (HFPPV) during transthoracic resection of tracheal stenosis and during preoperative bronchoscopic examination. Acta Anaesthesiol Scand 19:113–119, 1975.

144. Eriksson I, Sjostrand U. High-frequency ventilation (HFPPV) during laryngoscopy. Opuscula Med 19:2768–2786, 1974.

145. Eriksson, Heijneman L, Sjostrand U. High-frequency positive-pressure ventilation (HFPPV) in bronchoscopy during anesthesia. Opuscula Med 19:14–24, 1974.

146. Babinski M, Smith R, Klain M. High-frequency jet ventilation for laryngoscopy. Anesthesiology 52:178–180, 1980.

147. Sternbach G. Sven Ivar Seldinger: Catheter introduction on a flexible leader. J Emerg Med 8:635–637, 1990.

148. Horner J, Brazer SR, Massey EW. Aspiration in bilateral stroke patients: A validation study. Neurology 43:430–433, 1993.

149. Horner J, Massey EW, Brazer SR. Aspiration in bilateral stroke patients. Neurology 40:1686–1688, 1990.

150. DeVita MA, Spierer-Rundback L. Swallowing disorders in patients with prolonged orotracheal intubation or tracheostomy tubes. Crit Care Med 18:1328–1330, 1990.

151. Hollge J. Effect of abnormal gagging reflex on the possibility of aspiration in mentally retarded children. Sb Lek 92:18–22, 1990.

152. Luker J, Scully C. The lateral medullary syndrome. Oral Surg Oral Med Oral Pathol 69:322–324, 1990.

153. Jacobs CJ, Harnsberger HR, Lufkin RB, Osborn AG, Smoker WR, Parkin JL. Vagal neuropathy: evaluation with CT and MR imaging. Radiology 164:97–102, 1987.

154. Martin KM. Predicting short term outcome in comatose head-injured children. J Neurosci Nurs 19:9–13, 1987.

155. Craig TJ, Richardson MA, Pass R, Haugland G. Impairment of the gag reflex in schizophrenic inpatients. Compr Psychiatry 24:514–520, 1983.

156. Craig TJ, Richardson MA, Pass R, Haugland G. Impairment of the gag reflex in schizophrenic patients [letter]. Am J Psychiatry 140:950–951, 1983.

157. Foster WM, Hurewitz AN. Aerosolized lidocaine reduces dose of topical anesthetic for bronchoscopy. Am Rev Respir Dis 146:520–522, 1992.

158. Valley MA, Kalloo AN, Curry CS. Peroral pharyngeal block for placement of esophageal endoprostheses. Reg Anaesth 17:102–106, 1992.

159. Clark GD, Pond C. Adaptation of the de Vilbis atomizer for the delivery of topical anesthesia. Nurse Anesth 3:20–24, 1992.

160. Hudson C, Thornton J, OKeefe G. The effect of neuroleptic and antiparkinsonian medication on the gag reflex. Schizophr Res 3:283–285, 1990.

161. Wu TJ, Liu CC, Lin SY, Jiang CJ, Chen CL, Hou WY, Liang HC, Lee TS, Huang CH, Hong PY. Comparison of lower concentrations of lidocaine to suppress bucking before extubation during recovery of general anesthesia. Ma Tsui Hsueh Tsa Chi 28:279–283, 1990.

162. Callison GM. A modified edentulous maxillary custom tray to help prevent gagging. J Prosthet Dent 62:48–50, 1989.

163. Fleece L, Linton P, Dudley B. Rapid elimination of a hyperactive gag reflex. J Prosthet Dent 60:415–417, 1988.

164. Kaufman E, Weinstein P, Sommers EE, Soltero DJ. An experimental study of the control of the gag reflex with nitrous oxide. Anesth Prog 35:155–157, 1988.

165. Meeker HG, Magalee R. The conservative management of the gag reflex in full denture patients. N Y State Dent J 52:11–14, 1986.
166. Van Overvest Eerdmans GR, Slop D. Dental treatment in patients with a severe gag reflex (as applied to complete dentures). Rev Belge Med Dent 40:148–154, 1985.
167. Conny DJ, Tedesco LA. The gagging problem in prosthodontic treatment. II: Patient management. J Prosthet Dent 49:757–761, 1983.
168. Klepac RK, Hauge G, Dowling J. Treatment of an overactive gag reflex: Two cases. J Behav Ther Exp Psychiatry 13:141–144, 1982.
169. DeMeester TR, Skinner DB, Evans RH, Benson DW. Local nerve block anesthesia for peroral endoscopy. Ann Thorac Surg 24:278–283, 1977.
170. Cunningham ET, Ravich W, Jones B, Donner M. Vagal reflexes referred from the upper aerodigestive tract: An infrequently recognized cause of common cardiorespiratory responses. Ann Intern Med 116:575–582, 1992.
171. Taryle DA, Chandler JE, Good JT Jr, Potts DE, Sahn SA. Emergency room intubations—complications and survival. Chest 75:541–543, 1979.
172. Matsushima Y, Jones RL, King EG, Moysa G, Alton JD. Alterations in pulmonary mechanics and gas exchange during routine fiberoptic bronchoscopy. Chest 86:184–188, 1984.
173. Slogoff S, Keats AS. Does perioperative myocardial ischemia lead to postoperative myocardial infarction? Anesthesiology 62:107–114, 1985.
174. King DB, Harris LC, Greifenstein FE. Reflex circulatory responses to direct laryngoscopy and tracheal intubation performed during general anesthesia. Anesthesiology 12:556, 1951.
175. Stoelting RK. Circulatory changes during laryngoscopy and tracheal intubation: Influence of duration of laryngoscopy with and without prior lidocaine. Anesthesiology 17:381, 1977.
176. Derbyshire DR, Smith G. Sympathoadrenal responses to anesthesia and surgery. Br J Anaesth 56:725, 1984.
177. Bullington J, Mouton-Perry SM, Rigby J, Pinkerton M, Rogers D, Lewis TC, Preganz P, Wood AJ, Wood M. The effect of advancing age on the sympathetic response to laryngoscopy and tracheal intubation. Anesth Analg 68:603–608, 1989.

CHAPTER 20

The Laryngeal Mask and Perioperative Airway Management

George D. Shorten, M.B., F.F.A.R.C.S.(I.), F.C.Anaes.,
and James T. Roberts, M.D., M.A.

In 1983, A.I.J. Brain[1] described the laryngeal mask as an alternative means of airway maintenance during spontaneous or positive pressure ventilation in the anesthetized patient. Brain reasoned that gas flow continuity might be achieved by placing two tubes end to end (if the seal were airtight) as well as by inserting one in the other, as in conventional endotracheal intubation. Examination of cadaver airways revealed that such a seal may be produced if an elliptical cuff is inflated in the hypopharynx overlying the glottis. A prototype was constructed, made of the rubber cuff of a pediatric Goldman mask stretched over the diagonally cut distal end of a Portex (10 mm) endotracheal tube. Brain's initial evaluation identified five important points. First, the idea was feasible and warranted further investigation. Second, although positive pressure ventilation was possible, a leak around the cuff develops with higher inflation pressures. Third, correct placement was technically easy and did not require laryngoscopy. Fourth, a large epiglottis may be responsible for partial obstruction. Finally, a laryngeal mask was easily placed in patients in whom moderate difficulty at intubation would have been anticipated.

The laryngeal mask is easily inserted in most cases. The insertion technique is illustrated in Figures 20–1 to 20–8. First, the cuff is fully deflated. Lubricant is liberally applied to the dorsal surface of the mask and cuff. The patient's head and neck are positioned as for endotracheal intubation (partial cervical flexion and complete atlanto-occipital extension).[1-3] The mask tip should be flattened against the hard palate; at this stage, the anesthesiologist should look in the oral cavity to ensure correct placement.[4]

The laryngeal mask is advanced over the dorsum of the tongue.[5] An attempt should be made to avoid downfolding of the epiglottis by pressing the mask against the posterior pharyngeal wall. The laryngeal mask is correctly placed when resistance is encountered as the mask tip reaches the base of the hypopharynx.[6] The cuff is inflated and a slight bulging forward of the larynx is noted.[7] Manual ventilation is performed to confirm correct placement and to measure the pressure at which an audible leak occurs.[8] In adults, using the larger sizes, it is possible to ventilate the lungs at airway pressures up to 3.0 kPa.[5] Patency of the airway must now be checked, and the criteria used by Broderick and associates[2] serve as useful

Text continued on page 224

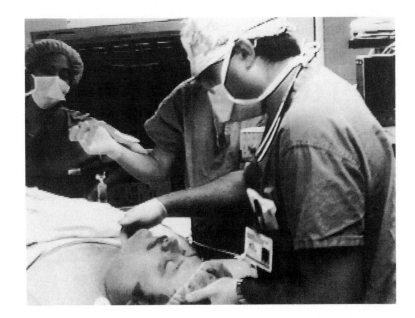

Figure 20–1. The nondominant hand pushes the head from behind, flexing the neck and extending the head.

Figure 20–2. An assistant passes the prepared laryngeal mask.

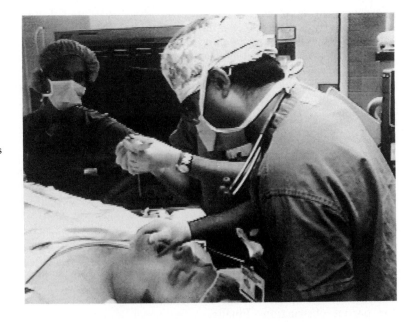

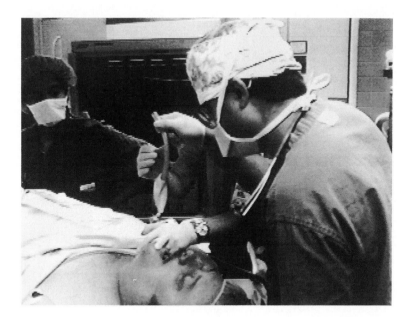

Figure 20–3. The tube of the laryngeal mask is held like a pen. Surgical gloves should be worn for insertion.

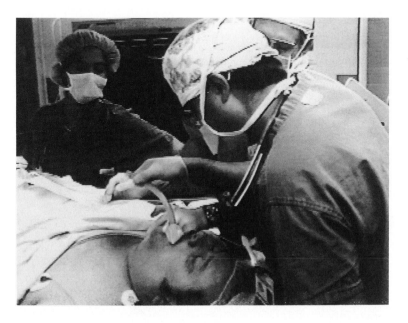

Figure 20–4. The laryngeal mask is inserted through the mouth with the aperture facing forward. The mask tip may be pressed upward against the hard palate.

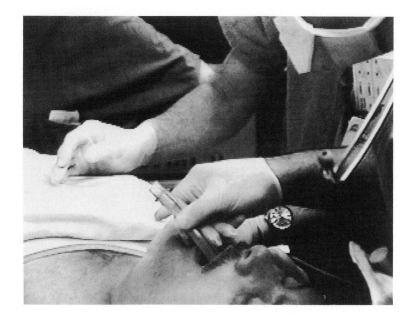

Figure 20–5. The mask is advanced over the hard palate into the laryngopharynx.

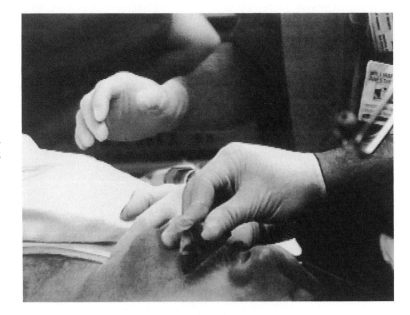

Figure 20–6. Resistance is encountered as the tip of the mask enters the upper esophagus.

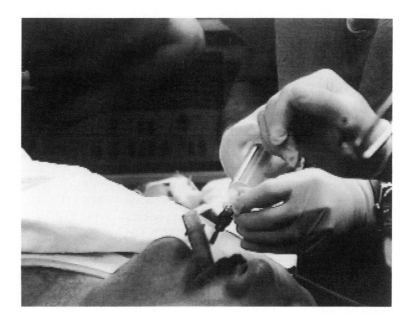

Figure 20–7. A little outward movement may be noted as the cuff is inflated.

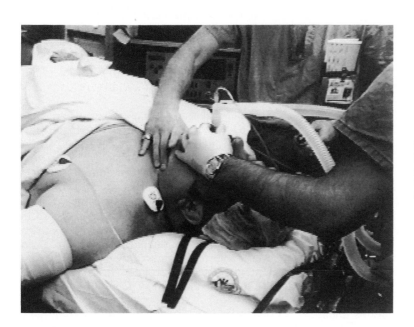

Figure 20–8. The anesthetic breathing circuit is connected, and the inflation pressure at which an audible leak occurs is detected.

guidelines; namely, the absence of extraneous airway sounds, a normal pattern of excursion of the reservoir bag, and the absence of any out-of-phase respiratory movements of the chest and abdomen. With respect to insertion of the laryngeal mask, a number of practical points should be borne in mind. First, an adequate depth of anesthesia should be achieved before insertion is attempted. This is probably deeper than the anesthetic depth at which a patient tolerates introduction of an oral airway.[2] Laryngospasm may occur and has been attributed to attempting laryngeal mask insertion at too light a level of anesthesia.[4] Interestingly, each of these patients had received sodium thiopental and it has been emphasized that, following thiopental, anesthesia should be deepened with a volatile agent before insertion is attempted.[5] Second, if difficulty is encountered on insertion, repeated attempts may traumatize the oropharynx. A laryngoscopy should be performed, any anatomic obstacle noted (eg, large tonsils), and the laryngeal mask placed under direct vision. Third, if the airway is not patent, the laryngeal mask should be removed and reinserted. Repositioning the patient's head, adding or removing air from the cuff, or the application of continuous positive airway pressure (CPAP) may be helpful.[9] Kinking of the size 2 laryngeal mask, when a flexion force is applied, has also been described.[10] In general, little practice is required to become proficient at placement of the laryngeal mask. Broderick and colleagues[2] gave each of the 18 anesthetists involved in their evaluatory study no more than general guidelines on the technique of insertion. The mask was passed easily in 92 of the 100 patients studied (80% at the first attempt). Three anesthesiologists, without prior experience in its use, inserted the laryngeal mask "easily" in 187 of 250 attempts.[4] In only two cases was insertion impossible.

In preliminary trials, patients were returned to the recovery room with the laryngeal mask in place.[6] The recovery nurses quickly gained confidence in caring for patients breathing through the laryngeal mask. A Venturi T-piece system has been described as a means of delivering supplementary oxygen through the laryngeal mask to patients in the recovery room.[11] When the patient responds to the command "open your mouth," the cuff may be deflated and the laryngeal mask withdrawn gently. The onset of swallowing is a useful predictor that such a level of wakefulness is imminent.[6] On withdrawal, the patient usually continues to breathe without interruption of the respiratory pattern. In one series, 6% of patients coughed and 4% clenched their teeth during removal of the airway, and 2% developed a short-lived stridor.[2] An oral airway,[7] a bite block,[8] and a bite guard for a fiberoptic gastroscope[12] have all been recommended in preventing patients from biting on and thus occluding the laryngeal mask.

One fundamental point must be emphasized in any discussion of the laryngeal mask. This device may not be relied on to protect the upper airway in the anesthetized patient. There have been several case reports of pulmonary aspiration of gastric contents in "fasted" patients with the laryngeal mask in place.[13, 14] Elective use should therefore be confined to patients who are not at risk of regurgitation or vomiting of gastric contents. With this important point in mind, certain partially protective features do exist. In the awakening patient, coughing is more likely to be effective because vocal cords may be apposed in order to generate the necessary expulsive pressure. The mucociliary transport system of the trachea and larynx is not impaired. The mask may be easily inserted with the patient in the lateral position, and may remain correctly placed if the patient is turned laterally after insertion. In his original description, Brain[1] indicated that during a difficult dental extraction, the laryngeal mask appeared to offer greater protection from debris, blood, and teeth than would an endotracheal tube. When methylene blue dye was placed in the pharynx of anesthetized patients with the laryngeal mask in place, no dye was detected when the larynx and trachea were examined fiberoptically.[11]

The laryngeal mask has proven useful both when a difficult intubation is anticipated and when it is unexpectedly encountered. Brain[1] noted that in two of the original 23 insertions described, the patients' anatomy suggested that endotracheal intubation would be difficult. Later, he reported three cases in which difficult or failed intubation was managed successfully using the laryngeal mask.[15] Airway management problems associated with severe facial burns,[16] Pierre Robin syndrome,[17] ankylosing spondylitis,[18] and juvenile chronic arthritis[19] have been overcome by using the laryngeal mask.

Even more importantly, the laryngeal mask has secured the airway in patients who have received a muscle relaxant and thereafter prove impossible to intubate. Several authors have described its use under these circumstances in elective or emergency caesarean section.[19–21] Although, unquestionably, it is not ideal in the presence of a full stomach, it has proven life saving in several "can't intubate, can't ventilate" situations. Although designed to meet the needs of the anesthesiologist during elective cases, its potential for use in emergency resuscitation has been recognized.[23] It has been used on two separate occasions to emergently secure the airway of a patient who had previously been difficult to intubate.[24]

Because the laryngeal mask does not provide airway protection, it may be advisable in the emergency situation to use it to facilitate endotracheal intubation once the airway has been secured. This may be accomplished either by passing an endotracheal tube blindly through the lumen of the laryngeal mask[15] or by first passing a gum elastic bougie into the trachea and thereafter using this to guide the endotracheal tube into place.[18, 25] An alternative is to guide an endotracheal tube into the trachea over a flexible fiberscope.

The laryngeal mask has three major advantages that are particularly useful in the management of emergency airway problems. First, the technique is simple, and even those with little or no experience in its use are usually successful at inserting it correctly. Thus, it is likely to be useful in the hands of paramedical personnel and those who undertake airway management infrequently. In field conditions, nonanesthetists who were given a single demonstration of its use correctly placed the laryngeal mask at each of 23 attempts.[26] Second, there appears to be little overlap between the anatomic features that are associated with difficult intubation and with difficult insertion of the laryngeal mask. Although poor incisor separation and possibly macroglossia impede both, the presence of an anterior larynx may actually facilitate insertion of the laryngeal mask.[1] Third, in the "can't intubate, can't ventilate" situation, the morbidity associated with tracheotomy or cricothyroidotomy is avoided.

In 1989, Braude and colleagues[27] noted the lesser cardiovascular response to laryngeal mask placement compared with that following laryngoscopy and endotracheal intubation. Patients in whom the laryngeal mask is used demonstrate an attenuated response compared with those who are intubated. Although mean heart rate changes were similar in the two groups, the increase in mean arterial pressure is less and of shorter duration in the laryngeal mask group. The laryngeal mask thus offers "some limited advantages" in patients in whom a pressor response is undesirable. The cardio-vascular response to laryngeal mask insertion is similar to that following placement of a Guedel oral airway.[28] It is widely held that direct laryngoscopy is mainly responsible for the pressor response to the laryngoscopy/intubation sequence. This is presumably due to "stimulation of the supraglottic region by tissue tension."[29] This does not explain the finding of Knight and associates[30] that intubation with or without laryngoscopy (ie, using a lighted stylet) produces similar cardiovascular responses. The increase in hypopharyngeal tissue tension associated with laryngeal mask placement and cuff inflation probably accounts for the responses seen.

Three of the 23 patients in whom Brain[1] originally evaluated the laryngeal mask complained of a mild sore throat. The incidence of this problem in his next large series ($n = 118$) was 6.8% (or 3.9% of cases in which other factors likely to cause a sore throat were excluded). Twelve percent of patients in one series[2] and 8% of another[3] had a temporary sore throat postoperatively. This incidence is similar to that reported in nonintubated patients following general anesthesia[31] and less than that following endotracheal intubation.[32] Postoperative sore throat results from oro- or hypopharyngeal trauma during insertion, especially if the tip of the deflated cuff impinges on the posterior pharyngeal wall. In one case at least, a severely bruised uvula has been found to be responsible.[33]

It is reasonable to expect that laryngeal mask insertion might precipitate airway problems in patients with hyperactive upper airway reflexes. Insertion of the laryngeal mask has provoked coughing, straining, or bronchospasm in patients with chronic respiratory disease.[34] In contrast, Brain[6] found no association between the use of the laryngeal mask in patients with chronic obstructive airway disease and airway problems.

The laryngeal mask is now manufactured in four sizes. Mask sizes 1 (neonates to 6.5 kg) and 2 (6.5 kg to 25 kg) are specifically intended for pediatric use. Large tonsils or a large, floppy epiglottis may present problems with placement and airway patency in children. Because an airway of larger internal diameter than the internal diameter of the trachea is used, resistance is less than with endotracheal intubation. A lower dead space results when a laryngeal mask is used compared with that with an oral Guedel airway. Perhaps the greatest advantage lies in obviating the need for multiple intubations when repeated anesthetics are necessary. Grebenik and associates[34] have reported their favorable experience in using the laryngeal mask in 312 consecutive anesthetics for infants and young children undergoing radiotherapy. This is especially useful when multiple procedures are required, because the repeated laryngeal trauma of endotracheal intubation is avoided. A similar advantage applies to magnetic resonance imaging (MRI), a procedure for which the laryngeal mask has been used with success both in adults[35] and in children.[36] It provides an excellent alternative to the conventional nasal mask for children undergoing outpatient dental anesthesia[37] and has been used for upper airway endoscopy.[38] Johnston and colleagues[39] compared the use of the laryngeal mask with a standard facemask in children aged 2 to 10 years who were undergoing otologic surgery. The laryngeal mask provided a satisfactory airway in all children, and hypoxia occurred less frequently when it was used. In only five of the 200 children studied by Mason and Bingham[9] did problems arise that were serious enough to warrant abandonment of the laryngeal mask. These included coughing, vomiting, laryngospasm, and complete airway obstruction. Another series of 200 children included only one in whom it was necessary to replace the laryngeal mask with an endotracheal tube.[40] Laryngeal mask insertion appears to be as technically simple in children as in adults. In children, approximately three quarters (78%, 67%, or 89.5%) of all insertions are successful at the first attempt.[9, 39, 40] Because in children, and especially in infants, the epiglottis is relatively large and floppy, the likelihood of a downfolding of this structure that results in partial or complete obstruction is greater. Flexible laryngoscopy carried out in 24 children revealed that the epiglottis was downfolded in eight.[9] Interestingly, none showed clinical evidence of airway obstruction. In another series, airway obstruction was detected clinically in only 2% of cases, but partial airway obstruction was demonstrable fiberoptically in a further 17%.[41] Denman and associates[36] have studied the position of the laryngeal mask in children using MRI. In two of the 28 patients studied, the laryngeal mask cuff was found to lie in the oropharynx. The epiglottis was seen to be posteriorly deflected in most (82%) cases. Again, irrespective of the position of the epiglottis or the laryngeal mask, the airway was clinically judged to be adequate in each case.

The laryngeal mask is a new and revolutionary concept in airway management. As experience with the use of this device increases, new indications for its use are being described.

Perhaps the most exciting of these is its role in the management of the difficult or failed intubation. With the exception of pulmonary aspiration, the complications to date are minor and are easily avoided or corrected. Correct placement of the laryngeal mask in most patients is easily achieved and its role in emergency airway management in the hands of trained paramedical personnel remains to be evaluated. Identification of incomplete airway patency is the most important skill necessary for its safe use.

References

1. Brain AIJ. The laryngeal mask–A new concept in airway management. Br J Anaesth 55:801–805, 1983.
2. Broderick PM, Webster NR, Nunn JF. The laryngeal mask airway: A study of 100 patients during spontaneous breathing. Anaesthesia 44:238–241, 1989.
3. Maltby JR, Loken RG, Watson NC. The laryngeal mask airway: Clinical appraisal in 250 patients. Can J Anaesth 37:509–513, 1990.
4. Maltby JR. The laryngeal mask airway. Anesthesiology Review 18:55–57, 1991.
5. Brain AIJ. Further developments of the laryngeal mask. Anaesthesia 44:530c, 1989.
6. Brain AIJ, McGhee TD, McAteer EJ, Thomas A, Abu-Saad MAW, Bushman JA. The laryngeal mask airway—Development and preliminary trials of a new type of airway. Anaesthesia 40:356–361, 1985.
7. Alexander CA, Leach AB, Thompson AR, Lister JB. Use your Brain! Anaesthesia 43:893–894c, 1988.
8. Brain AIJ, Simmonds D. Using the Intavent laryngeal mask. Product information sheet. London: Colgate Medical, 1989.
9. Mason DG, Bingham RM. The laryngeal mask in children. Anaesthesia 45:760–763, 1990.
10. Goldberg PJ, Evans PF, Filshie J. Kinking of the laryngeal mask airway in children. Anaesthesia 45:487–488c, 1990.
11. Broadway PJ, Royle P. Supplementary oxygen and the laryngeal mask airway. Anaesthesia 45:792–793c, 1990.
12. Marks L. Protection of the laryngeal mask airway. Anaesthesia 43:259c, 1988.
13. Griffin RM, Hatcher IS. Aspiration pneumonia and the laryngeal mask airway. Anaesthesia 45:1039–1040, 1990.
14. Cyna AM, McLeod DM. The laryngeal mask—Cautionary tales. Anaesthesia 45:167c, 1990.
15. Brain AIJ. Three cases of difficult intubation overcome by the laryngeal mask airway. Anaesthesia 40:353–355, 1985.
16. Thomson KD, Ordman AJ, Parkhouse N, Morgan BDG. Use of the Brain laryngeal mask airway in anticipation of difficult tracheal intubation. Br J Plast Surg 42:478–480, 1989.
17. Beveridge ME. Laryngeal mask anaesthesia for repair of cleft palate. Anaesthesia 44:656–657, 1989.
18. Chadd GD, Ackers JWL. Bailey PM. Difficult intubation aided by the laryngeal mask airway. Anaesthesia 44:1015c, 1989.
19. Smith BL. Brain airway for anaesthesia in patients with juvenile chronic arthritis. Anaesthesia 43:421–422c, 1988.

20. McClune S, Regan M, Moore J. Laryngeal mask for Caesarean section. Anaesthesia 45:227–228, 1990.
21. Chadwick IS, Vohra A. Anaesthesia for emergency caesarean section using the Brain laryngeal mask. Anaesthesia 44:261–262c, 1989.
22. deMello WF, Kocan M. The laryngeal mask in failed intubation. Anaesthesia 45:590–591c, 1990.
23. Brain AIJ. The laryngeal mask airway–A possible new solution to airway problems in the emergency situation. Arch Emerg Med 1:229–232, 1984.
24. Calder I, Ordman AJ, Jackowski A, Crockard HA. The Brain laryngeal mask—An alternative to emergency tracheal intubation. Anaesthesia 45:137–139, 1990.
25. Allison A, McCrory J. Tracheal placement of a gum elastic bougie using the laryngeal mask airway. Anaesthesia 45:419–420c, 1990.
26. de Mello WF, Ward P. The use of the laryngeal mask airway in primary anesthesia. Anaesthesia 45:793–794c, 1990.
27. Braude N, Clements EAF, Hodges UM, Andrews BP. The pressor response and laryngeal mask insertion—A comparison with tracheal intubation. Anaesthesia 44:551–554, 1989.
28. Hickey S, Cameron AE, Asbury AJ. Cardiovascular response to insertion of Brain's laryngeal mask. Anaesthesia 45:629–633, 1990.
29. Shribman AJ, Smith G, Achola KJ. Cardiovascular and catecholamine responses to laryngoscopy with and without tracheal intubation. Br J Anaesth 59:295–299, 1987.
30. Knight RG, Castro T, Rastrelli AJ, Maschke S, Scavone KA. Arterial blood pressure and heart rate response to lighted stylet or direct laryngoscopy for endotracheal intubation. Anesthesiology 69:269–272, 1988.
31. Jensen PJ, Hommelgaard P, Sondegaard D, Eriksen S. Sore throat after operation: Influence of tracheal intubation, intracuff pressure and type of cuff. Br J Anaesth 54:453–456, 1982.
32. Brindle GF, Soliman MG. Anaesthetic complications in surgical outpatients. Can Anaesth Soc J 22:613–618, 1975.
33. Lee JJ. Laryngeal mask and trauma to the uvula. Anaesthesia 44:1014c, 1989.
34. Grebenik CR, Ferguson C, White A. The laryngeal mask in pediatric radiotherapy. Anesthesiology 72:474–477, 1990.
35. Rafferty C, Burke AM, Cossar DF, Farling PA. Laryngeal mask and magnetic resonance imaging. Anaesthesia 45:590–591c, 1990.
36. Goudsouzian NG, Denman W, Cleveland R, Shorten G. Radiologic localization of the laryngeal mask airway in children. Anesthesiology 77:1085–1089, 1992.
37. Bailie R, Barnett MB, Fraser JF. The Brain laryngeal mask—A comparative study with the nasal mask in paediatric dental outpatient anaesthesia. Anaesthesia 46:358–360, 1991.
38. Maekawa N, Mikawa K, Tanaka O, Goto R, Obara H. The laryngeal mask airway may be a useful device for fiberoptic airway endoscopy in pediatric anesthesia. Anesthesiology 75:169–170c, 1991.
39. Johnston DF, Wrigley SR, Robb PJ, Jones HE. The laryngeal mask airway in pediatric anesthesia. Anaesthesia 45:924–927, 1990.
40. Ravalia A, Fawcett W, Radford P. The Brain laryngeal mask airway in pediatric anaesthesia [abstract]. Anesth Analg 72:S220, 1991.
41. Rowbottom SJ, Simpson DL, Grubb D. The laryngeal mask airway in children—A fiberoptic assessment of position. Anaesthesia 46:489–491, 1991.

Bibliography

John RE, Hill S, Hughes TJ. Airway protection by the laryngeal mask. Anaesthesia 46:366–367, 1991.

CHAPTER 21

Fiberoptic Laryngoscopes

Stephen F. Dierdorf, M.D.

Direct laryngoscopy as performed with the traditional laryngoscope has been a standard technique for tracheal intubation for decades. Using this technique, the vast majority of surgical patients can be intubated rapidly and atraumatically. Patients with abnormal airways, however, frequently present a significant obstacle to direct laryngoscopy and visualization of the glottis. A number of indirect techniques (eg, blind nasotracheal intubation, retrograde wire insertion) have evolved in order to achieve tracheal intubation in patients with anatomically altered airways. These techniques are often time consuming, unpredictable, and traumatic. The development of flexible fiberoptic laryngoscopes in the 1970s and 1980s has provided the anesthesiologist with a tool to manage abnormal airways with predictability and minimal trauma. The flexible fiberoptic laryngoscope is an instrument with which every modern anesthesiologist should be familiar (Figs. 21–1 and 21–2).

Although it was conclusively demonstrated by John Tyndall in 1854 that light could travel in a curved line, it was not until the 1950s that practical application of this discovery was initiated for medical purposes. Hopkins and Kapany[1] reported the development of a flexible fiberoptic unit that could convey images. Prior to the development of fiberoptics, endoscopes relied on a series of lenses, which resulted in a poor-quality image. Poor illumi-

nation permitted very little magnification; endoscopy was tedious and required a certain amount of good fortune to locate and examine a suspected lesion. Fiberoptic technology, however, soon provided the necessary components for quality image transmission. Soon after the report by Hopkins and Kapany, the first fiberoptic endoscope was introduced.[2] This first fiberoptic endoscope was a gastroscope and was introduced by Hirschowitz in 1957, but it was not enthusiastically accepted by medical practitioners. The first report of a

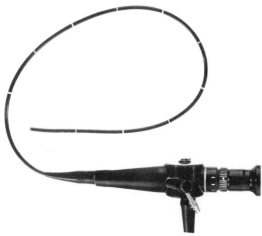

Figure 21–1. Olympus LF-1 flexible fiberoptic laryngoscope. This laryngoscope has an outstanding reputation for durability.

229

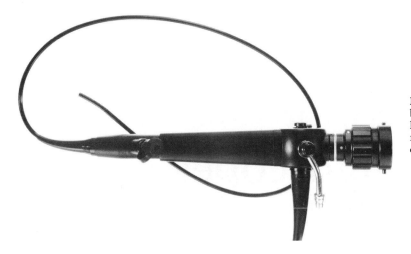

Figure 21–2. Pentax FI-10P flexible fiberoptic laryngoscope. This laryngoscope features high visual resolution and excellent optical qualities.

successful flexible fiberoptic tracheal intubation was in 1967; a choledoscope was used as the endoscope for a nasotracheal intubation.[3] In 1972, a bronchoscope was used for awake tracheal intubations.[4] Since that time, there have been dramatic improvements in the design and manufacture of fiberoptic endoscopes. Several manufacturers now produce high-quality, flexible, fiberoptic laryngoscopes for use by anesthesiologists. Fiberoptic technology has wide application not only for flexible bronchoscopy, but also has been incorporated into rigid bronchoscopes and traditional laryngoscopes as well.

An appreciation of the physical principles of fiberoptic light and image transmission in conjunction with the knowledge of how a fiberscope is constructed provides a better understanding of the capabilities and limitations of fiberoptic endoscopes. This understanding enhances the ease of learning techniques of fiberoptic laryngoscopy and tracheal intubation and minimizes the risk of damage to the equipment. This chapter conveys in an understandable manner those physical principles essential to fiberoptic image transmission.

PHYSICS OF FIBEROPTIC IMAGE TRANSMISSION

The critical physical principle that governs image transmission via flexible fiberoptic bundles is that light can be totally reflected internally by a fiberoptic strand (law of total internal reflection). Relative to the transmission medium (eg, fiberoptic strand), light rays can be termed as meridional or skew. Meridional rays pass through the axis of the conducting fiber without being reflected, whereas skew rays do not intersect the fiber axis and can be internally reflected.[5] Normally, as a ray of light traverses the boundary between two media (eg, air and glass), the light ray is split into two parts; most of the light passes into the air and is refracted, but part of the light is reflected back into the glass (Fig. 21–3). Light refraction occurs because the speed of light in material is less than the speed of light in air. The higher the refractive index of a material, the slower the speed of light in that material. The degree of reflection depends on the angle of incidence of the light and the refractive indices of the two transmission media. As the angle of incidence is increased, a point will be reached where the refracted light travels parallel to the boundary surface. The angle at which parallel transmission occurs is termed the "critical angle" (Fig. 21–4). If the incident angle is, however, increased beyond the critical angle, then total internal reflection of the light is achieved (Fig. 21–4). A simple example of total internal reflection is the prism system in

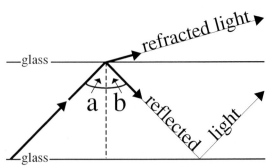

Figure 21–3. As light meets a glass–air interface, most of the light is refracted, but some is reflected. Angle a, the angle of incidence; angle b, the angle of reflection.

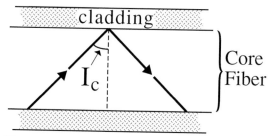

Figure 21–4. Light striking the boundary of a clad glass fiber is internally reflected. I_c, the critical angle. Light rays striking the boundary at an angle greater than the critical angle undergo total internal reflection.

the surface of the fiber with a material with a lower index of refraction. The sudden difference in refractive indexes produces the interface that allows total internal reflection along the glass fiber.[7] A fiber consists of two cylinders. The inner cylinder, or core, transmits the light; the outer cylinder, composed of cladding material, maintains the integrity of the internal reflective surface (Fig. 21–6). The internal boundary surface between the core and the cladding, which is then protected from damage, becomes the reflection surface. It is the cladding of the glass bundle that has been responsible for the wide medical application of flexible fiberoptics. Current materials and technology permit total internal reflection with only 0.001% light loss per reflection. There is, however, a limit to what light will be accepted by the fibers for transmission. Light entering the bundle at an angle smaller than the critical angle for the interface will not be reflected and consequently is lost. Other factors that reduce the amount of light accepted by the fiber include light scatter at the interface, light absorption by the core glass, and packing fraction loss. For endoscopes, fibers are arranged in bundles. The core or light transmission fibers are each surrounded by the cladding material. The cladding material does not transmit light, and any light striking the cladding material is lost. The packing fraction is the ratio between the cross-sectional area of the cladding material and the cross-sectional area of the core

a pair of binoculars. Binoculars, however, require only four reflections, whereas a fiberoptic bundle requires numerous reflections. Total internal light reflection is the underlying physical principle that governs light transmission through flexible glass fibers. A waveguide is constructed when a transparent material is layered between a material with a lower index of refraction.[6] Within the waveguide it is then possible for a light ray to be reflected numerous times and to zigzag along the entire course of the fiber (Fig. 21–5). Early practical attempts at total internal light reflection were frustrated because damage or contamination of the boundary surface with debris allowed light leakage through the fiber walls, resulting in transmission of a poor-quality image. This problem was overcome by coating (cladding)

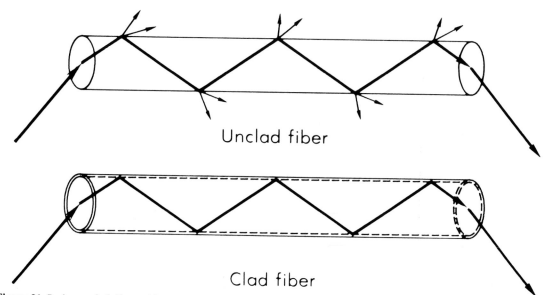

Figure 21–5. An unclad fiber with a contaminated surface loses light throughout its length. Cladding protects the interface surface and increases transmission efficiency. (From Barlow DE. Fiberoptic instrument technology. In Tams TR (ed). Small Animal Endoscopy. St. Louis: Mosby-Year Book, 1990; with permission.)

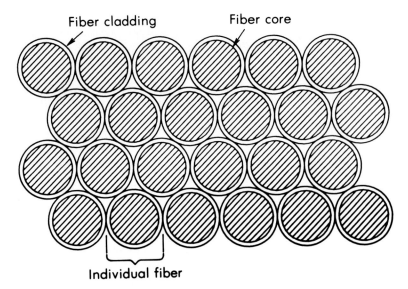

Figure 21–6. Individual fibers are grouped into a bundle in a honeycomb pattern. Only the light falling on the core glass (shaded area) is transmitted. (From Barlow DE. Fiberoptic instrument technology. In Tams TR (ed). Small Animal Endoscopy. St. Louis: Mosby-Year Book, 1990; with permission.)

material. In order to improve image resolution, a large number of small fibers is desirable; however, fiber density is limited because the packing fraction loss increases as fiber density increases.

The other essential practical factor important to fiberoptic light transmission was the development of glass of high purity and transparency. Glass with impurities is unsuitable for light transmission. For all practical purposes, current manufacturing techniques are producing silica-based glass that is at the theoretic limit of its transparency. Consequently, other materials with higher degrees of transparency are being developed. These newer materials are of special importance for the transmission of laser energy. Infrared fiberoptic light transmission in particular is of special interest for the communication industry. Fiberoptic signals transmitted by silica-glass fibers must be reamplified every 10 to 50 kilometers. Infrared signals, however, only require reamplification every hundreds or thousands of kilometers.[8] Infrared signal transmission does require fibers of a material different from silica glass. Current research interest has been focused on production of metal fluoride glass fibers.

FIBERSCOPE COMPONENTS

There are three basic parts of a fiberoptic endoscope: (1) the body, (2) the insertion cord, and (3) the light transmission cord[9] (Table 21–1; Fig. 21–7). The components of the insertion cord are of special importance, because it is these components that give the instrument flexibility while at the same time transmitting a high-quality image. The components of the insertion cord can be subdivided into the fiberoptic bundles, the optical system, and the mechanical system.

Fibers and Bundles

A single glass fiber can transmit light, but not an image. Image transmission requires a large number of bundles arranged in a coherent bundle.[10] A coherent bundle is constructed by precisely arranging the individual fibers so that fibers at one end of the bundle are perfectly arranged in the same relative location at the other end of the bundle. Incoherent bundles have fibers arranged in random order and can transmit light, but not an image (Fig. 21–8). Incoherent bundles are easier and less expensive to construct and are generally used as light conduits, referred to as light guide (LG) bundles, in endoscopes. The resolution power of the endoscope is determined by the

Table 21–1. COMPONENTS OF A FLEXIBLE FIBEROPTIC LARYNGOSCOPE

Body
  Tip deflection control lever
  Eyepiece
  Focusing ring
  Working channel sleeve
Insertion cord
  Working channel
  Image transmission bundle
  Light transmission bundle
Light transmission cord

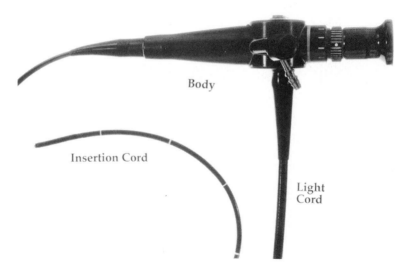

Figure 21–7. Photograph of the Olympus LF-1 laryngoscope showing the three parts: (1) body, containing the eyepiece, working channel port, and tip deflector (behind); (2) insertion cord, containing the image and light guide fiber bundles and angulation wires; and (3) light cord for transmitting light from the light source to the laryngoscope.

density of the fibers in the bundle; the higher the density, the better the resolution. The diameter of the basic fiber elements of most imaging fiberscopes is 8 to 10 μ. The cladding material surrounding each fiber is 0.5 μ thick. Bundles used for fiberoptic laryngoscopy contain 4000 to 6000 of these individual fibers. Fiberoptic fibers can be made from glass or plastic. Because of the light transmission qualities of glass and the resistance of glass to deterioration, glass fibers are preferred for high-quality applications, such as medical fiberoptics.

Excessive bending and acute angulation of the insertion cord will break individual fibers within the cord. Each broken fiber appears as a black dot in the ocular piece. As more and more fibers are broken, the visual field is distorted by the increasing number of black dots. The ultra-thin endoscopes (eg, Olympus PF-18M, Lake Success, NY) are especially vulnerable to bundle fracture at the junction of the insertion cord and the body. In order to minimize the risk of bundle breakage, a short piece of plastic tubing can be placed on the endoscope at this junction point. This prevents overbending of the fiberscope.

Optical System

Because the actual image transmitted by the fiberoptic bundle is quite small (0.3 to 5 mm

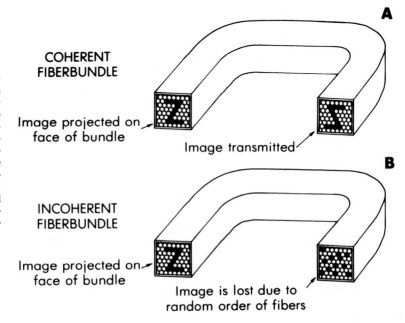

Figure 21–8. In a coherent fiberbundle, the arrangement of fibers in one end of the bundle exactly matches the arrangement in the opposite bundle face (*A*). An incoherent bundle exhibits no correlation between the fiber arrangements in the two bundle faces (*B*). (From Barlow DE. Fiberoptic instrument technology. In Tams TR (ed). Small Animal Endoscopy. St. Louis: Mosby-Year Book, 1990; with permission.)

COHERENT FIBERBUNDLE

Image projected on face of bundle

Image transmitted

INCOHERENT FIBERBUNDLE

Image projected on face of bundle

Image is lost due to random order of fibers

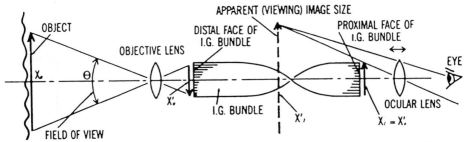

Figure 21–9. A basic fiberscope optical system. I.G., image guide. (From Sivak MV Jr. (ed). Gastroenterologic Endoscopy. Philadelphia: W. B. Saunders, 1987; with permission.)

in diameter), the image must be magnified for the endoscopist by a lens system. An objective lens is placed at the distal end of the fiberscope; this lens forms an image on the distal end of the image bundle. Because the objective lens inverts the image, the fiberoptic bundle is internally rotated 180 degrees, which compensates for the image inversion (Fig. 21–9). Because the image projected by the objective lens is limited by the size of the image bundle, the image is then magnified by an ocular lens placed in the eyepiece.[11] The eyepiece also contains a diopter adjustment, to compensate for any visual abnormality of the endoscopist. The result is a well-illuminated and magnified image of high resolution. The image presented at the eyepiece is a composite image that can be likened to the image formed on a television screen.[12] Magnification does have a practical limitation, in that with increasing magnification, the individual fibers within the bundle are magnified, become visible, and distort the object image.

The range of focus (or depth of field) is determined by the distance from the objective lens to the image bundle. For most fiberoptic laryngoscopes, the depth of field is 3 to 50 mm. The practical significance of this is that the fiberscope can be focused on objects between 3 and 50 mm from the tip of the laryngoscope.

In addition to the size and quality of the image, the field of view is also an important feature of the fiberscope. A wider field of view permits a better visual field of orientation for the endoscopist. However, increasing the field of view decreases the size of the primary image. The proper combination of field of view and the image size requires a set of compound lenses in the objective lens and illumination lenses at the distal end of the fiberscope.

Mechanical System

The modern fiberoptic bronchoscope appears deceptively simple in construction, but in reality is a complex structure containing image bundles, illumination bundles, working channels, angulation control wires, and a flexible distal joint system, all ensheathed in a tough, durable outer covering (Fig. 21–10). The endoscope must have a certain degree of rigidity for easy passage, but still have flexibility, particularly at the distal end, for smooth movement. The distal end of bronchoscopes and laryngoscopes, because they must be of a small diameter, typically have a two-way angulation system. Two-way angulation means that the tip can be deflected in two directions (up and down). In a two-way angulation system, movement of the tip to the right or left must be achieved by rotation of the proximal body of the scope. By combining up and down deflection with right and left rotation, movement of the tip in all four quadrants of the viewing field can be achieved. Gastroscopes and colonoscopes, because they can be of larger diameter, have four-way angulation systems, which permit movement in four directions with the hand controls of the fiberscope body. The flexible section of the distal end of the fiberscope is constructed of a series of metal bands attached together by flexible joints (Fig. 21–11). An angulation wire runs the length of the fiberscope from the control knob through the metal bands and is fixed at the distal end of the endoscope. Tip deflection is produced by rotating the control knob, which exerts tension on the angulation wire, which in turn flexes the metal bands (Fig. 21–12). When the fiberscope is extended, tip deflection occurs in the up and down directions when the control knob is manipulated. However, if the fiberscope is bent upon itself (flexed), tip de-

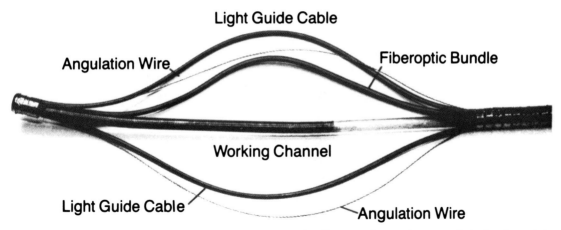

Light Guide Cable

Angulation Wire

Fiberoptic Bundle

Working Channel

Light Guide Cable

Angulation Wire

Figure 21–10. Inside of a fiberoptic bronchoscope insertion tube. Two angulation wires control the bending of the tip of the fiberscope. Two light guide cables contain fiberoptic bundles (incoherent), which bring light to the tip of the fiberscope. The fiberoptic bundle contains the coherent bundle, which transmits images from the objective lens at the tip of the fiberscope to the eyepiece of the fiberscope. The working or suction channel is used for suctioning of secretions and instillation of local anesthetics. (From Ovassapian A. Fiberoptic Airway Endoscopy in Anesthesia and Critical Care, p. 2. New York: Raven Press, 1990; with permission.)

flection may occur at a 90-degree angle to the up and down plane (Fig. 21–13). This altered directional response is most likely a result of internal twisting of the angulation control wire. This is of significance to the endoscopist, because as the direction of tip deflection becomes unpredictable, orientation is lost. There is considerable variation between fiberscopes as to the degree of altered movement that occurs. This variability is a function of the degree of stretching of the angulation control wire that occurs with use and aging of the fiberscope. The problem of altered tip deflection can be avoided if the fiberscope remains extended

during endoscopy. Improvements in the engineering and construction of the angulation system in recent years have resulted in an increase in the degree of tip deflection and smoothness of manipulation.

The working channel runs the length of the endoscope and can be used for a variety of functions (Fig. 21–14). Suction can be applied for clearing of secretions, and medications can be instilled into the airway. For routine tracheal intubation, insufflating oxygen at 4 to 7 L per minute will keep the objective lens dry and clear of secretions. The working channel of most laryngoscopes is 1.2 mm in diameter.

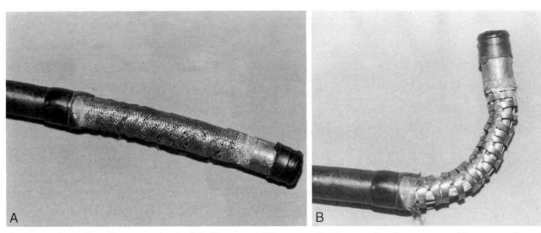

Figure 21–11. *A,* Distal section of a flexible fiberscope. The outer plastic cover has been removed to expose the wire mesh surrounding the flexible joints. *B,* Flexible metal bands and joints of the distal end of the fiberscope. The wire mesh has been removed.

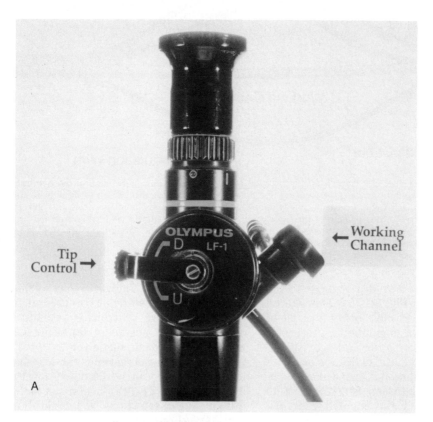

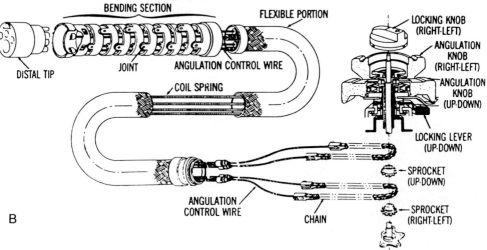

Figure 21–12. *A,* Body of a flexible laryngoscope, demonstrating the tip control lever and the working channel sleeve. *B,* Bending section and angulation system of a fiberoptic endoscope. (From Sivak MV Jr. (ed). Gastroenterologic Endoscopy. Philadelphia: W. B. Saunders, 1987; with permission.)

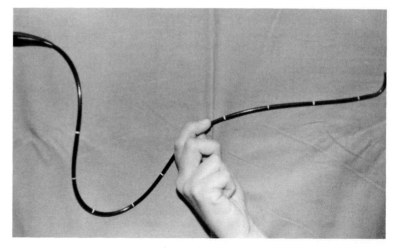

Figure 21–13. Photograph of a flexible laryngoscope. When the insertion cord is bent upon itself, as in this photograph, tip deflection may be at an abnormal angle, producing a loss of visual orientation. To avoid altered tip control, the insertion cord should remain extended.

Suction applied to a channel this small is seldom as effective for clearing of secretions as oxygen insufflation. The working channels of bronchoscopes are 2 to 4 mm in diameter, which accommodates suction for clearing of secretions, as well as the use of biopsy instruments for diagnostic procedures.

Light Sources

Two basic types of light sources are in widespread clinical use today (Fig. 21–15). A low-power halogen light source provides only adequate illumination, but is relatively compact and inexpensive. A halogen light source provides adequate illumination for still photography via the endoscope. High-power xenon light sources are also available that provide excellent illumination and are necessary if a video image display is used. The xenon light source, however, costs five to ten times more than a halogen light source. The light guide connector that inserts into the light source becomes quite hot and can produce a third-degree burn if it contacts the skin of the patient or the endoscopist. Care must be exercised after the light cord is detached from the light source so that an accidental burn does not occur. Some fiberoptic laryngoscopes have been manufactured that have the light source in the handle of the endoscope and employ "C" batteries as a power source (Fig. 21–16). Although the laryngoscope is small, the illumination is poor

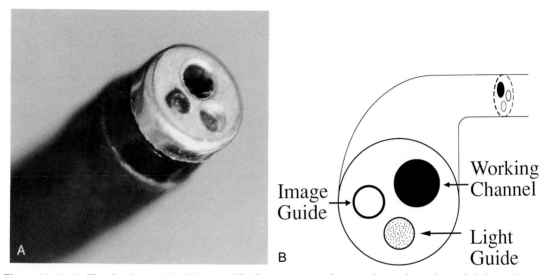

Figure 21–14. *A*, The distal tip of the Olympus LF-1 laryngoscope, showing the working channel, light guide, and objective lens. *B*, Schematic diagram of the distal tip.

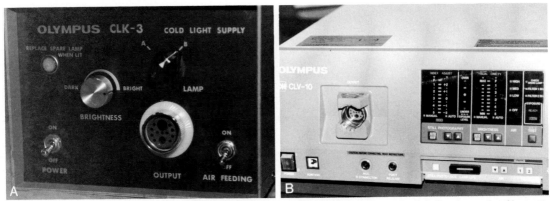

Figure 21–15. *A,* Halogen light source (Olympus model CLK-3). This is the standard light source for fiberoptic laryngoscopy. *B,* Olympus xenon light source for fiberscopes. The cost of this unit is several times that of the halogen light source.

and imaging is often inadequate. The production of a self-contained laryngoscopic unit may be feasible in the near future, but the illumination intensity must be increased.

Photographic Systems

A visual record of different phases of the tracheal intubation process may be required for teaching purposes or as part of the patient record. Patients that need frequent airway examination for therapeutic reasons or as a means of tracking the progress of a pathologic condition may require a video recording of the examination for future reference and comparison to subsequent examinations. Pentax and Olympus (Orangeburg, NY) devices also have adaptors for 35-mm still cameras. The correct light source with a flash device is necessary for color photographs. Videotaping is also possible; video equipment, however, more than doubles the cost of the flexible fiberoptic system (Fig. 21–17). The increased investment may be acceptable for large teaching programs, but is generally not cost effective for the private practitioner. However, many hospitals already have sophisticated endoscopic video equipment that may be adapted to the anesthesiologist's flexible fiberoptic laryngoscope. Computer systems that digitally store video images that may be quite useful for maintain-

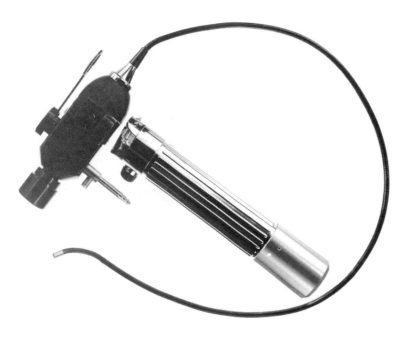

Figure 21–16. A fiberscope with a self-contained light source. The handle contains three "C" batteries. Light intensity of this unit is poor as compared with independent halogen or xenon light sources.

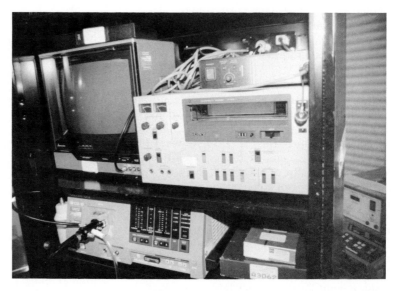

Figure 21–17. Flexible fiberoptic system with videotape capability. Included in the system are a video monitor, videotape recorder, xenon light source, and fiberscope.

ing a record of endoscopic images are near completion of development.

TYPES OF FIBERSCOPES

A variety of medical-grade fiberscopes are commercially available. The size of the endoscope and its features depend on the intended application. The diameter of the light and image bundles is actually quite small. Consequently, the size of the endoscope depends on the additional components that are required (Fig. 21–18).

Gastrointestinal Endoscopes

Gastroscopes and colonoscopes are much larger than bronchoscopes and laryngoscopes because the gastrointestinal tract accommodates larger instruments. A typical colonoscope contains 40,000 fibers and is 12 to 20 mm in diameter. There are also a number of therapeutic procedures that can be performed with these devices. In addition to the illumination and imaging bundles, gastroscopes and colonoscopes have working channels for suction, air insufflation, and biopsy instruments. The diameter of these endoscopes are substantially greater than endoscopes designed for the airway.

Airway Endoscopes

The number of ancillary components and ultimately the size of the airway endoscope depends on whether the scope is designed for

Figure 21–18. Comparative photograph of the distal ends of four different fiberscopes. As more channels are constructed in the scope, the greater the scope's diameter. *A,* Olympus CF colonoscope, 15 mm diameter; *B,* Olympus LF-1 laryngoscope, 4 mm diameter; *C,* Olympus LF-P pediatric laryngoscope, 2.2 mm diameter, two-way directional control but no working channel; *D,* Olympus PF-18M ultra-thin bronchoscope, 1.8 mm diameter, no working channel, and no directional control.

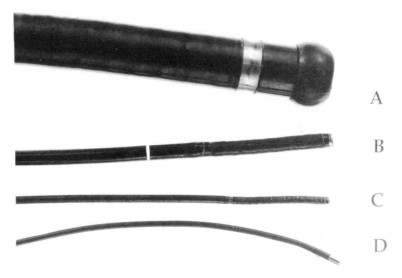

diagnostic or therapeutic procedures. Bronchoscopes with an external diameter as small as 1.8 mm that pass easily through a tracheal tube of 2.5-mm internal diameter are available (Olympus PF-18M). Fiberscopes this small, however, have no directional control apparatus or working channels and are suitable for diagnostic purposes only. As directional controls and working channels are added, the diameter of the scope increases. The Olympus LF-P scope is only 2.2 mm in diameter and is designed for pediatric applications; this scope has a directional control mechanism, but no working channel. The standard adult laryngoscopes, such as the Olympus LF-1 (4.0 mm diameter) or Pentax FI-10P (3.5 mm diameter), contain light guides, image bundles, two-way directional control, and one working channel. The Olympus LF-1 and the Pentax FI-10P are the predominant laryngoscopes in use by anesthesiologists in the United States (Table 21–2). Both instruments are quite durable and function in comparable fashion. The differences are subtle, and the endoscopist's personal preferences will determine which instrument is used. The FI-10P has a larger field of view (90 degrees, versus 75 degrees for the LF-1) and a slightly greater range of motion. The larger field of view is secondary to the fact that the FI-10P has two light guide bundles, whereas the LF-1 has one. The FI-10P is also totally immersible for cleaning purposes; the body of the LF-1 is not immersible. The LF-1 has been used extensively and is very durable. The LF-1 has external white markings every 5 cm, which some endoscopists find useful; the LF-1 is also slightly stiffer. Some endoscopists believe that the increased stiffness increases the ease of insertion of the LF-1, whereas others think that the increased flexibility of the FI-10P enhances insertion. Both the LF-1 and the FI-10P are high-quality instruments that transmit a good image and, with proper care, will

provide many years of reliable service for the anesthesiologist.

Flexible nasopharyngoscopes are of comparable diameter to flexible laryngoscopes. The nasopharyngoscopes, however, have a short working length (25 to 30 cm) and generally do not have a working channel (eg, Machida ENT-3L and 4L; Olympus ENF-P2). Because of the short length, these nasopharyngoscopes are not suitable for tracheal intubation.

ADDITIONAL MEDICAL APPLICATIONS

Fiberoptic technology has many other medical applications besides flexible diagnostic endoscopy and tracheal intubation.[13] Fiberoptic light and image transmission devices have been incorporated into rigid bronchoscopic instruments, as well as into flexible ones. The newer generations of rigid bronchoscopes (eg, Storz bronchoscopic systems, Storz Instrument Co., St. Louis, MO) employ fiberoptic illumination devices. The advantages include excellent illumination and accurate image transmission with appropriate magnification. The high-intensity illumination provided by fiberoptic bundles permits magnification of the image. This equipment permits controlled diagnostic and therapeutic procedures via rigid endoscopy for infants and small children, as well as for adults.

Optical fibers are also used for measurement of physiologic and chemical parameters. This type of device is made up of an optical fiber within a catheter that is inserted into the desired part of the body. At the distal end of the catheter is a miniature sensor (optode), and at the proximal end is an optical processor. Light is transmitted via the fiber to the optode. Reflected light is then transmitted back to the processor. Physiologic alteration of the reflected light is processed and a measurement value determined. This technique can be used to measure arterial and intracranial pressures. For pressure measurement, the sensor consists of a small tube at the distal end of the optical fiber; the end of the tube in contact with the patient is sealed with a reflective membrane. If the pressures are equal on both sides of the membrane, the light is reflected straight back through the optical fiber to the processor. Pressure changes distort the membrane and alter the light reflection from the membrane. Blood velocity can also be measured with a fiberoptic apparatus. Blood velocity is determined when laser light is transmitted through

Table 21–2. SPECIFICATIONS OF OLYMPUS LF-1 AND PENTAX FI-10P FLEXIBLE LARYNGOSCOPES

Specification	LF-1	FI-10P
Angle of viewing field (degrees)	75	90
Range of tip deflection (degrees)	Up–down, 120	Up–down, 130
External diameter (mm)	4.0	3.5
Working length (cm)	60	60
Totally immersible	No	Yes

a fiber and scatters off moving red blood cells. As the speed of the red cell increases, the wavelength of the reflected light decreases. The processor can analyze the wavelength differences and compute the blood velocity. Optical fibers are also used to measure the oxygen saturation of hemoglobin. Oxygenated hemoglobin reflects more red light than desaturated hemoglobin, whereas infrared light is reflected equally by saturated and desaturated hemoglobin. By transmitting both red and infrared light through an optical fiber in the blood, the total hemoglobin and ratio of saturated hemoglobin can be determined by analyzing the amount of reflection of red and infrared light. Optical sensors that can measure blood chemistries have also been developed. For many physiologic measurements, fiberoptic systems are more sensitive, reliable, and less expensive to manufacture than microelectronic sensors.

One of the most promising applications of fiberoptic technology has been the ability to transmit laser energy inside the body for therapeutic procedures. The type of laser employed depends on the therapeutic goal. For destruction of tissue, higher energy levels are required than for coagulation of blood and proteins. Significant technologic problems must be resolved in order to deliver the proper energy level to the tissue without heat damage to the fiberoptic guide. Laser applications have necessitated the use of materials other than glass for the manufacture of optical fibers. For example, quartz fibers are used for transmission of argon and yttrium aluminum garnet (YAG) lasers. Research is continuing in the search for an efficient fiber that will transmit radiation from carbon dioxide lasers. Optical transmission of laser energy is being used for relieving obstruction of coronary arteries (laser angioplasty) and holds promise of much wider application in the near future.

SUMMARY

Fiberoptic endoscopes, seemingly simple devices, are complex instruments that required significant research and development to achieve the current level of sophistication. Fortunately for the medical profession, fiberoptic light transmission is an important principle with wide applications in the communi-cation industry. For this reason, research and development continues at a rapid pace. This research is then readily applicable to medical instrument technology. The benefit for the physician is a wide variety of reliable, high-quality fiberoptic instruments. The union of fiberoptic medical technology with sophisticated video and computer equipment has enhanced our ability to diagnose, treat, and record pathologic conditions in many previously inaccessible areas of the body.

Fiberoptic endoscopy has become an integral part of anesthesiology practice as well. Anesthesiologists are now routinely using fiberscopes for tracheal intubation and examination of the airway. This equipment allows the anesthesiologist to manage with increased facility patient airways that were extremely difficult to manage without fiberoptics. Fiberoptic technology will continue to be of increased importance in the practice of anesthesiology and critical care medicine; knowledge of the principles of fiberoptics aid in understanding its medical applications.

References

1. Hopkins HH, Kapany NS. A flexible fiberscope, using static scanning. Nature 173:39, 1954.
2. Hirschowitz BI. A personal history of the fiberscope. Gastroenterology 76:864, 1979.
3. Murphy P. A fibre-optic endoscope used for nasal intubation. Anaesthesia 22:489, 1967.
4. Taylor PA, Towey RM. The broncho-fiberscope as an aid to endotracheal intubation. Br J Anaesth 44:611, 1972.
5. Welford WT. Optics, 3rd ed. Oxford: Oxford University Press, 1988.
6. Yariv A. Guided-wave optics. Sci Am 240:64, 1979.
7. Seippel RG. Fiber Optics. Reston, Virginia: Reston Publishing, 1984.
8. Drexhage MG, Moynihan CT. Infrared optical fibers. Sci Am 259:110, 1988.
9. Ovassapian A, Dykes MHM. The role of fiberoptic endoscopy in airway management. Semin Anesth 6:93, 1987.
10. Barlow DE. Fiberoptic instrument technology. In Tams TR (ed). Small Animal Endoscopy. St. Louis: Mosby-Year Book, 1990; p. 1.
11. Kawahara I, Ichikawa H. Fiberoptic instrument technology. In Sivak MV (ed). Gastroenterologic Endoscopy. Philadelphia: W. B. Saunders, 1987; p. 20.
12. Sloan TB, Ovassapian A. The principles of flexible fiberoptic endoscopes. In Ovassapian A (ed). Fiberoptic Airway Endoscopy in Anesthesia and Critical Care. New York: Raven Press, 1990; p. 1.
13. Katzir A. Optical fibers in medicine. Sci Am 260:120, 1989.

CHAPTER 22

The Role of Fiberoptic Bronchoscopy in Thoracic Anesthesia

William E. Hurford, M.D.

The necessity for skill in endobronchial intubation has grown with increased activity in thoracic and tracheal surgery. Complex surgical procedures such as bronchoplasty or tracheal or carinal resections have mandated the development of reliable techniques to ensure and protect the airway during surgery. Selective endobronchial intubation now is used routinely to provide a quiet field for the thoracic surgeon, to maintain continuity of the airway during tracheal and bronchial resections, and to limit the spread of secretions, infection, or pulmonary hemorrhage.[1]

Historically, endobronchial intubation has been performed by anesthesiologists in a blind manner, relying on physical signs such as breath sounds and chest movements to confirm proper placement of the endobronchial tube. Although this has been satisfactory in most cases, sometimes blind endobronchial intubation is difficult or impossible. As a result of a poorly positioned endobronchial tube, oper-

ating conditions may suffer or a variety of life-threatening complications may occur (see Complication of Endobronchial Intubation, below). In addition, recent studies have demonstrated that the physical signs used to confirm endobronchial tube placement can be unreliable.[2–6] Upper lobe obstruction may commonly occur despite apparently proper positioning of the tube when blind techniques are used.[2]

Fiberoptic bronchoscopy has become increasingly popular for aiding endobronchial intubation.[6,7] Several authors have argued that the technique should be used routinely for endobronchial intubation.[3,6] Although this position remains controversial, it is clear that the thoracic anesthetist needs to be skilled in fiberoptic bronchoscopy. Besides aiding and confirming the placement of double-lumen endobronchial tubes, fiberoptic bronchoscopy is useful for placing endobronchial blockers, removing secretions, changing the position of the endotracheal or endobronchial tube intraoperatively, and assessing airway patency during and after surgical repair (Table 22–1). The

Portions of this chapter are adapted from Anesthesiology Clinics of North America 9(1):97–109, 1991.

Table 22–1. ROLE OF FIBEROPTIC BRONCHOSCOPY IN THORACIC ANESTHESIA

1. Placement of double-lumen endobronchial tubes.
2. Confirmation of double-lumen endobronchial tube placement.
3. Placement of endobronchial blockers.
4. Removal of secretions.
5. Changing position of endobronchial tube intraoperatively.
6. Intraoperative endobronchial intubation.
7. Assessment of airway patency after surgical repair.

From Hurford, WE. Fiberoptic endobronchial intubation. Anesth Clin North Am 9(1):97–109, 1991.

thoracic anesthetist should, therefore, have a thorough knowledge of tracheobronchial anatomy and the techniques of fiberoptic-assisted endotracheal and endobronchial intubation.

TRACHEOBRONCHIAL ANATOMY

The adult trachea is approximately 10 to 13 cm long (mean, 11 cm) and composed anteriorly and laterally of approximately 20 U-shaped cartilaginous rings and posteriorly by the trachealis muscle.[8, 9] The internal diameter of the trachea averages 2.3 cm laterally and 1.8 cm anteroposteriorly.

At the carina, the trachea divides into right and left mainstem bronchi, which in turn branch into 18 segmental bronchi (Fig. 22–1).[10] The right mainstem bronchus divides at an angle of approximately 20 degrees from vertical, as opposed to 50 degrees for the left mainstem bronchus, and has an average length of 1.2 cm (approximate range, 1 to 4 cm). The bronchus to the right upper lobe takes off laterally and superiorly from the right mainstem bronchus and then divides into bronchi supplying the apical, anterior, and posterior segments of the right upper lobe. The bronchus intermedius extends 2 to 4 cm distal to the take-off of the right upper lobe bronchus. At this point, the middle lobe bronchus opens anteriorly, dividing into medial and lateral segmental branches. Almost immediately distal and posterior to the middle lobe bronchus is the opening to the superior segment of the lower lobe and then the confluence of the four bronchi to the medial, anterior, lateral, and posterior basal segments.

The left mainstem bronchus is narrower and longer than the right. It averages 5 cm in length (range, 3 to 7 cm) and bifurcates into upper and lower lobe bronchi, which are nearly equal in size. This bifurcation usually lies obliquely. The bronchus to the upper lobe divides almost immediately into the lingular bronchus, which supplies the superior and inferior segments of the lingula, and the upper lobe bronchus, which supplies the anterior and combined apical–posterior segments. The bronchus to the lower lobe is a continuation of the left mainstem bronchus and divides into the bronchus to the superior segment and the confluence of the anterior, lateral, and posterior basal segments.

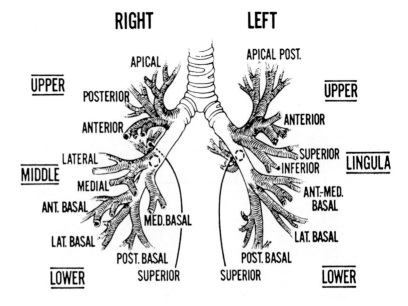

Figure 22–1. Tracheobronchial anatomy. (From Miller JI. Thoracic Surgery. In Kaplan JA (ed). Thoracic Anesthesia, p. 11. New York: Churchill Livingstone, 1983; with permission.)

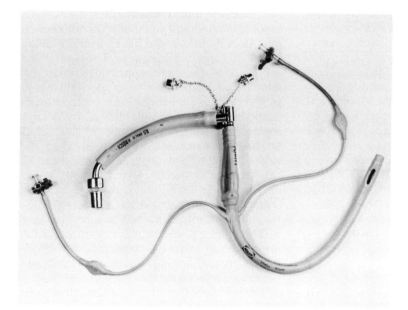

Figure 22–2. Lateral view of right-sided Leyland Robertshaw double-lumen tube with Cobb connector attached. (From McKenna MJ, Wilson RS, Botelho RJ. Right upper lobe obstruction with right-sided double-lumen endobronchial tubes: A comparison of two tube types. Journal of Cardiothoracic Anesthesia 2:734–740, 1988; with permission.)

ENDOBRONCHIAL TUBES

These specialized tubes were initially developed for differential bronchospirometry and the control of unilateral pulmonary hemorrhage and secretions. In current use, they permit selective ventilation of each lung, providing a quiet, collapsed lung upon which to operate while isolating the nonoperative lung from blood and secretions.[1] Most importantly, endobronchial tubes maintain an intact airway during unilateral bronchial resection.

Robertshaw Double-Lumen Tubes

Robertshaw tubes are made of red rubber and are available in left- or right-sided versions.[11] The right-sided version has a slotted bronchial cuff to accommodate the bronchial

orifice to the right upper lobe (Fig. 22–2). The tubes have large diameter, low-resistance lumens, and no tracheal hook. Small, medium, and large sizes are available, corresponding to 8, 9.5, and 11 mm endotracheal tubes.

Disposable, polyvinyl chloride versions of the Robertshaw tube are available from several manufacturers in 35, 37, 39, and 41 French sizes (Fig. 22–3). The greater variety of sizes may permit a better fit. These tubes are, however, expensive, not reusable, and more difficult to place correctly.

Insertion of Robertshaw Tubes

Prior to intubation, the cuffs of the tube are checked for leaks, the tube is lubricated, and a stylet is placed in the bronchial lumen. At our institution, the nonoperative or dependent lung is chosen as the lung to be selectively

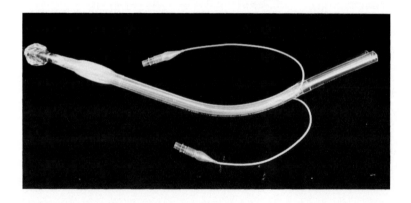

Figure 22–3. Lateral view of right-sided Mallinckrodt double-lumen tube. (From McKenna MJ, Wilson RS, Botelho RJ: Right upper lobe obstruction with right-sided double-lumen endobronchial tubes: A comparison of two tube types. Journal of Cardiothoracic Anesthesia 2:734–740, 1988; with permission.)

intubated. If this is done, the endobronchial tube does not interfere with resection of the mainstem bronchus, should this be necessary. If the nondependent lung is intubated, mediastinal compression or surgical manipulation may displace the bronchial limb and interrupt isolation of the operative lung. Mediastinal compression may also push the tracheal lumen against the tracheal wall, creating a ball-valve obstruction to ventilation.

For laryngoscopy, a Macintosh blade is preferred over a Miller blade, because it provides more room for manipulating the tube within the pharynx. Double-lumen tubes have a compound curve: the upper shaft of the tube curves anteriorly, whereas the distal tip curves laterally. Intubation must therefore be systematic. First, the tube is placed in the oropharynx with the concavity of the distal tip facing anteriorly. Once the tip of the tube has passed through the cords, the tube is gently rotated so that the concavity of the main shaft faces anteriorly. The tube then is slid off the stylet until it is seated with its tip in the bronchus and its bite block at the patient's incisors.

Confirming Position of the Tube

The position of the tube must be checked carefully after insertion and again after positioning the patient to ensure that the correct lung can be isolated. Even if the placement of the endobronchial tube is to be confirmed with the bronchoscope, the following four maneuvers should be performed to ensure proper lung isolation and function of the bronchial and tracheal cuffs (Table 22–2):

1. Chest movements should be observed and breath sounds auscultated bilaterally prior to inflation of the cuffs. A moderate leak around the tube should be detectable.

2. The tracheal limb of the Cobb connector is clamped, the cap of the tracheal limb is removed, and the bronchial cuff is inflated to produce an airtight seal with minimal cuff volume (3 to 5 mL of air). Lung compliance should not decrease excessively, assuming that the compliance of each lung is relatively equal.

3. The tracheal limb is then recapped, the clamp is removed and placed on the connector to the bronchial limb, and the cap on the bronchial limb is removed. Next, the patient is ventilated only through the tracheal side of the Robertshaw tube. Inflation of the tracheal cuff with 5 to 10 mL of air should produce an airtight seal. The chest should move, and breath sounds should be heard only on the

Table 22–2. BLIND CONFIRMATION OF DOUBLE-LUMEN TUBE PLACEMENT

1. Confirm tracheal placement of tube:
   Observe chest rise and fall.
   Auscultate chest and stomach.
   Monitor end-tidal CO_2.
2. Inflate and check bronchial cuff:
   Clamp tracheal limb of Cobb connector, uncap tracheal port.
   Apply positive pressure.
   Slowly inflate bronchial cuff until air leak from tracheal port disappears.
   Leak should disappear with 3 to 5 mL air.
   If minimal leak—tube may be too large or inserted too far.
   If >5 mL air required—cuff torn or tip of tube may be in trachea.
3. Confirm endobronchial placement:
   Apply positive pressure.
   Observe chest rise and fall.
   Auscultate chest, assess compliance.
   Wrong side intubated—withdraw tube and gently re-advance.
   If compliance is low—tube may be kinked; try withdrawing slightly, then readvance if necessary.
4. Confirm patency and position of tracheal lumen:
   Recap tracheal port and unclamp tracheal limb of Cobb connector.
   Clamp bronchial limb of Cobb connector and uncap bronchial port.
   Apply positive pressure.
   Slowly inflate tracheal cuff until air leak around tube disappears.
   Leak should disappear with <10 mL air.
   If minimal leak—tube may be too large.
   If >10 mL air required—cuff torn or tip of tube may be in trachea.
   Continue ventilation.
   Observe chest rise and fall.
   Auscultate chest, assess compliance.
   Wrong side intubated—withdraw tube and gently re-advance.
   If compliance is low—tube may be kinked; try withdrawing slightly, then readvance if necessary.

From Hurford, WE. Fiberoptic endobronchial intubation. Anesth Clin North Am 9(1):97–109, 1991.

nonintubated side. No air should leak from the open bronchial port. Again, lung compliance should not decrease excessively.

4. Finally, ventilation through both lumens is checked once again. The bronchial cuff should be left inflated from the time of insertion until differential ventilation is no longer needed. Keeping this cuff inflated minimizes changes in the tube's position. We have not observed airway trauma from keeping the bronchial cuff inflated during this limited time, probably because the cuff is inflated only to minimal occlusion pressure and intraoperative movement of the tube is minimized.

Carlens and White Double-Lumen Tubes

The Carlens tube is designed for left-sided endobronchial intubation; the White tube is a right-sided version. Carlens and White tubes are constructed of red rubber and are available in 35, 37, 39, and 41 French sizes. They have lumens of smaller internal diameter than the Robertshaw tubes and a carinal hook. The hook, although increasing the stability of the tube, makes the tube difficult to insert. Also because of the hook, the tube must be withdrawn back into the trachea before carinal surgery or pneumonectomy can be performed.

Insertion of the Carlens or White Tube

After laryngoscopy, the tube is placed in the oropharynx so that the concavity of the distal tip is anterior. Once the tip passes between the cords, the tube is rotated so that the carinal hook is anterior and can pass between the cords. Once the hook is beyond the larynx, the tube is rotated back 90 degrees, so that the concavity of the shaft is anterior. The tube is then slid off the stylet and advanced until its hook engages the carina. The position of the tube is checked using the procedure outlined previously for the Robertshaw tube.

Bronchial Blockers

When endobronchial intubation is difficult, as in pediatric or some laryngectomized patients, a number 8-14 Fogarty catheter (10 mL balloon volume), placed with the aid of a fiberoptic bronchoscope and then inflated, may be used to selectively occlude a mainstem or lobar bronchus. To do this, a standard endotracheal tube is first placed. Under direct vision, a Fogarty catheter is then passed between the vocal cords, alongside the endotracheal tube. The tip of the catheter is positioned using the fiberoptic bronchoscope and inflated under direct vision until the bronchus is seen to be occluded. Once one-lung ventilation is no longer necessary, the Fogarty catheter balloon may be deflated without disturbing the endotracheal tube.

Single-Lumen Endobronchial Tubes

If ventilation or suctioning of the operative lung is unnecessary or unwise (ie, the pneu-monectomized patient or a patient with a bronchopleural fistula or massive intrapulmonary hemorrhage), endobronchial intubation with a single-lumen tube may be desirable. Specialized single-lumen endobronchial tubes, such as the Macintosh-Leatherdale tube for left-sided intubation or the Gordon-Green tube for right-sided intubation, have been developed but are rarely used in current practice. Long polyvinyl chloride or flexible armored tubes are usually used instead. A fiberoptic bronchoscope should be used to place these tubes, in order to simplify placement and avoid obstruction of an upper lobe bronchus.

COMPLICATIONS OF ENDOBRONCHIAL INTUBATION

Poor positioning of the endobronchial tube with failure to isolate the operative lung is the most common problem of endobronchial intubation (Fig. 22–4). Usually the endobronchial tube has not been passed far enough into the bronchus. This problem may occur when an inappropriately small tube is selected or when bronchial or tracheal narrowing prevents passage of an appropriately sized tube. The inflated bronchial cuff then rests at or above the level of the carina, producing partial or complete obstruction of the nonintubated bronchus. Gas trapping with inability to deflate the operative lung may occur. The tube also may be passed too far down a mainstem bronchus, resulting in obstruction of an upper lobe and hypoxemia. The wrong side may also be intubated. When the position of the tube is in doubt, it should be withdrawn and replaced.

The "margin of safety," or the distance between the most proximal and distal acceptable positions for placing double-lumen tubes, is relatively small and varies with the manufacturer and type of tube.[4, 5, 12] For left-sided Mallinckrodt (Broncho-Cath; Glens Falls, NY), Rüsch (Bronchial Double-Lumen Tubes; New York, NY), and Sheridan (Broncho-Cath; Argyle, NY) tubes and medium left-sided Leyland Robertshaw tubes (London, England), the margin of safety is approximately 16 to 19 mm. For right-sided double-lumen tubes, the margin of safety varies greatly with the manufacturer's design. For medium Leyland, all Mallinckrodt, and large and small Rüsch double-lumen tubes, the margin of safety is 11, 7, 4, and 1 mm, respectively. Although the Leyland double-lumen tube has

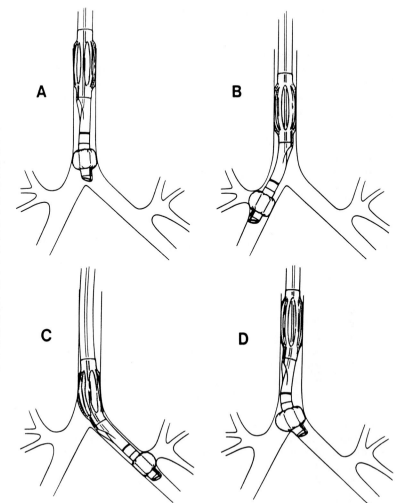

Figure 22–4. Malpositioned left-sided double-lumen tubes. *A,* The endobronchial portion is above the carina. *B,* The wrong mainstem bronchus has been intubated. *C,* The endobronchial portion has been passed too far into the left main bronchus, placing the tracheal lumen past the carina. *D,* The endobronchial portion is not placed far enough into the left main bronchus. Bronchial cuff inflation will obstruct ventilation to the right lung. (From Katz JA, Fairley HB. Pulmonary surgery. In Marshall BE, Longnecker DE, Fairley HB (eds). Anesthesia for thoracic procedures, p. 384. Boston: Blackwell Scientific 1988. Reprinted by permission of Blackwell Scientific Publications, Inc.)

the largest margin of safety, blind insertion of the tube is still associated with a 10% incidence of right upper lobe obstruction.[2] This incidence is much lower than the 89% incidence of right upper lobe obstruction noted after blind endobronchial intubation using right-sided Mallinckrodt tubes. Bronchoscopic confirmation of the position of the tube theoretically should permit ideal placement of the tube in nearly all cases. But the placement of the tube needs to be reconfirmed after patient positioning, because movement of the patient's neck may alter the position of the tube. Saito and coworkers,[13] for example, reported that left-sided Mallinckrodt tubes moved approximately 28 mm when the neck was flexed or extended.

Laryngeal trauma and tracheal and endobronchial rupture, although rare, have been reported, presumably secondary to the large size of the endobronchial tube or overinflation of the cuffs.[14–16]

TECHNIQUES FOR FIBEROPTIC BRONCHOSCOPY

Ideally, the fiberoptic bronchoscope chosen should have an insertion cord with a diameter of 4 mm or less. The small diameter of the insertion cord enables it to pass through both lumens of either small Robertshaw tubes or 35 French disposable double-lumen tubes such as the Broncho-Cath. Bronchoscopes with larger diameter insertion cords may be used with larger endobronchial tubes. For fiberoptic-assisted intubation, a long insertion cord is necessary. Several suitable bronchoscopes are available.[6] For our purposes, a bronchoscope such as the Olympus LF-1 (Olympus Corp., Lake Success, NY) is ideal. The insertion cord is 4 mm in diameter, 60 cm long, and has a 1.2-mm working channel which, although small, may be used to clear secretions or insufflate oxygen. This bronchoscope also has an extra-long fiberoptic cable that leads to the light source. This feature is especially convenient when using the bronchoscope intraoperatively under the surgical drapes.

Fiberoptic Confirmation of Endobronchial Tube Position

Fiberoptic bronchoscopy may be used to confirm the position of the endobronchial tube or to assist with diagnosis of positioning problems in difficult cases. Although the Leyland Robertshaw tubes used at our institution may be placed blindly with an acceptable degree of accuracy, disposable double-lumen tubes tend to be more difficult. The position of this type of tube probably should be confirmed with the bronchoscope in all cases. Certainly, the small margin for error in the placement of currently available disposable right-sided tubes mandates bronchoscopic confirmation.

The procedure for confirming tube position with the bronchoscope is simple (Table 22–3). Ventilation can be continued during bronchoscopy, because the bronchoscope may be inserted through an open port after the Cobb connector is clamped or through a bronchoscopic swivel adaptor. For left endobronchial intubation, after blind placement of the tube, the fiberoptic bronchoscope is inserted into the tracheal lumen. The patency of the tracheal lumen is assessed while the insertion tube of the bronchoscope is advanced under direct vision toward the carina. The main carina should be clearly visible distal to the end of the tracheal lumen. The right mainstem bronchus should be clear and unobstructed. The proximal end of the endobronchial cuff of the tube should be barely visible at the carina. The fiberoptic bronchoscope is next removed and inserted into the bronchial lumen. The patency of the bronchial lumen should be confirmed as the insertion tube of the bronchoscope is advanced. The secondary carina and the left upper and lower mainstem bronchi should be clearly visible and unobstructed.

The procedure is similar for right-sided endobronchial intubation. After inserting the bronchoscope through the tracheal lumen, the main carina should be identified. Again, the proximal edge of the endobronchial cuff should be barely visible. The bronchoscope is then withdrawn and inserted through the bronchial lumen. On passing the bronchoscope through the bronchial lumen, the patency of the lumen is confirmed. The secondary carina of the right middle and lower lobes should be clearly visible beyond the end of the tube. On withdrawing the bronchoscope slowly, the slot for the right upper lobe should be visualized. The right upper lobe bronchus should be centered in the slot.

The abnormality most often encountered is that the tracheal lumen is partially kinked (see Fig. 22–4 and Table 22–4). It is difficult to pass the bronchoscope, and the right mainstem bronchus is not well visualized. If this is the case, then the wrong side may have been intubated, or the tube may not have been passed beyond the carina. Slowly withdrawing the endobronchial tube under direct vision usually is sufficient to make the proper diagnosis. Reassessing the chosen size of the endobronchial tube may be necessary. Another common problem is failure to visualize the

---

Table 22–3. FIBEROPTIC CONFIRMATION OF ENDOBRONCHIAL TUBE POSITION

After insertion of endobronchial tube and confirmation of position using blind technique:
For left endobronchial intubation:
1. Insert fiberoptic bronchoscope into tracheal lumen.
2. Assess patency of tracheal lumen.
3. Identify main carina and left mainstem bronchus. Proximal end of bronchial cuff should be barely visible.
4. Remove fiberoptic bronchoscope and insert into bronchial lumen.
5. Confirm that the endobronchial portion of the tube terminates before the secondary carina of the left lung.
6. Adjust tube as necessary.
For right endobronchial intubation:
1. Insert fiberoptic bronchoscope into tracheal lumen.
2. Assess patency of tracheal lumen.
3. Identify main carina and right mainstem bronchus. Proximal end of bronchial cuff should be barely visible.
4. Remove fiberoptic bronchoscope and insert into bronchial lumen.
5. Confirm that the endobronchial portion of the tube terminates before the secondary carina of the right middle and lower lobes.
6. Slowly withdraw the fiberoptic bronchoscope until the slot for the right upper lobe is visualized.
7. Check for patency of the right upper lobe. Adjust tube as necessary.

From Hurford, WE. Fiberoptic endobronchial intubation. Anesth Clin North Am 9(1):97–109, 1991.

Table 22–4. TROUBLE-SHOOTING WITH THE FIBEROPTIC BRONCHOSCOPE

Problem	Cause

1. Fiberoptic bronchoscope cannot be passed through tracheal lumen	1. Fiberoptic bronchoscope too large or not well lubricated
	2. Wrong side intubated
	3. DLT kinked
	   a. DLT too large
	   b. DLT impacted on carina
	   c. DLT not inserted far enough

2. Operative lumen not visualized	1. Wrong side intubated 2. DLT impacted on carina
3. Bronchial cuff not observed	DLT advanced too far
4. Bronchial lumen kinked	DLT impacted on carina
5. Wrong side seen	Wrong side intubated
6. Right upper lobe orifice not seen during right-sided endobronchial intubation	DLT inserted too far (common) or not far enough (uncommon)

From Hurford, WE. Fiberoptic endobronchial intubation. Anesth Clin North Am 9(1):97–109, 1991.
DLT, double-lumen tube.

upper lobe bronchus. This may occur with either left- or right-sided intubations and is generally due to the tube being passed too far distally.

Fiberoptic-Assisted Endobronchial Intubation

The fiberoptic bronchoscope may also be used for initial placement of the endobronchial tube (Table 22–5). For this, the trachea is intubated with the endobronchial tube using either direct or fiberoptic laryngoscopy. If the trachea is to be intubated initially with the fiberoptic bronchoscope, the insertion cord is best placed through the bronchial lumen of the double-lumen tube. After confirmation of tracheal placement and adequate ventilation, the fiberoptic bronchoscope is inserted through the bronchial lumen of the endobronchial tube and the main carina is identified. For left endobronchial intubation, the tip of the insertion tube is advanced to a point just proximal to the secondary carina of the left upper and lower lobe bronchi (Fig. 22–5). The double-

Table 22–5. FIBEROPTIC-ASSISTED ENDOBRONCHIAL INTUBATION

1. Intubate trachea with endobronchial tube.
2. Confirm placement of tube within the trachea using standard techniques.
3. Insert fiberoptic bronchoscope through bronchial lumen of endobronchial tube.
4. Identify main carina.
5. For left endobronchial intubation:
   a. Advance fiberoptic bronchoscope to just proximal to the secondary carina of the left lung.
   b. Advance double-lumen tube over the bronchoscope until tube just comes into view or resistance is felt.
   c. Confirm that the endobronchial portion of the tube terminates before the secondary carina of the left lung.
   d. Remove fiberoptic bronchoscope and insert into tracheal lumen.
   e. Assess patency of tracheal lumen. Identify main carina and right mainstem bronchus. Proximal end of bronchial cuff should be barely visible.
   f. Adjust tube as necessary.
6. For right endobronchial intubation:
   a. Advance fiberoptic bronchoscope into the bronchus intermedius.
   b. Advance double-lumen tube over the bronchoscope until tube just comes into view or resistance is felt.
   c. Confirm that the endobronchial portion of the tube terminates before the secondary carina of the right middle and lower lobe bronchi.
   d. Slowly withdraw the fiberoptic bronchoscope until the slot for the right upper lobe is visualized.
   e. Check for patency of the right upper lobe. Adjust tube as necessary.
   f. Remove fiberoptic bronchoscope and insert into tracheal lumen.
   g. Assess patency of tracheal lumen. Identify main carina and left mainstem bronchus. Proximal end of bronchial cuff should be barely visible.
   h. Adjust tube as necessary.

From Hurford, WE. Fiberoptic endobronchial intubation. Anesth Clin North Am 9(1):97–109, 1991.

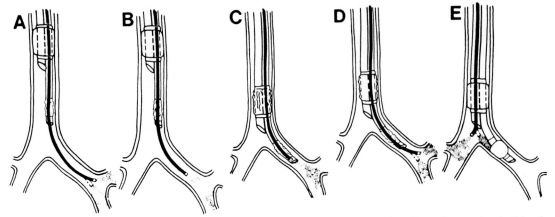

Figure 22–5. Fiberoptic placement and positioning of a left-sided double-lumen tube. (From Ovassapian A, Schrader SC. Fiber-optic-aided bronchial intubation. Seminars in Anesthesia 6:133–142, 1987; with permission.)

lumen tube is then advanced over the bronchoscope until the tip of the tube just comes into view or until resistance is felt. The endobronchial position of the tube is then confirmed. The bronchoscope is then removed and reinserted into the tracheal lumen. After assessing the patency of the tracheal lumen, the main carina and right mainstem bronchus are identified. The proximal edge of the endobronchial cuff should be barely visible.

Fiberoptic-assisted right-sided endobronchial intubation is similar (Fig. 22–6). In this case, the tip of the bronchoscope is positioned within the bronchus intermedius and the tube is advanced until it just comes into view or resistance is felt. After confirming that the endobronchial portion of the tube terminates proximal to the secondary carina of the right

middle and lower lobe bronchi, the bronchoscope is slowly withdrawn until the slot for the right upper lobe is visualized. The tube is then adjusted so that the right upper lobe bronchus is positioned in the center of the slot. The bronchoscope is then removed and reinserted into the tracheal lumen. After assessing the patency of the tracheal lumen, the main carina and left mainstem bronchus are identified. The proximal end of the endobronchial cuff should be barely visible.

Other Uses for Fiberoptic Bronchoscopy

Using similar techniques and landmarks, the fiberoptic bronchoscope can be invaluable in

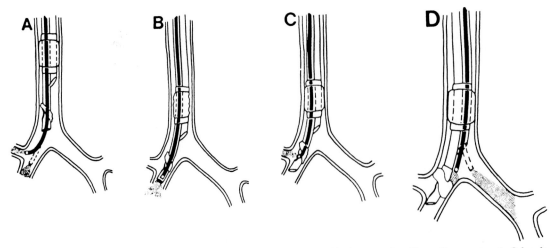

Figure 22–6. Fiberoptic placement and positioning of a right-sided double-lumen tube. (From Ovassapian A, Schrader SC. Fiber-optic-aided bronchial intubation. Seminars in Anesthesia 6:133–142, 1987; with permission.)

placing bronchial blockers and single-lumen endobronchial tubes.[17] Endobronchial tubes and blockers displaced during surgery may be replaced with accuracy. Bronchoscopy also permits secretions to be removed and can provide a direct assessment of endobronchial anatomy both intraoperatively and prior to extubation. Such an assessment of airway anatomy may be especially important after carinal resection and reconstruction or bronchoplasty.

References

1. Wilson RS. Endobronchial intubation. In Kaplan JA (ed). Thoracic Anesthesia. New York: Churchill Livingstone, 1983; pp. 389–402.
2. McKenna MJ, Wilson RS, Botelho RJ. Right upper lobe obstruction with right-sided double-lumen endobronchial tubes: A comparison of two tube types. Journal of Cardiothoracic Anesthesia 2:734–740, 1988.
3. Benumof JL. Fiberoptic bronchoscopy and double-lumen tube position. Anesthesiology 65:117–118, 1986.
4. Benumof JL, Partridge BL, Salvatierra C, Keating J. Margin of safety in positioning modern double-lumen endotracheal tubes. Anesthesiology 67:729–738, 1987.
5. Benumof JL. Improving the design and function of double-lumen tubes. Journal of Cardiothoracic Anesthesia 2:729–733, 1988.
6. Ovassapian A, Schrader SC. Fiber-optic-aided bronchial intubation. Seminars in Anesthesia 6:133–142, 1987.
7. Slinger PD. Fiberoptic bronchoscopic positioning of double-lumen tubes. Journal of Cardiothoracic Anesthesia 3:486–496, 1989.
8. Grillo HC, Dignan EF, Miura T. Extensive resection of mediastinal trachea without prosthesis or graft: An anatomical study in man. J Thorac Cardiovasc Surg 48:741–749, 1964.
9. Smith TC. Functional anatomy of the respiratory system. In Marshall BE, Longnecker DE, Fairley HB (eds). Anesthesia for Thoracic Procedures. Boston: Blackwell Scientific, 1988; pp. 1–37.
10. Miller JI. Thoracic surgery. In Kaplan JA (ed). Thoracic Anesthesia. New York: Churchill Livingstone, 1983; pp. 9–32.
11. Robertshaw FL. Low resistance double lumen endobronchial tubes. Br J Anaesth 34:576–579, 1962.
12. Keating JL, Benumof JL. An analysis of margin of safety in positioning double-lumen tubes. Anesthesiology 63:A563, 1985.
13. Saito S, Dohi S, Naito H. Alteration of double-lumen endobronchial tube position by flexion and extension of the neck. Anesthesiology 62:696–697, 1985.
14. Guernelli N, Bragaglia RB, Briccoli A, Mastrorilli M, Vecchi R. Tracheobronchial ruptures due to cuffed Carlens tubes. Ann Thorac Surg 28:66–68, 1979.
15. Heiser M, Steinberg JJ, MacVaugh H III, Klineberg PL. Bronchial rupture, a complication of use of the Robertshaw double-lumen tube. Anesthesiology 51:88, 1979.
16. Burton NA, Fall SM, Lyons T, Graber GM. Rupture of the left mainstem bronchus with a polyvinylchloride double-lumen tube. Chest 83:928–929, 1983.
17. El-Baz N, Faber LP, Kittle F, Warren W, Ivankovich AD. Bronchoscopic endobronchial intubation with a single lumen tube for one-lung anesthesia. Anesthesiology 65:A480, 1986.

CHAPTER 23

Teaching Fiberoptic Laryngoscopy and Intubation

Calvin Johnson, M.D., and Abdel R. El-Ganzouri, M.D.

Fiberoptic intubation is a technique in which every anesthesiologist should be competent. In experienced hands, the technique has been proven to be lifesaving when managing patients with compromised airways.[1-4] In a recent study, Spielman and associates[5] surveyed 110 private practice anesthesiologists, 76 chairpersons of anesthesiology, and 138 members of the Society for Education in Anesthesia as to which procedural skills were necessary for a resident to be considered competent as a "consultant in anesthesiology." The procedure that received the highest endorsement from these groups was fiberoptic laryngoscopy and intubation. However, a survey of 90 anesthesia residency programs in the United States[6] revealed that only three of these institutions had initiated fiberoptic training programs, and no program had a written protocol or established criteria with which to evaluate residents' performance. In addition, several recent studies have demonstrated that the most effective method of teaching or learning fiberoptic intubation is via a formal training program.[7-9]

GOAL OF TEACHING/ TRAINING FIBEROPTIC ENDOSCOPY

The training necessary for a novice anesthesiologist to become proficient in flexible fiberoptic endoscopy has not been standardized because the end point, a "qualified endoscopist," has never been defined. The lack of concordance in defining the exact qualifications of a "qualified endoscopist" has led to discrepancies between investigators as to the number of fiberoptic intubations practices necessary to become proficient in fiberoptic endoscopy. In a monograph on the role of fiberoptic endoscopy in airway management, Ovassapian and Dykes[3] did not objectively define the number of attempts necessary to attain the skills required to reach their end point. Johnson and Roberts[8] claim that technical expertise in fiberoptic intubation is acquired by residents after they perform 20 successful fiberoptic intubations. However, Sia and Edens[2] imply that at least 30 successful fiberoptic intubations are required before an endoscopist can be confi-

Table 23–1. CLEANING THE FIBEROPTIC SCOPE

All cleaning is done at the field with suction still attached. The fiberscope is cleaned with a series of three solutions:

A. ⅓ soap and ⅔ sterile water
B. Cidex 2% (Surgihos Company, Arlington, TX)
C. Sterile water
   1. Immediately after removing the fiberscope from the patient, gently wipe all debris from the insertion tube with a gauze moistened with soap and water.
   2. Aspirate soap and water through suction channel of the scope.
   3. Follow with Cidex, wiping first outside of the scope with Cidex, then aspirate all of the solution in the container.
   4. Follow with sterile water, repeating Step 3.
   5. Aspirate air to dry the channel.
   6. Gently dry all external surfaces of the scope with a soft gauze. Do *not* put tension on the insertion tube of the fiberscope while drying, because the outer cover of the bending section may be excessively stretched.

The scope is now clean and is prepared for reuse or for storage. Alternatively, a scope can be ethylene oxide gas sterilized. Make sure to follow the manufacturer's recommended procedures if disinfection or sterilization is needed.

dent of his or her ability to solve the problems encountered in an unexpected difficult intubation. We believe that the completion of at least 50 successful fiberoptic intubations is required to develop the anesthesiologist's confidence in his or her ability to manage the patient with a difficult airway and to be sufficiently proficient in the procedure without expert assistance. This higher number is in accordance with the guidelines established by the American College of Chest Physicians (ACCP)[10] for proficiency in fiberoptic endoscopy.

Setting strict criteria for competence in fiberoptic endoscopy is not the goal of this chapter. Rather, the goal is to establish methods to ensure a safe and effective resident training program, as well as a training method for practicing anesthesiologists in their own hospitals.

As with any psychomotor skill, in order to become skillful at fiberoptic intubation, the anesthesiologist must first know what to do, how to use his or her hands properly, and be able to adapt these skills to a specific airway problem. The modeling of these motor skills should be based on observation of an expert "instructor" who performs the skill that trainees are about to learn. Frequent practice of the skills is necessary until mastery is achieved. Finally, supervision by qualified instructors to evaluate the trainees' skills guarantees accurate feedback about their performance, thereby improving the training process.

In order to obtain a high success rate in training anesthesiologists in fiberoptic endoscopy, definite goals have to be established for the training, and all elements of the curriculum must be readily available to all participants—both trainees and instructors.

REQUIREMENTS FOR TRAINING

Establishing a Protocol

Prior to establishing a fiberoptic training program, a protocol that specifies the steps needed for trainees to become certified in fiberoptic intubation should be developed. The protocol presented in this chapter is based on that established for the Department of Anesthesiology at Rush-Presbyterian-St. Luke's Medical Center in Chicago, Illinois.[7] These training steps include:

A. Reading and demonstrating proficiency in topics such as endobronchial anatomy; physical characteristics, cleaning, and care of the fiberscope (Table 23–1); and other pertinent references.
B. Attendance at a workshop on the care and cleaning of the scope, as well as practice on intubation models under the supervision of an experienced instructor.
C. Training on patients with normal airways scheduled for general anesthesia and endotracheal intubation.
D. Completion of gradual stepwise practice on patients with compromised airways (Note: steps C and D are performed under direct supervision of instructors).
E. Program evaluation and feedback are done by answering a fiberoptic questionnaire and post-training test.

Equipment

Fiberscopes

Several fiberoptic laryngoscopes and bronchoscopes are available (Table 23–2). The fi-

Table 23–2. FIBEROPTIC LARYNGOSCOPES AND BRONCHOSCOPES

Manufacturer	Insertion Cord Length (cm)	Insertion Cord Diameter (mm)	Working Channel Diameter (mm)	Tip Deflection		Field of View	Depth of View
American Optical laryngoscope Model LS-8	50	6.2	2.6	Up Down	140° 60°	80°	5–70 mm
Machida intubation scope Model FLS-6-50	50	6.0	2.0	Up Down	120° 120°	70°	5–50 mm
ACMI bronchoscope Model F-3	60	5.3	1.8	Up Down	135° 135°	67°	3 mm–∞
Olympus bronchoscope Model BF-4B2	59.5	4.9	2.0	Up Down	180° 60°	70°	3–50 mm
Pentax bronchoscope Model FB-15A	58.0	4.9	2.0	Up Down	180° 100°	85°	3–50 mm
Olympus bronchoscope Model BF-3C4	59.5	3.6	1.2	Up Down	160° 60°	55°	3–50 mm
Pentax fiberscope Model FB-15H	60	4.8	2.0	Up Down	180° 130°	100°	3–50 mm
Pentax fiberscope Model FB-19H	55	6.3	2.6	Up Down	160° 100°	90°	3–50 mm
Olympus fiberscope Model LF-2	60	4.0	1.5	Up Down	120° 120°	90°	3–50 mm

berscopes most widely used in clinical anesthesia are the Olympus (Tokyo, Japan) model LF-2, and the Pentax (Tokyo, Japan) models FB-15H Slim and FB-19H multipurpose large-channel bronchofiberscopes. Finding a fiberscope that can fulfill all the requirements for training, versatility, and utility for both adults and pediatric patients is difficult. The Olympus LF-2 is 60 cm long, with an insertion tube outer diameter (OD) of 4.0 mm. This fiberscope is longer and stiffer than other 4.0-mm diameter scopes, which allows it to pass through all double-lumen endobronchial and endotracheal tubes as small as 5 mm inner diameter (ID). With practice, manipulation of the Olympus LF-2 can be easily mastered. It can be used in adult and pediatric patients as young as 3 to 4 years of age. However, it may be difficult for the novice anesthesiologist to learn quickly with this scope due to its small visual field, its small channel diameter (1.2 mm), and the difficulty that can be encountered when threading a large diameter tube (8 mm or more ID). The Pentax FB-19H, with its large visual field, big insertion tube diameter of 6.3 mm, and large working channel of 2.6 mm, is ideal for training; however, the smallest size endotracheal tube that can be used with it is 7.5 mm ID, limiting its use to adult patients only.

As a general rule, the ID of the smallest endotracheal tube through which a fiberscope can easily pass must be at *least* 1 mm larger than the largest diameter of the insertion cord. The fiberscope is a delicate instrument that must be handled with care. The insertion tube should *never* be subjected to severe bending, nor should any sharp or heavy objects be placed on it.

Early in our experience, we found that improper storage of these instruments was responsible for a significant number of cases of fiber damage. A practical way of storing these fiberscopes is to hang them straight in cabinets designed especially for them (Fig. 23–1). Entrusting the keys to these cabinets only to qualified anesthesiologists prevents their use by unqualified personnel and reduces the possibility of damage.

Fiberoptic Carts

Organizing the equipment for fiberoptic intubation on a mobile cart aids in the training process, as well as increases its usefulness in emergency situations. Fiberoptic carts should ideally be equipped with a light source, cleaning solutions, and ancillary equipment stored in an organized fashion. In our institution, these carts are maintained in a fashion similar to our anesthesia carts in that it is the responsibility of a fiberoptic technician to check the

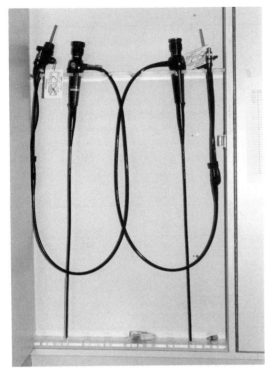

Figure 23–1. Fiberoptic cabinet with hanging fiberscopes.

scope before and after its use, and to restock the used ancillary equipment. A practical and useful way to store the fiberoptic scope on these carts is to hang it straight in a plastic tube attached to the cart. The use of two tubes helps to distinguish a dirty scope from a clean scope (Fig. 23–2). An oxygen source separate from the O_2 supply of the anesthesia machine should also be attached to the cart for O_2 insufflation.

Funding

A budget is needed to purchase the above equipment and to fund maintenance, due to the inevitable need for repair to keep the scopes in optimal condition. For a typical academic department with three fiberoptic scopes, the initial cost of the scopes, carts, training materials, and supplies can easily exceed $35,000, with an annual cost of repair of $5000 or more. Hospital administration and department chairpersons should be aware that the primary importance of this equipment is to ensure patient safety while training in fiberoptic techniques. Money spent on equipment and maintenance is of little consequence when compared with the greatly increased probability of saving a human life.

Communication

Effective communication between anesthesiologists, surgeons, and other health care providers is essential in achieving the necessary environment for effective fiberoptic intubation training. The anesthesiologist must outline the merits of fiberoptic endoscopy and the need for training in order to ensure competence in its practice. This cooperation and understanding are vital in order to keep these programs strong and to avoid any potential misunderstandings or problems that might arise between the anesthesiologist and surgeon.

PRACTICAL POINTS FOR SUCCESSFUL TRAINING IN FIBEROPTIC ENDOSCOPY

Since the establishment of a fiberoptic intubation training program at Rush-Presbyterian-St. Luke's Medical Center in 1986, we believe that two steps in our training protocol—attendance at a hands-on workshop in order to practice on fiberoptic intubation training models and training on patients with normal airways under general anesthesia—have led to the success of the program.

Hands-on Workshop

Studies have shown that practice on intubating models leads to statistically significant higher success rates when residents begin intubating surgical patients.[12, 13] Therefore, practice on models under the supervision of experienced instructors is the first element in our training curriculum. Also, because repairs of fiberscopes can be extremely expensive, care and cleaning of the fiberscope is reinforced at these sessions.

Practicing anesthesiologists can also benefit from training in fiberoptic training by attending an American Society of Anesthesiologists (ASA) sponsored workshop on fiberoptic endoscopy that is held each year in conjunction with its annual meeting, or they can attend workshops held at other medical centers. Practice on intubation models while under expert supervision in workshop settings pinpoints areas needing improvement and considerably enhances the trainee's learning process.

Training on Patients with Normal Airways

After successfully attaining necessary skills from practice on fiberoptic intubation models, training continues with practice on patients with normal airways under general anesthesia with muscle relaxation. These are optimal conditions to ensure fiberoptic intubation training that involves minimal risk or unpleasantness to the patient. Because this procedure is not outside the normal practice of anesthesia, there is no need to obtain the consent of the patient to an awake intubation. The time to perform the procedure is short, usually 1 to 2 minutes[7]; therefore, surgery is not delayed and the surgeons tend to be willing to cooperate with this training. Optimal training results require that two anesthesiologists work together: the trainee, and an assistant who both supervises the trainee and monitors the patient during the intubation. This team approach may be difficult to achieve in a community hospital; however, an experienced anesthesiologist who has completed workshop training in fiberoptic intubation can usually get another anesthesiologist or nurse anesthetist to play the assistant's role during the training process. As discussed previously, preliminary preparation of the equipment, the patient, and the environment are all essential to making the learning process successful.

Problems Encountered During Fiberoptic Intubations and Their Solutions

A checklist needs to be followed before each fiberoptic intubation attempt to ensure that all equipment is available before the procedure is begun (Table 23–3). The use of this checklist should be instituted early in the training period in order to establish it as a routine procedure.

The most common problems encountered in teaching fiberoptic intubation techniques are the failure of the trainee to introduce the scope at the midline and the inability to advance the endotracheal tube over the scope into the trachea. To ensure a midline insertion during an oral intubation, the fiberscope is initially inserted into the center of the tongue and the oral airway for a distance of 8 cm in the adult patient. After advancing the fiberscope 8 cm, the trainee looks into the eyepiece of the scope for the first time. When the vocal cords are visualized, the tip of the scope is adjusted by the control lever to enter the center of the glottis. If the tip of the scope is *not* in the middle line, or if the anatomy is distorted, the trainee should look to the right or left by rotating the head of the scope clockwise or counterclockwise, respectively. The combination of anteroposterior rotation and tip flexion

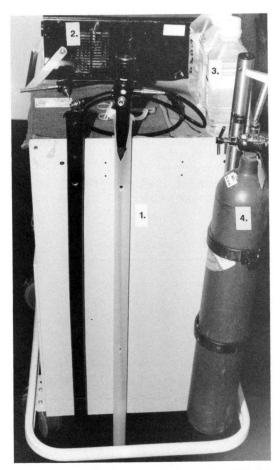

Figure 23–2. Fiberoptic cart, including *1*, two gold club tubes, one for clean scope (white) and one for used scope (black); *2*, light source; *3*, cleaning solutions (soap, Cidex, and water); and *4*, oxygen tank.

Table 23–3. FIBEROPTIC CHECKLIST

1. Light source and fiberoptic scope
2. Endotracheal tube and syringe
3. Bottle of hot water (endotracheal tube softening)
4. Stack of 4 × 4 gauze pads
5. Lidocaine 2% jelly
6. Orange plastic forceps
7. Oral airways, normal and Ovassapian
8. Tongue depressor
9. Gloves
10. Containers (soap, Cidex, water)

Table 23–4. CAUSES OF FAILURE OF
FIBEROPTIC INTUBATION

1. Lack of training and experience
   Solution: Practice, practice, practice
2. Secretions blind you
   Solution: blow or suck secretions away
3. Don't know where you are
   Solution: withdraw scope until you do
4. Image blurred
   Solution: clean the lens
5. Image does not change
   Solution: tip not flexed
6. O_2 saturation drops
   Solution: ventilate by mask, 100% oxygen
7. Endotracheal tube will not advance
   Solution: rotate counterclockwise 90 degrees
8. Assurance of intubation
   Solution: verify with end-tidal CO_2, ascultate
   epigastrium and upper chest
9. Laryngospasm (no vocal cords in view)
   Solution: Succinylcholine 20 mg
10. Resident breaks scope
    Solution: guess?

allows the operator to visualize any of the four
quadrants in the target area.

Problems may be encountered by trainees
when advancing the endotracheal tube over
the scope into the trachea, especially with the
oral approach. The endotracheal tube may
hang up at the level of the epiglottis, arytenoid,
or cords. Usually pulling the endotracheal tube
back up the fiberscope, rotating it 90 degrees
counterclockwise, and then advancing it allows
the endotracheal tube to follow the scope into
the trachea.[14] Sometimes a twisting motion of
the tube is needed to thread it over the scope.

If this fails, then the tongue and epiglottis need
to be elevated by one of several maneuvers:
an assistant can do a jaw-thrust maneuver; he
or she can pull the tongue forward by grasping
it with a gauze pad with the aid of a drape
forceps; or, on rare occasions, the base of the
tongue and epiglottis may need to be elevated
with the aid of a rigid laryngoscope to allow
the endotracheal tube to advance into the
trachea.

The foremost cause of failed fiberoptic intubation is *inexperience*—in preparation of the
trainee, the equipment, the patient, or the
environment. Experience can be gained only
through practice. Trainee residents and practicing anesthesiologists should participate in
practice with models and with patients with
normal airways in order to gain confidence and
skill. With experience, most of the problems
encountered in fiberoptic intubation are easily
overcome (Table 23–4). We have experienced
an unexpected outcome of this practice: trainees sometimes develop an overconfidence syndrome. After completion of training, trainees
sometimes think they can intubate *any* patient
with a fiberscope, no matter how difficult the
airway. For the patient's convenience, these
trainees have the tendency to put patients to
sleep and try to perform fiberoptic intubation
using the fiberscope even though a life-threatening situation may result: the time-limiting
factor in an asleep and paralyzed patient is
definitely a disadvantage in this situation. Continuous supervision is necessary in order to
protect against this syndrome, because its consequences could be disastrous. Trainees should

Table 23–5. PREOPERATIVE ASSESSMENT OF THE AIRWAY

To eliminate the concept of "unanticipated airway difficulty"
To move accurately, identify patients in whom fiberoscopy will facilitate intubation
To intubate all patients *with ease* in whom intubation is originally scheduled

Preoperative assessment to include		(circle one)	
1. Thyromental distance	6.5 cm	6.0–6.5 cm	6.0 cm
2. Mallampati classification	Class I	Class II	Class III
3. Head/neck movement	90°	−90°	90°
4. Body weight	90 kg	90–110 kg	100 kg
5. Jaw movement (interincisor gap)	5 cm	5 cm	
6. Buck teeth	Can prognath	Can approximate	Cannot approximate
7. History of difficult intubation	No	Yes	

All adult patients
Based on above assessment, classify expected difficulty as:
   0 (none)   *1* (possibly some)   *2* (probably some)   *3* (difficulty predicted)
   For *0*: proceed as usual
   For *1*: check scope availability; proceed as usual
   For *2*: scope in room: rigid laryngoscopy × 1 *or* asleep fiberoscopy
   For *3*: awake fiberoscopy
   At any time, only three attempts at rigid laryryngoscopy allowed, with minimal trauma, then
      fiberscope either asleep or awake

Table 23–6. INTUBATION ALTERNATIVES

DIFFICULT AIRWAY ALGORITHM

1. Assess the likelihood and clinical impact of basic management problems:

A. Difficult Intubation

B. Difficult Ventilation

C. Difficulty with Patient Cooperation or Consent

2. Consider the relative merits and feasibility of basic management choices:

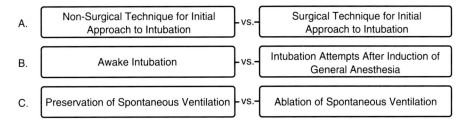

A.	Non-Surgical Technique for Initial Approach to Intubation	vs.	Surgical Technique for Initial Approach to Intubation
B.	Awake Intubation	vs.	Intubation Attempts After Induction of General Anesthesia
C.	Preservation of Spontaneous Ventilation	vs.	Ablation of Spontaneous Ventilation

3. Develop primary and alternative strategies:

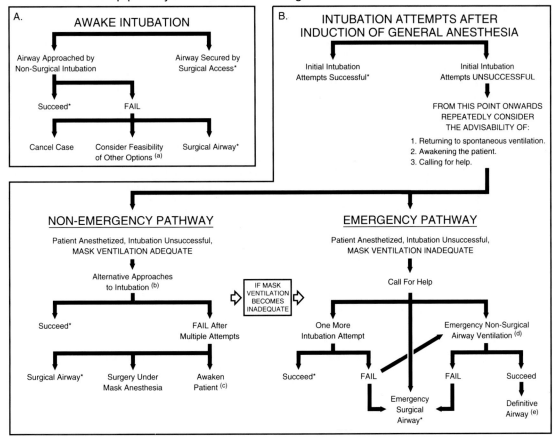

A. AWAKE INTUBATION

- Airway Approached by Non-Surgical Intubation
- Airway Secured by Surgical Access*

- Succeed*
- FAIL

- Cancel Case
- Consider Feasibility of Other Options (a)
- Surgical Airway*

B. INTUBATION ATTEMPTS AFTER INDUCTION OF GENERAL ANESTHESIA

- Initial Intubation Attempts Successful*
- Initial Intubation Attempts UNSUCCESSFUL

FROM THIS POINT ONWARDS REPEATEDLY CONSIDER THE ADVISABILITY OF:

1. Returning to spontaneous ventilation.
2. Awakening the patient.
3. Calling for help.

NON-EMERGENCY PATHWAY

Patient Anesthetized, Intubation Unsuccessful, MASK VENTILATION ADEQUATE

- Alternative Approaches to Intubation (b)

- Succeed*
- FAIL After Multiple Attempts

- Surgical Airway*
- Surgery Under Mask Anesthesia
- Awaken Patient (c)

IF MASK VENTILATION BECOMES INADEQUATE

EMERGENCY PATHWAY

Patient Anesthetized, Intubation Unsuccessful, MASK VENTILATION INADEQUATE

Call For Help

- One More Intubation Attempt
- Emergency Non-Surgical Airway Ventilation (d)

- Succeed*
- FAIL

- FAIL
- Succeed

- Emergency Surgical Airway*
- Definitive Airway (e)

---

* CONFIRM INTUBATION WITH EXHALED CO_2

(a) Other options include (but are not limited to): surgery under mask anesthesia, surgery under local anesthesia infiltration or regional nerve blockade, or intubation attempts after induction of general anesthesia.

(b) Alternative approaches to difficult intubation include (but are not limited to): use of different laryngoscope blades, awake intubation, blind oral or nasal intubation, fiberoptic intubation, intubating stylet or tube changer, light wand, retrograde intubation, and surgical airway access.

(c) See awake intubation.

(d) Options for emergency non-surgical airway ventilation include (but are not limited to): transtracheal jet ventilation, laryngeal mask ventilation, or esophageal-tracheal combitube ventilation.

(e) Options for establishing a definitive airway include (but are not limited to): returning to awake state with spontaneous ventilation, tracheotomy, or endotracheal intubation.

ASA practice guidelines for management of the difficult airway. Anesthesiology 78:597–602, 1993.

be reminded to routinely assess the airway (Table 23–5) in order to avoid encountering a patient with a difficult airway without proper fiberoptic preparation.

An algorithm of delineating the various intubation alternatives is shown in Table 23–6 and should be followed closely. The clear message in this algorithm is that, after proper assessment of airway, the patient with a documented difficult airway should be fiberoptically intubated *awake*. Fiberoptic intubation after general anesthesia should be done only by experienced personnel or by trainees under the supervision of instructors. If an unanticipated difficult intubation is encountered, experienced personnel should be called. It is important to avoid too much trauma when using a rigid laryngoscope, because the presence of secretions or bleeding makes fiberoptic intubation difficult even in the most experienced hands. It is a good idea to affix this algorithm to the fiberoptic cart in a readily available position. In our experience, the necessity of performing cricothyrotomy or tracheostomy or of canceling surgery because of the inability to intubate patients is significantly reduced if this algorithm is followed.

CONCLUSION

Practical experience by residents and attending anesthesiologists is the most important condition for acquiring expertise in the performance of fiberoptic intubation. Developing skill and confidence requires considerable experience and practice with both fiberoptic models and patients with normal airways, followed by training on patients with difficult airways. It has been our experience that a training program such as the one outlined in this chapter provides the necessary curriculum to ensure mastery of this vital anesthetic procedure.

References

1. Delaney KA, Hessler R. Emergency flexible nasotracheal intubation: A report of 60 cases. Ann Emerg Med 17:919–926, 1988.
2. Sia RL, Edens ET. Flexible fiberoptic endoscopy in difficult intubation. Ann Otolaryngol 90:308–309, 1981.
3. Ovassapian A, Dykes M. The role of fiberoptic endoscopy in airway management. Semin Anesth 6:93–104, 1987.
4. Ovassapian A, Land P, Schafer MF, Cerullo L, Zalkind MS. Anesthetic management for surgical corrections of severe flexion deformity of the cervical spine. Anesthesiology 58:370–372, 1983.
5. Spielman FJ, Levin KJ, Matherly JA, et al. Which procedural skills should be learned by anesthesiology residents. Anesthesiology 69(Suppl):72S, 1988.
6. El-Ganzouri A, El-Baz N, Ford E. A survey of fiberoptic endoscopy utilization and training in anesthesia residency program. Presented at the Midwest Anesthesia Residents Conference, Chicago, IL, March 1987.
7. El-Ganzouri A, El-Baz N, Ford E, Murphy P, Badrinath S, Braverman B, Ivankovich A. Training residents in fiberoptic intubation in the operating room. Anesthesiology 69:A805, 1988.
8. Johnson C, Roberts J. Clinical competence in the performance of fiberoptic laryngoscopy and endotracheal intubation: A study of resident instruction. J Clin Anesth 1:344–349, 1989.
9. Ovassapian A, Dykes M, Golmon M. A training program for fiberoptic nasotracheal intubation use of model and live patients. Anaesthesia 38:795–798, 1983.
10. Guidelines for competency and training in fiberoptic bronchoscopy. Section on Bronchoscopy. American College of Chest Physicians. Chest 81:739, 1982.
11. Rothenberg D, Parnass S, El-Ganzouri A. A new method for oxygen insufflation during fiberoptic intubation. J Clin Anesth 1:472–473, 1989.
12. Ovassapian A, Yelich S, Dykes M, Golmon ME. Fiberoptic nasotracheal intubation: Stepwise training versus traditional teaching. Anesthesiology 55:A347, 1981.
13. Dykes M, Ovassapian A. Dissemination of fiberoptic airway endoscopy skills by means of a workshop utilizing models. Br J Anaesth 63:595–597, 1989.
14. Schwartz D, Johnson C, Roberts J. A maneuver to facilitate flexible fiberoptic intubation. Anesthesiology 71:470–471, 1989.
15. ASA. Practice guidelines for management of the difficult airway. Anesthesiology 78:597–602, 1993.

CHAPTER 24

Complications of Endotracheal Intubation

Pamela Angle, M.D., and Steven Elia, M.D., F.R.C.P.C.

Endotracheal intubation is a commonly performed procedure that is used to obtain emergent or elective control of the airway. Although the life-saving and life-sustaining merits of endotracheal intubation are clear, its use is not without the potential for serious morbidity or mortality.

Transtracheal approaches to securing the airway are less commonly used than endotracheal intubation. They are usually performed in the setting where endotracheal intubation is impossible and rapid control of the airway is mandated (ie, cricothyroidotomy or emergency tracheotomy) or for elective tracheotomy, where the patient requires prolonged ventilatory support. Complications of transtracheal intubation include pneumomediastinum, pneumothorax, recurrent laryngeal nerve palsy, obstruction of the tracheostomy tube, tracheoesophageal fistulae, and failure due to unfamiliarity with the procedure during a crisis. High-frequency ventilation has been discussed elsewhere in this book (see Chapter 33).

The complications of endotracheal intubation are most conveniently categorized into those associated with mechanical trauma, physiologic/reflex responses, pharmacologic side effects, or technical difficulties. The na-

ture of these complications may then be considered as they occur in the context of intubation itself (Table 24–1).

The overall incidence of complications secondary to endotracheal intubation is not known with certainty in the medical literature. The broad diversity of patients undergoing intubation for both elective and emergency airway control, as well as varying durations of ventilation, makes such a study difficult.

It is clear, however, that even short periods of intubation with a cuffed endotracheal tube cause local irritative effects on the underlying tracheal mucosa.[1, 2] Intubation for greater than 48 hours results in at least minor sore throats and nonobstructive edema of the glottis in almost all patients.

PREDISPOSING FACTORS

Difficult Airway/Traumatic Intubation

Although for the most part the majority of endotracheal intubations are achieved with relative ease by persons skilled in airway management, on occasion, even in the most opti-

Table 24–1. COMPLICATIONS OF ENDOTRACHEAL INTUBATION

Intubation	Tube in Situ	Extubation
Eye trauma	Eye trauma	
Cervical spine injury	Cervical spine injury	
Dental damage		
Truama to mouth, lips, oropharynx, glottis	Ulceration of mouth, oropharynx, posterior cords, anterior trachea	Vocal cord damage
Epistaxis		
Tracheal perforation	Tracheal perforation	
Pneumothorax	Pneumothorax	
Laryngospasm		Laryngospasm
Esophageal perforation		
Endobronchial intubation	Endobronchial intubation	
Aspiration	Aspiration	Aspiration
	Tube obstruction	Tube obstruction
Glottic edema	Glottic edema	Glottic edema
Sinusitis		
Failed intubation	Disconnect	Croup
Aspiration of the tube	Accidental extubation	Sore throat
Cardiovascular instability		Laryngeal and tracheal damage
	Ignition of the tube during laser surgery	
	Bronchospasm	
	Sinusitis	

mal setting, a difficult airway is encountered. Repeated and often traumatic attempts at direct laryngoscopy and intubation may lead to oral buccal, pharyngeal, tracheal, or laryngeal swelling, laceration, or dental injury. Excessive force during tube insertion may lead to perforation of the pyriform sinus or cervical esophagus or dislocation of the arytenoid cartilages. Difficult laryngoscopy may be predictable based on the history of past intubations (if available), underlying medical problems, and evaluation of the airway. Careful examination of the airway includes range of motion during flexion and extension of the cervical spine (where not contraindicated); jaw mobility; and noting the presence of prominent incisor or loose teeth, receding chin, or high arched narrow palate. In addition, visualization of the oropharynx to identify the faucial pillars, the base of the uvula, and the soft palate must be performed. Lack of visualization of the pillars and uvula has been shown to correlate with increased difficulty during laryngoscopy and intubation.[3] A medical history of conditions that produce difficulty in opening of the mouth or extending the head at the atlanto-occipital joint, such as rheumatoid arthritis, ankylosing spondylitis, scleroderma, or cervical spondylosis or fusion, forewarn the anesthesiologist of probably increased difficulty during laryngoscopy. Conditions producing obstruction of the upper airway, such as tumors, infection, burns, trauma, and inflammatory or congenital malforma-

tions, may complicate airway management and often require awake sedated fiberoptic intubation with surgeons skilled in emergency tracheotomy as back-up. Table 24–2 lists condi-

Table 24–2. CONDITIONS ASSOCIATED WITH DIFFICULT INTUBATION

Congenital
  Pierre Robin
  Down's syndrome
  Cleft lip/palate
  Hurler's syndrome
  Macroglossia
  Mediastinal mass
  Tracheal webs
  Vascular rings
  Micrognathia
Traumatic
  Burn contractures
  Fractured mandible/maxilla
  Fractured cervical-spine, trachea, larynx
Infectious/neoplastic/inflammatory
  Ludwig's angina
  Epiglottitis
  Retropharyngeal
  Abscess
  Neck mass
  Laryngeal polyps
  Epiglottic cyst
  Mediastinal lymphadenopathy
Arthritic
  Rheumatoid arthritis
  Ankylosing spondylitis
  Cervical spine fusion
Endocrinologic
  Goiter
  Acromegaly

tions commonly associated with difficulty during laryngoscopy and intubation.

Endotracheal Tube Size, Type, and Cuff Pressure

Several risk factors for long-term tracheolaryngeal sequela following endotracheal intubation have been reported in the medical literature. These include high cuff pressure, oral intubation, and difficulty and duration of intubation. High cuff pressure (above tracheal capillary mucosal pressure [>25 mm Hg]) seems to be the most significant predisposing factor for the development of tracheomucosal injury. Use of an appropriately sized endotracheal tube with a low-pressure, high-volume cuff (see Chapter 12), frequent monitoring of cuff pressure during anesthesia (particularly during protracted cases where the diffusion of nitrous oxide into the air-filled tracheal cuff raises the pressure), and long-term stay in the intensive care unit help to prevent tracheal wall ischemia and possible resulting tracheal stenosis. Cuff pressure may be easily measured during expiration by use of a water manometer attached via a three-way stopcock to the cuff. Pressures should be kept at 20 to 25 cm H_2O pressure to avoid tracheal mucosal ischemia. For prolonged intubation in the intensive care unit, nasotracheal intubation affords greater patient comfort and tube stability, and therefore probable diminished laryngeal trauma. In children under the age of 8 years, cuffless endotracheal tubes are most commonly used. An air leak at a peak airway pressure of less than 25 cm H_2O indicates a reasonable tube fit without applying undue pressure to the subglottic/cricoid area, the area most at risk in children for the development of tracheal stenosis.[4]

The material with which an endotracheal tube is made is also important in determining the type and frequency of complications secondary to endotracheal intubation. Polyvinyl chloride endotracheal tubes (in common use today) become more pliable with warming and exert less pressure over time on areas of contact in the posterior larynx and anterior tracheal wall, the areas most prone to ulceration. Latex and red rubber tubes may initiate an inflammatory response in areas of tissue contact.

Full Stomach

Patients with bowel obstruction, symptomatic hiatus hernia, recent meal, recent trauma, abdominal masses, scleroderma, collagen vascular diseases, pregnancy, advanced age, or gastroparesis are considered at high risk for aspiration of gastric contents during unconscious intubation.[5] Aspiration of gastric fluids with a pH of less than 2.5 and a volume greater than 25 mL may produce a severe pneumonitis and death.[6]

Aspiration of acidic gastric content first manifests itself by tachypnea, tachycardia, hypoxemia, and progressive worsening of lung compliance. Chest radiograph findings usually show diffuse, patchy infiltrates in dependent areas. The mainstay of treatment includes maintenance of arterial oxygenation and ventilation. The use of prophylactic antibiotics and steroids have not been show to be useful in these patients.[7-10] Aspiration of feculent material secondary to bowel obstruction is associated with an almost 100% mortality. Gastric prophylaxis includes the use of H2 blockers the night prior to and morning of surgery, if possible, or parenterally 1 hour prior to intubation, as well nonparticulate antacids such as citric acid suspensions. The use of metoclopramide can improve gastric emptying and increase lower esophageal sphincter tone in high-risk patients.[11, 12] Regional rather than general anesthesia may be used where feasible to decrease the risk of pulmonary aspiration.

In the setting where the patient has a "good airway," a rapid-sequence induction may be used. If there is doubt about ability to secure the airway, then careful, mild sedation and topical local anesthetic to the airway may facilitate the use of a blind nasal approach, direct laryngoscopy, or fiberoptic intubation.

Complications of endotracheal intubation may be most conveniently considered by dividing them into those occurring during:

1. Placement of the endotracheal tube
2. The period when the tube is *in situ*:
   a. Short duration (<24 h)
   b. Prolonged (>24 h)
3. Extubation.

INTUBATION: EARLY COMPLICATIONS

The act of laryngoscopy and the placement of an endotracheal tube may be complicated by many and various adverse mechanical or traumatic outcomes.

Positioning/Unstable Cervical Spine

Patients with conditions associated with underlying cervical spine instability (Table 24–3) or those with traumatic cervical spine injuries are at increased risk of spinal cord damage as a result of positioning for standard laryngoscopy. In the setting where obtaining control of the airway is nonemergent, these patients should undergo radiographic evaluation of cervical spine stability and receive clearance prior to intubation. Essential radiographic examination includes a lateral radiograph of the cervical spine, including the junction of C7–T1 (often difficult to visualize), an anteroposterior view, and an odontoid view. A normal cross-table lateral radiograph does not ensure an uninjured cervical spine. Further examination of the cervical spine by oblique views as well as pleuridirectional tomography (PT), computed tomography, or magnetic resonance imaging (MRI) may be required to determine the extent of injury to the cervical spine.[13]

In the patient with a possible acute cervical spine injury requiring emergent control of the airway, intubation should take place with a person designated to provide manual in-line stabilization.[14] In all other patients with potential cervical spine injury, further evaluation should proceed (as discussed previously) prior to attempted intubation. The patient with a "stable" cervical spine (best declared by concurrence among a group of radiologists and physicians) may be intubated in a standard fashion. Patients with suspected or known cervical spine instability should be intubated with great care not to move the neck. Intubation may be achieved in many different ways, including awake blind or fiberoptic placement of the tube, by orotracheal intubation via direct laryngoscopy, retrograde intubation, or by transtracheal methods. The use of cricoid pressure and muscle relaxants in this group of patients is controversial.

Esophageal Intubation

Esophageal intubation is best ruled out by direct visualization of the vocal cords as the endotracheal tube is passed through them. This, however, is not always possible secondary to difficult patient anatomy or blockage of the view by the endotracheal tube itself. The tube may be dislodged during taping or during positioning of the patient as well. Spontaneously breathing patients should demonstrate tidal breathing in the reservoir bag. Typical signs of esophageal intubation include the absence of chest excursion and bilateral breath sounds in the lung apices during positive pressure ventilation, as well as increased gurgling of gastric juices as air is forced into the stomach and the absence of condensation within the tube lumen during expiration. In some patients, however, these clinical signs may not be immediately clear. The use of a colorimetric device, which attaches to the endotracheal tube and has pH-sensitive paper that changes color in the presence of CO_2, or a typical CO_2 waveform on the capnograph are the most reliable indicators of successful endotracheal intubation when they are detected for more than the first few breaths. Clinical signs such as good bilateral breath sounds in axillae, symmetric chest excursion with ventilation, and the maintenance of satisfactory arterial oxygen saturation following intubation are reassuring. Late signs of esophageal intubation include cyanosis, bradycardia, and cardiac arrest.

Ventilation through the endotracheal tube should be ceased immediately after recognition of esophageal intubation or where serious doubt exists about the correct placement of the tube, in order to prevent further gastric distension predisposing to pulmonary aspiration. The stomach should be suctioned if oxygenation status permits. If not, cricoid pressure should be maintained during mask ventilation and any subsequent attempts at reintubation. Once the airway has been secured, stomach contents or air should be removed via a nasal or orogastric tube. Acceptance of the premise that esophageal intubation is a risk during any tracheal intubation, no matter how routine it appears, should enhance vigilance and timely treatment of this complication. Knowledge of possible difficult intubation in the past, abnormal airway anatomy, or the presence of medical conditions predisposing to difficulty during endotracheal intubation should lead to more extensive preparation prior to attempts at intubation. Multiple laryngoscopy blades and handles should be available for intubation of the difficult airway, as well as equipment for fiberoptic intubation and tracheotomy and

Table 24–3. CONDITIONS ASSOCIATED WITH CERVICAL SPINE INJURY DURING INTUBATION

Ankylosing spondylitis
Rheumatoid arthritis
Down's syndrome
Trauma

other available persons skilled in airway management.

Endobronchial Intubation

Overadvancement of the endotracheal tube or flexion of the head after intubation (in the setting of a low-lying tube) may lead to a mainstem endobronchial intubation. In general, women tend to require an endotracheal tube advanced to around 21 to 22 cm in length at the lips, whereas men require a length of approximately 23 to 24 cm.

Endobronchial intubation, in and by itself, is not a major problem. However, failure to recognize and treat it appropriately may have serious consequences. Endobronchial intubation may lead to hypoxemia, increased inspiratory pressures, atelectasis, and obstruction of the right upper lobe that leads to right upper lobe collapse and/or collapse of the entire nonventilated lung. Breath sounds should be assessed bilaterally after intubation and following repositioning of the patient in order to detect this situation early. Assessment includes clinical findings, assuring proper length of the tube measured at the teeth, an arterial blood gas compatible with a large pulmonary shunt fraction, and possible fiberoptic evaluation and chest radiograph. Treatment is provided by placing the patient on 100% oxygen, carefully retracting the tube (while checking breath sounds bilaterally, under direct laryngoscopy or with the aid of a fiberoptic bronchoscope), and using hand ventilation or positive end-expiratory pressure (PEEP) to reexpand the atelectatic lung. Decreasing peak inspiratory pressures, improving arterial oxygen saturation and Po_2, suggest improved ventilation to the previously nonventilated lung. Chest radiograph (showing the tip of the tube at T2, between the glottis at C4 and the carina at T6) and/or fiberoptic evaluation may be used to confirm placement if any doubt remains.[15] In adults, the cuff of the endotracheal tube should pass only 1 cm below the cords. In children, the tip should pass 2 to 3 cm below the cords to assure proper placement.

Dental Trauma

Damage to dentition is one of the most common causes of litigation after endotracheal intubation. A history of loose, capped, or broken teeth should be elicited when possible prior to intubation and the risk of damage or loss of teeth explained prior to laryngoscopy. Risk of damage may be reduced by careful laryngoscopy technique. Oral airways should be avoided in patients with very fragile front teeth. In this setting, rolled gauze inserted between the teeth (molars) bilaterally may function adequately as protection for the endotracheal tube during emergence from anesthesia. Care must be exercised to remove these at the time of extubation.[16]

Magill forceps should be available for retrieving any dislodged teeth. Inhaled teeth require bronchoscopic removal if possible or thoracotomy to prevent lung abscess. A lateral chest radiograph, and perhaps an abdominal radiograph, may be necessary to differentiate between the aspirated versus swallowed tooth—the swallowed tooth may be allowed to pass through the gastrointestinal tract without further intervention. Any dental damage resulting from airway management should be discussed with the patient, and a consultation with an oral surgeon may be warranted.

Eye Trauma

Corneal abrasions and chemical irritation of the eyes secondary to scrub solutions may be prevented by carefully closing the patient's eyes with a bio-occlusive dressing. Blindness has been reported as a rare complication resulting from orbital or periorbital compression during mask anesthetics or those conducted in the prone position. Attention to the position of the patient's eyes, particularly during anesthetics, where it is not easy to monitor them (eg, surgical procedures requiring the prone position), and in particular, where the patient's head is not stabilized in pins, requires "eye checks" at short and regular intervals to rule out possible change in head position with resulting ocular compression. The complaint of postoperative eye pain warrants consultation with an ophthalmologist.

Epistaxis

Epistaxis is the most common complication of nasal intubation.[17] Prior use of vasoconstrictor or analgesic agents such as topical cocaine (4% solution) or phenylephrine/xylocaine solution, as well as adequate use of lubrication on the endotracheal tube and an appropriately sized endotracheal tube (usually one half size smaller than the required size for oral intubation) may reduce the risk of epistaxis. In the situation where brisk bleeding occurs in the patient unable to protect his or her airway, the larynx should be held in an anterior position as the nasotracheal tube is passed into the position in order to prevent blood aspiration. If bleeding is slower, the tube may be left in place to tamponade it.

Continued bleeding requires consultation with an otolaryngologist, cauterization with silver nitrate, nasal packing, or, in the case of submucosal dissection, surgical repair. Coagulopathy and hypertension promote epistaxis. In severe cases, interventional radiologic embolization of the offending bleeding vessel may be life saving.

Reflex Responses to Laryngoscopy

Intubation may also be complicated by three reflex responses to laryngoscopy: the laryngosympathetic, laryngovagal, and laryngospinal responses.[18]

The laryngosympathetic response to laryngoscopy generally results in hypertension and tachycardia. These responses may be blunted pharmacologically by the judicious use of sedatives, hypnotics, narcotics, antihypertensives, or beta-blockers prior to intubation in patients where this response may be particularly deleterious.

The laryngovagal response during laryngoscopy may result in the production of excessive bradycardia, cardiac arrhythmias, and hypotension from increased vagal response. This response is seen less commonly in adults than the laryngosympathetic response and occurs more frequently in children due to increased parasympathetic tone.

Laryngospasm, bronchospasm, and apnea may also be seen as part of this response. Laryngospasm results from reflex closure of the glottis secondary to contracture of one or more of the three sets of intrinsic muscles of the larynx—the cricothyroids, the thyroarytenoids, and the lateral cricoarytenoids.[19] Laryngospasm may be initiated by secretions, blood, saliva in the airway, premature use of an oral airway, attempted endotracheal intubation, airway irritation by pungent volatile anesthetics, or noxious stimuli such as placement of a Foley catheter or surgical incision during "light" anesthesia.

Prevention of laryngospasm may be achieved by ensuring adequate anesthetic depth prior to attempted intubation and the use of neuromuscular blocking agents such as succinylcholine to facilitate intubation. In the setting where an awake intubation is required (ie, full stomach and difficult airway), prevention of laryngospasm may be achieved by anesthetizing the oral cavity and trachea with topical local anesthetics and the use of superior laryngeal nerve blocks. Treatment of laryngospasm includes administration of 100% FIO_2 by positive pressure mask ventilation. Occasionally, a vigorous "jaw thrust" maneuver is all that is required. Succinylcholine (10 to 20 mg intravenously) may be required to break laryngospasm and permit ventilation. Bronchospasm is manifested by wheezing, increasing difficulty in ventilation and, in severe cases, decreasing arterial oxygen saturation and poor arterial blood gases similar to laryngospasm, it may be prevented by intubating under a "deep" level of anesthesia, use of neuromuscular blockers, continuing steroids and beta-adrenergic inhalers prior to intubation in patients predisposed to bronchospasm, as well as by avoiding elective intubation in the presence of active wheezing or pulmonary infection. Where possible, the use of a mask anesthetic or regional anesthesia as an alternative to general anesthesia with endotracheal intubation may avoid precipitating an attack of bronchospasm in susceptible individuals. Stimulation of the carina from a low-lying endotracheal tube is an easily correctable cause of bronchospasm, resolving with careful withdrawal of the tube more proximally. Intraoperative bronchospasm may be treated by the administration of volatile agents, metered dose inhalers, steroids and, in the presence of continued bronchospasm, may require the administration of epinephrine 0.3 mg subcutaneously every 15 min or by low-dose intravenous infusion (usually 0.25 to 1.0 µg/min). Increasing the tidal volume and expiratory phase of the ventilator is important to avoid air trapping and possible barotrauma in these patients.

The laryngospinal reflex may lead to coughing and vomiting in the inadequately anesthetized patient during laryngoscopy. Technical difficulties encountered during intubation may range from equipment failure (such as a cuff or pilot balloon leak that requires reintubation) to swallowed or aspirated laryngoscopy bulbs to failure to intubate. Failure to both mask ventilate and intubate occurs in up to 2/10,000 cases.

Failed Intubation

In the setting where induction has proceeded and translaryngeal intubation is impossible, hand ventilation with 100% oxygen and allowing the patient to regain consciousness and spontaneous respiration is ideal. If ventilation by mask with an oral or nasal airway is impossible, the use of a 14-gauge angiocatheter, inserted through the cricothyroid membrane, attached to the barrel of a 3 mL syringe with the adapter of a 7.5 endotracheal tube, may allow apneic oxygenation to take place until further intervention takes place.

INTUBATION: THE TUBE
IN SITU

The three most common problems encountered during endotracheal intubation are obstruction of ventilation, disconnection of the tube from the ventilator or oxygen source, and displacement of the tube. Ventilatory obstruction may be secondary to extra-luminal compression of the tube (eg, kinking of the tube at the endotracheal adaptor or in the pharynx, or biting on the tube by the patient) or by intraluminal obstruction secondary to secretions or mucous plugging, tissue, foreign body, or cuff herniation. Pediatric endotracheal tubes (particularly small tubes) are susceptible to obstruction. In the spontaneously breathing intubated patient, obstruction of ventilation leads to paradoxic breathing (chest wall retractions and abdominal excursions), use of accessory muscles of respiration, and diminished or absent breath sounds with ventilatory efforts. In the fully ventilated patient, the presence of increased peak inspiratory pressures (particularly if abrupt in onset) with diminished breath sounds should alert one to the possibility of tube obstruction. Visual (and manual) inspection of the endotracheal tube should be undertaken to rule out kinking or biting of the tube. A suction catheter should be passed through the endotracheal tube to assess patency, as well as to remove secretions. If there is any suspicion that the ventilatory obstruction is cuff related, the cuff should be deflated and ventilation assessed. In the event that these maneuvers do not relieve the obstruction (and there is no concern that difficulty in ventilation is not secondary to very severe bronchospasm), the tube should be changed. If there is total obstruction to ventilation, the replacement of the tube should be considered an emergency.

If there is only a partial obstruction but adequate ventilation and oxygenation are being maintained, then the tube should be changed as safely and expeditiously as possible.

Kinking of the endotracheal tube may be prevented by proper support of the tube and airway circuit, cutting the endotracheal tube to the appropriate length, and where longer term intubation is required, the use of nasotracheal tubes. Proper cuff function should be established prior to intubation and caution should be taken during orotracheal intubation to avoid tearing the cuff on teeth. Humidification of gases and the use of low gas flows during long cases help to prevent drying of secretions and subsequent obstruction of the endotracheal tube. Small amounts of sterile normal saline (2 mL) may be necessary to loosen dried secretions prior to suctioning in some patients.

Disconnection from the airway may occur at any connection point between the endotracheal tube and the ventilator. Most commonly, disconnects take place between the endotracheal tube adaptor and the airway circuit. In the spontaneously breathing patient, a disconnect at this point may not have serious consequences. In the apneic patient, an unrecognized disconnection may result in serious morbidity or death.

Signs of disconnection include lack of tidal breathing in the reservoir bag in the spontaneously breathing patient or the fully ventilated patient, failure of the chest to rise with ventilation, absent breath sounds and CO_2 waveform on the capnograph, and sounding of the low pressure alarm on the ventilator.

Displacement of the endotracheal tube may range from inadvertent movement of the tube into the right mainstem during head flexion, placement of the patient in Trendelenberg or lithotomy position, to accidental extubation of the patient. Accidental extubation of the patient may occur during manipulation of the patient's head or extension of the neck in the presence of a high-riding tube. Signs of inadvertent extubation include those of a disconnect, except that in some cases where the patient is spontaneously breathing and the tube is poised above the vocal cords there may be some evidence of CO_2 production on the capnograph. Examination of the position of the endotracheal tube should reveal that the tube has moved cephalad.

Direct laryngoscopy should be used to evaluate tube position and, if necessary, to reintubate the patient. Prevention may be achieved by firmly taping tubes into position using adhesive substances such as benzoin. This is particularly important in children (where the margin for error is much smaller than for adults) or in cases where the patient will be in the prone position and the tube tape will be exposed to secretions. The use of drying agents and frequent suctioning (where possible) may help to prevent loosening and destabilization of the tube.

EXTUBATION

The period of extubation may be complicated by many of the same hazards encountered during intubation, with the additional consideration that these patients should have demonstrated the ability to protect their airway (especially in intensive care unit patients) and maintain adequate ventilation on their own. Trauma during extubation may occur to the teeth (particularly loose teeth in children), the mouth, pharynx, and vocal cords. Inspiratory stridor secondary to glottic or subglottic edema may be present and require prompt treatment with racemic epinephrine nebulizers.

Administration of potent steroids, such as dexamethasone (4 to 10 mg) intravenously may help to prevent further airway edema. Reintubation may be required for increasing difficulty in ventilation secondary to inadequate reversal of neuromuscular blockade, airway edema, or fatigue (increased respiratory rate, use of accessory muscles of respiration, low tidal volumes, and later with increasing CO_2 or worsening oxygenation). Glottic and subglottic edema may be minimized by careful intubating technique, use of the proper endotracheal tube size, attention to cuff pressure (or the presence of an air leak at 20 to 25 cm H_2O pressure in children with cuffless tubes), and by limiting movement of the tube.

Other difficulties specific to extubation include inability to deflate the cuff or a retained cuff or foreign body such as a throat pack. Inability to extubate secondary to failure to deflate the balloon cuff may be remedied by cutting the pilot balloon (not 100% effective) or pulling the endotracheal tube gently up to the larynx and deflating it via a needle placed through the cricothyroid membrane. Unrecognized retention of a throat pack in the pharynx may lead to complete airway obstruction and death. Great care should always be taken to ensure that these are removed at the end of surgery, prior to extubation.

Sore throat is a common complaint postextubation and may be treated by administration of throat lozenges. Sore throat occurs secondary to instrumentation of the airway, oropharynx, and the use of throat packs during surgery. It may be minimized by careful technique.

Aspiration may be avoided by suctioning the stomach (where possible) and oropharynx prior to extubation, waiting for the patient to demonstrate a cough or gag or an adequate level of alertness prior to extubation. In addition, high-risk patients may be extubated in the lateral position.

Extubation may also be complicated by laryngospasm or hypertension and tachycardia. Laryngospasm is unlikely to occur if extubation takes place under an adequate plane of anesthesia (in patients with good airways and a low risk for postoperative respiratory compromise or pulmonary aspiration) or when the patient is awake. Treatment consists of administration of 100% oxygen by mask with continuous positive airway pressure (taking care not to overdistend the stomach). In the event that this does not work, a small dose of succinylcholine (10 to 20 mg) may be necessary to achieve adequate ventilation.

Hypertension and tachycardia may be blunted by judicious use of narcotics, betablockers, or antihypertensives (particularly important in patients with cardiac disease) prior to and during emergence from anesthesia.

Postextubation croup manifests itself by inspiratory stridor secondary to glottic or subglottic edema. It is seen most commonly in the pediatric population secondary to trauma at the subglottic level by an improperly sized endotracheal tube. Treatment includes the use of aerosolized racemic epinephrine. Reintubation may be required if the patient is not able to adequately ventilate despite these therapies.

Laryngeal trauma usually presents postoperatively as hoarseness. This condition (induced at any point during the intubation process) usually is self-limiting (lasting <7 days). In cases where hoarseness persists longer, consultation with an ear, nose, and throat specialist is warranted to evaluate possible structural change to the larynx. Use of the appropriate size of endotracheal tube, minimizing motion of the tube during the period it is *in situ*, and ensuring full deflation of the cuff prior to extubation help to minimize laryngeal damage.

Tracheomalacia/Tracheal Stenosis

Damage to the tracheal mucosa may lead to the more serious complications of tracheomalacia or tracheal stenosis. This is seen more commonly after more prolonged intubation than that occuring in the operating room. Patients present with symptoms of upper airway obstruction. Diagnosis may require the use of flow volume loops, tracheal tomograms and, ultimately, bronchoscopy during spontaneous ventilation. Tracheomalacia and tracheal stenosis result from mucosal ischemia leading to infarction. Prevention may be achieved with the use of low-pressure, high-volume cuffs, as well as only a brief period of intubation. In patients requiring longer term intubation, meticulous attention to cuff pressure may help to avoid this complication.

Vocal Cord Granulomas

Granuloma formation occurs more frequently in women than men, and rarely in children. Symptoms include hoarseness, cough, and throat discomfort secondary to overgrowth of granulation tissue, usually on the posterior laryngeal wall. Prevention may be achieved by minimizing trauma during laryngoscopy and intubation. Surgical removal is generally required.

Vocal Cord Paralysis

This complication is thought to be secondary to pressure exerted on the recurrent laryngeal nerve and is usually self-limited. Symptoms of respiratory obstruction occur with bilateral recurrent laryngeal nerve involvement. Complete respiratory obstruction requires reintubation and possible tracheotomy.

References

1. Campbell D. Trauma to larynx and trachea following intubation and tracheotomy. J Laryngol 82:981–986, 1968.
2. Baron SH, Kohlmoos HW. Laryngeal sequellae of endotracheal anesthesia. Ann Otol Rhinol Laryngol 60:767–791, 1961.
3. Mallampati SR, Gatt SP, Gugino LD, Desai SP, Waraksa B, Freiberger D, Liu PL. A clinical sign to predict difficult tracheal intubation: A prospective study. Can J Anaesth 32:429–434, 1985.
4. Cote CJ, Todres ID. The pediatric airway. In Ryan JF (ed). A Practice of Anesthesia for Infants and Children. Philadelphia: WB Saunders, 1986.
5. Pontoppidan H, Beecher HK. Progressive loss of protective reflexes in the airway with the advance of age. JAMA 174:2209, 1960.
6. Mendelson CL. Aspiration of stomach contents into the lungs during obstetrical anesthesia. Am J Obstet Gynecol 52:191, 1946.
7. Downs JB, Chapman RL Jr, Modell JH, Hood CI. The ineffectiveness of steroid therapy in treating aspiration of hydrochloric acid. Arch Surg 108:858, 1974.
8. Downs JB, Chapman RL Jr, Modell JH, Hood CI. An evaluation of steroid therapy in aspiration pneumonitis. Anesthesiology 40:129, 1974.
9. Cameron JL, Mitchell WH, Zuidema GD. Aspiration pneumonia: Clinical outcome following documented aspiration. Arch Surg 106:49, 1973.
10. Bynum LJ, Pierce AK. Pulmonary aspiration of gastric contents. Am Rev Respir Dis 114:1129, 1976.
11. Dilaawri JB, Misiewicz JJ. Action of oral metaclopromide on the gastroesophageal junction in man. Gut 14:380, 1973.
12. Stanciu C, Bennett JR. Metoclopromide in gastroesophageal reflux. Gut 14:275, 1973.
13. Crosby ET, Lui A. The adult cervical spine: Implications for airway management. Can J Anaesth 37:1, 77–93, 1990.
14. Lanza DC, Parrnes SM, Koitni PJ, Fortune JB. Early complications of airway management in head-injured patients. Laryngoscope 100:958–961, 1990.
15. Owen RL, Chensy FW. Endobronchial intubation: A preventable complication. Anesthesiology 67:255–257, 1987.
16. Chidyllo SA. Dental examination prior to elective surgery under anesthesia. NY State Dent J 56:69–70, 1990.
17. Dauphinee F, Zukaitis JA. Nasotracheal intubation. Emerg Med Clin North Am 6:715–723, 1988.
18. Blanc VF, Tremble NAG. The complications of tracheal intubation. Anesth Analg 53:202–213, 1974.
19. Roberts JT. Fundamentals of Tracheal Intubation. Orlando, FL: Grune & Stratton, 1983.

CHAPTER 25

Extubation Following Anesthesia and Surgery

William Panza, M.D., and James T. Roberts, M.D., M.A.

EXTUBATION

Prior to anesthetizing a patient, the anesthesiologist develops a plan. Part of this plan should be the conclusion of the anesthetic, which includes the patient's disposition, extubation, and postoperative pain control. Once intubated, the airway is secured for the surgery. However, at the end of the surgery one must decide if extubation is feasible. If so, then one must decide when and how to extubate the patient. These decisions depend on several factors, including the patient's preoperative status, the intraoperative course, and expected postoperative recovery. Among the considerations given to the intraoperative course are the operative procedure itself, the anesthetic used, the response of the patient to the anesthetic, the hemodynamic response to blood loss and fluid replacement, and the patient's condition at the end of surgery. Ideally, one wishes to return the patient to his or her preoperative status. The goal is a smooth awakening and extubation without complications.

Anesthetic Level and Extubation

Because most patients come to us unintubated, our goal is to extubate them in the operating room postoperatively, prior to transport to the postanesthetic care unit. The patient can be extubated either when he or she is "awake" or anesthetized. These two terms refer to the depth of anesthesia to which the patient is subjected when the endotracheal tube is removed.

Usually, the patient is extubated when he or she is awake. That is, the patient can maintain and protect his or her airway. Coughing is not considered awake, because this may occur during stage II anesthesia, when the patient is not responsive to verbal stimuli, has deviated eyes, may undergo periods of breath-holding, but is responding to laryngeal stimulus of the endotracheal tube. During this time period premature extubation and unnecessary stimulation may precipitate laryngospasm. Coughing and bucking may show the ability to maintain an airway and the return of protective reflexes, but often the patient becomes re-anesthetized once the noxious stimulus of the endotracheal tube is removed. The degree to which a patient is awake may vary with the desired goals of the anesthetist. In any case where there is a question of the patient's ability to maintain a patent airway, the patient should be sufficiently awake to follow simple commands and comprehend his or her surroundings. This applies in the case of a patient with full stomach precautions, emergent surgery, airway surgery, or suspected airway disfunction. In an electively scheduled patient with a preoperative fast, the patient can be extubated just before awakening. At this point in stage I anesthesia, the laryngeal reflexes have returned, as shown by swallowing. However, the patient is not awake to remember the extubation, and the hypertension and bucking associated with an awake extubation may be avoided. Of course, scrupulous maintenance of the airway is required until the patient is wide awake.

Extubation of the trachea while the patient is deeply anesthetized presents several advantages: (1) reduced coughing on the endotracheal tube, because the airway reflexes are still anesthetized; (2) less chance of laryngeal trauma; (3) fewer hemodynamic swings; and (4) less tensing of abdominal musculature against a new suture line. To perform such a maneuver requires full reversal of muscle relaxants with the patient spontaneously breathing. Secretions are suctioned from the patient's oropharynx. The cuff is deflated at peak inspiration after a positive pressure breath, and the endotracheal tube is removed in one smooth motion during expiration. The patient is still deeply anesthetized, so he or she must then be mask ventilated until sufficiently awake to protect his or her airway. Maintenance of the airway is paramount, because it is the conduit for uptake of oxygen and elimination of anesthetic gases.

Contraindications to deep extubation are difficult mask airway; difficult intubation; increased risk of aspiration; or surgical positioning that predisposes to airway edema or that puts the respiratory muscles, especially the diaphragm, at a mechanical disadvantage. Postextubation airway obstruction must be avoided, because it can lead to lack of gas exchange with resultant hypoxemia and hypercarbia. Without an airway, emergence will be delayed because breathing off the anesthetics is not possible. Even partial obstruction will have the significant consequences of delayed awakening due to slower exhaust of anesthetic. Inspiration against a closed or obstructed glottis may lead to negative pressure pulmonary edema. Secretions in the oropharynx may lead to tracheal stimulation, which can cause coughing and laryngospasm. Suction should always be available to clear the oropharynx, because the patient may vomit on emergence. Many practitioners believe that deep extubation is premature because it risks laryngospasm, aspiration, and loss of the airway. Also, there is

no way to guarantee that coughing will be eliminated.

Position for Extubation

Extubation of the trachea can be performed with the patient in any of several different positions: supine, lateral, head up (reverse Trendelenburg), Trendelenburg, or prone. All have advantages and disadvantages. The supine position is most commonly used for routine extubation. This position allows ease of access to the mouth, and is convenient if re-intubation is necessary. In the supine position, the tongue has a tendency to be displaced backward by gravity, thus obstructing the airway. Also, secretions pool in the posterior pharynx. This could lead to aspiration, especially if the patient vomits after extubation. The lateral position allows ease of extubation and, in the case of postextubation vomitus, allows drainage of the stomach contents anteriorly. Also, gravity holds the tongue anteriorly, thus maintaining the patent airway. If re-intubation becomes necessary, the tongue in the right lateral position would obstruct the view of the cords. Extubation in the Trendelenburg position provides good drainage for vomitus, but this position puts the diaphragm at a mechanical disadvantage for breathing, because the abdominal contents are thrust against the diaphragm. The head-up or Fowler's position allows patients to breath more easily postoperatively because it reduces the mechanical resistance of abdominal viscera against the diaphragm. This facilitates deep breathing, which increases the functional residual capacity (FRC) and the buffer for the development of hypoxia after extubation. A disadvantage of this position is that it allows secretions or stomach contents in the case of vomiting to track down the trachea into the lungs.

The prone position presents special challenges. After neurosurgery or spinal surgery, one goal of anesthesia is to have the patient awake for a neurologic examination. However, in turning the patient to the supine position, the endotracheal tube provides a strong trachea stimulus to cough. To avoid this, the patient may be extubated in the prone position. Prior to prone extubation, several factors must be assessed. Significant facial edema can develop during prolonged surgery in the prone position or after administration of large fluid volumes. This correlates with the development of tracheal edema, which would make prone extubation contraindicated. Re-intubation is possible in the prone position, but is more difficult due to the infrequency of our familiarity with it. The other advantage of the prone position is the tendency of tongue to fall forward with gravity, so that the airway is maintained naturally.

Factors Necessary for Extubation

Prior to extubation, one must decide if all of the conditions for extubation have been met. Unfortunately, there is no one number, parameter, or test that can determine whether or not a patient is ready for extubation. One must look at the whole patient to decide. Among the factors that the anesthetist must decide on are the following: the patient's intraoperative course, including (1) the procedure—length, type, location; (2) the patient's underlying conditions—such as lung or heart disease; and (3) the patient's current status—the fluid balance, current pulmonary function, hemodynamic stability, level of consciousness, muscle strength–degree of reversal, temperature. If the patient has had a labile intraoperative course or problems in any of the above areas, then the patient should not be extubated in the operating room immediately at the end of surgery. Instead, he or she should be brought to the postanesthetic care unit or an intensive care unit for further stabilization prior to extubation.

If the patient has had a stable intraoperative course and the conditions are optimal, then he or she may be extubated in the operating room. Vital signs should be stable. The heart rate and blood pressure should be in the patient's usual range, in order to ensure adequate tissue perfusion. Also, stability of vital signs allows the patient to tolerate the stress of extubation better.

The patient must have a core temperature greater than 35.5 to 36.0°C prior to extubation. As a patient warms, many physiologic changes occur. Shivering may increase oxygen demand up to 400 times the normal requirement. This puts an enormous strain on the cardiopulmonary system for transport of oxygen and elimination of carbon dioxide which, if unmet, can lead to tissue hypoxia, anaerobic metabolism, hypercarbia, and acidosis.

The level of consciousness should be adequate to maintain a patent airway and clear secretions. The gag reflex and an adequate cough should have returned. If the plan was for an awake patient at the end of a procedure, the inhalation anesthetic should have been turned off early enough to allow elimination via the lungs. This is dependent on the characteristics of the anesthesia circuit, the gas flows, mode of ventilation, and the anesthetic used.

The ventilatory status of the patient should be assessed. Once spontaneously breathing, the patient should be able to maintain an airway for adequate gas exchange. If necessary, an oral or nasal airway may be needed to facilitate this. The respiratory pattern should be observed for rate, depth, and characteristics. One learns more about the adequacy of ventilation by looking at the patient than by relying on a single number. Some pulmonary mechanics that are often used as criteria for extubation follow. Vital capacity should be 10 to 20 mL/kg: This assesses the patient's respiratory reserve. It requires that the patient is able to cooperate. Successive measurements may be performed to determine a trend of patient reserve and fatiguability. Maximum negative inspiratory force of ≥ 20 to 30 cm H_2O is an indicator of the patient's ability to clear secretions and cough. Tidal volume (5 to 8 mL/kg) must be greater than dead space for ventilation to be effective. Sedation and splinting from postoperative pain can be treated to improve tidal volume. Respiratory rate should be 10 to 25 breaths per minute (for adults). Lower rates may be a result of narcosis, inadequate reversal of muscle relaxant, and may contribute to inadequate minute ventilation, hypoxia, and hypercapnia. Higher rates may be a result of pain or agitation from hypercarbia. Tachypnea results in a higher ratio of dead space ventilation and the possibility of muscle fatigue with respiratory failure. Minute ventilation should be less than 10 L/min to maintain a normal Pa_{CO_2}. This factor is dependent on both respiratory rate and tidal volume being adequate and is a measure of the body's respiratory requirements. Higher minute ventilation could lead to respiratory failure due to fatigue. Many other criteria have been put forth as possible criteria for weaning from mechanical ventilation; these are listed in the Table 25–1. However, none is sufficient alone to guarantee the success of an extubation.

Aids to Extubation

The local anesthetic lidocaine is frequently given intravenously to attenuate coughing by

Table 25–1. CRITERIA FOR WEANING AND EXTUBATION

Pulmonary mechanics	
Breathing pattern	Uniform, unlabored
Vital capacity	>10 to 15 mL/kg
Tidal volume	>5 to 8 mL/kg
Maximal negative inspiratory force	< -20 to -30 cm H_2O
Respiratory rate	12 to 25/min
FEV_1	> 10 mL/kg
Functional residual capacity	>50% predicted
Minute ventilation	<10 L/min
Dead space/tidal volume ratio	<0.6
Reversal of neuromuscular blockade	>90%
Sustained head lift	5 sec
Train of four twitches	Four twitches without fade
Posttetanic facilitation	None
Tetanic stimulation	No fade
Arterial blood gas parameters	
	Back to preoperative room air baseline and/or
pH	>7.30
Pa_{CO_2}	<50 mm Hg
Pa_{O_2} on Fi_{O_2} of .40 or less	>60 mm Hg
Level of consciousness	Awake, following simple commands
Gag reflex	Intact

a central effect in doses of 1 to 1.5 mg/kg. This may prolong wake up; in some studies, it has not been uniformly effective.[1–3] Another drug that has been shown to decrease the hemodynamic effect of intubation can also be used to prevent the same effects on extubation is esmolol, the short-acting β_1 selective beta-blocker. It has been shown in doses of 50 to 100 mg to decrease hypertension and tachycardia associated with laryngoscopy. Caution must be exercised because rapid hypotension may develop after such a bolus dose. Sodium nitroprusside and nitroglycerin (as an infusion and as a transdermal ointment) have also been shown to attenuate the hypertension associated with airway manipulation. Narcotics play an important role in the anesthetic management of the patient. They provide anesthesia for the surgery and analgesia for the postoperative period. Prior to planned extubation, the anesthesiologist can titrate a narcotic to effect a smooth wake up from inhalation anesthesia. Titrating a narcotic to a respiratory rate of 10 to 12 usually provides sufficient analgesia to suppress the laryngeal reflex to cough during extubation.

Extubation Preparation

Prior to extubation, one should have a strategy. Just as one prepares for induction, one has emergency medications drawn up and available for extubation in case an unexpected complication occurs. These include atropine, succinylcholine, and an induction agent such as thiopental sodium. A functioning laryngoscope, an endotracheal tube, stylet, suction catheter hooked to wall suction, oral airways, and syringe to deflate the endotracheal tube cuff should be within reach, in case rapid reintubation is necessary. One may reuse the prior endotracheal tube in an emergency, so do not discard it on extubation. Remember that the used endotracheal tube may have a damaged cuff or a collection of secretions after extubation. Have the appropriate size mask and anesthesia circuit (or Ambu bag) to provide positive pressure ventilation and oxygen after extubation.

One extubation sequence begins with the anesthesiologist turning off the inhalation agent sufficiently in advance to allow the patient to awaken in a timely fashion. With the patient still anesthetized, the stomach is suctioned via an orogastric or nasogastric tube. Suctioning the stomach empties contents that may have accumulated during surgery. Surgical stress is a potent stimulus for increased gastric secretions and decreased gastrointestinal motility. Removing these secretions and gas may decrease postoperative nausea and vomiting, thus lessening the risk of aspiration and discomfort. In those patients who do not require postoperative nasogastric drainage, the gastric tube is removed prior to extubation. This decreases the risk of regurgitation, because it prevents the gastric tube from serving as a conduit that makes the esophageal gastric junction incompetent. This should be done with the patient adequately anesthetized, so that there is no unnecessary bucking and coughing with the posterior pharyngeal stimulation. If indicated, the endotracheal tube is suctioned of any secretions. The use of sterile saline may be needed to loosen secretions. The endotracheal tube is suctioned in a sterile fashion so as not to introduce any pathogens into the tracheobronchial tree unnecessarily. Again, this is done while the patient is adequately anesthetized to prevent unwanted coughing due to tracheal stimulation. The oropharynx is suctioned to remove secretions and prevent their aspiration during the first few breaths immediately after extubation of the trachea. Removing the secretions removes a potent stimulus to the development of laryngospasm in the immediate postextubation period.[6] Either a soft-tipped flexible suction catheter, a stiff Yankauer suction tip, or a blunt-tipped tubing may be used. The soft catheter may cause less pharyngeal trauma, but it has a smaller lumen and may be more difficult to manipulate into the desired location. A Yankauer tip may have a larger suction lumen and be more easily directed; however, it may cause more laryngeal trauma. The blunt end of a suction hose has the largest suction diameter, but because it has no side ports, it may suck soft tissue into the opening, thus being ineffective, and exposing the tissue to high wall-suction pressures. In the pediatric patient, the nasopharynx is suctioned to provide a patent airway, because the pediatric patient is dependent on the nasal passage as an airway. This may be done with either a soft suction catheter or the tip of a Yankauer suction catheter. Next, peripheral items such as a temperature probe and esophageal stethoscope are removed so that they do not interfere with extubation or an emergent re-intubation attempt. A precordial stethoscope may be placed so that breath sounds and heart rate can be continuously monitored. Assessment of adequate reversal of neuromuscular blockade was already discussed. The patient is spontaneously breathing with assisted ventilation. During assisted ventilation, the anesthesiologist learns many clinical factors about the patient's status. One can discern the pattern of ventilation, the rate, the depth, the regularity. All are clues as to the degree of neuromuscular reversal and depth of anesthesia. The quality of lung compliance can also be assessed by the feel of the bag. The assisted ventilation should not be so vigorous as to decrease the P_{CO_2} and

deprive the patient of respiratory drive. Assisted ventilation may help to speed the pulmonary exchange of alveolar gases. It also allows for full expansion of the lungs, with elimination of atelectasis. If used, the nitrous oxide is discontinued and 100% oxygen at high flows is maintained for sufficient time for the nitrous oxide to be expelled. The high-flow oxygen turns the standard, semi-closed circle system into an open circuit. This flushes the anesthetic gases out of the circuit and carries off exhaled gases more quickly, in order to prevent rebreathing. Fully deflating the bag also hastens awakening by eliminating a reservoir of anesthetic gases. Also, 100% oxygen is used in order to fill the FRC with oxygen. This allows the patient a longer period of adequate oxygenation in case the airway becomes obstructed after extubation. This gives the anesthesiologist more time to recognize and effectively treat the airway obstruction. The most common causes of such obstruction are mechanical obstruction due to posterior displacement of the tongue, laryngospasm, and inspissated secretions.

During the awakening from the anesthetic, the anesthetist should always have a hand on the endotracheal tube to stabilize it against inadvertent extubation. As the patient proceeds through stage II anesthesia, he or she may become excited; during this time period, stimulation should be kept to a minimum. Background noise should be minimized, someone should stand beside the operating table to prevent the patient from rolling off and from thrashing his or her extremities and being hurt. During this excitatory phase, the patient may suddenly move and dislodge the endotracheal tube despite the securing tape. Therefore, the anesthesiologist should hold the tube at the base against the face to prevent its dislodging. Just prior to extubation, the endotracheal tube tape is peeled off the face to facilitate removal. When the desired level of alertness has been attained, the patient is instructed as to the upcoming events both as a calming and instructional exercise. The patient is instructed to open his or her mouth. After a large positive pressure breath to inflate the lungs to maximal FRC, the cuff is fully deflated with a syringe, and the endotracheal tube is removed in a smooth continuous motion. The large breath also serves to expel secretions pooled above the cuff when the endotracheal tube is removed. A syringe is used to deflate the cuff, rather than pulling off the pilot balloon, for several reasons. First, the tube can be reused emergently, if needed. Second, this ensures that the endotracheal tube cuff is fully deflated more quickly, and thus minimizes the risk of vocal cord damage by the passing of a partially inflated cuff. If tolerated, the oral airway is left in place. It is not pushed back into the mouth unless needed to maintain a patent airway, because the added stimulation can induce laryngospasm or vomiting. If needed, a well-lubricated nasal trumpet airway can be placed to ensure the patency of the patient's airway. Jaw thrust by lifting at both mandibular angles is usually sufficient to clear an airway obstructed by the tongue. Once the endotracheal tube is removed, an oxygen mask that is connected to the anesthesia machine circuit is placed over the patient's face to provide additional oxygen and positive pressure ventilation. This is useful in the treatment of apnea, desaturation, and laryngospasm. Once the patient demonstrates that he or she can adequately maintain respiration, his or her airway monitoring can be disconnected and he or she can be readied for transport to the postanesthetic care unit. Throughout this period, the anesthesiologist must maintain contact with the patient and ensure that the patient maintains his or her airway. Airway obstruction can lead to hypoxia, hypercarbia, and acidosis that may cause hypertension and tachycardia, then bradycardia, hypotension, and subsequently arrhythmias and cardiac arrest. In children, airway obstruction can lead to these complications very quickly, because children have a small FRC for oxygen storage and a higher weight-based oxygen consumption and cardiac output.

Assessment of Reversal of Neuromuscular Blockade

During anesthesia, neuromuscular blockade is usually used to facilitate endotracheal intubation and maintain good muscular relaxation to facilitate surgery. Prior to extubation, the neuromuscular blockade should be reversed so that the patient has sufficient strength for breathing, coughing to clear secretions, and to maintain an airway. The anesthesiologist can determine that the degree of blockade is sufficiently reversed by physical examination and by the use of a peripheral nerve stimulator. There are several simple clinical tests that can be performed in the operating room prior to extubation. The patient should respond to simple commands such as squeezing your fingers with his or her hand. This ensures that his or

her level of consciousness is adequate, and also gives a qualitative measure of muscle strength. During a sustained head lift, the patient should be able to lift his or her head off the pillow for 5 seconds. This indicates that adequate return of muscular strength after the use of muscle relaxants and inhalation anesthetics. The patient may be asked to open his or her mouth and stick out his or her tongue. This is an assessment of the patient's ability to clear and maintain an airway. A maximum negative inspiratory force may be performed, as well as other tests of pulmonary function to determine adequacy of ventilation. The return of the patient's gag reflex is demonstrated by the patient swallowing on the endotracheal tube or coughing with oropharyngeal suctioning. The return of the gag reflex signals that the patient can clear his or her airway of secretions.

Reversal of muscle relaxant blockade may be shown electrophysiologically with a peripheral nerve stimulator. Monitoring neuromuscular blockade with a peripheral nerve stimulator during surgery allows one to adjust the dose of relaxant according to patient response without overdosing. At the end of surgery, nerve stimulation confirms that adequate strength for sustained respiration has returned, thus eliminating suspicion of residual blockade as a cause for postoperative respiratory depression. Any neuromuscular unit can be monitored. Most frequently used are ulnar nerve stimulation of the adductor pollicis longus at the wrist and facial nerve stimulation of the orbicularis oculi. By measuring the amplitude of the muscle tension developed during successive twitches and the fade of muscle tension with tetanic stimulus, the degree of muscular blockade can be estimated. Determining the degree of single-twitch suppression may vary clinically with the examiner. Single-twitch monitoring is not well suited for demonstrating conditions best suited to extubation, because there can be significant fade even when the return of a single twitch is 100% of preoperative status. Train-of-four twitch monitoring gives a more reliable indicator of clinical recovery of neuromuscular function. When the ratio of the fourth to the first twitch of a train of four twitches is 60%, patients are able to sustain head lift for at least 3 seconds. At a 75% ratio, head lift is sustained for 5 seconds, maximum negative inspiratory force is at least -25 cm H_2O and, although slightly decreased, vital capacity is 15 to 20 mL/kg.[7–10] Tetanic stimulation at 50 Hz for 5 seconds without fade of the amplitude is a good sign that reversal is adequate. However, tetanic stimulation is painful in the awake patient and repeated tetanic stimulation can induce recovery in the stimulated muscle not representative of the rest of the body. Post-tetanic stimulation of muscle is another method of determining the adequacy of reversal. There should be no increase in the amplitude of a single twitch 10 seconds after a 5-second 50 Hz tetanic stimulus. However, nerve stimulator testing is only an adjunct to the clinical examination and never replaces good clinical judgment.

Endotracheal Tube Changes

Problems may develop with the endotracheal tube intraoperatively or in the intensive care unit. Sometimes the problems can be temporarily fixed to allow the conclusion of surgery. However, if surgery is to be prolonged or the endotracheal tube is to be left in for prolonged mechanical ventilation in the intensive care unit, the most prudent and safest course of action is changing the endotracheal tube.

Endotracheal Tube Problems

Types of problems with endotracheal tubes can be divided into two categories: airway obstruction and mechanical failure.

Airway obstruction may be noticed when peak inspiratory pressures rise or when full exhalation does not occur. It may be due to kinking of the tube in the airway or the patient biting on the tube. It may be caused by the tip of the tube against the carina or side wall of the trachea. Secretions or blood may obstruct the lumen. Trouble shooting involves auscultation of the chest for breath sounds. Bag ventilate by hand to test lung compliance. Pass a suction catheter to ensure patency and remove secretions. If time allows, pass a fiberoptic bronchoscope to check position.

Mechanical failure includes disconnect of the breathing circuit from the endotracheal tube, which may be ascertained by loss of breath sounds in the precordial/esophageal stethoscope, low pressure, disconnect alarm, a drop in airway resistance, or the inability to keep the bag filled.

Mechanical failure also may be due to a cuff leak. Cuff leak is detected by the sound of escaping air on inspiration, by failure to return the entire tidal volume given, and the require-

ment of high gas flows to keep the positive pressure bag filled. An endotracheal tube may leak due to improper positioning; this can be diagnosed clinically by observing the markings at the lips, by chest radiograph, or by direct vision with a laryngoscope or fiberoptic scope. On an adult chest radiograph, the glottis is at the level of the fifth cervical vertebrae, so the cuff of the endotracheal tube should be below this level. The correct position for the tip of the endotracheal tube is in the mid-trachea at least 2 cm above the carina in adults, because with movement of the head the position of the endotracheal tube changes in the trachea. Flexion of the neck can move the tip of the tube down 2 cm, and extension of the neck can move the tip of the tube up 2 cm. If the tube is too high in the subglottic region such that the cuff impinges on the vocal cords, a leak may be present. Such a leak may persist despite a large volume of air injected into the cuff. This should be corrected by advancing the endotracheal tube to the proper position. Failure to correct this problem can lead to continued leak around the cuff, resulting in less than full expansion of the lungs, aspiration, aerophagia with stomach distention, and trauma to the vocal cords and larynx that may lead to edema, hoarseness, granulation tissue, or eventually to stenosis. The endotracheal tube is advanced after appropriate suctioning of the pharynx to prevent aspiration of secretions pooled above the cuff or in the posterior pharynx. The lungs are inflated, and at peak inflation the cuff is let fully down. The tube is then advanced and the cuff is reinflated until the leak is sealed.

A cuff leak may be due to other problems intrinsic to the endotracheal tube itself. The cuff or pilot balloon may be defective from the manufacturing process. This can be avoided by inspecting all endotracheal tubes and by test inflating the cuffs prior to use. Most cuff leaks cause slow deflation of the cuff, requiring periodic reinflation to maintain a seal. There may be a leak in the cuff caused by careless placement, during which the cuff was torn on the teeth; this can be avoided by careful technique during placement. Recently, a temporary solution to such a cuff leak has been described. Inflation of the cuff with saline or lidocaine jelly provides a temporary seal for short-term use. The pilot balloon valve may become incompetent. This can be temporarily fixed by clamping the pilot tubing distal to the pilot balloon or by placing a three-way stopcock on the end of the pilot balloon. During surgery, the pharynx may be packed to minimize leak. Vigilance must be maintained and the pack removed prior to extubation in order to prevent postextubation obstruction by the foreign body. One such reminder is to leave the tail of the pack hanging out of the side of the mouth. This serves as a reminder and allows one to pull the pack out more easily.

Procedure for Changing Endotracheal Tubes

All of the same precautions made for intubation and extubation must be maintained when an elective endotracheal tube change is planned. First, the patient status and the airway are evaluated and the record is reviewed in order to ascertain the degree of difficulty involved with the previous intubation. All necessary drugs and equipment are assembled (see previously in this chapter). Adequate anesthesia is provided. This may involve either general anesthesia or local/regional anesthesia, including xylocaine ointment, benzocaine spray, superior laryngeal nerve block, and transtracheal lidocaine injection. It may be done with the patient relaxed or spontaneously breathing. The use of relaxants facilitates placement of the endotracheal tube by preventing patient movement and ensuring that the vocal cords are abducted. Doing a tube change during spontaneous respiration may be technically more difficult, because the vocal cords are moving with respiration. However, spontaneous respiration may provide an additional margin of safety if placement of the tube is initially unsuccessful. The patient is put in the optimal head position for intubation (see Chapter 16). The endotracheal tube that is in place is suctioned to clear secretions. The oropharynx and gastric tube are suctioned as noted previously to prevent aspiration. The patient is ventilated with positive pressure ventilation for several minutes with 100% oxygen to increase the margin of safety during the apneic period of the tube change and to expand the FRC. Then the anesthesiologist can proceed with the endotracheal tube change.

There are several methods to change the endotracheal tube. In the first, the patient with an easy airway to ventilate by mask and no history of difficulty with intubation, the endotracheal tube may be removed as described previously, not under direct vision. Then a laryngoscope may be inserted into the mouth and a new endotracheal tube inserted under direct vision, as described previously. This technique has a severe disadvantage in that sight of the patent airway is lost prior to re-intubation. Second, an existing endotracheal tube may be replaced orally under direct vision. Under direct laryngoscopy, the vocal cords and endotracheal tube are located. An assistant is instructed to deflate the cuff, and the initial tube is removed under direct vision. A second endotracheal tube is immediately placed under direct vision. Third, sometimes an oral tube is changed to a nasal endotracheal tube in order to improve patient tolerance of the tube. The nares are anesthetized with either 4% cocaine (200 mg) or 4% lidocaine and vasoconstricted with either phenylephrine or oxymetazoline 0.05% (Afrin spray; Schering, Kenilworth, NJ). An endotracheal tube is passed through the nostril back into the posterior pharynx. A laryngoscope is inserted into the mouth and, under direct vision with the aid of Magill forceps, the nasal endotracheal tube is passed anteriorly to the *in situ* oral tube. Then, under direct vision, the oral tube is removed and the nasal tube is inserted. In some cases direct vision is not possible. Then the endotracheal tube may be changed either over a bronchoscope or over a tube-changing stylet. A standard, flexible fiberoptic laryngoscope is not of sufficient length to facilitate a tube change. If a bronchoscope is available, it should be used because it gives a direct view of the trachea, thus confirming proper placement of the tube. It also allows oxygen to be insufflated through the suction port during the tube change. The new endotracheal tube is prepared and placed over the bronchoscope. The bronchoscope is then guided down the *in situ* endotracheal tube and into the trachea. The cuff on the tracheal tube is deflated and the tube is withdrawn carefully, so as not to dislodge the bronchoscope. As the tube is removed from the trachea, it is sliced along its length so that it can be removed from the bronchoscope. The new endotracheal tube is advanced over the bronchoscope into position in the trachea. Finally, use of a tube-changing stylet does not allow visualization of the airway, but the stylet should maintain a path for the new endotracheal tube to follow. The stylet can be any of several different types. It can be a plastic stylet specifically designed for endotracheal tube changes. It can be a urethral Foley catheter or a orogastric tube with the end cut off. It should not be a rigid wire stylet, because they are usually too short and they can damage the airway. It should not be a Seldinger flexible wire, because they are too flimsy and may lose the path to the airway.

The stylet is passed down the *in situ* endotracheal tube, which is then removed over the stylet. With the stylet still in place in the trachea, a new endotracheal tube is slid down the stylet into the trachea. Occasionally, there is difficulty passing the new endotracheal tube past the glottis. Rotating the tube 90 degrees in either direction usually allows the new tube to pass.

Complications of Intubation Discovered at Extubation

The endotracheal tube is a foreign body in the natural airway. As such, it may cause a number of complications to the airway. Most of these complications are not discovered until after the endotracheal tube is removed. Some complications that may be found include but are not limited to aspiration; hoarseness; dysphagia; inability to cough; laryngeal edema at the epiglottis, vocal cords, or subglottic area; laryngospasm; dislocation of the arytenoid cartilages; mucosal ulceration of the epiglottis, vocal cords, or trachea; granuloma or granulation tissue in the subglottic region or vocal cords; stenosis of the trachea or larynx; and sinusitis or epistaxis (from nasal endotracheal tube).

Laryngospasm

Laryngospasm is a reflex closure of the vocal cords that may cause partial or total glottic obstruction. As noted in Chapter 1 on airway anatomy, the larynx derives sensory innervation from two branches of the vagus nerve. The superior laryngeal nerve innervates the glottis and supraglottic airway, including the base of the tongue, the vallecula, the epiglottis, and the epiglottic folds. The recurrent laryngeal nerve supplies sensation to the tissue below the glottis, the trachea. The motor function is controlled by the external branch of the superior laryngeal nerve to the cricothyroid muscle, and the recurrent laryngeal to the rest of the intrinsic muscles of the larynx. Under normal conditions, the reflex arc associated with laryngeal stimulation can close the glottis at three levels to prevent aspiration. The cricothyroideus, the lateral cricoarytenoids, and the transverse interarytenoids act to close at the level of the true cords. The false cords are closed by action of the lateral thyroarytenoids. Most superiorly, the aryepiglottic folds are closed by the contraction of the arytenoepiglottic and the oblique arytenoid muscles. Stimulation of the supraglottic region initiates the afferent limb of the reflex pathway through the superior laryngeal nerve to the central vagal nuclei. Motor impulses return via the efferents of the superior laryngeal to the cricothyroideus and via the recurrent laryngeal to the thyroarytenoids and lateral cricoarytenoids.[5] Spasm of the true cords alone prevents inspiration, but not expiration, whereas spasm of the false cords prevents all air flow. Anything that irritates the structures of the airway from the nares to the pharynx, larynx, trachea, or bronchi can be the stimulus for laryngospasm. Stimulation of the vagally innervated structures of the abdomen can also precipitate laryngospasm. Laryngospasm usually occurs during the excitatory phase of stage II anesthesia. Any foreign body, including secretions (mucus, saliva, blood), or an airway, laryngoscope, endotracheal tube, or suction catheter, may precipitate laryngospasm. Irritation of the airway by inhalation anesthetics or by excessive manipulations, such as jaw thrust, can also cause laryngospasm.

Prevention is the best treatment of laryngospasm. Premedication with a vagolytic such as atropine, glycopyrrolate, or scopolamine (especially after the use of neostigmine) decreases secretions. Suctioning and other airway manipulation should be done when the patient is sufficiently anesthetized to blunt laryngeal stimulation, thus preventing laryngeal reaction. If laryngospasm develops, it is manifest as stridor in cases of partial obstruction. Complete obstruction demonstrates a "rocking" pattern of breathing, such that the abdomen rises and the chest falls on inspiration, and the abdomen falls and the chest recoils on expiration, with no gas exchange or breath sounds. The goal of treatment is to restore ventilation quickly and calmly. The stimulus is removed, and positive pressure ventilation with 100% oxygen should be instituted immediately.[4] This delivers some oxygen in the case of partial obstruction and may be sufficient to "break" the laryngospasm. Presumably, this stretches the intrinsic muscles of the larynx and allows them to relax, thus opening the true cords. In the case of complete obstruction, it may be impossible to ventilate the patient by mask. If quick, intermittent positive pressure breaths do not relieve the laryngospasm, deepening the anesthesia intravenously and succinylcholine may be used to facilitate muscle relaxation (10 to 20 mg in adults).

Transport to the Postanesthesia Care Unit

The anesthesiologist's responsibility to the patient does not stop at the end of the operation. The goals during the immediate postoperative period are the prevention of complications, pain control, maintenance of a stable patient, and timely transfer of the patient to the recovery room. The vigilance of the anesthesiologist should not be compromised by distractions, because several complications can occur during this time period. Some of the possible complications include airway obstruction, vomiting and aspiration, hemodynamic instability, bleeding, arrhythmias, and postoperative delirium with uncontrolled motor function. Monitoring should be maintained until the patient is stable enough for discontinuation and until the patient is ready to be moved to the stretcher for transfer. When all preparations for transfer have been made, the patient is moved from the operating table, with particular attention paid to the extremities, head, and neck to prevent jostling. Awake patients may be laid supine, but the head of the stretcher should be raised to make breathing easier (see Position for Extubation in this chapter). Patients with blunted airway reflexes are placed in the lateral decubitus position to facilitate patency of the airway and drainage of secretions and vomitus, thus lowering the risk of aspiration. All patients have a oxygen mask placed for transport to the recovery area to prevent hypoxia. After all, the goal of the anesthesiologist is the comfort and safety of the patient.

References

1. Baraka A. Intravenous lidocaine controls extubation laryngospasm in children. Anesth Analg 57:506–507, 1978.
2. Bidwai AV, Bidwai VA, Rogers CR, Stanley TH. Blood pressure and pulse rate responses to extubation with and without prior injection of lidocaine. Anesthesiology 51:171–173, 1979.
3. Gefke L, Andersen LW, Friesel E. Lidocaine given intravenously as a suppressant of cough and laryngospasm in connection with extubation after tonsillectomy. Acta Anesthesiol Scand 27:111–112, 1983.
4. Dehaven CB, Hurst JM, Branson RD. Postextubation hypoxemia treated with a continuous positive airway pressure mask. Crit Care Med 13:46–48, 1985.
5. Rex M. A review of the structural and functional basis of laryngospasm and a discussion of the nerve pathways involved in the reflex and its clinical significance in man and animals. Br J Anaesth 42:891–899, 1970.
6. Jamil AK. Laryngotracheal toilet before extubation. Anaesthesia 29:630–631, 1974.
7. Lareng L, Cathala B, Vaysse C. Criteres d'extubation en salle de reveil. Ann Fran Anesth Reanim 35:887–896, 1978.
8. Prakash O, Jonson B, Meij S, Egbert B, Hugenholtz P, Nauta J, Hekman W. Criteria for early extubation after intrracardiac surgery in adults. Anesth Analg 56:703–708, 1977.
9. Shoults D, Clarke TA, Benumof JL, Mannino FL. Maximum inspiratory force in predicting successful neonatal tracheal extubation. Crit Care Med 7:485–486, 1979.
10. Tahvanainen J, Salmenpera M, Nikki P. Extubation criteria after weaning from intermittent mandatory ventilation and continuous positive airway pressure. Crit Care Med 11:702–707, 1983.

MANAGING
SPECIFIC
AIRWAY
PROBLEMS

CHAPTER 26

Establishing an Airway Outside the Hospital

Charles J. McCabe, M.D.

PREHOSPITAL EMERGENCY MEDICAL SERVICES

Prehospital management of the injured and acutely ill patient has undergone dramatic change in the last two decades. In 1965, the now landmark paper entitled "Accidental Death and Disability, the Neglected Disease of Modern Society" pointed out the existing deficiencies in the delivery of prehospital emergency care.[1] Since then, stimulated by the Emergency Medical Services Act of 1973, the care of patients before they reach the hospital has greatly improved. Emergency medical technicians (EMTs) are now formally trained in basic life support, and paramedics have been further educated to perform invasive advanced life support airway procedures. It is now common to receive patients into the hospital after they have already been intubated.

In most areas, an emergency medical system (EMS) has developed. An integral part of this system is a communication network. Using well-defined and previously arranged protocols, advanced life support measures are carried out under the remote advice and supervision of medical control personnel (physicians and registered nurses).

This chapter is concerned with the methods and techniques that can be used to provide a patent airway and adequate ventilation in the prehospital setting.

THE ENVIRONMENT AND THE EMERGENCY MEDICAL TECHNICIAN

The physician will find the prehospital environment very foreign. It is essential to ride on the ambulance and respond to emergency calls in order to appreciate the physical obstacles (road traffic, stairwells) and the associated time constraints involved in providing prehospital care. The setting of the patient must always be considered, because the potential diagnosis may vary accordingly.

Advances in prehospital services have paralleled the development of skilled and educated EMTs. In 1966, the Department of Transportation was given the task to formulate a curriculum and training standards for ambulance personnel. At that time, "50% of the ambulance drivers were morticians driving a hearse which fulfilled the single ambulance requirement at the time, the ability to trans-

Table 26–1. BASIC EMERGENCY MEDICAL TECHNICIAN CURRICULUM

Introduction to emergency care
Anatomy, physiology, and patient assessment
Airway obstruction and respiratory arrest
Cardiac arrest
Manikin practice and cardiopulmonary resuscitation
Practical use of airway adjuncts
Bleeding and shock
Wounds and soft-tissue injuries
Principles of musculoskeletal care; fractures of the
    upper extremity, pelvis, hip, and lower extremity
Fracture management
Injuries of the head, eye, face, neck, and spine
Injuries to the chest, abdomen, and genitalia
Medical emergencies
Emergency childbirth
Pediatric emergencies
Burns and hazardous materials
Environmental emergencies
Psychologic aspects of emergency care
Lifting and moving patients
Principles of extrication
Eight to ten hours of clinical observation

---

port a patient in the supine position."[1] Since then, ambulances are required to meet specific standards, and EMT training has undergone significant changes.

There are two broad categories of emergency medical care that can be provided: (1) basic life support (BLS), and (2) advanced life support (ALS). The training requirements, skill capabilities, and continuing education requirements for the EMT who provides this care are markedly different.

Basic Life Support

The didactic and practical training emphasize the principles and skills of cardiopulmonary resuscitation (CPR), oxygen support, emergency child birth, fracture immobilization, wound care, patient assessment, and communications (Table 26–1). After 10 hours of clinical observation, the student must successfully complete a written and practical examination in order to practice as an EMT. Continuing education and recertification of CPR techniques are usually required.

Advanced Life Support

Variable levels of life support training have been established; the titles may be different, but they are basically (1) paramedic, (2) car-

diac, and (3) intermediate. All are an attempt to bring the invasive, therapeutic techniques normally used in the emergency room into the field. The individuals are trained in the application of the military antishock trousers (MAST), advanced airway support (esophageal obturator airway [EOA], endotracheal intubation), as well as intravenous cannulation. At the cardiac and paramedic levels, individuals receive instruction in defibrillation and the administration of pharmacologic agents. In addition, the paramedic is trained in psychiatric, pediatric, and obstetric emergencies (Table 26–2). Education is divided into three phases: (1) didactic and laboratory, (2) clinical internship, and (3) field internship. The didactic provides presentation of anatomy and

Table 26–2. LEVELS OF ADVANCED TRAINING

Program development
  Uses the U.S. Department of Transportation
    National Training Course for Advanced Life
    Support
  Curriculum includes 15 modules
   1. Role and responsibility of the EMT
   2. Human systems & patient assessment
   3. Shock & fluid therapy
   4. General pharmacology
   5. Respiratory system
   6. Cardiovascular system
   7. Central nervous system
   8. Soft-tissue injuries
   9. Musculoskeletal system
  10. Medical emergencies
  11. Obstetric/gynecologic emergencies
  12. Pediatric and neonatal
  13. Management of the emotionally disturbed
     patient
  14. Rescue techniques
  15. Telemetry and communications
Levels of training will vary with specific needs (basic
  EMT training required for all levels)
EMT—intermediate training program
  Length: 125–250 hours
  Includes: Modules 1, 2, 3; parts of 5, 15
         Classroom
         Clinical
         Field internship
EMT—cardiac training program
  Length: 300–400 hours
  Includes: Modules 1–6, 15
         Classroom
         Clinical
         Field internship
EMT—paramedic training program
  Length: 500–1500 hours
  Includes: Modules 1–15
         Classroom
         Clinical
         Field internship

EMT, emergency medical technician.

physiology and the physiologic alterations caused by diseases. In the laboratory, technical skills are practiced on manikins. The student then performs on live patients in the controlled hospital environment, and then finally in the prehospital setting. At each level of training, greater clinical responsibility is developed under careful supervision. The length of time at each phase is divided into thirds, with a total time commitment different for each of the three levels. The average paramedic program would require 500 to 1500 hours; the cardiac level, 300 to 400 hours; and the intermediate level, 125 to 250 hours. Ordinarily, the skill capabilities and training can be adjusted to the needs of the region served. Before being certified to practice, a written and a practical examination must be successfully completed. Continuing education and skill maintenance are required.

THE PATIENT AND BASIC LIFE SUPPORT

The approach to the patient must be organized and standardized. The mental status is assessed first. The conscious patient who is able to respond provides good evidence of adequate cerebral perfusion and, presumably, tissue oxygenation. The unconscious patient, conversely, requires rapid examination and perhaps intervention. A patent airway must always be established. This is followed by an examination of chest wall motion with respiration, and finally by a search for and control of any external hemorrhage and palpation of a pulse. These pieces of information determine the urgency of the situation and the need for intervention.

Establishing a patent airway is based on the anatomy described in Chapter 1. The tongue is the most common cause of airway obstruction. In addition, blood, vomitus, and foreign bodies can all lead to occlusion of the airway. Suctioning and positioning of the mandible forward usually provides a patent upper airway. The most successful technique is to perform a "jaw lift" maneuver (Fig. 26–1). The angles of the mandible are grasped bilaterally and drawn forward; at the same time, the neck is slightly hyperextended. In a patient with no gag reflex, an oropharyngeal airway can then be inserted to maintain the tongue in a forward position. After these maneuvers, inability to ventilate the patient indicates lower airway obstruction (aspirated food, foreign body).

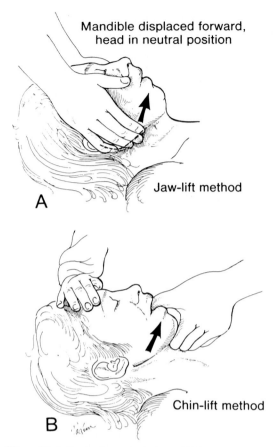

Figure 26–1. Basic airway technique. With anterior traction on the mandible, the tongue is displaced from occluding the airway. (From McCabe CJ. In *Emergency Medicine, Scientific Foundations and Current Practices*, 3rd ed. © 1989, the Williams & Wilkins Co., Baltimore.)

The apneic patient requires artificial ventilation. A face mask with an Ambu bag are ideal, but a good mask seal is *essential*. The respiratory rate should initially be rapid and then be at about 16 per minute in the adult. The chest wall must be exposed in order to observe its motion with respiration. This also allows identification of any chest wall defects or wounds. A carotid pulse should be palpated and, if absent, full CPR is required. If a face mask and Ambu bag are not available, then mouth-to-mouth ventilation is required. This technique is esthetically difficult, particularly in the presence of blood and vomitus.

The problems with the previously described techniques are that they require an absolutely perfect face mask seal and will fully occupy the efforts of the person administering ventilation. Aspiration of vomitus can occur, and the airway is never secure. When using the Ambu bag, good ventilation may actually re-

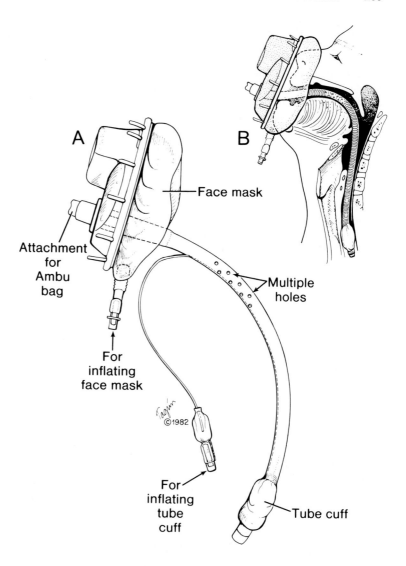

Figure 26–2. Esophageal obturator airway. Oxygen is forced into the oropharynx through the multiple side holes in the proximal portion of the tube. (From McCabe CJ. In *Emergency Medicine, Scientific Foundations and Current Practices,* 3rd ed. © 1989, the Williams & Wilkins Co., Baltimore.)

Face mask

Attachment for Ambu bag

Multiple holes

For inflating face mask

For inflating tube cuff

Tube cuff

quire two sets of hands in order to simultaneously obtain a good face mask seal and use the Ambu bag.

PREHOSPITAL ADVANCED LIFE SUPPORT

There are a number of advanced life support procedures that may be used in order to provide a patent and more secure airway in the prehospital arena. These include the esophageal obturator airway (EOA), the esophageal gastric tube airway (EGTA), and the endotracheal tube (orotracheal or nasotracheal).

The Esophageal Obturator Airway

This device has become popular with some prehospital emergency medical systems (Fig. 26–2). The tube has the appearance of an endotracheal tube, but is occluded distally and is meant to be inserted into the esophagus. It has an inflatable balloon around its distal end. Once it is inserted and its position is confirmed, the balloon is inflated with 30 mL of air in order to totally occlude the esophagus. The intent is to prevent regurgitation and aspiration. Ventilation is provided by forcing oxygen through the attached face mask and proximal patent portion of the esophageal obturator airway. The oxygen then flows into the tube and out of the appropriately fashioned side holes in the pharyngeal portion of the tube. With a good face mask seal, the preferential direction of oxygen flow is into the trachea.

Insertion is performed using a chin-lift maneuver (see Fig. 26–1). The thumb grasps the jaw behind the lower teeth; with the index finger supporting the chin, the mandible is pulled anteriorly. The EOA is then inserted, with the face mask attached, gently into the oropharynx and advanced into the esophagus. If there is any difficulty, the tube should be removed, rather than forcefully advanced. Successful insertion is possible in approximately 80% of the cases. Once fully inserted, a quick ventilation is performed to verify position by listening over the chest wall for breath sounds. If breath sounds are audible, the balloon is inflated with 30 mL of air. If breath sounds are not heard, the tube is in the trachea and should therefore be removed.

Good ventilation requires an excellent face mask seal. If there is any leak around the face mask, poor gas exchange occurs. The device should not be used in children and cannot be used in conscious patients.

Tube removal depends on the patient's level of consciousness. If the patient becomes conscious, the tube will probably need to be removed because of poor patient tolerance. The patient commonly vomits on removal, so precautions must be taken to prevent aspiration. The patient must be placed on his or her side; suction should be immediately available. The balloon is then deflated and the tube removed. In the unconscious patient, the EOA must remain in place until an endotracheal tube is inserted. This is normally done in the hospital's emergency department. If an attempt is performed in the field, the patient should be hyperventilated prior to endotracheal intubation. The face mask on the EOA is removed, and the esophageal obturator airway is drawn to one side of the mouth. Laryngoscopy is performed with the EOA in place. The endotracheal tube is then positioned into the trachea and the balloon inflated. Once its position is confirmed as being in the trachea, the esophageal obturator balloon may be deflated and the tube removed, but leaving the EOA in place is also acceptable.

The EGTA (Fig. 26–3) is similar in design to the EOA, with two exceptions. The device has a central lumen so that a tube can be inserted into the stomach to prevent gastric dilatation. The face mask has an inlet for the tube and a separate area for ventilation.

The popularity of the EOA and the EGTA is based primarily on the ease with which the emergency medical technician can be taught to use the device. The skill can be learned and practiced on a manikin. Although the initial use was tested in the hospital environment on live patients in the operating room, it is clearly an inferior airway to the endotracheal tube, and it would not be responsible to provide live patient training. In the usual circumstance, the only clinical use of this device is during the field training experience.

The initial hospital trials of the EOA were excellent, with good oxygenation. Unfortunately, very few studies have been done on the field use since it was approved. In some recent work, its use in the prehospital setting has not been satisfactory, and vigorous criticism has been voiced. It is clear that use in the prehospital area must be studied more carefully.

The Oro- and Nasotracheal Airway

Endotracheal intubation is the best method of providing ventilation or airway protection. This is possible with insertion of either a nasal or an oral endotracheal tube. The training requires more extensive didactic and skill practice on manikins, as well as insertion on actual patients, in order to attain mastery. Maintenance of this skill requires an active advanced life support system.

The nasotracheal method is ideal in the conscious patient who may not tolerate laryngoscopy, and it is more easily performed on a patient that is tachypneic or panting. Some difficulty usually occurs while passing the tube through the nasal turbinates; generously lubricating the tube and using a smaller size tube is often helpful. The tube is advanced through the nose to just above the epiglottis. At this time, further advancement is timed with inspiration. The natural curve of the pharynx helps to direct the tip into the larynx. As the patient inspires, the epiglottis should move anteriorly and the tube can be advanced through the larynx. Timing and advancing may be difficult, and the tube will often pass into the esophagus. If insertion is successful, the patient will cough and be unable to speak. This procedure is usually performed without visualizing the vocal cords. Rarely, if laryngoscopy is tolerated, the tip of the tube can be directed into the trachea under direct vision with the assistance of McGill forceps.

Orotracheal intubation has become the standard of ideal airway management in the prehospital setting. It requires in-depth knowledge of airway anatomy and, certainly, laboratory practice on the intubation manikin. An animal laboratory experience is also beneficial. Development of the technique is fostered with live intubations of patients prior to

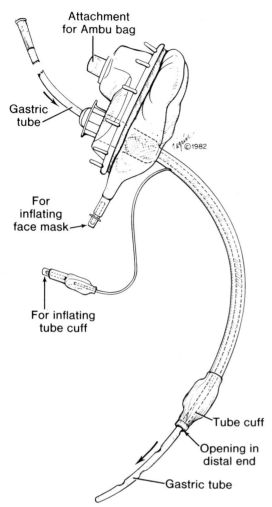

Figure 26–3. Esophagogastric tube airway. A central lumen permits insertion of a tube into the stomach. Oxygen is placed into the pharynx through a separate port on the face mask. (From McCabe CJ. In *Emergency Medicine, Scientific Foundations and Current Practices*, 3rd ed. © 1989, the Williams & Wilkins Co., Baltimore.)

Attachment for Ambu bag

Gastric tube

For inflating face mask

For inflating tube cuff

Tube cuff

Opening in distal end

Gastric tube

surgical operation. This technique should be the method used in most advanced life support systems. Placement requires visualization of the vocal cords and passage of the appropriate-sized tube. The laryngoscope blades commonly used are the Miller (straight) and Macintosh (curved). The blade selection depends upon the EMT's preference and on patient anatomy. On very difficult intubations, the Miller blade may be more useful.

Using the Macintosh blade, the blade tip is inserted into the vallecula and, with a force applied at 45 degrees to the horizontal, the cords are seen as the epiglottis is drawn anteriorly. With the Miller blade, the tip of the blade is actually placed on the epiglottis and

is used to retract the epiglottis out of the line of sight.

If secretions are present, they are suctioned using a portable suction device; any foreign body in the trachea is removed using the McGill forceps. The endotracheal tube is inserted such that the balloon rests just below the vocal cords. The tube is then secured in place. Good breath sounds should be auscultated. If the tube is inserted too deeply, it will enter the right main stem bronchus and result in absent breath sounds on the left. This should be recognized and corrected by pulling the tube back until breath sounds are audible bilaterally.

The Trauma Patient

The causes of inadequate ventilation in the injured patient are (1) airway obstruction, and (2) altered chest wall mechanics. Airway obstruction is most commonly caused by the tongue, but maxillofacial injuries, dentures, blood, vomitus, and foreign bodies are other common causes. The altered chest wall mechanics result from an open or tension pneumothorax, a hemothorax, or a flail chest. An open, sucking chest wound must be sealed with the hand, a rubber glove, or a vaseline gauze pack. Taping the gauze in place on three quadrants creates a one-way flap that allows escape of air from the pleural space with exhalation and prevents inhalation into the pleural space with inspiration. Paradoxic motion secondary to a flail chest is apparent with observation of the chest wall; the flail segment is managed by either lying the patient on the affected side or by placing sandbags on the chest wall segment.

It is sometimes difficult to differentiate a massive hemothorax from a tension pneumothorax. Both can cause a shift of the mediastinum and cardiovascular collapse. Massive hemothorax usually presents with flat neck veins and a dull chest to percussion. The tension pneumothorax causes neck vein distention and a hyperresonant chest to percussion.

In emergency medical systems that permit it, once a tension pneumothorax is diagnosed, a needle may be placed into the pleural space in order to equalize intrapleural pressure with atmospheric pressure. This eliminates the mediastinal shift and circulatory compromise. There is very little that can be done in the prehospital setting in order to treat a massive hemothorax. Volume resuscitation and rapid transport to a hospital are recommended.

Airway obstruction must be relieved immediately. The airway should be opened and the oropharynx suctioned; any foreign body, vomitus, and fractured teeth or dentures are removed. The mandible is then drawn forward. If the patient is without a gag reflex, an oropharyngeal airway is placed and oxygen is supplied. If ventilation must be assisted, an Ambu bag and face mask are initially used.

The advanced life support options in the apneic patient are similar to those in the nontrauma victim; that is, using the EOA or the endotracheal or nasotracheal tubes. Unlike the nontrauma patient, cervical manipulation must be avoided on patients suspected of having a cervical spine fracture. Any trauma patient who is unconscious or who has an injury above the clavicle must be treated as if a cervical fracture is present. Laryngoscopy in these patients can result in spinal cord transection. The experienced laryngoscopist may, however, be able to visualize the vocal cords and intubate without neck extension. In the breathing patient, the nasotracheal tube is an alternative to laryngoscopy and oral endotracheal intubation.

Direct tracheal trauma occurs infrequently, and is most commonly secondary to penetrating trauma to the neck. These patients present with obvious subcutaneous air, and upper airway obstruction is always a threat. Normally, a large quantity of blood accumulates in the airway and frequent suctioning is a necessity. An open wound leads to noisy respirations, and air and blood bubble from the wound. Injuries to the neck with hematoma formation may also cause airway compromise because of the mass effect, with compression or displacement of the trachea. If respiratory distress is severe, oro- or nasotracheal intubation is required. It must be understood that if there is a total transection of the trachea, intubation from above the injury will be unsuccessful and a direct surgical airway will most surely be necessary.

Blunt trauma to the area is not rare. Attempted suicides (hanging) or assaults can result in severe damage to the larynx and trachea. There is not much that can be done in the prehospital setting, except to administer oxygen and suction the oropharynx. The airway is tenuous, and laryngoscopy may precipitate total occlusion. These patients commonly require a tracheostomy and repair of the injury surgically.

Nontraumatic Airway Obstruction

There are very few causes of nontraumatic airway obstruction. The most common are foreign body aspiration and epiglottitis. The latter has been discussed. The so-called "café coronary," secondary to food aspiration, is the cause of approximately 2500 deaths per year. In many states, this problem is recognized and restaurants are required to have at least one employee working who is familiar with this entity and trained in the appropriate therapy. Normally in these cases, the patient fails to adequately chew his or her food and swallows, perhaps while laughing or talking; aspiration results. This causes either partial or complete airway obstruction. The patient becomes immediately anxious. Therapy must be rapid and accurate. The differential diagnosis from an acute myocardial infarction is sometimes difficult, particularly if the patient should become unconscious. With airway obstruction, the patient usually reaches for his or her throat and is unable to speak. The patient must be approached as any patient in acute distress, by attempting to establish a patent airway, observing the chest wall for motion, and palpating a carotid pulse.

Therapy of this entity depends on the patient's level of consciousness and physical position. The conscious patient may be anxious and fearful and may attempt to flee. The initial attempts at clearing the airway should be to calm the patient and to encourage him or her to cough. The force generated by a cough usually clears the bolus of food from the airway. If this is unsuccessful, the patient may be assisted in his or her efforts by a number of maneuvers. In the seated or standing patient, four sharp and forceful back blows should be applied between the scapulas, followed by four abdominal thrusts. The abdominal thrusts are performed by wrapping both arms around the patient and clasping one hand with the other just above the mid abdomen. The soft portion of the palm should be facing the patient and four quick upward and inward compressions are performed. If the patient is pregnant, a similar maneuver is applied to the mid sternal area. After these procedures, an attempt may be made to manually clear the pharynx of the foreign body. If these attempts are unsuccessful, the techniques are repeated.

If the patient is unconscious, similar techniques are recommended, but the differential diagnosis from the acute myocardial infarction is more difficult. Once again, the patient evaluation begins with the determination of upper airway patency, followed by observing the chest wall for motion with respiration, and then by checking for a pulse. Attempts at providing ventilation should make the diagnosis apparent. The therapy in the seated, unconscious patient is the following: lean the patient forward and then perform four sharp back blows, followed by four abdominal thrusts, as described in the conscious patient. If the patient is supine, the therapy is slightly different; first, roll the patient to the side and perform four back blows between the scapulas. The patient is then rolled supine, and four abdominal thrusts are performed. This is done with one hand placed on the other midway between the xiphoid process and the umbilicus. Four upward and inward thrusts are administered. Again, in the pregnant patient these maneuvers are applied to the mid sternal area. After these two technical maneuvers, a sweep of the oropharynx is made to clear the bolus of food from the pharynx. Ventilation is then attempted. Successful ventilation means that the airway is patent; if not, the maneuvers are repeated.

If the airway is unsuccessfully cleared with these techniques, there are very few options. If equipment is available, laryngoscopy should be performed and the bolus of food removed using McGill forceps. If this is unsuccessful, the only other option is to perform either a needle or a surgical cricothyrotomy. In general, this requires the presence of a physician. In some EMS, however, these procedures are permitted after proper training. The needle cricothyrotomy is performed by placing a 14- or 12-gauge needle into the trachea through the cricothyroid membrane. Oxygen is then supplied under pressure (50 psi), and intermittent boluses of air are insufflated into the tracheal passage. The normal sequence is to insufflate for 1 second and then allow for exhalation for 4 seconds. Usually, the obstruction of the airway is not complete and the carbon dioxide and oxygen are expelled on exhalation through the normal tracheal passage. The force used to inject the oxygen into the tracheal passage is enough to expand the lungs. Normal chest wall and lung collapse provides the force for exhalation. In experimental studies, it has been shown that adequate oxygenation and ventilation can be provided using these techniques. If, however, the needle cricothyrotomy is unsuccessful, the only option available is to perform a surgical cricothyrotomy. Using any sharp instrument (such as a pocket knife), an incision is made transversely through the skin, subcutaneous tissue, and cricothyroid membrane into the trachea. Once the cricothyroid membrane has been opened, the patient will be able to inspire. The opening must then be maintained by obturating the lumen. This provides a temporary airway until the hospital setting can be reached. This procedure has some risk of complication, particularly for the nonsurgeon. The technique should be practiced in the animal laboratory setting before clinical use.

THE PEDIATRIC PATIENT

A young infant or child commonly places objects into his or her mouth. As a result, foreign body obstruction of the airway in this age group is not an uncommon event. The therapy depends on the age and size of the patient. The infant should be placed face down over the forearm with the head in the dependent position and supported by the hand. Four back blows are then administered (with appropriate force); after this, the infant is turned supine, supported by the forearm, and then given four chest thrusts using two fingers to push in on the mid sternal area. Abdominal thrusts are not used, because damage to the intra-abdominal viscera is likely to occur. A finger sweep of the oropharynx may be necessary to clear the bolus from the pharynx. With the older child, the back blows may be given with the patient supported on the thigh and the head dependent. The chest thrusts are performed with the child supine on the floor. The force used should depend on the age and size of the patient.

SUMMARY

There is no doubt that we have vastly improved prehospital care and capabilities. It is important to realize, however, that the pharmacology, the cardiac defibrillator, and the antishock garments will be unsuccessful unless the airway and ventilation is properly cared for. The establishment of a patent airway must be the first goal in any therapy administered in the prehospital setting.

References

1. Accidental Death and Disability, the Neglected Disease of Modern Society. National Academy of Science/National Research Council, 1966.

Bibliography

Adler J, DyKan M. Gastric rupture: An unusual complication of the esophageal obturator airway. Ann Emerg Med 12:224–225, 1983.

Auerbach PS, Geehr EC. Inadequate oxygenation and ventilation using the esophageal gastric tube airway in the prehospital setting. JAMA 250:3067–3071, 1983.

Bass RR, Allison EJ, Hunt RC. The esophageal obturator airway: A reassessment of use by paramedics. Ann Emerg Med 11:358–360, 1982.

Branigan CO, Grow JB. Cricothyroidotomy: Elective use in respiratory problems requiring tracheotomy. J Thorac Cardiovasc Surg 71:72–81, 1976.

Elling R, Politis J. An evaluation of emergency medical technicians ability to use manual ventilation devices. Ann Emerg Med 12:765–768, 1983.

Hoffman JR, Pietrafesa CA, Orban DJ. Esophageal perforation following use of esophageal obturator airway (EOA). Am J Emerg Med 3:282–287, 1983.

Jacobs LM, Barrizbeitia L, Bennett B, Madigan C. Endotracheal intubation in the prehospital phase of emergency medical care. JAMA 250:2175–2177, 1983.

McGill J, Clinton J, Ruiz E. Cricothyrotomy in the emergency department. Ann Emerg Med 11:36–38, 1982.

Neff CC, Pfeister RC, Van Sonnenberg E. Percutaneous transtracheal ventilation: Experimental and practical aspects. J Trauma 23:84–90, 1983.

Smith JP, Bodai BI, Aubourg R, Ward R. A field evaluation of the esophageal obturator airway. J Trauma 23:317–321, 1983.

Smith JP, Bodai BI, Seifkin A, et al. The esophageal obturator airway—a review. JAMA 250:1081–1085, 1983.

CHAPTER 27

Management of the Acute Airway in the Emergency Department

Louis P. Bucky, M.D., Mark S. Allen, M.D., and Charles J. McCabe, M.D.

The management of the airway is the first priority in the evaluation of every emergency department patient. In patients with potential airway compromise, appropriate management is essential in order to prevent a solvable problem from developing into a life-threatening disaster. The physician who cares for patients in the emergency department must be familiar with the various conditions that lead toward ventilatory disturbances, the signs and symptoms of respiratory compromise, the principles of management, and the fundamental procedures in order to achieve a successful outcome. Familiarity with emergency laryngoscopy, naso- and orotracheal intubation, bronchoscopy, and emergency cricothyrotomy or tracheotomy equips the physician to control any airway problem encountered.

The trauma patient who presents to the emergency department with ineffective breathing is most likely suffering from airway obstruction. However, one should be familiar with other causes of inadequate ventilation that require immediate recognition and treatment. Open pneumothorax, tension pneumothorax, massive hemothorax, and flail chest should be considered in the patient with a history of trauma who demonstrates poor ventilation. Patients who present in respiratory distress without trauma must be evaluated for ventilatory disturbances secondary to asthma, pneumonia, pulmonary edema, spontaneous pneumothorax, pulmonary embolism, or pleural effusion, as well as airway obstruction from infection (epiglottitis, croup) or neoplasms.

UPPER AIRWAY OBSTRUCTION

Clinical Presentation

In general, the patient with an upper airway obstruction and *hypoxia*, with or without a history of trauma, is anxious (air hungry) and appears ashen, cyanotic, or gray. Auscultation of the chest reveals gurgling or crowing sounds, and there is ineffective respiratory excursion,

291

constriction of the cervical muscles, and retraction of the suprasternal, intercostal, and epigastric regions. The hypercarbic patient is somnolent and difficult to arouse.

In any emergency situation, the airway must be assessed for patency. The appropriate treatment for the various causes of airway obstruction, both traumatic and nontraumatic, depends on the level of obstruction. Food (the "café coronary"), vomitus, dentures, blood, and secretions that cause upper airway obstruction should be removed manually under direct vision with the physician's gloved finger and a tonsil-tip sucker. In the patient with altered consciousness, the tongue and soft tissues are common causes of obstruction at the hypopharynx. Attempts at an anterior jaw thrust or placement of an oropharyngeal airway should be made to resolve the obstruction caused by the tongue. If these maneuvers are unsuccessful, then laryngoscopy with direct visualization of the vocal cords and removal of the obstructing agent is the preferred maneuver in most instances. Distal tracheal obstruction may require bronchoscopy and subsequent intubation with a long endotracheal tube.

Endotracheal intubation is the most commonly employed method for airway management in the patient with ineffective ventilation. If the patient requires intubation for longer than 24 hours, nasotracheal intubation may be preferred. Nasotracheal intubation allows more comfort for the patient and less motion of the tube, which decreases the risks of injury to the tracheal mucosa. However, use of aspirin or warfarin, or suspected thrombocytopenia, precludes attempting this route.

Expeditious airway control is the emergency department physician's first priority, but repeated attempts at intubation either nasally or orally can be dangerous. Furthermore, there are situations when endotracheal intubation is either impossible or contraindicated. Generally, in those instances where visualization is difficult, anatomy is distorted, or positioning for endotracheal intubation is impossible, emergent cricothyrotomy is necessary. In the extreme situation of airway obstruction, or in patients less than 14 years old, a temporary life-saving alternative is the placement of a 15-gauge needle through the cricothyroid membrane and oxygenation via jet insufflation using oxygen under 50 psi. All surgical cricothyrotomies should be converted to formal tracheotomies within 24 hours to prevent glottic or subglottic injury.

TRAUMA

Facial Fractures

The most common airway problems seen in the emergency department are trauma related. Primary injury to the airway itself or the structures adjacent to the upper airway dictate management and the specific techniques employed for airway control. The patient with severe facial fractures poses several problems for adequate airway management. Not only is normal anatomy distorted, but bone fragments, blood, and teeth can directly lead to airway occlusion. In the patient with distorted facial anatomy or suspected cribiform plate fracture, nasotracheal intubation is contraindicated. Concomitant bleeding, bony instability, and local debris may portend impending obstruction that should be relieved by emergent tracheostomy or cricothyrotomy. Furthermore, repair of facial fractures and facial soft-tissue injuries is enhanced with the placement of the endotracheal tube away from the field of injury.

Head Injury

Patients who present with head injuries need prompt airway security for adequate ventilation, protection from airway obstruction, and the production of secondary brain injury from hypoxia. Any patient with a gunshot wound to the head is at risk for massive oropharyngeal bleeding. Early intubation, before significant bleeding and "hemic drowning" occurs, is essential.

Cervical Spine Injury

In trauma patients, the status of the cervical spine is always in question. Those patients with suspected spinal injuries pose a difficult problem in the management of the airway. A lateral cervical spine radiograph should be obtained immediately in all patients who do not require emergent intubation. A normal lateral neck radiograph does not exclude a cervical fracture. Fortunately, 90% of unstable fractures are demonstrated on a lateral cervical spine radiograph that visualizes all seven vertebrae. If a cervical spine injury is discovered, positioning for intubation must be carefully performed. In the breathing patient, nasotracheal intubation may be possible, or the experienced endoscopist may attempt intubation with in-line immobilization of the neck. Flexible bronchoscopy with an endotracheal tube threaded over the bronchoscope is an alternative technique. If a bronchoscope is unavailable or airway access is urgent, cricothyrotomy may be indicated.

LARYNGOTRACHEAL TRAUMA

Trauma to the larynx and trachea may occur from either penetrating or blunt injuries. The diagnosis of a primary injury to the airway requires a high index of suspicion based on the mechanism of injury, familiarity with the manifestations of laryngotracheal trauma, and a knowledge of the potential associated injuries. The patient with an airway injury and impending obstruction displays restlessness, tachycardia, a decreased level of consciousness, and arterial blood gases that reveal hypoxemia and hypercapnea. Without prompt intervention, respiratory arrest and death are imminent. The key to effective management in the emergency department is prompt control of the airway. Definitive treatment of the injured respiratory tract is reserved for the experienced surgeon in the operating room.

Blunt Trauma

The injuries that are most likely to be evaluated in the emergency department are the result of direct blows to the neck from dashboards, strangulations, or hyperextension injuries. The mechanism of injury in automobile accident victims is the compression of the larynx, hyoid bone, and upper trachea between the dashboard and the cervical spine. Blunt injuries to the larynx are less common in children due to the higher positioning of the larynx in the neck and the subsequent protection provided by the mandible. However, severe injuries have occurred in children while riding bicycles, off-road vehicles, and snowmobiles. Significant upper airway injury has been reported from striking a horizontal cable or a fall against the handlebars. The spectrum of presentation ranges from minor complaints of hoarseness or pain to an open laceration with visible damage to cervical contents. Clinical findings in blunt laryngotracheal trauma include (1) subcutaneous emphysema or crepitus, (2) dysphonia, (3) loss of the laryngeal prominence, (4) dysphagia, (5) stridor,

(6) hemoptysis, (7) cough, or (8) localized tenderness.

The most common blunt injury to the larynx is a vertical fracture of the thyroid cartilage, with or without fracture of the cricoid cartilage. The cricoid cartilage is the only complete cartilaginous ring, and its stability is critical to maintain a patent airway. Another common injury occurs at the laryngotracheal junction via hyperextension that results in separation of the larynx from the relatively fixed trachea. Lacerations of the trachea between the vocal cords and the carina can occur as a result of blunt trauma with acceleration/deceleration or compression types of forces. In addition, this mechanism can result in avulsion fractures of the bronchus just distal to the carina. Prolonged radiographic evaluation of these injuries can be dangerous, with an unstable airway converting to an occluded airway in the radiography suite. Initially, a lateral neck radiograph of C1 through C7 should be obtained to search for vertebral fractures, subcutaneous emphysema, or loss of the tracheal air column. In the more stable patient, full cervical radiographs can be undertaken, along with contrast studies of the esophagus. Direct endoscopic evaluation of the airway and the esophagus should be performed in the operating room.

The potential injuries to the cervical spine, esophagus, and neurovascular structures in the neck after blunt trauma cannot be ignored. As mentioned previously, cervical spine injuries require immobilization and stabilization. Obviously, failure to suspect injury to the cervical column can result in permanent paralysis. Furthermore, undetected esophageal tears with subsequent leakage of its contents can result in a tracheo-esophageal fistula, failed tracheal repair, and life-threatening mediastinitis. Arterial injuries are fraught with complications from an expanding hematoma, stroke, or fatal hemorrhage.

It is critical in the management of direct airway trauma to achieve complete airway security. If the physician has any question about the integrity of the airway, intubation should be performed. In the difficult case, repeated attempts at intubation should be avoided and emergency tracheostomy or cricothyrotomy performed. In the stable patient, endoscopic evaluation of the airway and alimentary tract should occur in the operating room with the ability to perform emergent tracheostomy available. Even the apparently stable airway can rapidly obstruct if mucosal swelling, bleeding, secretions, or separation of transected ends of the airway occurs. In the severe case of the patient with an open transected trachea, the distal segment may retract into the mediastinum. The physician should try to locate the distal trachea with digital exploration, grasp the segment, and bring the orifice of the distal component into the wound for intubation. The patient should be stabilized for transfer to the operating room or appropriate facility where primary repair of the trachea can occur.

Penetrating Trauma

The incidence of penetrating trauma involving the upper airway is dependent on the demographics of the patient population. Studies of penetrating neck wounds have revealed injury to the upper airway in as many as 25% to 40% of patients.[1, 2] Respiratory compromise may result from direct injury to the airway or to an adjacent vascular structure with subsequent hematoma formation and airway compression. Life-threatening obstruction or massive hemorrhage can result from stab wounds, gunshot wounds, or shrapnel from an explosion. In these instances, airway obstruction occurs from a bullet lodging in the airway itself, extrinsic compression from adjacent soft-tissue injury, or intrinsic compression from fractures and displacement of the hyoid or thyroid cartilage and concomitant edema formation. Furthermore, the communication of a major blood vessel and the airway can result in death from "hemic drowning." Any patient who presents to the emergency room with a penetrating injury to the neck should be considered to have an injury to the airway until proven otherwise. Precautions to avoid airway obstruction are immediately necessary. Unlike blunt trauma, penetrating trauma to the upper airway is usually obvious. Although the wound site itself (stab wound, gunshot) may be deceptively benign in appearance, the concomitant symptoms of cough, stridor, dysphonia, and the presence of subcutaneous emphysema should suggest that a serious injury has occurred. Subcutaneous emphysema has been reported in 75% of patients with airway penetration.[3] If the distal trachea is involved, air may dissect into the mediastinum and a Hamman's sign (mediastinal crunch) may be present. Furthermore, if the pleura are involved, a pneumothorax must be suspected and treated.

Penetrating cervical trauma requires early evaluation of the aerodigestive (respiratory, alimentary), the neurologic and the vascular systems. Furthermore, removal of foreign bodies in the cervical region should be performed in the controlled setting of the surgical suite. In the stable patient with a penetrating wound to the neck, nonsurgical exploration of the neck may be used to exclude serious injury. Bronchoscopy, laryngoscopy, esophagoscopy, and radiologic evaluation should be considered to rule out a significant laryngotracheal injury. Angiography and barium swallow can detect the precise location of a vascular or esophageal injury. The patient who presents with signs of partial airway obstruction requires expeditious management in the emergency ward. A lateral neck radiograph should be obtained to check for air in the soft tissues. Orotracheal intubation can normally be performed in patients with stab and gunshot wounds; however, neck immobilization is necessary until all views of the neck are obtained (lateral, anteroposterior, and open mouth odontoid). An emergency cricothyrotomy kit should be on hand in case the patient shows signs of complete airway obstruction or attempts at endotracheal intubation are unsuccessful. Repeated attempts at oral or nasotracheal intubation are contraindicated. If the patient has a cervical spine fracture and a compromised airway from a penetrating injury, cricothyrotomy may be necessary. These patients require diagnostic bronchoscopy and esophagoscopy in the operating room, after control of the airway has been obtained.

BURNS

Inhalation/Ingestion Injuries

The emergency department physician will be exposed to patients who have sustained thermal injuries. A significant aspect of the treatment of any patient sustaining a burn injury involves the initial management of the airway. Pulmonary injury caused by smoke inhalation is a principal cause of early mortality in burn patients. The term inhalation injury refers to damage to the respiratory tract caused by the products of combustion. Many of these agents not only cause local pulmonary insult, but have severe systemic toxicity when absorbed. The nature and severity of these injuries are determined by the chemical composition of the smoke and the extent of the victim's exposure.

Damage to the respiratory tract can range from erythema and mild edema to frank necrosis and mucosal sloughing. Like other injuries to the airway, this process can slowly lead to total airway obstruction. The key to management in the emergency department entails a high index of suspicion, early detection of potential injury, and securing the airway via endotracheal intubation before respiratory decline ensues.

Thermal Injury

Among the mechanisms of inhalation injury, true thermal injury is uncommon. The amount of thermal damage is proportional to the temperature of the inhaled gas at the time it makes contact with the respiratory mucosa. Dry air has a low heat capacity and, with the exception of steam and soot particles, most of the thermal energy is dissipated in the upper respiratory tract. Severe thermal burns of the intrathoracic airway are found in less than 5% of cases, and are caused by steam, soot, and fumes from combustible materials.

Chemical Inhalation

The dangers with chemical inhalation lie not only with local irritation, but systemic poisoning as well. Many of the common chemical irritants—chlorine, phosgene, ammonia, nitrogen oxide, and sulfur dioxide—cause direct damage to the mucous membranes. Soluble agents (chlorine, ammonia, sulfur dioxide) are easily recognized by their pungent odor. The noxious nature of these gases leads to a short exposure time, and damage is usually limited to a tracheobronchitis of the upper airway. Poorly soluble agents, conversely, are less noxious and often lead to damage of the distal airway, which may be manifested by pulmonary edema.

Several gases do not exert their toxic effect on the lungs, but are deleterious once systemically absorbed. Carbon monoxide, which is produced by the incomplete combustion of carbon-containing material, is the prime example of a gas that acts as a systemic poison. Cyanide, hydrogen sulfide, methyl bromide, and arsenic are systemic poisons that are produced in household fires via the combustion of synthetic materials.

Caustic Ingestion

The ingestion of caustic substances can result in damage to the airway in addition to the esophagus and stomach. Solid caustics, particularly alkali agents (Draino), can cause inflammation and necrosis of the oropharynx with edema formation and early airway obstruction. Liquid caustics, more commonly acids, can erode through the esophagus into the trachea and cause severe destruction of the mediastinal structures. All patients who present with a history of a caustic ingestion should be considered for laryngoscopic and bronchoscopic evaluation. Direct visualization of the upper airway is important due to the high likelihood of damage and subsequent scar formation.

Diagnosis

The diagnosis of an inhalation or ingestion injury requires knowledge of the pathophysiology of the injury and a high index of suspicion. The history of exposure to fire and gas in an enclosed space, loss of consciousness or ingestion of a caustic agent are significant details when obtaining the history. Even in the absence of any physical signs of injury, one must suspect an occult pulmonary injury in these patients. The physical findings of facial burns, hoarse voice, singed nasal hairs, and carbonaceous deposits in the pharynx are further indications of a respiratory injury. Certainly, patients presenting with cough, dyspnea, cyanosis, wheezes, rales, or rhonchi have sustained an injury and treatment measures should quickly ensue. Routine chest radiograph, arterial blood gas, carboxyhemoglobin level, and an electrocardiogram should be obtained. Commonly, the significant findings on chest radiograph lag behind the auscultatory signs of pulmonary injury.

Treatment

The treatment in the emergency department is primarily supportive. Appropriate therapy is based on careful diagnosis and understanding the timing of the manifestations of the various pulmonary injuries. Airway control via endotracheal intubation during the early presentation period is performed to protect the airway from the manifestations of thermal injury. Laryngeal edema typically develops within the first 2 to 8 hours. Any evidence of edema of the upper portion of the airway is manifested by labored respirations, activation of the accessory respiratory muscles, and deteriorating arterial blood gases. Direct laryngoscopy can be performed to confirm the diagnosis, and early endotracheal intubation is indicated if there is any sign of compromise. Tracheotomy should be avoided if at all possible in patients with inhalation injury and burns of the face and neck. The high bacterial counts in these burned areas can lead to local infection at the incision and subsequent respiratory infections. Distal airway burns are usually manifested within 12 to 92 hours and resemble the findings of pulmonary edema. If there is progressive respiratory insufficiency with hypercapnia, hypoxemia, and a widened alveolar–arterial oxygen gradient, then the patient should be intubated and treatment with positive end-expiratory pressure (PEEP) begun. Other indications for endotracheal intubation include difficulty handling secretions, respiratory compromise from circumferential deep burns of the chest, and protection from aspiration in the comatose patient. In summary, the exact diagnosis of the multiple agents involved in an ingestion or inhalation injury is unnecessary for proper initial management. Whether damage is due to local thermal or chemical irritation, the basic tenets of airway control and oxygen support should be heeded. A careful history and a high index of suspicion for an airway burn can lead to early prophylactic intubation and prevention of complications.

NONTRAUMATIC AIRWAY OBSTRUCTION

Epiglottitis

Nontraumatic causes of airway obstruction that dictate emergency management are primarily infections, neoplasms, and aspiration of foreign bodies. Infections cause 80% of airway obstructions in children and can occur in adults as well. Epiglottitis, or supraglottitis, is a fulminant, rapidly progressing bacterial inflammation of the supraglottic structures that is infamous for its potential to cause rapid, complete upper airway obstruction in the pediatric population. It is less commonly recognized that epiglottitis occurs in adults, and has a reported mortality of almost 6%, largely due to misdiagnosis and inappropriate treatment.[4] Acute epiglottitis represents 0.1% to 0.3% of pediatric hospital admissions. It usually occurs in children between 2 and 6 years old and is more common in males than in females. It is more commonly found in drier, temperate regions, and most cases tend to appear during the winter months. The incidence of the disease appears to be increasing in both children and adults.

The clinical presentation of acute epiglottitis differs slightly between the pediatric and adult population. The classic pediatric patient presents appearing acutely ill, with the abrupt onset of high fever, a rapidly progressing sore throat over the preceding few hours, and may be irritable or lethargic. As the supraglottic edema progresses, the patient reveals signs of dysphagia, dysphonia, drooling (it hurts to swallow), and respiratory distress. The characteristic "airway preserving" position of the child with acute epiglottitis is characterized by a sitting position with forward flexion at the waist, slight cervical flexion, forward chin thrust, with a protruding tongue and saliva drooling from the mouth. This child is on the verge of complete airway obstruction, and all maneuvers that can lead to a change in the position of the child should be avoided until the airway is secured. Specifically, radiographs, venipuncture, and arterial blood gases should be performed in this position or not at all. In adults, the manifestations of epiglottitis are more variable than in children; and the diagnosis is more difficult. Adult patients with epiglottitis complain of a sore throat and dysphagia out of proportion to the physical findings. However, the sore throat may be present for several days prior to presentation or may begin only several hours before complete obstruction. At presentation, symptoms of airway obstruction are less obvious than with children. Absence of stridor does not rule out the diagnosis. Airway obstruction is thought to be less likely in adults because they have a larger, more rigid upper airway with less reactive lymphoid tissue. Recent literature indicates, however, that sudden airway obstruction can occur without any preceding signs of deterioration.[5] This factor leads to minimizing all diagnostic tests in the patient with an unprotected airway. Clearly, all radiographs performed should occur in the emergency department with the patient accompanied by personnel capable of managing acute airway occlusion. These investigations, however, should not delay the definitive management of the airway in any patient who exhibits respiratory distress. There are characteristic changes on lateral neck and chest radiographs in patients with epiglottitis (Fig. 27–1). Soft-tissue radiographs of the neck usually reveal swelling of the epiglottis (thumb printing) and dilatation of the hypopharynx. It is important to note that if the radiographs are negative and epiglottitis is suspected clinically, the epi-

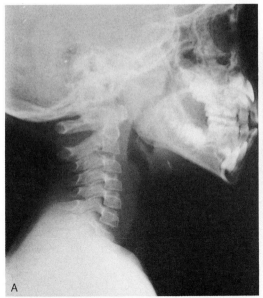
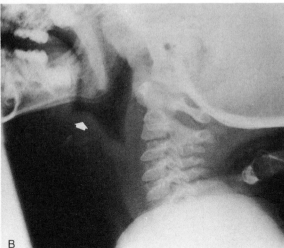

Figure 27–1. *A,* Lateral view of a normal airway. *B,* Lateral view of epiglottitis. "Thumbprint" *(arrow)* and hypopharyngeal dilatation are consistent with epiglottitis. (Courtesy of Johan G. Blickman, MD.)

glottis should be visualized laryngoscopically in the operating room in order to definitely exclude epiglottitis. *Hemophilus influenzae* type B is usually the responsible organism, but streptococcus species (Pneumococcus) and *Staphylococcus aureus* have been implicated. Intravenous antibiotics should be started immediately in the stable patient (ampicillin, chloramphenicol).

The management of the airway in children with epiglottitis has become well standardized. Nasotracheal intubation performed in the operating room is now considered the procedure of choice. Experienced personnel should be on hand in order to perform an emergency tracheotomy, if necessary. Furthermore, inhalation induction with halothane and 100% oxygen is optimal in order to prevent laryngospasm. This aggressive approach has reduced mortality from 6% to less than 1%. Currently, the mortality in adults is approximately 6%.[5] Many of these deaths occur in patients considered stable and treated without intubation. Furthermore, it has not been possible to identify risk factors that separate those who may develop sudden airway obstruction from those who may not. Therefore, a trend toward early intubation via the oral or nasal route to secure the airway should be initiated in all adults with epiglottitis. Once again, trained personnel should be available to perform emergency tracheostomy. *No attempt should be made to visualize the epiglottis in the*

emergency ward. An examination should be performed in the operating room, where adequate support is available.

Croup

Croup is the most common infectious form of acute and subacute upper airway obstruction in infants and children. It accounts for about 70% of all pediatric stridor.[6] Like epiglottitis, it is more common in males than females, but occurs in a younger age group (3 months to 3 years of age). Unlike epiglottitis, croup is caused by a virus and has an associated prodrome of gradual onset over 1 to 7 days. The child is usually able to swallow and there is no drooling. The child commonly presents with malaise, temperature less than 38°C, mild leukocytosis, coryza, hoarseness, and a high-pitched "barking cough." Of note, a decrease in stridor or coughing as the child fatigues may indicate respiratory failure, rather than an improvement of symptoms. Radiographically, the characteristic unique features of croup are symmetric narrowing of the subglottic air shadow on an anteroposterior radiograph, known as the "church steeple" sign (Fig. 27–2), and blurring of the tracheal air shadow laterally (Fig. 27–3). Radiographic findings do not correlate with the severity of croup, but radiologists can make the diagnosis with 90% accuracy.[6]

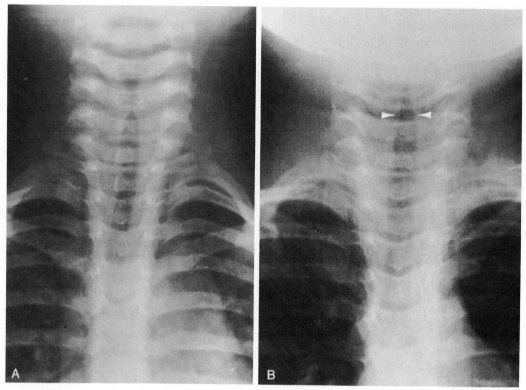

Figure 27–2. Anteroposterior views of *A,* normal subglottic region, and *B,* "church steeple" *(arrows)* appearance of subglottic region consistent with croup. (Courtesy of Johan G. Blickman, MD.)

Understanding the pathogenesis of croup is important in making the correct diagnosis and implementing the appropriate treatment. Croup produces a slowly progressive inflammatory edema of the subglottic larynx, trachea, and bronchi. Progressive narrowing of

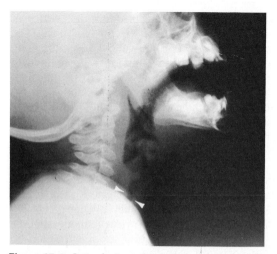

Figure 27–3. Lateral view of subglottic narrowing *(arrows)* consistent with croup. (Courtesy of Johan G. Blickman, MD.)

the lower airway at the cricoid level produces the inspiratory stridor of croup. The slower progression of croup versus epiglottitis allows more time for accurate diagnosis and appropriate medical management. The principles of initial medical management of croup include (1) oxygen administration, (2) intravenous hydration, and (3) humidification of the tracheobronchial tree. Nebulized racemic epinephrine has shown some early transient improvement. Antibiotics are not indicated, and the use of steroids is controversial. The vast majority of treated patients improve and can be managed as outpatients. However, those few patients who have a worsening clinical picture and who are refractory to medical treatment may require intubation. In these cases, nasotracheal intubation with a smaller than predicted endotracheal tube is recommended. The early conversion to a tracheostomy is indicated if longer intubation is required in order to prevent the complications of subglottic stenosis.

Tracheal Tumors and Tracheal Stenosis

Primary neoplasms of the trachea are rare and can cause acute airway obstruction. More commonly, these tumors gradually cause increasing dyspnea, stridor, and wheezing. Ideally, they should be managed by a thoracic surgeon well versed in the methods of tracheal resection and reconstruction. Occasionally, an emergency physician sees chronic tracheal stenosis that has resulted from trauma, infection, or previous intubation. Like tumors of the trachea, these rarely present with acute distress. In some cases, intubation with a small endotracheal tube to temporarily control ventilation is possible. One must not be lulled into a false sense of security by placing the endotracheal tube just past the vocal cords. Often the stenosis is distal to the vocal cords, and airway patency is not provided by placement of a tube above the narrowed trachea. Furthermore, an emergency cricothyrotomy does not solve the problem if the stenosis or tumor is in the distal airway. Rigid bronchoscopy by a qualified endoscopist may be necessary to control the airway or dilate the stenosis. A helium–oxygen mixture with a lower viscosity than room air may be used to attempt to decrease the viscosity of the air as a temporary treatment in the patient with severe tracheal stenosis.

Foreign Bodies

Aspiration of foreign bodies is more frequent in children than adults. Presentation ranges from a barely audible wheeze to total airway obstruction. Initiation of therapy depends on the degree of obstruction. Obviously, for complete obstruction, the treatment is immediately performed. Initially, the hypopharynx should be visualized and swept clean. If this maneuver does not clear the airway, the Heimlich maneuver is performed. Laryngoscopy and removal using a McGill forceps is often successful. If this procedure fails, a needle or surgical cricothyrotomy may be necessary. For lesser degrees of obstruction, a careful physical examination of the oral cavity and a mirror examination of the larynx should be performed. Radiographs can occasionally be helpful in localizing the foreign body or demonstrating air trapping. The object can then be removed in the operating room. Radiologic extraction of foreign bodies is mentioned only to be condemned. A failed extraction in a dark, isolated radiology suite leaves one in a dangerous environment to attempt emergency access. Foreign bodies are best removed in the operating room where adequate light, equipment, and assistance are available.

Peritonsillar Abscess

Peritonsillar abscess usually presents in patients with a history of a sore throat for 5 to 10 days, and frequently after the patient has been taking oral antibiotics. The patient presents with a very sore throat and complains of pain when swallowing. Dysphagia is accompanied by fever and trismus. Examination of the pharynx, which may be difficult secondary to the patient's pain, reveals a bulge at the superior pole of the tonsillar fossa and displacement of the uvula. The examiner should determine if there is actual fluctuance at the superior tonsillar pole. The physician should use a needle to aspirate the area. After confirming the diagnosis, intravenous antibiotics should be initiated and the abscess should be drained.

Retropharyngeal Abscess

Retropharyngeal abscess typically occurs in children less than 3 years old with a history of a progressive upper respiratory infection, but can also occur in adults. The child appears ill, has tachycardia and fever, and may be drooling. The child holds his or her head still and complains of severe pain when it is moved. Oral examination reveals a bulge in the posterior pharyngeal wall. A lateral radiograph demonstrates an increased distance between the posterior pharyngeal wall and the vertebral column, straightening of the cervical spine and, occasionally, a gas pocket in the superior aspect of the abscess. Proper treatment includes admission to the hospital for intravenous antibiotics and drainage under general anesthesia.

Ludwig's Angina

Ludwig's angina is an uncommon cause of airway obstruction. It is characterized by a very tense and diffuse swelling of the submandibular space, which causes intense pain, compression of the trachea, and airway obstruction. The cause of this infection is normally periodontal infection as a result of mouth organisms (Streptococcus, Staphylococcus, mixed aerobes and anaerobes). The patient normally presents with neck pain and difficulty breathing. Physical examination reveals a very tense neck area with brawny induration. High doses of intravenous antibiotics are essential in the management of these patients. Incision and drainage of the soft-tissue space and tracheostomy is at times necessary.

References

1. Ashworth C. Penetrating wounds of the neck. Am J Surg 121:387–391, 1971.
2. Hermon A. Complete cricotracheal separation following blunt trauma to the neck. J Trauma 27:1365–1367, 1987.
3. Fitchett VH. Penetrating wounds of the neck. Arch Surg 99:307–314, 1969.
4. Baxter FJ. Acute epiglottitis in adults. Can J Anesth 35:428–435, 1988.
5. Mayo Smith MF. Acute epiglottitis in adults: An eight year experience in the state of Rhode Island. N Engl J Med 314:1133–1139, 1986.
6. Brenner BE. Comprehensive Management of Respiratory Emergencies. Gaithersburg, MD: Aspen Systems Corp., 1985; pp. 1–13, 241–247.

Bibliography

Beall AC. Surgical management of tracheal trauma. J Trauma 7:248, 1967.
Benumof J. Anesthesia for Thoracic Surgery. Philadelphia: W. B. Saunders, 1987; pp. 264–285.
Diaz JH. Croup and epiglottitis in children: The anesthesiologist as diagnostician. Ann Anesth 64:621–633, 1985.
Eckhauser FE. Tracheostomy complicating massive burn injury. Am J Surg 127:418–423, 1974.
Grillo HC, Mathisen DJ. Current Therapy in Cardiothoracic Surgery. St. Louis: C. V. Mosby, 1989; pp. 51–52, 63–64.
Le May SR. Penetrating wounds of the larynx and cervical trachea. Arch Otolaryngol 94:558–565, 1971.
Mace SE. Acute epiglottitis in adults. Am J Emerg Med 3:543–550, 1985.
Mathisen DJ. Thoracic trauma. Current Reviews in Respiratory and Critical Care 9:19–23, 1986.
Mathisen DJ, Grillo HC. Laryngotracheal trauma. Ann Thorac Surg 43:254–262, 1987.
McGill J. Cricothyrotomy in the emergency department. Ann Emerg Med 11:361–364, 1982.
Myers EM. The management of acute laryngeal trauma. J Trauma 27:448–452, 1987.
Ordog GJ. Bullet wounds to the neck. J Trauma 25:238–246, 1985.
Roberge RJ. Tracheal transection following blunt trauma. Ann Emerg Med 17:47–52, 1988.
Selbst SM. Epiglottitis. Am J Emerg Med 3:342–350, 1983.
Sahn SA. Pulmonary emergencies. New York: Churchill Livingstone, 1982 pp. 61–75, 375–386.
Sofferman RA. Management of laryngotracheal trauma. Am J Surg 141:412–417, 1981.
Stair TO. Adult supraglottitis. Am J Emerg Med 3:512–518, 1985.
Thom SR. Smoke inhalation. Emerg Med Clin North Am 7:371–385, 1989.
Wilkins E Jr. MGH Textbook of Emergency Medicine: General Thoracic Emergencies. Baltimore: Williams & Wilkins, 1989; pp. 609–627, 650–652.
Wood J. Penetrating neck injuries: Recommendations for selective management. J Trauma 29:602–605, 1989.

CHAPTER 28

Airway Considerations for Ear, Nose, and Throat Surgery

Michael P. Joseph, M.D.

The ear, nose, and throat surgeon has a special interest in the anatomy and physiology of the upper airway. This chapter offers some thoughts about the airway.

OTOLOGY

Some middle ear surgery (eg, stapedectomy) is done with local anesthesia and sedation. Mastoid surgery requires general anesthesia with no paralysis, because monitoring of the facial nerve is important. Controlled hypotension should be maintained until any packing of the cavity has been completed. Placing the mastoid dressing requires head motion; the patient must not wake up too soon. The surgeon should request that nitrous oxide be stopped before a tympanic membrane graft is placed into position.

NASAL, SINUS, AND ORBITAL SURGERY

Many nasal and sinus procedures can be done with local anesthesia and intravenous sedation. When general anesthesia is required, a local anesthesia with epinephrine is frequently used to minimize blood loss. Bleeding from mucosal surfaces can be decreased with topical vasoconstriction; eg, oxymetazolone. Controlled hypotension is also helpful. Packing, frequently placed in the nose, creates partial or complete nasal obstruction.

Surgical access to the orbit can be gained through the paranasal sinuses. Once the sinuses and orbit have been opened, it is inappropriate to place packs, because the packs would push against the orbit and optic nerve. In these cases, it is especially important that the emergence from anesthesia be gentle and controlled. Sudden or violent awakening can result in increased bleeding and more coughing, and also bleeding into the orbit.

When there has been loss of bone (by accident or surgery) in the sinuses (particularly ethmoid or sphenoid) or along the orbit, great care must be taken in the introduction of catheters or tubes into the nose, because there is risk of intracranial or intraorbital damage.

When there is an opening in the skull base

(eg, severe head trauma) topical vasoconstrictors (which might enter the cerebrospinal fluid) and positive pressure ventilation should be avoided. In cases of pneumocephalus, nitrous oxide must not be used.

HEAD AND NECK SURGERY

Oral Cavity, Oropharynx, and Nasopharynx

The lesion and the planned procedure determine whether nasotracheal or orotracheal intubation is preferable. When there is likely to be great difficulty with intubation or the possibility of bleeding or aspiration of pus from an abscess that ruptures, an awake intubation (with a fiberoptic endoscope) and/or a tracheostomy should be considered. The surgeon should be able to describe in detail the extent of the lesion.

If postoperative airway compromise is expected, a nasal airway or prolonged intubation or tracheotomy should be considered.

Hypopharynx and Larynx

Large tumors of the larynx and hypopharynx may necessitate awake fiberoptic intubation or tracheotomy. If debulking of the tumor at biopsy will improve the airway, intubation is reasonable. If there will be compromise of the airway even after biopsy and debulking, then tracheotomy is preferable. When there is a small lesion of the true vocal cord, a small endotracheal tube should be used, so there is room to work around it. If the carbon dioxide laser is used, burning of the endotracheal tube must be avoided. Usually, a metal tube is used.

Superior laryngeal nerve block can make endoscopic laryngeal procedures more comfortable in awake patients. Even when the endoscopic laryngeal procedure is being done with general anesthesia, superior laryngeal nerve block may be of use in reducing the bradycardiac stimulus that accompanies suspension of the larynx.

Surgery for vocal cord paralysis (Teflon injection or laryngoplasty) moves one vocal cord toward the midline to improve the voice. It is done with topical anesthesia and intravenous sedation, because the patient's voice is monitored to determine the appropriate vocal cord position.

When there has been radiation for laryngeal or hypopharyngeal cancer, edema and airway obstruction can follow even gentle endoscopy and biopsy. Intravenous steroids and careful observation are important.

Neck

For may procedures in the neck, the location of nerves is confirmed by stimulation; paralysis should be avoided. After radiation therapy, a neck dissection may result in laryngeal edema; a tracheostomy should be considered. Loss of both jugular veins (even staged bilateral neck dissections) leads to facial and cerebral edema. When a procedure includes bilateral neck dissection, it is usual that one or both jugular veins be preserved. Because neck dissections may injure the vagus or phrenic nerves, one may anticipate tachycardia or paralysis of the diaphragm. Bradycardia or hypotension (or both) may accompany a dissection at the carotid bifurcation.

CHAPTER 29

Airway Management of Tracheal Stenosis

Douglas J. Mathisen, M.D., and Hermes C. Grillo, M.D.

Tracheal stenosis resulting from trauma, neoplasm, or postintubation injury often presents as a life-threatening emergency. Physicians involved with airway management should be well versed in the management of these most difficult problems. A thorough understanding of presenting signs and symptoms of tracheal stenosis is necessary to promptly recognize the problem, and an awareness of the pitfalls that may be encountered is necessary to avoid loss of life or serious complications. Proper anesthetic technique is crucial to the successful management of these problems. The rigid bronchoscope remains a crucial instrument in the management of these difficult airway problems, and surgeons should continue to be adept at using it.

TRACHEAL STENOSIS

The compromised airway presents a formidable challenge to physicians caring for such problems. Few other emergencies require such prompt recognition of the problem and need for effective immediate action as the compromised airway. The ability to identify the problem and secure an airway quickly often is the difference between life and death for the patient. Surgeons and anesthesiologists should be well versed in the recognition of the problem and the methods needed to secure airways in

these difficult circumstances. The ability to skillfully secure the airway may not only be life saving, but ultimately avoids the need for lifelong, permanent tracheostomy in some patients.

Tracheal stenosis can be thought of in three broad categories: post-traumatic, postintubation, and neoplastic. Many of the principles of airway management are common to all three, but because of subtle differences, it is important to discuss each separately.

Post-traumatic

Laryngotracheal trauma may be life threatening. These injuries can occur in the most remote area or in the busiest metropolitan setting. Emergency ward physicians, general surgeons, thoracic surgeons, anesthesiologists, and otolaryngologists should be well versed in the manifestations and management of these injuries. Successful outcome demands prompt recognition, skillful and expeditious management of difficult airways, careful evaluation of associated injuries, and careful planning of the proper treatment of each injury. Failure to accomplish each of these considerations properly may result in death, multiple reoperations, or lifelong tracheostomy or gastrostomy.

Etiology

Damage in blunt cervical injury may occur in the airway at any level from the hyoid bone, through the larynx, into the cervical trachea. The pharyngoesophageal junction or upper esophagus may also be injured and partially or totally disrupted. Motor vehicle accidents that result in rapid deceleration, which causes the passenger to strike the extended neck against the dashboard or steering wheel, produce the majority of laryngotracheal injuries. This has been referred to as the "padded dashboard syndrome." Direct injury to the laryngotracheal area compresses the airway against the vertebral bodies, resulting in a crushing injury. Hyperextension of the neck causes an avulsion injury by pulling the larynx away from the distal trachea, which is restricted in its excursion by surrounding tissue and the left mainstem bronchus beneath the aortic arch. Striking the neck against an unseen wire or chain while riding a motorcycle or snowmobile accounts for a number of these injuries. Penetrating trauma from knife or gunshot wounds occurs much less frequently.

Signs and Symptoms

Acute Cervical Tracheal Injury. Acute cervicotracheal injuries produce a spectrum of signs and symptoms. A high index of suspicion is imperative to avoid catastrophic consequences. Presentation may range from no visible external signs of trauma, to abrasion and contusion, to extensive laceration that exposes cervical structures. The airway may appear to be completely patent or may be absent in an apneic patient. The combination of the type of accident and signs or symptoms of hemoptysis, localized pain, local contusion, subcutaneous emphysema, a change in voice, hoarseness, inspiratory stridor, or respiratory distress should alert one to the possibility of laryngotracheal injury.

Chronic Cervical Tracheal Injury. Failure to recognize injuries immediately may result in progressive airway obstruction as cicatrization occurs and stenosis develops. The rapidity with which these injuries develop depends on the extent of the initial injury. Progressive respiratory distress or stridor in a patient who has sustained recent trauma in the area should alert one to the possibility of laryngotracheal injury.

Acute Intrathoracic Tracheobronchial Injury. Major pneumothorax, unilateral or bilateral, associated with a large air leak in which the lung fails to reexpand completely after placement of a chest tube warns of the likely presence of a significant tracheobronchial injury. The presentation may be more subtle, with pneumothorax responding to pleural suction and cessation of air leak. In patients with the pleura obliterated, there may be no pneumothorax. Subcutaneous or mediastinal emphysema, with or without pneumothorax, may be the only finding present with a major intrathoracic airway injury. However, respiratory distress may be present secondary to complete transection of the airway or to tension pneumothorax. A high degree of suspicion is necessary to diagnose correctly the more subtle presentations. Bronchoscopy should be performed whenever suspicion exists.

Chronic Intrathoracic Tracheobronchial Injury. In addition to signs of progressive respiratory distress that may be seen in patients with laryngotracheal injuries, patients with injuries at the carina or mainstem bronchi level may have air trapping in one lung, with total atelectasis, or obstructive pneumonitis. The history of a recent chest injury and these findings should raise the suspicion of this type of injury.

Associated Injuries

Injuries of the magnitude suficient to cause severe laryngotracheal damage may also cause injury to the esophagus, cervical spine, or vascular structures. If time and circumstances permit, each patient should be carefully examined for these injuries. If there is a stable airway, a soft collar should be placed and cervical spine roentgenograms obtained to search for fractures or subluxation. Cervical spine injuries may threaten the spinal cord and dictate the course of surgical management. In such a case, the first step, excluding the possible need for urgent tracheostomy, may be the placement of tongs to provide cervical traction stabilization. Extension of the neck for intubation, bronchoscopy, or esophagoscopy or flexion to relieve tension on the anastomosis must be avoided; the cervical esophagus is frequently injured in accidents of this nature. Contrast studies of the upper esophagus are helpful, but sometimes are difficult to interpret. Esophagoscopy and direct inspection of the esophagus at the time of surgery should be carried out when the possibility exists that the esophagus was involved. Cervical spine injury obviously demands special caution and probably the omission of esophagoscopy. Failure to recognize an esophageal injury may lead to mediastinal sepsis, tracheo-esphageal fistula, and disruption of airway repair.

Vascular injuries may occur; the carotid artery, innominate artery, or the aorta itself may be injured. Careful search should be made for differential pulses, localized bruits, or radiographic signs of aortic tears. Angiography may be required to evaluate these injuries.

Radiologic Assessment

Acute Injuries. Depending on the severity of the injury and the status of the airway, radiologic assessment of these injuries may be helpful. Plain roentgenograms of the neck may reveal distortion or disruption of the tracheal airway. Most commonly, air is seen dissecting cervical planes, with extension up to the base of the skull. Cervical spine radiographs, contrast studies of the esophagus, chest roentgenograms, and angiograms may be required to assess associated injuries. Tomograms of the larynx and trachea may be helpful in evaluating less emergent injuries. Computed tomography (CT) may be valuable in certain circumstances, but is generally not necessary. Intrathoracic tracheal disruption most often leads to mediastinal emphysema or unilateral or bilateral pneumothoraces, with or without evidence of mediastinal displacement. Excessive time should not be spent in preoperative studies, because there may be acute obstruction of an apparently stable airway.

Airway Management. The most crucial aspect of laryngotracheal trauma after its recognition is the management of the airway. Apneic patients should be managed by thrusting the jaw forward and holding the patient in the "sniffing position." This may help align a transected airway. Endotracheal intubation can be attempted while preparations are being made for emergency tracheostomy. Repeated attempts at intubation should be avoided. Whenever doubt exists as to the status of the airway, emergency tracheostomy should be performed. If the patient has a compromised airway, but is still breathing, attempts at intubation or inspection of the airway with a flexible bronchoscope should be done in the operating room with everything set to perform emergency tracheostomy. An endotracheal tube can be placed over a flexible bronchoscope and guided into place over the flexible bronchoscope. Repeated attempts at intubation should be avoided and emergency tracheostomy performed without hesitation; this is best done

under local anesthesia with the patient breathing spontaneously. In the totally separated trachea, the distal end may retract into the mediastinum and may be difficult to locate. It is best found by inserting a finger in the area where the trachea should have been, locating the distal trachea by palpation, and grasping it with a clamp to bring it to the surface of the wound. An endotracheal tube can then be inserted and the airway secured. If repair is not contemplated, the divided distal end of the trachea can be sewn to the skin. In this circumstance, the proximal end can be sewn to the skin as a separate stoma or closed and a drain placed next to it. If the trachea is partially disrupted, a tracheostomy tube inserted through the damaged area is the best alternative to repair and should not under any circumstance be placed through noninjured, viable trachea. Every attempt should be made to conserve viable trachea, whether securing or repairing an airway.

Management of the airway of injuries of the distal trachea, carina, or proximal mainstem bronchi can be very difficult. Awareness of the injury allows the anesthetist and the surgeon to plan accordingly. Use of double-lumen tubes should be avoided because of the possibility of extending the injury. A long endotracheal tube could be positioned beyond the injury or into the appropriate mainstem bronchus to provide single-lung ventilation. This should be done very carefully with the aid of the flexible bronchoscope to serve as a guide and to check final position. Great care must be taken not to extend the injury. A long, uncut endotracheal tube or, preferably, a more flexible Tovell tube with a proximal extension may allow the surgeon to manipulate the tube into the appropriate bronchus at the time of operation. If available, a high-frequency ventilation catheter can be passed through an endotracheal tube and placed in proper position.

For those situations in which a long endotracheal tube was not used or cannot be positioned properly, a sterile endotracheal tube (preferably, a Tovell tube) with appropriate connecting tubing can be used to intubate the opposite lung across the wound itself. The connecting tube is then passed off the operating field to the anesthetist. Repair of the injury is by intermittent removal of the endotracheal tube and individual placement of the sutures. After all of the sutures are placed, the tube is removed, the airway approximated, and ventilation continued through the original endotracheal tube.

Results

It is beyond the scope of this chapter to present details of surgical repair or detailed analysis of results of treatment. Interested readers are referred elsewhere. Suffice it to say that, if properly managed, most traumatic airway injuries can be managed satisfactorily with restitution of a normal airway and voice. We have treated 10 patients with acute injuries. All had successful repair of their airways and preservation of their voice. Seventeen patients have been treated for delayed traumatic laryngotracheal stenosis; vocal cord paralysis was documented in 14. Concomitant esophageal injury was repaired in four patients. Eight required intralaryngeal procedures prior to repair of the laryngotracheal stenosis. All patients except one have a good airway, and 16 of 17 have a good voice.

Airway Obstruction Due to Neoplasm

Primary or secondary neoplasms of the trachea (the latter include principally thyroid carcinoma, laryngeal carcinoma, carcinoma of the lung and, less commonly, of the esophagus or metastasis from a distance) may cause acute airway obstruction. With secondary tumors, the patient frequently has a history related either to the concurrent presence of the primary tumor or to a previous history of tumor. With occult secondary tumors like thyroid cancer or with primary tumors of the trachea, there may be history of hemoptysis, dyspnea on exertion, wheezing, cough, hoarseness, or dysphagia. Patients with primary tumors of the trachea who have only shortness of breath and wheezing are often diagnosed late because chest radiographs show normal lung fields. The diagnosis of "adult-onset asthma" is frequently made. Such patients may already be on high doses of steroids when organic obstruction is finally diagnosed.

Diagnostic Studies

The presence of any of the above symptoms or signs without adequate explanation is justification for simple but careful radiologic studies. These studies define the presence and extent of tumor in almost every case. The use of an intratracheal contrast medium is generally unnecessary. The following studies are helpful:

1. Chest film (posteroanterior, lateral, and oblique) centered high enough to obtain good views of the trachea.
2. Anteroposterior overpenetrated high-kilovolt view including the larynx and trachea to the carina.
3. Lateral view of the neck in extension with swallowing to elevate the upper trachea.
4. Fluoroscopy of the larynx and trachea with necessary spot radiographs and opacification of the esophagus with barium.
5. Anteroposterior, lateral, and oblique linear laminagraphy of the trachea, if necessary, following the prior views.

The overpenetrated anteroposterior view is often the most useful view in obtaining a general picture of the extent of the tumor and its involvement of the trachea, its extension into the mediastinum, and its relationship to the normal portions of the airway. The fluoroscopic views provide information on the involvement of the recurrent laryngeal nerves, any variability in the airway, and involvement of the esophagus. Laminagraphy may give additional precise information about invasion of tracheal and laryngeal walls and the extent of mediastinal and carinal involvement. Some patients may be nearly obstructed, and thus the use of even a topical anesthetic and liquid contrast medium may be contraindicated. Although insufflated tantalum studies may be useful, in general the quality of the information obtained from the simple radiographic studies described is such that no further data are required to plan the next diagnostic and therapeutic steps. Xeroradiography studies provide very much the same information that radiographic studies do, but are often dramatic in quality. If there is a question of involvement of the superior vena cava, innominate artery, or pulmonary arteries, angiography occasionally becomes helpful. CT has thus far added little additional information to the examination of the trachea. It does, however, add valuable information about the extraluminal extent of tumor and enlarged lymph nodes. Magnetic resonance imaging (MRI) has not yet been fully evaluated in tracheal pathology. It does offer the advantage of sagittal and coronal views, which may prove helpful in evaluating the extent of involvement of neoplasms.

Anesthesia

The anesthetic management of patients with a compromised airway is crucial to a successful outcome. We have employed in virtually every case the same technique used for patients with tracheal stenosis. This has been described in detail by Wilson.[1] Deep halothane inhalation anesthesia has been the technique used. This allows the patient to maintain spontaneous ventilation throughout the procedure. Induction can be time consuming and requires patience on the part of the anesthesiologist and surgeon. Any disadvantage this may impose is greatly outweighed by the tremendous advantage of having the patient spontaneously ventilating throughout the procedure. This is especially important initially, before the exact nature of the obstruction is known. The surgeon has more time to establish an airway in this circumstance than in the apneic patient. During the course of tumor removal, difficulties in maintaining the airway may be encountered, and the patient's ability to breathe is often times the only thing that carries him or her through a rather difficult period. We have deliberately avoided the use of muscle relaxants and agents that depress the respiratory drive. Patients need to be able to clear secretions, debris, and blood from their airways postoperatively. Anesthetic agents that interfere with this function should obviously be avoided.

It is important that the surgeon be in attendance during the induction of anesthesia. Sudden compromise of the airway may occur and immediate insertion of a rigid bronchoscope may be required to secure the airway. This implies that the surgeon and his or her assistants be prepared to have all of the instruments available to establish an emergency airway. We had no occasions to perform emergency tracheostomy, because all patients could be intubated with a rigid bronchoscope. Knowledge of the location of the tumor makes this task much easier.

The technique of inserting a rigid bronchoscope should be familiar to all. It is important to have available rigid bronchoscopes of graded sizes (3.5 to 9 mm). A small pediatric rigid bronchoscope is often the only bronchoscope that can be inserted through very proximal, tight malignant strictures. This allows establishment of an airway; subsequently, larger bronchoscopes can be inserted. For more distal tumors, insertion of a larger bronchoscope in the proximal airway allows careful inspection and suctioning of any secretions. It is possible in most tumors to pass a #8 rigid bronchoscope along one side of the tumor to establish an airway and remove retained secretions. It is important to establish an airway

initially and clear the airway of any retained secretions before proceeding with removal of the tumor. This allows the patient to be maximally ventilated at the start of the procedure. Inspection of the distal airway will aid the bronchoscopist in reestablishing the airway once the actual procedure has started. It is important to establish the axis of the airway when the coring out of the tumor commences. The endoscopist should stay parallel to the axis at all times to avoid penetrating the wall and creating a pneumothorax or injuring the pulmonary artery. It is important to first biopsy the tumor to determine its consistency and vascularity. Once this has been established, a decision can then be made whether repeated removal of the tumor with bronchoscopic forceps should be attempted or to use the tip of the bronchoscope to "core out" the tumor. If the tumor is thought to be of sufficient consistency and vascularity to allow a large portion of it to be removed, the rigid bronchoscope is then used in a corkscrew-type fashion. The beveled tip of the bronchoscope is used to shave off a large piece of the tumor. Most tumors are of such consistency that this is easily accomplished and does not require excessive force. The anesthesiologist should stop any assisted ventilation of the patient to avoid forcing debris and tissue more distally into the airway. The piece of tumor can then be grasped with forceps and removed, or may be aspirated. Occasionally, it is necessary to remove large pieces of tumor and bronchoscope at the same time from the airway. The endoscopist should intermittently cease removing tumor, reestablish the airway, and allow the anesthesiologist to ventilate the patient. This also allows the bronchoscope to tamponade any bleeding that might be occurring from the surface of the tumor. Once sufficient amounts of tumor have been removed, it is important to clean the airway of debris; this may be aided by irrigation. The use of the flexible bronchoscope through the rigid bronchoscope allows suctioning at the subsegmental level.

Control of Hemorrhage

The misconception of the likelihood of major hemororhage remains the single greatest obstacle to widespread acceptance of the technique of endoscopic removal of obstructing malignancies of the airway. This misconception stems from experiences in the early days of endoscopy, chiefly from the rare hypervascular carcinoid, and has been perpetuated. In reality, major hemorrhage is uncommon. Minor bleeding is easily controlled with simple measures. Irrigation with saline is the first maneuver to diminish bleeding. This is frequently all that is necessary. Diluted epinephrine (1 to 10,000 per 1 mL) or epinephrine-soaked pledgets on long applicators will stop persistent oozing. Various methods of tamponade are also successful in managing any persistent bleeding that does not respond to the previous methods. The use of the rigid bronchoscope to tamponade the raw surface of the tumor is effective. For bleeding from the mainstem bronchus or more distal airway, dental packs or Fogarty venous occlusion catheters can be used to tamponade bleeding. Fogarty venous occlusion balloons can be left in place if necessary. The use of a carefully placed endotracheal tube is also effective in controlling bleeding that persists beyond the previously mentioned measures. Placing the endotracheal tube so that the balloon is resting against the raw surface and then inflating the balloon serves to tamponade and control any active bleeding. This measure has rarely been necessary. Insulated electrodes are available to coagulate bleeding points if needed. It goes without saying that any abnormalities in coagulation should be corrected prior to the procedure itself. The use of fresh-frozen plasma and platelets at times may be necessary to correct these abnormalities.

Tumors that may be dangerously vascular are some carcinoid tumors and hemangiomas or arteriovenous malformations presenting in the tracheal wall. Obviously, biopsy of these must be avoided. Examination with Storz-Hopkins telescopes should permit identification of such tumors. In such cases, an endotracheal tube may be slipped past the lesion and surgical resection performed.

Once the airway is established, further workup of the patient may be done in a leisurely way and, if the patient is an appropriate candidate for surgery, elective operation may be planned in deliberate fashion.

During the past 8 years, we have treated 56 patients with obstructing neoplasms of the airway. The location of the obstructing neoplasm have been as follows: trachea, 16; carina, 14; and bronchus, 16. A single bronchoscopy was sufficient to establish the airway in 96%. There were four deaths within 2 weeks of core-out. All four occurred in patients with extensive disease and postobstructive pneumonia. Two of the patients had failed radiation therapy. Nineteen complications occurred in 11 patients, including intraoperative arrhythmias requiring prolonged treatments, 6; pneumonia,

6; mild hypoxia/hypercarbia, 2; bleeding (500 mL), 3; pneumothorax, 2; and laryngeal edema, 1. There were *no* episodes of major hemorrhage and *no* intraoperative deaths. Most patients went on to definitive resection or radiation therapy.

Although the laser can be used similarly to open an obstructed airway, it is more time consuming, tedious, and accomplishes nothing more than the procedure described in the majority of cases. Because of the amount of tumor to be removed, it is frequently necessary to repeat laser treatments to achieve a patent airway. The underlying cost of the laser must be taken into account and the cost of repeat treatments that may be necessary. Indeed, some physicians who regularly use the laser through the rigid bronchoscope employ it to clear the tumor so it can be removed by the rigid bronchoscope or to "touch-up" bleeding points. Neither of these are generally necessary with the technique described.

Postintubation Injuries

Wide spread use of "low-pressure" cuffs on endotracheal tubes and tracheostomy tubes has not eliminated postintubation tracheal stenosis. The low-pressure cuff that is overinflated to provide a seal quickly becomes a high-pressure cuff because of inherently limited extensibility of the plastic material from which it is made. The cuffs have obviously not eliminated the other causes of postintubation stenosis, specifically prolonged endotracheal intubation, tube tip injuries, excessively large tracheostomy tubes, improper technique of tracheostomy, and excessive leverage by the tracheostomy tube on the stomal margin.

Signs and Symptoms

The patient has a history of intubation, often a recent one, and presents with signs of upper airway obstruction, namely progressive dyspnea on exertion, wheeze and stridor, and possibly intermittent obstruction with mucus plugs. Such symptoms appear at rest when the airway is under 6 mm in diameter. Sometimes the patient is found to have an airway diameter of only 3 to 4 mm, a point at which obstruction can easily occur due to a mucus plug.

Radiologic Assessment

Radiographs of the trachea reveal the lesion in every case. Overpenetrated films and tomograms are of use. Usually, bronchoscopy does not have to be done until definitive treatment is given. In an extreme emergency, an endotracheal tube may be inserted above the lesion, the airway suctioned, and forced ventilation given. This, of course, is not possible if the obstruction is in the immediate subglottic level. No attempt should be made to force the tube blindly through the stenosis. A word of caution should be mentioned about flexible bronchoscopy in this setting. The unsuspecting endoscopist may encounter critical airway stenosis and precipitated obstruction from secretions, blood, edema, or by occluding the narrow opening with the flexible bronchoscope. *For this reason, flexible bronchoscopy under local anesthesia should rarely be done in the presence of severe obstruction.* The patient should be taken to the operating room immediately and given inhalation anesthesia, as described for tumor management. The surgeon must be immediately at hand with emergency bronchoscopic equipment laid out on the table in case acute airway obstruction occurs during induction of anesthesia. One should not attempt to dilate an obstructed airway under local anesthesia.

The best method of emergency management is to dilate the obstructed airway under direct vision, using a rigid bronchoscope. The Jackson type of bronchoscope with a somewhat rounded and beveled tip is preferrable to the sharper tip of a Storz bronchoscope for this purpose. A flexible bronchoscope is useless. Frequently, the obstruction is visualized through an adult-size rigid bronchoscope and an initial dilatation made with a Jackson plastic-tipped or woven-tipped esophageal bougie through the bronchoscope. Once initiated, dilatation is continued by sequential placement of pediatric rigid bronchoscopes (selecting from the 3.5-, 4-, 5-, and 6-mm sizes, then progressing to adult sizes 7, 8, or 9 if the lesions can be dilated to this size). These bronchoscopes are introduced with a corkscrewing motion, taking care not to use excessive force, which can rupture the normal tissue more easily than a firm stenosis. As each bronchoscope is passed, the patient is suctioned and ventilated until stable before the next size bronchoscope is passed. Introduction of the bronchoscope is facilitated by the use of a Jackson laryngoscope with the metal slide removed, because the smaller diameter bronchoscopes are shorter.

Once the lesion is dilated, there is no urgent need to proceed to emergency operation, because the patient will maintain an airway from this point on for days to weeks. It is now possible to study the patient in detail, correct serious medical problems, wean him or her from steroids, if he or she is on high doses, or otherwise prepare him or her for elective tracheal reconstruction under optimal conditions. The laser generally adds nothing, either in the emergency treatment or as definitive treatment. Only a few web-like stenoses, a rare occurrence, or granulomas can be effectively treated with long-term results by lasering.

If the patient with stenosis who has been dilated to relieve the acute emergency must be maintained for a long period prior to primary repair, a tracheostomy tube or T-tube may be placed. If it is possible to fashion the stoma through the already damaged segment of trachea, this is optimal. It is preferable not to damage more trachea by placing a stoma either just above or below the area of injury. In a low retrosternal stenosis, the stoma may safely be put in the upper trachea at the usual point in the second and third tracheal rings and a long tracheostomy tube inserted to traverse the dilated stenosis. It is dangerous to place a tube above a stenosis, because the patient can obstruct below the tracheostomy tube tip, despite an illusion of security.

Familiarity with the presentation of tracheal stenosis is important to all who may care for airway problems. Knowledge of how to secure the airway is crucial to the successful management of these most difficult airway problems.

References

1. Wilson RS. Tracheostomy and tracheal reconstruction. In Kaplan JA (ed). Thoracic Anesthesia. New York: Churchill Livingstone, 1983; pp. 421–445.

Bibliography

Dumon JF. YAG Laser Bronchoscopy, vol. 5. New York: Praeger, 1985.
Dumon JF, Reboud E, Garbe L, Aucomte F, Meric B. Treatment of tracheobronchial lesions by laser photoresection. Chest 81:278–284, 1982.
Dumon JF, Shapshay S, Bourcereau J, Cavaliere S, Meric B, Garbi N, Beamis J. Principles for safety in application of neodymium-YAG laser in bronchology. Chest 86:163–168, 1984.
Mathisen DJ, Grillo HC. Laryngotracheal trauma. Ann Thorac Surg 43:254–262, 1987.
Mathisen DJ, Grillo HC. Laryngotracheal trauma—Acute and chronic. In Grillo HC, Eschapasse H (eds). International Trends in General Thoracic Surgery, vol. 2. Philadelphia: W. B. Saunders, 1987; pp. 117–123.
Mathisen DJ, Grillo HC. Emergency and palliative relief

of airway obstruction due to neoplasm or inflammation. In International Trends in General Thoracic Surgery, vol. 4. Philadelphia: W. B. Saunders, 1989; pp. 48–51.

Mathisen DJ, Grillo HC. Endoscopic relief of malignant airway obstruction. Ann Thorac Surg 48:469–475, 1989.

McElvein RB, Zorn GL Jr. Indications, results, and complications of bronchoscopic carbon dioxide laser therapy. Ann Surg 199:522–525, 1984.

Montgomery WW. Management of glottic stenosis. Otolaryngol Clin North Am 12:841, 1979.

Sessions DG, Ogura JH, Heeneman H. Surgical management of bilateral vocal cord paralysis. Laryngoscope 86:559, 1976.

Shapshay SW, Healy GB, Davis RK, Strong MS. Endoscopic management of airway obstruction from tracheo-bronchial neoplasia: Use of the carbon dioxide laser. Lahey Clinic Foundation Bulletin 32:29–38, 1983.

Toty L, Personne C, Colchen A, LeRoy M, Vourc'h G. Laser treatment of postintubation lesions. In Grillo HC, Eschapasse H (eds). Internation Trends in General Thoracic Surgery, vol. 2. Philadelphia: W. B. Saunders, 1987; pp. 31–37.

Vourc'h G, Fischler M, Personne C, Colchen A. Anesthetic management during Nd-YAG laser resection for major tracheobronchial obstructing tumors. Anethesiology 61:636–637, 1984.

Vourc'h G, Tannieres ML, Toty L, Personne C. Anesthetic management of tracheal surgery using the neodymium-YAG laser. Br J Anaesth 52:993–997, 1980.

CHAPTER 30

Hemoptysis, Minor and Massive

Ashby C. Moncure, M.D.

ETIOLOGY

Minor Hemoptysis

Coughing up small amounts of blood is fairly common. It may result in blood-streaked sputum, or there may be gross hemoptysis of small quantities of blood. In this clinical setting, after excluding the nasopharynx and the gastrointestinal tract as a source, one must consider a number of possible causes of hemoptysis. Many of these patients are also found to be hypertensive. Other frequent causes of minor hemoptysis include bronchitis, bronchiectasis, carcinoma of the lung, and tuberculosis. Less common causes are inflammatory processes, such as a lung abscess or necrotizing pneumonia; other neoplasms, such as bronchial adenoma or metastatic tumor; and vascular disorders, such as pulmonary embolism, diseases causing pulmonary hypertension, conditions causing pulmonary vasculitis, arteriovenous malformations (AVMs), pulmonary hemosiderosis and amyloidosis of the respiratory tract; and traumatic causes, such as pulmonary contusion, fractured bronchus, or aspiration of a foreign body. Finally, hemorrhagic disorders, such as a complication of anticoagulation therapy or a hemorrhagic diathesis, may present as minor hemoptysis.[1–4]

Massive Hemoptysis

Massive hemoptysis, generally defined as the loss of 600 mL or more of blood in 24 hours, fortunately is a much less common clinical event. In several series of patients who underwent surgical intervention for massive hemoptysis, bronchiectasis, pulmonary abscess, pulmonary tuberculosis, and primary or metastatic pulmonary neoplasms proved to be the leading causes.[5–7] In recent years, massive hemoptysis has complicated the use of balloon-tipped, flow-directed pulmonary artery (Swan-Ganz) catheters used in monitoring left-sided cardiac filling pressures. This apparently occurs secondary to injury of the pulmonary arterial branch by the pressure of the balloon. Less common causes for massive hemoptysis include rupture of a thoracic aortic aneurysm into the left lung; erosion of the vascular suture lines placed in repair of myocardial or thoracic aortic defect, usually into the left lung; and massive hemorrhage from necrotic excavating lesions such as those seen in Wegener's granulomatosis.

DIAGNOSIS AND MANAGEMENT

Minor Hemoptysis

The clinician's concerns in the event of minor hemoptysis are to define the disease process that is causing the hemoptysis and, if possible, to identify the precise site of the bleeding in the event of the onset of superimposed massive hemoptysis with the threat of asphyxiation or exsanguination. A careful and detailed history and physical examination may suggest the diagnosis, but radiographs of the chest, including conventional films and computed tomography (CT) scanning (with "pulmonary windows"), and ultimately the bronchoscopic examination, are usually necessary in confirming the diagnosis and determining the precise site of bleeding.

The initial management of the patient with gross, but not massive, hemoptysis should include admission to the hospital, bed rest with the affected side, if known from the symptoms or radiographic studies of the chest, kept dependent to minimize aspiration of blood to the opposite normal side, and the administration of cough suppressants and the treatment of bronchopulmonary infection and systemic hypertension, if present. Tracheal intubation and suctioning equipment must be readily available nearby. Bronchoscopic examination is best done soon after the bleeding has subsided in order to allow identification of the anatomic source of the hemorrhage.[8]

Approximately 30% of patients presenting with gross hemoptysis have no abnormalities demonstrable on radiographs of the chest,[9] and even with careful fiberoptic bronchoscopic study (which may allow examination to fifth-order bronchi), the cause of the hemoptysis cannot be determined in 15% of patients. Studies of sputum, including cytologic examination, Ziehl-Neelsen staining for acid-fast bacilli, and cultures for acid-fast bacilli, other bacteria, and fungi may be unrevealing. Pulmonary tomographic and fluoroscopic examinations, and particularly CT scanning and magnetic resonance imaging (MRI), may be helpful in further evaluation of the thorax. Follow-up studies of patients in whom the cause for the hemoptysis is not clear should include serial radiographs of the chest, even though the likelihood of detecting the evolution of a small carcinoma or tuberculosis is small. If there is recurrent hemoptysis, the evaluation should be repeated, including careful fiberoptic bronchoscopic study with selective segmental bronchoscopic washings; if the diagnosis is in doubt, repeat CT and MRI studies, bronchographic examination, pulmonary and selective bronchial arteriographic examination, and cardiac evaluation.

In the 15% of patients in whom the exact cause of the hemoptysis cannot be determined, termed "essential hemoptysis," usually individuals who experience single episodes of bleeding and who have minimal or no respiratory symptoms, normal chest radiograph findings and totally normal bronchoscopy examination and in whom bronchial washings reveal no evidence of infections or malignancy, it is rare to subsequently identify the precise cause. In follow-up of a series of 81 patients for 1 to 10 years after the episode of hemoptysis, in only three patients with "essential hemoptysis" was the cause later identified, all secondary to pulmonary vascular disease.[10]

Massive Hemoptysis

Massive hemoptysis must be approached as a clear-cut medical emergency, because acute asphyxiation secondary to aspirated blood and exsanguination threaten the patient's life. A thoracic surgeon must be an integral member of the professional group caring for the patient. Massive bleeding from the tracheobronchial tree mandates immediate endoscopic identification of its source, which is best accomplished with a large, rigid bronchoscope (Fig. 30–1). This instrument not only permits the efficient use of suction and thereby increases the likelihood of lateralizing the source of the hemorrhage as well as identification of the precise bronchus from which the hemorrhage issues, but also allows placement of a bronchial

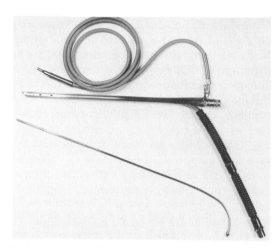

Figure 30–1. A 9-40 Jackson bronchoscope with side-ventilating portal and a metal suction device. The use of this instrument, rather than the fiberoptic bronchoscope, is necessary in determining the appropriate diagnosis of massive hemoptysis and in achieving its temporary control with placement of a bronchial blocker (see text).

blocker (inflated endobronchial Fogarty embolectomy catheter balloon).[11] This maneuver may allow prevention of aspiration of blood into the uninvolved side with its attendant gas-exchange problems. Subsequent operative management is indicated to control the hemorrhage, the procedure to be done being dictated by the causative disease process and its distribution.[12, 13]

The usual indications for emergency thoracotomy in this setting are (1) life-threatening hemoptysis in excess of 600 mL/24 hours, (2) accurate localization of the bleeding source, (3) adequate pulmonary reserve (ie, FEV_1 greater than 40% to 50% of predicted values), and (4) failure of medical therapy. Failing the above, repeated attempts at endobronchial tamponade or bronchial arterial embolization may be the more appropriate approach.[14]

In accomplishing thoracotomy and the pulmonary resection or vascular procedure necessary to control the hemorrhage, the anesthesiologist and surgeon must be ever mindful of the necessity to prevent the aspiration of blood into the unaffected bronchial tree, which is the "down lung" in the lateral decubitus position the patient assumes when positioned for posterolateral thoracotomy. Hence, a double-lumen endotracheal tube must be accurately placed, or failing this, a "bronchial blocker" must be placed in the affected main stem bronchus to assure that the down lung is protected from aspiration of blood during the conduct of the operation. Assiduously clearing the bronchial tree of the down lung prior to the conclusion of the operation is also important in achieving the goal of adequate gas exchange in a spontaneously ventilating postoperative patient.

References

1. American Thoracic Society. The management of hemoptysis. Am Rev Respir Dis 93:471–474, 1966.
2. Lyons HA. Differential diagnosis of hemoptysis and its treatment. ATS News 26–30, 1976.
3. Sonders CR, Smith AT. The clinical significance of hemoptysis. N Engl J Med 247:790–793, 1952.
4. Pursel SE, Lindskog GE. Hemoptysis. Am Rev Respir Dis 84:329–336, 1961.
5. Crocco JA, Rooney JJ, Fankushen DS, DiBenedetto RJ, Lyons HA. Massive hemoptysis. Arch Intern Med 121:495–498, 1968.
6. Gourin A, Garzon AA. Operative treatment of massive hemoptysis. Ann Thorac Surg 18:56–60, 1974.
7. Mattox KL, Guinn GA. Emergency resection for massive hemoptysis. Ann Thorac Surg 17:377–383, 1974.
8. Selecky PA. Evaluation of hemoptysis through the bronchoscope. Chest 73:741–745, 1978.
9. Jackson CL, Diamond S. Haemorrhage from the trachea, bronchi and lungs of nontuberculous origin. Am Rev Tuberc 46:126–138, 1942.
10. Barrett RJ, Tuttle WM. A study of essential hemoptysis. J Thorac Cardiovasc Surg 40:468–474, 1960.
11. Gottlieb LS, Heilberg R. Endobronchial tamponade for intractable hemoptysis. Chest 67:482–483, 1975.
12. Garzon AA, Cerruti MM, Golding ME. Exsanguinating hemoptysis. J Thorac Cardiovasc Surg 84:829–833, 1982.
13. Conlan AA, Hurwitz SS, Krige L, Nicolaou N, Pool R. Massive hemoptysis. J Thorac Cardiovasc Surg 85:120–124, 1983.
14. Porter DK, Van Every MJ, Mack JW Jr. Emergency lobectomy for massive hemoptysis in cystic fibrosis. J Thorac Cardiovasc Surg 86:409–411, 1983.

CHAPTER 31

Drug Interactions and the Airway

Harold J. DeMonaco, M.S.

Although the anatomy and physiology of the airway have been described in previous chapters, a brief review from the pharmacologic perspective is in order.

The human airway anatomically consists of the trachea and mainstem bronchi. The airway is further branched out to the level of the alveolar sac. The airway wall is composed of an epithelial layer, a smooth muscle layer, and a connective tissue sheath. Within the epithelium is an array of ciliated columnar cells, mucous-secreting goblet cells, neuroendocrine cells, and brush cells. Deep within the epithelium of large bronchi are mucous glands that connect to the bronchial surface via narrow channels or ducts. These mucous glands extend to the level of small bronchi where, along with goblet cells, they produce a thin mucous layer that covers the airway. This thin mucous layer or blanket serves to trap large foreign particles, which in turn are moved upward through ciliary action. The smooth muscle layer extends from the bronchi to the bronchioles in a continuous sheath. The outer connective tissue layer includes the cartilaginous rings to the level of small bronchi. From this level and below, connective tissue is replaced by a more fibrous sheath.[1]

Neural control of the airways is governed by a variety of mediators that interact with specialized receptors and nerves to determine bronchial tone and mucous gland secretion.[1, 2]

Three afferent receptors have been identified with their fibers travelling via the vagus nerve.[3] Stretch receptors are mechanoreceptors that are affected by changes in tension within the airway. Irritant receptors are found in the upper airways, where they produce the cough reflex, and distally, where they produce bronchoconstriction. These irritant receptors react to a variety of noxious stimuli, including ammonia, sulfur dioxide, and ozone, as well as to histamine, serotonin, and prostaglandin F_{2a}. The third and final subtype of afferent receptor is unmyelinated nerve endings. Like irritant receptors, they respond to histamine, prostaglandin F_{2a}, and sulfur dioxide. Additionally, they respond to bradykinin, capsaicin, and prostaglandins E_2 and I_2. These unmyelinated nerve endings (C fiber endings) effects may be caused by the release of substance P and other neurosensory peptides (Table 31–1).

Efferent innervation is sympathetic, cholinergic, and nonadrenergic noncholinergic in nature.[1, 2] Bronchial tone at rest is mediated by cholinergic activity via the vagus nerve. Adrenergic control of the airways, conversely, is mediated through the actions of circulating catecholamine, such as epinephrine on β_2 adrenoreceptors. These β_2 receptors are found throughout the airway smooth muscle with their density inversely proportional to the size of the airway. The β_2 receptors are located on bronchial epithelial cells. Stimulation causes

Table 31–1. MEDIATORS INVOLVED IN
ASTHMATIC RESPONSE

Pathologic Changes	Mediators
Bronchospasm	Histamine
	Leukotrienes
	Prostaglandins and
	thromboxane
	Bradykinin
	Platelet activating factor
	Acetylcholine
Mucosal edema	Histamine
	Leukotrienes
	Prostaglandin E
	Bradykinin
Airway hyperreactivity	Eosinophil chemotactic
	factor
	Neutrofil chemotactic factor
	Leukotriene B4
Mucus secretion	Histamine
	Prostaglandins
	Acetylcholine

Adapted from Kaliner M. Mechanism of glucocorticosteroid action in bronchial asthma. J Allergy Clin Immunol 76:321–329, 1985; with permission.

active ion transport and water secretion, which decreases the viscosity of bronchial secretions. Additional β_2 receptors are found on mucous glands and on the surface of mast cells. Although beta-blockade has little or no effect on resting bronchial tone in normal individuals, it may produce bronchoconstriction in asthmatics. Because there is no significant direct sympathetic innervation, circulating epinephrine may regulate bronchial tone through inhibition of mast cell degranulation and the subsequent release of mediators.[2, 3] The role of alpha-adrenergic receptors in the human airway is incompletely understood.[4, 5]

The nonadrenergic, noncholinergic system exhibits a direct dilating effect on bronchial smooth muscle. Substance P has been impli-

cated as the major mediator of this pathway, in addition to vasoactive peptide and peptide histidine methionine. Figure 31–1 represents a schematic representation of the three separate efferent pathways of the human airway.[2]

THERAPEUTIC DRUG INTERACTIONS

Sympathomimetic Drugs

The sympathomimetic drugs, including the methylxanthines and beta-adrenergic agonists, cause a relaxation of bronchial smooth muscle. As previously noted, bronchial tone at rest is mediated by cholinergic activity.[2, 3] Adrenergic control of the airways is mediated through the actions of circulating catecholamines. Circulating catecholamines such as epinephrine interact with β_2 receptors located on the bronchial epithelial cells. Activation of β_2 receptors produce a rise in cyclic adenosine monophosphate (cAMP) levels in bronchial muscle cells and, in a dose-dependent fashion, determine bronchial tone. High levels of cAMP lead to reduced bronchial tone and relaxation of the airway. β_2-adrenergic agonists activate adenyl cyclase and indirectly increase cellular levels of cAMP.[6] Chronic use of beta-adrenergic agonists may lead to down regulation of receptors and resulting attenuation of clinical response.[2, 6]

Methylxanthines such as theophylline have previously been thought to produce a cellular increase in cAMP through the interruption of the actions of phosphodiesterase. This action of the methylxanthines has only been demonstrated at extremely high molar concentrations in *in vitro* preparations.[6] The actions of the-

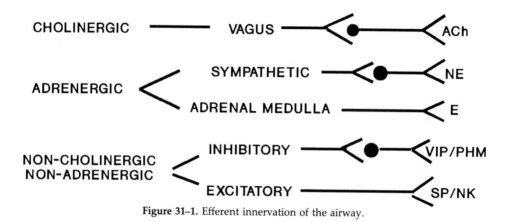

Figure 31–1. Efferent innervation of the airway.

ophylline at pharmacologic serum levels have not been demonstrated to have an impact on phosphodiesterase activity *in vivo*. Much speculation has been presented in the literature concerning the mechanism of bronchodilatation seen with theophylline, ranging from an interaction with adenosine receptors in the airway to increasing systemic levels of epinephrine. Both the methylxanthines and β_2 agonists increase clearance of mucus from the airway by enhancing ciliary function.[7] Table 31–2 lists the more commonly used beta-adrenergic agonists and their relative specificity and duration of action. Although many claims have been made concerning superiority of the newer members of this class, no convincing evidence exists either in efficacy or toxicity.

Anticholinergics

Bronchial tone at rest is dependent on cholinergic activity mediated by the vagus nerve. Acetylcholine released from preganglionic fibers activates nicotinic receptors, resulting in bronchoconstriction. Muscarinic receptors are target cells of postganglionic acetylcholine release.[8] Activation of muscarinic receptors in the airway leads to an inhibition of adenyl cyclase and a resultant fall in cellular cAMP levels. Nicotinic receptor activity may be blocked by hexamethonium, whereas muscarinic activity may be blocked by drugs like atropine and ipratropium. The density of muscarinic receptors is highest in the human lung in the central airways and in tracheal smooth muscle.[2, 3, 8] Cholinergic agonists are potent bronchoconstrictors both *in vivo* and *in vitro*. Maximal effect of cholinergic activity is seen when a minority of cholinergic receptors is occupied, suggesting a large reserve of receptor capacity.[8, 9] Muscarinic receptors are also located on submucosal glands in the airways. Activation of these receptors stimulates secretion of mucus and serous glands equally, resulting in an increase in the amount of secretion but no alteration in the viscosity. Allergen-induced bronchospasm occurs within 15 to 20 minutes of exposure in susceptible patients.[10] Preinhalation of anticholinergic drugs such as atropine has only a partial inhibitory effect on allergen-induced bronchoconstriction, with the maximum attenuation occurring within the first few minutes of challenge.[11, 12] Exercise-induced bronchospasm is likewise attentuated by administration of atropine or ipratropium.[10, 11] This effect is not consistent among patients, and considerable interpatient variability exists.[3] The response to anticholinergic drugs administered by inhalation is somewhat less then than that of β_2-adrenergic agonists.[10, 14]

Mucolytics

Tracheobronchial secretions originate from four main sources[14]: (1) submucosal glands in the cartilaginous airways, (2) goblet cells, (3) Clara cells, and (4) tissue fluid transudate.

Under normal physiologic conditions, approximately 10 to 100 mL of mucus is produced

Table 31–2. BETA-ADRENERGIC AGONISTS

Beta Agonist	Relative Affinity	Usual Adult Dose	Duration of Action (h)
Isoproterenol	B_1, B_2		
Sublingual		10–20 µg	3–4
Intravenous		5–10 µg/min	
Inhalation		1–2 inhalations	3–4
Epinephrine	A_1, A_2, B_1, B_2		
Subcutaneous		0.1–0.5 mg	4
Intravenous		0.25–4 µg/min	
Inhalation		150–250 µg	3–4
Metaproterenol	B_2		
Oral		20 mg	6–8
Inhalation		1.3–1.8 mg	3–4
Terbutaline	B_2		
Oral		2.5–5 mg	6–8
Subcutaneous		0.25 mg	4–6
Inhalation		400 µg	4–6
Albuterol	B_2		
Oral		2–4 mg	6–8
Inhalation		180 µg	6–8

and transported. In patients with bronchitis, this quantity may increase to 200 to 300 mL. Mucus flow in the human trachea varies from 5 to 20 cm/min and diminishes toward the lung periphery. Pulmonary secretions in the periphery are thought to be more watery in nature, and reabsorption takes place rather than movement. In healthy airways, mucus is composed primarily of water (95%), along with a variety of glycoproteins (2%), various proteins (1%), lipids (1%), and inorganic salts (1%). This thin blanket of mucus may be thought of as a sol layer, which lies directly above and bathes the cilia, and a gel layer, which in turn lies directly above the sol layer. The sol layer, which is thin and watery, allows the cilia to beat and thereby sweep the overlying gel layer in a cephalic direction.[14] Although this is an oversimplification, it represents a working model that is useful in defining the role of mucolytic drugs (Fig. 31–2). The efficiency with which the cilia function is dependent on their frequency of beating, the gel layer thickness and viscoelasticity, biochemical properties, consistency, and thickness of the sol layer.

The effects of pharmacologic agents on airway secretions remain clouded. Although mucolytics and expectorants are frequently prescribed, there is little objective evidence to suggest that they in fact work. Part of the difficulty in evaluating the efficacy of mucolytic drugs is the lack of a standardized measure of mucus clearance. Although changes in viscosity have frequently been used as an outcome measure, it is only one component of a somewhat more complicated scheme. Changes in elasticity, spinnability, adhesiveness, and tackiness all play an important but as yet undefined role in secretion clearance. A variety of compounds have been used clinically to loosen secretions and improve their clearance. These drugs have been administered both locally (in the form of aerosols) and systemically.[16]

Acetylcysteine

Compounds containing free sulfhydryl groups such as acetylcysteine and S-carboxy-methylcysteine are capable *in vitro* of splitting the disulfide bonds of the glycoproteins of mucus and reducing viscosity. Acetylcysteine is frequently used as an adjunct in the management of patients with thick or insippated secretions associated with pneumonia, bronchitis, tracheobronchitis, bronchiectasis, and a wide variety of other pulmonary conditions. Although there is widespread belief that aerosolized acetylcysteine is efficacious in enhancing mucus clearance, there is no demonstrable evidence to suggest that this is so.[16] Although acetylcysteine may reduce sputum viscosity with *in vitro* application, pulmonary function does not improve substantially with *in vivo* administration. It has not been established that acetylcysteine offers any advantages over properly performed saline instillation or adequate hydration. Although acetylcysteine has a wide margin of safety, it is not benign and aerosol administration is not without risk. The more common adverse effects of acetylcysteine are nausea (probably related to the very disagreeable odor), stomatitis, severe rhinorrhea, fever, and chills. Chest tightness and bronchoconstriction have been reported with the aerosol administration of acetylcysteine. It has been suggested that this is more commonly seen with the use of the 20% solution, especially in the undiluted form.

Acetylcysteine is commercially available in both a 10% and a 20% solution. It is usually administered three or four times a day as a nebulized aerosol in a dose of 3 to 5 mL of the 20% solution or 6 to 10 mL of the 10% solution. The 10% strength is preferable in order to reduce the risk of bronchospasm. Beta-adrenergic stimulants such as isoproterenol may be administered either prior to or simultaneously with acetylcysteine in order to reduce the likelihood of bronchospasm.[16] In patients with very thick mucous plugging, acetylcysteine may be of use through direct instillation, rather than by aerosolization.

Deoxyribonuclease

Pancreatic dornase contains deoxyribonuclease, an enzyme that degrades deoxyribonucleoprotein and deoxyribonucleic acid. Deoxyribonuclease depolymerizes DNA *in vitro* and has been shown to reduce the viscosity of purulent sputum *in vitro*. This effect has not been demonstrated on nonpurulent sputum. It has been speculated that the polymerization of DNA by deoxyribonuclease allows for the activation of protease in the sputum. Because

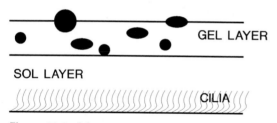

Figure 31–2. Schematic representation of pulmonary secretions.

DNA is only released from frank pus, this effect is not seen in normal sputum. Aerosolization of deoxyribonuclease has been reported to cause bronchoconstriction and pharyngeal irritation. Because of the relatively high incidence of adverse effects, deoxyribonuclease has been replaced in clinical use by acetylcysteine. Pancreatic dornase is no longer commercially available in the United States.[16, 17]

Water, Saline, and Other Agents

As noted previously, a major determinant of mucus clearance is the viscosity of the sol layer. It has been demonstrated both clinically and experimentally that unhumidified air decreases mucociliary clearance.[16] Aerosolization of water and saline has been used clinically to improve ciliary function. The inhalation of water, saline, and hypertonic saline has been shown to have a small effect on mucus clearance in both healthy subjects and in patients with chronic bronchitis.[18, 19] Mist therapy has not been shown to be of value in patients with cystic fibrosis and may induce bronchospasm in patients with asthma or acute bronchitis.

A variety of systemically administered drugs have been used clinically to improve mucociliary clearance. Guaifenesin has been used for many years as an aid to mucus clearance. To date, no study has provided convincing evidence for its efficacy in a variety of patients with pulmonary disease. Bromhexine, a synthetic derivative of vasicine, is claimed to have an effect on both the structure and volume of secretions in patients with bronchitis and other pulmonary diseases. At least one clinical study in patients with chronic bronchitis showed subjective and objective improvement in sputum volume, quality, and ease of clearance and in pulmonary function.[16] Ambroxol, a metabolite or bromhexine, has been shown to produce subjective improvement in mucus clearance in patients with chronic obstructive pulmonary disease in at least one double-blind study. Studies measuring the retention of technetium-99m–labeled Teflon particles in the lungs of patients with chronic bronchitis have, however, failed to show a difference between placebo and ambroxol. Neither bromhexine nor ambroxol is available in the United States.[16]

Corticosteroids

Corticosteroids have been recognized as valuable adjuncts to therapy for a variety of diseases involving airways, including asthma, cystic fibrosis, and bronchitis. Considerable controversy exists, however, as to their precise indications, dosage, and methods of administration. Given the plethora of uses of corticosteroids in modern medicine, this discussion is limited to those involving the respiratory airways.[20]

The most complete data exist for the use of glucocorticoids in the management of asthma. Airway obstruction in asthma is related to the inhalation of antigens into the airways which then interact with sensitized mast cells. Antigen complexes on the surface of the mast cells stimulate the synthesis and release of mediators that initiate the allergic response. As a result of mast cell stimulation, the classic asthmatic response of bronchial smooth muscle is spasm, mucosal edema, increased airway responsiveness, and mucosal secretion. A variety of mediators have been implicated in the development of the symptoms[21] (Table 31–3). The pharmacologic effects of corticosteroids in diseases of the airway are complex and highly interrelated. It is unlikely that one of the myriad of effects is critical to a positive therapeutic outcome; rather, the effects are all contributory.

The corticosteroids have a defined and well-described effect on β_2-receptor activity. As was noted previously, β_2 stimulation causes an inhibition of mast cell and basophil mediator release, an increase in the water content of airway secretion, and smooth muscle relaxa-

Table 31–3. PHARMACOLOGIC ACTIONS OF CORTICOSTEROIDS IN ASTHMA

General Actions	Specific Actions
A. Beta-adrenergic receptors Increase population Increase adenyl cyclase activity Increase protein kinase activity B. Distribution of leukocytes C. Decrease inflammatory process	A. Lower IgG levels B. Stabilize mast cells, basophils, and neutrophils Inhibition of mediator release Inhibition of histamine release Inhibition of eicosanoid release C. Vasoconstriction D. Decrease vascular permeability E. Decrease late phase reactions F. Decrease mucus secretion

From Kaliner M. Mechanism of glucocorticosteroid action in bronchial asthma. J Allergy Clin Immunol 76:321–329, 1985; with permission.

tion. β_2-adrenergic activity has been demonstrated to be reduced in patients with asthma.[21] It is reasonable then to assume that pharmacologic alterations in β_2 function using agonists and antagonists would have a positive or negative impact, respectively, on symptomatology. Pharmacologic alteration of adrenergic function may be the result of changes in receptor sensitivity, in the number of functional receptors, or both.[20] Tissue cultures of human embryonic lung tissue incubated with hydrocortisone have demonstrated an increase of β_2 receptors of 100% over baseline.[20, 21] Maximal effect requires 24 hours. This effect has also been demonstrated with human lymphocytes and granulocytes *in vivo*. Administration of cortisone acetate to human subjects has been shown to dramatically increase the granulocyte beta-adrenergic receptors. These effects peak at 4 hours and 24 hours, respectively. Within 24 hours, both lymphocytes and granulocytes have the same number of receptors.[21]

There is considerable *in vitro* evidence that the administration of corticosteroids also increases adenylate cyclase responsiveness to β_2 agonists such as isoproterenol.[22] The addition of hydrocortisone to leukocytes from normal volunteers causes an immediate increase in cAMP levels. Leukocytes from patients with asthma fail to respond in a similar fashion, however, to beta-adrenergic stimulation unless a corticosteroid is added to the preparation concomitantly.[22] The exact clinical significance of this immediate effect is unclear, because most patients do not derive any meaningful clinical benefit from corticosteroid administration for 4 to 24 hours after administration.

Stimulation of beta-adrenergic receptors has been shown to increase cAMP production, the action of which is mediated by a variety of protein kinases. Corticosteroids may enhance the actions of these protein kinases and thereby increase the actions of cAMP.[22]

It would appear then that the actions of corticosteroids on the beta-adrenergic system in the airway are highly complex. Corticosteroids affect the number of receptors in the same manner in which adenyl cyclase is coupled and in protein kinase activation. These actions have been demonstrated in normal volunteers, as well as in patients with asthma. It is clear that the effects of corticosteroids on the airways of patients with asthma require from at least 4 hours to as much as 24 hours to reach maximal potential.

The effect of corticosteroids on the distribution of leukocytes has been studied in both human and animal models. In humans, corticosteroids reduce the number of circulating lymphocytes arriving at sites of inflammation. Additionally, corticosteroids decrease the number of monocytes, basophils, and eosinophils circulating, as well as increase the number of neutrophils.

Inflammation has classically been described as consisting of four components: heat, redness, swelling, and pain. This symptom set is the result of increased capillary permeability, vasodilation, cellular infiltration with neutrophils and, as the process matures, tissue destruction. Neutrophil migration is inhibited by the actions of corticosteroids to reduce chemotaxis, a reduction in the attachment of neutrophils to the endothelium, and reduced margination. Although corticosteroids have been demonstrated to affect each of these processes to a varying degree, it is likely that the effect on leukocyte infiltration is the major component.

In addition to the general effects of the corticosteroids, a number of more specific effects related specifically to asthma are noted. Corticosteroids have been demonstrated to reduce the elevated levels of gamma E immunoglobulin (IgE) associated with childhood asthma. Although chronic administration of pharmacologic doses of corticosteroids have demonstrated a dramatic drop in serum IgE, skin positivity and antigen inhalation challenge are maintained. It is, therefore, unlikely that this represents a clinically meaningful mechanism of action of the corticosteroids. Chronic corticosteroid administration has been demonstrated to reduce histamine synthesis and an inhibition of eicosanoid release. It is likely that, given the widespread actions of the arachidonic acid cascade, including the development of edema and increase in mucus production, suppression of release represents a major mechanism of action of the corticosteroids.

Although the role of corticosteroids in reducing airway lability in asthma is well established, their value in chronic obstructive pulmonary disease is uncertain.[23, 24] Clinical trials have all been subject to criticism for both methodologic flaws as well as diagnostic rigidity, which would exclude patients with asthma. It is clear that some patients with chronic obstructive pulmonary disease (COPD) respond to steroid administration. What is less clear is whether or not patients can be identified prior to therapy.[24] Duration and severity of illness, previous responsiveness to systemic corticosteroid administration, age, sex, and eosinophilia of both blood and sputum all fail as markers of responsiveness. It has been sug-

Table 31–4. SYSTEMICALLY ADMINISTERED CORTICOSTEROIDS

Drug	Dose	Anti-inflammatory Activity*	Half-life (h)
Short acting			
Cortisone	25 mg	0.8	8–12
Hydrocortisone	20 mg	1.0	8–12
Medium duration			
Methylprednisolone	4 mg	5	18–36
Prednisolone	5 mg	4	18–36
Prednisone	5 mg	4	18–36
Triamcinolone	4 mg	5	18–36
Long acting			
Betamethasone	0.6 mg	20–30	36–54
Dexamethasone	0.5–0.75 mg	20–30	36–54

*Relative potency as compared with hydrocortisone.

gested that patients who have failed to respond (less than a 10% increase in FEV_1) to inhaled bronchodilators are unlikely to respond to systemic corticosteroid administration. Although steroids may not be indicated in patients with stable COPD, a brief trial may be useful in patients with severe disease who fail to respond adequately to theophylline in adequate doses or to an inhaled or orally administered beta-adrenergic agonist. Alternate-day systemic corticosteroids are perhaps as effective as daily administration and may produce a lower incidence of side effects with prolonged therapy.

Steroid responders who cannot be managed on a chronic basis with theophylline and beta-adrenergic agonists may be managed with the use of inhaled corticosteroids. Clinical trials have demonstrated that the majority of such patients may have their dose of systemically administered corticosteroids reduced or even eliminated. Inhaled corticosteroids have the advantage of a reduced incidence of systemic side effects. The most commonly occurring side effects associated with inhaled corticosteroids are oropharyngeal candidiasis and hoarseness. No one corticosteroid aerosol has been shown to have superiority over the other members of the class in either asthma or COPD. Triamcinolone acetonide is the least expensive member of the group, an important consideration for chronic therapy. Table 31–4 lists the available corticosteroids for systemic administration; Table 31–5 lists those available for inhalation.

Miscellaneous Drugs

During the early 1980s, a number of investigators examined the utility of calcium channel blockers in the management of bronchospasm. The similarities between the pathophysiology of coronary artery vasospasm and bronchospasm are striking. Both may be precipitated by a variety of stimuli, such as exercise, methacholine, histamine, and ergonovine. Recent evidence suggests that calcium-dependent pathways may play a role in the development of bronchospasm.[25, 26] The calcium channels may play a role in mast cell degranulation, mucous gland secretion, smooth muscle contraction, and inflammatory cell infiltration. It seemed reasonable, therefore, to examine the effects of calcium channel blocking drugs in experimentally induced asthma. Nifedipine, verapamil, diltiazem, and gallapomil (a methoxy derivative of verapamil) have all been studied. The majority of studies to date have concluded that all of the above calcium channel blocking drugs have a small impact on airway reactivity.[25] There is insufficient evidence to suggest that the calcium channel blocking drugs provide a significant clinical benefit.

The loss of water and resulting hyperosmolarity of the fluid bathing the airway has been postulated as an initiator mechanism for exercise-induced bronchospasm.[27, 28] Based on experimental evidence, a variety of drugs, including furosemide, have been examined as possible therapeutic options for patients with exercise-induced bronchospasm. At least one randomized double-blind study has concluded

Table 31–5. CORTICOSTEROID AEROSOLS

Drug	Dose/ inhalation	Usual Dose
Beclomethasone	250 μg	500 μg 3–4 times daily
Flusinolide	250 μg	500 μg three times daily
Triamcinolone	200 μg	400 μg three times daily

that furosemide exerts a dose-dependent attenuation in exercise-induced drops in FEV_1.[28] Inhaled furosemide in a 28-mg dose appears to dramatically attenuate the fall in FEV_1, whereas orally administered furosemide does not. Smaller doses of furosemide by inhalation appear to have a dose-dependent response. Although the mechanism of action is unclear, it appears that local action is required, because systemically administered furosemide does not differ from placebo in this regard. Furosemide has also been shown to attenuate the bronchoconstrictive response to adenosine 5'-monophosphate, as well as a variety of antigens in susceptible patients.[29] Furosemide does not appear to have any clinically significant effects on methacholine-induced bronchospasm.

DRUG-INDUCED BRONCHOSPASM

Beta-Adrenergic Blockers

Bronchial tone is mediated by cholinergic pathways at rest. Adrenergic tone, mediated by the β_2 receptors in the airway, function to prevent cholinergically mediated bronchoconstriction. Loss of β_2 adrenergic tone in susceptible patients would, therefore, be expected to produce bronchospasm.[1]

In normal individuals, beta-adrenergic blocking drugs have few demonstrable effects on bronchial tone either at rest or at exercise, nor do they enhance bronchial reactivity to methacholine.[30] This is far different from the response seen with patients with previously documented airway reactivity. Although it is enticing to suggest that the bronchospasm noted is the result of unrestrained cholinergic activity, this may not be the sole mechanism and it does not explain why this effect is not seen in "normals." Beta receptors are located on the surface of mast cells. Although no evidence of a release of mediators from mast cells has been demonstrated with beta-adrenergic blockers, pretreatment with sodium cromoglycate blocks propranolol-induced bronchospasm in susceptible patients. The mechanism of beta-blocker–induced bronchospasm remains to be elucidated.[1, 30]

Although patients with reactive airway disease such as asthma have a clear predisposition to the development of bronchospasm, not all patients develop symptoms. When used in patients with asthma, beta-blockers should be used with caution and the risks weighed against the presumed benefits. Although beta-agonists have been used as direct antagonists to beta blockade, inhaled anticholinergics are the treatment of choice for drug-induced bronchospasm. Beta-blockers that are said to be specific for the β_1 receptor may be safer than nonselective drugs such as propranolol. It should be noted that the selectivity of drugs such as atenolol, metoprolol, and acebutolol is relative and dose related. Asthmatic patients requiring the use of beta-blockers should be managed on a selective agent at the lowest possible dose.

Aspirin and Related Nonsteroidal Anti-inflammatory Drugs

Sensitivity to aspirin and to nonsteroidal anti-inflammatory drugs (NSAIDs) may take the form of bronchospasm or uticaria and angioedema.[1, 31] In many patients, both manifestations of sensitivity are evident. It has been estimated that aspirin-induced bronchospasm occurs in 0.3% of the normal population and between 4% and 20% of asthmatics. The incidence of aspirin sensitivity in patients with both nasal polyps and asthma may be as high as 75%.[1]

Aspirin-induced bronchospasm is usually seen in the third to fourth decade of life and tends to be more common in women. Classically, susceptible patients who receive aspirin develop vasomotor rhinitis and nasal congestion prior to the development of bronchospasm. Patients may have been exposed to aspirin on numerous occasions prior to the development of rhinitis and nasal congestion or bronchospasm. The complete symptom set includes conjunctival irritation, rhinorrhea, and facial flushing, followed by bronchospasm.[32]

Although the exact mechanism of aspirin and NSAID-induced bronchospasm is unclear, two working hypotheses have been proposed. The development of bronchospasms is due to (1) the development of an imbalance in the production of bronchodilating and bronchoconstricting prostaglandins, or (2) a shunting of arachidonic acid through the lipogenase pathway with resulting increased production of leukotrienes. Although both mechanisms have experimental support, neither fully explain the reaction.[32]

Angiotensin-Converting Enzyme Inhibitors

Upper airway irritation and cough are well recognized side effects of angiotensin-converting enzyme (ACE) inhibitors captopril, lisinopril, and enalapril. The reported incidence of ACE inhibitor-related cough is 1% to 2% in most series for enalapril and captopril. Patients describe a dry, persistent, and, in some instances, disabling cough. Symptoms have been shown to develop within days of initiation of therapy with an ACE inhibitor and usually resolve within 2 to 3 weeks of discontinuation. The mechanism for ACE inhibitor-induced cough is unclear. Many mechanisms have been proposed, although it would appear that underlying airway hyperractivity may be a predisposing factor. Substance P and bradykinin have been implicated as having a role in ACE inhibitor-induced cough.[1]

Iodine-Containing Contrast Media

Adverse reactions to iodine-containing contrast agents have been recognized with both low-osmolarity and high-osmolarity drugs. The incidence of severe reactions is approximately 1 to 14,000 procedures with high-osmolarity contrast drugs and somewhat lower with the low-osmolarity types. Clinically significant bronchospasm occurs in approximately 10% of patients who experience a severe, contrast-related reaction. The mechanism of contrast-induced bronchospasm is unknown. It has been shown that a subclinical decline in FEV_1 develops in the majority of patients who receive high-osmolarity contrast agents, regardless of a prior history of contrast-related allergy. It is unclear whether or not this reaction is independent of the development of bronchospasm. It is clear that the reaction does not involve the development of antibodies and is, therefore, not a true allergic phenomenon. Mechanisms proposed have involved the activation of mast cells and the resulting release of histamine, increased leukotriene production, and an inhibition of the enzymes that normally degrade leukotriene. Although histamine may play a role, plasma histamine levels are increased in patients receiving contrast media, regardless of whether or not a reaction occurs. It is unclear whether pretreatment with antihistamines or corticosteroids reduce the likelihood of bronchospasm, although the incidence of severe contrast reactions is reduced.[1]

References

1. Meerer DP, Wiedemann HP. Drug induced bronchospasm. Clin Chest Med 11:163–175, 1990.
2. Barnes PJ. Neural control of human airways in health and disease. Am Rev Respir Dis 134:1289–1314, 1986.
3. Sant' Ambrogio G. Information arrising from the tracheobronchial tree of mammals. Physiol Rev 62:531–539, 1982.
4. Szentivanyi A. The beta adrenergic theory of the atopic abnormality in bronchial asthma. J Allergy 42:203–232, 1968.
5. Gabella G. Innervation of airway smooth muscle: Fine structure. Ann Rev Physiol 49:583–594, 1987.
6. Torphy TJ. Biochemical regulation of airway smooth muscle tone. Rev Clin Basic Pharm 6:61–103, 1987.
7. Pavia D, Sutton PP, Lopez-Vidriero MT, Agnew JE, Clarke SW. Drug effects on mucociliary function. Eur J Respir Dis 64(Suppl 128):304–317, 1983.
8. Barnes PJ. Muscarinic receptors in lung. Postgrad Med J 63(Suppl):13–19, 1987.
9. Grandoroy BM, Cuss FM, Sampson AS, Palmer BJ, Barnes PJ. Phosphatidylinositol response to cholinergic agonists in airway smooth muscle: Relationship to contraction and muscarinic receptor occupancy. J Pharmacol Exp Ther 238:273–279, 1986.
10. Holgate ST. Anticholinergics in acute bronchial asthma. Postgrad Med J 63(Suppl 1):35–39, 1987.
11. Cartier A, Thomson NC, Roberts R, Hargreave FE. Allergen induced increase in bronchial responsiveness to histamine: Relationship to the late asthmatic response and change in airway caliber. J Allergy Clin Immunol 70:170–177, 1982.
12. Fish JE, Rosenthal RR, Sommer WR, Menkes H, Normal PS, Permutt S. The effect of atropine on acute antigen mediated airway constriction in subjects with allergic asthma. Am Rev Respir Dis 115:371–379, 1977.
13. Godfrey S, Konig P. Inhibition of exercise induced bronchospasm by atropine. Am Rev Respir Dis 31:137–143, 1976.
14. Ziment I, Au JP. Anticholinergic agents. Clin Chest Med 7:355–366, 1986.
15. Clarke SW. Rationale of airway clearance. Eur Respir J 2(Suppl 7):599–604, 1989.
16. Lourenco RV, Contromanes E. Clinical aerosols. II: Therapeutic aerosols. Arch Intern Med 142:2299–2308, 1982.
17. Raskin P. Bronchospasm after inhalation of pancreatic Dornase. Arch Rev Respir Dis 98:597–598, 1968.
18. Foster WM, Bergofsky EH, Bohning DE, Lippman M, Albert RE. Effect of adrenergic agents and their mode of action on mucociliary clearance in man. J Appl Physiol 41:146–152, 1976.
19. Pavia D, Thomson ML, Clark SW. Enhanced clearance of secretion from the human lung after administration of hypertonic saline aerosol. Am Rev Respir Dis 117:199–203, 1978.
20. Siegel SC. Corticosteroid agents: Overview of corticosteroid therapy. J Allergy Clin Immunol 76:312–320, 1985.
21. Kaliner M. Mechanism of glucocorticosteroid action in bronchial asthma. J Allergy Clin Immunol 76:321–329, 1985.
22. Logsdon PF, Middleton E, Coffee RG. Stimulation of leukocyte adenyl cyclase by hydrocortisone and isoproterenol in asthmatic and non asthmatic subjects. J Allergy Clin Immunol 50:42–56, 1972.
23. Sahn SA. Corticosteroids in chronic bronchitis and pulmonary emphysema. Chest 73:389–396, 1978.

24. Mandella LA, Manfreda J, Warren CPN, Anthonsen NR. Steroid response in chronic stable obstructive pulmonary disease. Ann Intern Med 96:17–21, 1982.
25. Massey KL, Hendeles L. Calcium antagonists in the management of asthma: Breakthrough or ballyhoo? Drug Intell Clin Pharm 21:505–509, 1987.
26. Middleton E. Antiasthmatic drug therapy and calcium ions: Review of pathogenesis and role of calcium. J Pharm Sci 69:243–251, 1980.
27. Nichol GM, Alton EW, Nix A, Geddes DM, Chung KF, Barnes PJ. Effect of inhaled furosemide on metabisulfite and methacholine induced bronchospasm and nasal potential difference in asthmatic subjects. Am Rev Respir Dis 142:576–580, 1990.
28. Bianco S, Vaghi A, Robuschi M, Pasargiklian M. Prevention of exercise induced bronchoconstriction by inhaled furosemide. Lancet 2:252–255, 1988.
29. Polosa R, Lau LC, Holgate ST. Inhibition of adenosine-5-monophosphate and methacholine induced bronchoconstriction in asthma by inhaled furosemide. Eur Respir J 3:665–672, 1990.
30. Grieco MH, Pierson RN. Mechanism of bronchoconstriction due to beta adrenergic blockade. J Allergy Clin Immunol 48:143–152, 1971.
31. Slepian IK, Mathews KP, McLean JA. Aspirin sensitive asthma. Chest 87:386–391, 1985.
32. Ribon A, Parikh S. Drug induced asthma: A review. Ann Allergy 44:220–224, 1980.

CHAPTER 32

Airway Infections

Depak Soni, M.D., and Charles A. Hales, M.D.

Infections of the airway can be serious and potentially life threatening. Fortunately, the human airway is remarkably well equipped to defend itself against a variety of agents, including microbial pathogens. Minor viral infections of the nose and upper airways that cause nuisance illnesses are common. However, the relatively infrequent occurrence of serious airway infections in healthy persons is a tribute to the efficacy of these airway defense mechanisms. Only when exposed to a particularly virulent microbe, an unusually large inoculum, or in the setting of an impaired host are failures of the airway defense mechanisms documented. In this chapter, we describe in some detail these airway defense mechanisms. We then discuss two major upper airway infections (acute laryngotracheobronchitis and epiglottitis), and conclude with the important topic of airway colonization and its relationship to infection of the lower respiratory tract.

AIRWAY DEFENSE MECHANISMS

By the very act of breathing, the tracheobronchial tree is exposed to over 10,000 L of ambient air daily. This volume could fill a good-sized swimming pool. The airway is called on to defend itself against infectious agents, mineral dusts, chemical toxins, and immunogenic particles that are contained in this volume of air. In addition, it must defend against microbes in the naso-oropharynx,

which are ubiquitously present in human beings. The airway employs both nonspecific and specific defense mechanisms, the combination of which is wonderfully effective (Fig. 32–1).

Nonspecific Mechanisms

Nasopharynx. The nasal apparatus is designed chiefly to function as a filtration system. The narrow and tortuous passages near the front of the nose, where the hairs are located, trap most of the inhaled particulate matter. These particles, which are present anteriorly, can then be removed by sneezing or nose blowing. More posteriorly, the nasal turbinates are covered by ciliated, mucus-secreting epithelium. Particles depositing in this region are swept backward to the nasopharynx and swallowed. The nasopharynx traps particles greater than approximately 10 μ in size. The filtration function of the nose and nasal passages is eliminated by mouth breathing or placement of either an endotracheal or tracheostomy tube.

Cough. Cough serves an important function in the removal of inhaled foreign material or abnormal bronchial secretions. Cough receptors are located in many parts of the respiratory tract, including the oropharynx, larynx, trachea, and large bronchi. Topical anesthesia, inflammation, and irritation diminish the sensitivity of cough receptors. These receptors also adapt to stimuli, so that patients who

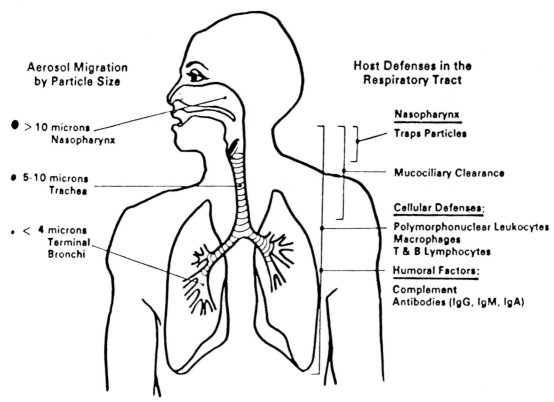

Aerosol Migration by Particle Size

● > 10 microns
   Nasopharynx

● 5-10 microns
   Trachea

· < 4 microns
   Terminal
   Bronchi

Host Defenses in the Respiratory Tract

Nasopharynx
Traps Particles

Mucociliary Clearance

Cellular Defenses:
Polymorphonuclear Leukocytes
Macrophages
T & B Lymphocytes

Humoral Factors:
Complement
Antibodies (IgG, IgM, IgA)

Figure 32–1. Schematic diagram of host defenses in the upper and lower respiratory tract. (From Craven DE, Driks MR. Semin Respir Infect 2:20–33, 1987; with permission.)

initially display cough paroxysms during intubation with cuffed endotracheal tubes lose the cough within a short period of time. The loss of cough and upper airway filtration with placement of an endotracheal tube makes intubated patients uniquely susceptible to environmental insults. In reponse to receptor stimulation, coughing begins with a rapid inspiration, followed by glottal closure, laryngeal smooth muscle constriction, and expiratory muscle contraction. Pleural pressure rises to 50 to 100 mm Hg. Sudden opening of the glottis allows explosive ejection of air. The cough event lasts for about 0.5 second, during which up to 1 L of air is expelled. The vigorous expiratory effort during cough causes central airways to be markedly compressed. This sufficiently increases the velocity of airflow to generate a shearing force that dislodges mucus and particles from the luminal surface, eventually leading to expectoration. Cough is highly effective predominantly in the central airways, and only when performed from high lung volumes. Cough becomes inefficient when secretions are excessive or highly viscid.

Mucociliary Clearance. The mucociliary apparatus of the airways provides an important host defense function by removing inhaled particulate matter from the tracheobronchial mucosa (Fig. 32–2). The mucosal surface covering the airways from the upper trachea down to the respiratory bronchioles consists of a pseudostratified, columnar, ciliated, mucus-secreting epithelium. A turnover of cells occurs approximately every 7 days. A film of mucus is continuously impelled proximally by the beating motion of the cilia, and has been termed the "ciliary escalator." Particles depositing on the mucous film are carried along with

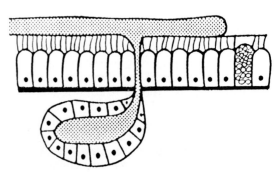

Figure 32–2. Schematic representation of the tracheal mucociliary apparatus.

it to the oropharynx, where they are swallowed or expectorated.

Particles are removed from the airstream the instant they contact any portion of the lining of the respiratory tract. The three principal forces governing deposition of particles in the airways are inertia, sedimentation, and diffusion. Deposition of particles in the nasopharynx and trachea is almost exclusively governed by inertial forces. The tortuous passages in the nasopharynx call for frequent changes in direction of inhaled particles. Once in motion, however, a particle tends to move in the same direction, owing to inertial forces. Thus, if a particle continues in its original direction when it should turn, it will impact and be deposited on the epithelial surface.

The surface of each ciliated columnar cell contains approximately 200 cilia, each with an average length of 6 μ and a diameter of 0.2 μ. Each cilium is a complex structure that contains longitudinal microtubules that represent contractile elements. Two microtubules form a central core, and nine doublets of microtubules are arranged in a circular fashion in the periphery of the cilium. Beating of cilia occurs in one plane with a fast effective stroke (power stroke) and a slow recovery stroke. The effective stroke is two to three times faster than the recovery stroke. Numerous mitochondria cluster beneath the basal bodies of cilia, furnishing the adenosine triphosphate required for ciliary activity. The motion among cilia of adjacent cells, although not anatomically connected, is coordinated so that a metachronal wave spreads in a cephalad direction. The mechanisms responsible for this coordination have not been elucidated. In humans, ciliary beat frequency ranges between 12 and 15 Hz. Ciliary beat frequency is exquisitely sensitive to variations in temperature. A slowing of ciliary beat frequency occurs at low temperatures and an increase occurs at supranormal temperatures.

The mucous lining is composed of a double (sol-gel) layer on the surface of the bronchial epithelium. The cilia are surrounded by a periciliary fluid layer (sol) and are covered by a mucous layer (gel). The mucous layer is 5 to 10 μ deep, is produced by goblet cells, is nonabsorbent to water and protects the sol phase from desiccation. In humans, the overlying mucous film moves at a rate ranging between 2 to 20 mm/min. Particle transport has been shown to fail in the absence of mucus. The clearance of particulate matter from the trachea is remarkably fast. Assuming a tracheal length of 12 cm and a mucous transport rate of 10 mm/min, it would take a particle deposited at the carina 12 min to reach the larynx.

In adults, mucociliary clearance decreases with age. Drying and possibly cooling of the tracheal mucosa impairs mucociliary clearance. Airway mucociliary clearance has been shown to be depressed in various types of airway disease (chronic bronchitis, cystic fibrosis, immotile cilia syndrome, asthma, acute respiratory infections), by cigarette smoke and air pollutants, and by anesthetic gases and oxygen. Bacterial products, such as a cilio-inhibitory factor, can affect mucociliary function in the presence of airway colonization or infection. Viral respiratory infections are known to damage the epithelium and impair airway mucociliary clearance. Interestingly, Battista and colleagues[1] have shown that at least 50% of the surface of the tracheal epithelium has to be devoid of cilia for mucus transport to decrease.

Specific (Immunologic) Defense Mechanisms

Secretory IgA. In the nasopharynx, oropharynx, and conducting airways, a complex mixture of mucus, bronchial gland secretions, and immunoglobulins coat the mucosal surface. Secretory IgA is the predominant immunoglobulin in samples from the upper respiratory tract. IgA is part of the protective coating that overlies the ciliated epithelial surface.

Secretory IgA differs from serum IgA in that the secretory immunoglobulin is a dimer of two IgA molecules linked by a secretory component and a joining chain. This confers a greater resistance to proteolysis compared with immunoglobulins of other classes. Monomeric IgA is synthesized by B lymphocytes located in the airway submucosa and then transported to the epithelial cells for assembly with secretory component. The precise role of secretory IgA in the defense of the lungs is not known; however, there are numerous postulated roles. IgA antibodies possess complement-independent neutralizing activity against a wide variety of respiratory viruses. IgA is a very efficient agglutinator of microbes; via this activity, it may enhance mucociliary transport of bacterial particles. This immunoglobulin has the ability to neutralize toxins such as diphtheria toxin. Also, IgA reduces the attachment of bacteria to mucosal surfaces, preventing the first stage of infection. Secretory IgA differs functionally from IgG and IgM in its relative inability to opsonize bacteria or to fix complement in the classic manner. Major phagocytic cells such as polymorphonuclear neutrophils (PMNs), monocytes, and macrophages do not have abundant cell-surface receptor sites for IgA. The contribution of IgA to antibacterial immunity remains unclear, although it has a well-established role in resistance to viral infections. The major biologic function of secretory IgA appears to be a regulation of microbial antigen entry. Secretory IgA is probably a more important immunologic defense in the nose, oropharynx, and trachea than in the peripheral airways and alveoli.

Immunoglobulin G. IgG is the predominant immunoglobulin found in lower respiratory tract secretions. Alveolar IgG undoubtedly plays an important role in local defense of the lower respiratory tract; however, serum IgG is also involved in defense of the upper respiratory tract. There is a strong correlation between serum IgG deficiency and chronic upper respiratory tract infections. Chronic inflammation that leads to bronchiectasis has been found in IgG-deficient patients. An IgG subclass deficiency alone can be associated with recurrent bacterial infections. A study has documented four patients with severe recurrent sinopulmonary infections and bronchiectasis who had virtually absent levels of IgG-4 in serum. These patients had total serum IgG levels within the normal range and no striking abnormalities of other IgG subclasses or other immunoglobulins. Thus, simple measurement of total IgG may not indicate the presence of a subclass deficiency. The combination of IgG-2 and IgG-4 subclass deficiency is also seen in patients with recurrent respiratory infections.

ACUTE LARYNGOTRACHEOBRONCHITIS

Acute laryngotracheobronchitis or croup is a viral infection of the upper and lower respiratory tract that produces inflammation in the subglottic area. Croup was derived from the old Scottish term "roup," which meant "to cry out in a shrill voice." Croup occurs mostly in children between the ages of 3 months and 3 years. It may be caused by a variety of viral agents, and occasionally by *Mycoplasma pneumoniae*. Parainfluenza type 1 and type 3 viruses are, respectively, the first and second most common causes of croup in the United States.

Influenza A is also a major cause of croup. Less common causes include respiratory syncytial virus, adenovirus, rhinovirus, enterovirus, and parainfluenza type 2 virus.

The viral infection initially affects the upper respiratory tract, usually producing inflammation of the nasal passages and nasopharynx. Subsequently, the infection moves downward, causing inflammation in the larynx and trachea, and giving rise to stridor, hoarseness, and cough. The inflammation and obstruction are greatest at the subglottic level. This is the least distensible part of the airway, because it is encircled by the cricoid cartilage. In addition, the negative intra-airway pressure relative to atmospheric pressure surrounding the neck causes airway narrowing during inspiration. Flow through this region is impeded and produces the classic high-pitched inspiratory vibratory sounds, or stridor. Involvement of the lower respiratory tract is also present in most cases that require hospitalization. Histologic sections reveal inflammatory changes in the linings of the bronchi, bronchioles, and even the alveoli.

Croup is preceded by a prodrome of several days' duration that consists of rhinorrhea, sore throat, mild cough, and fever. Hoarseness and a deepening cough signal the onset of croup. The cough is distinctive and reminiscent of a barking seal. Tachypnea and a characteristic inspiratory stridor accompany the cough. One of the hallmarks of croup is its fluctuating course. A child clinically may appear to worsen or improve within an hour. In most children, the course of croup is 3 to 4 days.

The diagnosis of croup is usually based on the characteristic clinical picture. The differential diagnosis for stridor includes foreign body aspiration, allergic reaction, and epiglottitis. The clinical history and anteroposterior and lateral roentgenograms of the neck can aid in distinguishing between these entities. In viral laryngotracheobronchitis, the anteroposterior view of the neck reveals the characteristic subglottic swelling, which has been described as the "hourglass" or "steeple" sign. Subglottic swelling is not present in epiglottitis. The cause of croup is determined in only approximately one third to two thirds of cases. Viral isolation has usually been accomplished from throat, tracheal, and nasal wash specimens. Serologic diagnosis is unreliable.

The mortality of croup ranges from 0 to 2.7% in different series. The major acute complication of ventilatory failure that necessitates tracheotomy varies between 0 and 13%. The severity of croup appears to be influenced by both virus and host factors. Some studies have reported croup caused by influenza A to be more severe than that caused by other viral agents. Boys are particularly prone to develop croup, for unclear reasons. Some children appear predisposed to croup, with repetitive episodes from a variety of agents. Children with recurrent croup tend to have lower serum IgA levels. Complications of croup include pneumonia, pneumothorax, pulmonary edema, and aspiration pneumonia.

The cornerstone of successful management is close observation and supportive care. Supplemental oxygen should be administered to children with hypoxemia. Humidification of the airway is of unproven benefit. Nebulized racemic epinephrine may result in clinical improvement of stridor. Use of corticosteroids remains controversial. Antibiotic therapy is not indicated for viral croup.

EPIGLOTTITIS

Acute epiglottitis or "acute supraglottitis" is a rapidly progressive cellulitis of the epiglottis and supraglottic structures, with the ever-present threat of complete airway obstruction. It is predominantly a disease of children 1 to 4 years of age, but some surveys have indicated that up to 12% of patients may be adults. It is of historical interest that George Washington probably died of epiglottitis. Sore throat is the most prominent symptom in older children and adults. Patients present with varying degrees of respiratory distress and prefer to sit leaning forward while drooling oral secretions. Fever is also usually present. Unlike croup, there is no prodrome, and symptoms develop rapidly over 6 to 12 hours. There is a report of a patient who progressed from being completely asymptomatic to complete airway obstruction in 30 minutes. Inspiratory stridor occurs frequently, but the barking cough of the croup syndrome is rare. Stridor results from swollen aryepiglottic folds that tend to move downward during inspiration, creating a ball–valve situation. Similarly, swollen supraglottic tissues cause dysphagia with pooling of secretions and saliva. Children with croup do not have the dysphagia and drooling that are characteristic of epiglottitis.

The diagnosis is confirmed by finding an edematous, "cherry red" epiglottis. A lateral neck roentgenogram that shows an enlarged epiglottis, ballooning of the hypopharynx, and normal subglottic structures strongly suggests the diagnosis. However, use of x-ray films in the diagnosis of acute epiglottitis suffers from poor sensitivity and specificity. *Haemophilus influenzae* type b is implicated most often as the etiologic agent. Positive cultures are obtained from blood or the epiglottis. Other agents occasionally implicated are pneumococci, staphylococci, streptococci, and *Haemophilus paraphrophilus*.

Maintenance of an adequate airway is the first priority in established or suspected cases of epiglottitis. Mortality ranges between 33% to 80% in children who develop airway obstruction. Most authors agree that immediate provision of an airway is the safest course to pursue, rather than placement after a period of observation. Most also prefer the use of an endotracheal tube rather than a tracheostomy. Inflammation and edema usually subside in 36 to 48 hours after institution of appropriate antimicrobial therapy. The pediatric airway is best managed in the controlled setting of the operating room. After obtaining appropriate cultures, antibacterial therapy should be directed at *H. influenzae*. In light of the increasing occurrence of ampicillin-resistant *H. influenzae*, intravenous cefuroxime or a third-generation cephalosporin such as cefotaxime can be used for initial therapy. Antibiotics should be continued for 7 to 10 days. Household contacts under age 4 years of patients with epiglottitis should receive rifampin prophylaxis. Second cases of epiglottitis are extremely rare. This is likely due to high levels of serum antibody to capsular polysaccharide following infection with *H. influenzae*.

AIRWAY COLONIZATION

Bacterial colonization of the tracheobronchial tree (Table 32–1) is the crucial first step in the pathogenesis of nosocomial pneumonia. Pneumonia is the leading cause of death from nosocomial infection. Understanding the biology of colonization may represent our best hope of someday intervening in the devastating problem of nosocomial pneumonia. In this section, we review the epidemiology and pathogenesis of bacterial colonization and its role in the development of nosocomial pneumonia.

With the exception of the gastrointestinal tract, Gram-negative bacteria are not considered part of the normal flora, and they infrequently colonize the upper respiratory tract of

Table 32–1. EPIDEMIOLOGIC RISK FACTORS FOR BACTERIAL COLONIZATION OF THE TRACHEOBRONCHIAL TREE

Hospital or institutional setting
Intubation, tracheostomy, mechanical ventilation
Underlying illness
   Chronic cardiopulmonary disease, diabetes,
     alcoholism, neurologic, renal or hepatic disease
Previous antibiotics
Recent surgery
   Thoracic or abdominal
Elderly
Bedridden
Neutropenia
Immunosuppressive illnesses and drugs
Malnutrition
Coma, hypotension, acidosis
Smoking
Viral infection

normal individuals. Studies of hospital personnel reveal no increase in colonization with Gram-negative bacilli, indicating direct patient contact has little effect on the frequency of colonization. There are numerous risk factors associated with the development of Gram-negative bacillary colonization of the tracheobronchial tree. Hospitalized patients experience increasing rates of colonization, associated with increasing severity of illness. For example, Johanson and associates[2] found 73% of severely ill patients colonized, versus 35% of moderately ill patients. Nursing home patients, bedridden patients, and patients with underlying pulmonary disease all have high rates of colonization. Broad-spectrum antibiotic therapy and malnutrition are risk factors for colonization.

A major risk factor for colonization is endotracheal intubation. This includes both short-term intubations for surgery and longer-term intubation for respiratory failure. The endotracheal tube eliminates the filtration function of the nose and conducting airways and impairs the mucociliary clearance system of the airways. In addition, mechanical irritation and injury of respiratory mucosa predisposes to local colonization with potential bacterial pathogens. In this setting, colonization may occur with Gram-negative bacilli or with *Staphylococcus aureus*. There is a four-fold increase in nosocomial pneumonia in patients who are intubated on ventilators.

The intensive care unit (ICU) setting predisposes to bacterial colonization independently of intubation. Colonization increases with time spent in the ICU. ICU patients are among the most compromised in the hospital, suffering from ailments that include major organ dysfunction, immunosuppression, and malnutrition. In addition, use of antacids and histamine type 2 receptor blockers has been associated with higher rates of colonization. Hands of ICU personnel are a common source of transfer of nosocomial pathogens between patients. Respiratory equipment itself may be a source of bacteria. Medication nebulizers inserted into the inspiratory limb of the mechanical ventilator circuit may produce bacterial aerosols. Condensate present in dependent regions of disposable ventilator tubing can also become contaminated. This contamination primarily originates from the patient. Interestingly, Craven and colleagues[3] found that 48-hour tubing changes result in lower risk of pneumonia than 24-hour changes. Presumably, this is due to less frequent manipulation of tubes. Simple procedures such as turning the patient or raising the bedrail may accidentally wash contaminated condensate directly into the patient's tracheobronchial tree. Bedside resuscitation bags are a potential source of bacterial contamination; these are used frequently to ventilate patients during chest physiotherapy, and may become contaminated with secretions. Spirometers and oxygen analyzers have also been implicated as sources of contamination.

Recent surgery is a major risk factor for developing Gram-negative colonization of the airway independent of intubation. Length of preoperative stay, duration of surgery, and site of surgery are variables that contribute to the risk. The highest risks for colonization are associated with thoracic surgery, and the lowest with gynecologic and obstetric surgery.

Bacteria gain access to the upper airway when host defenses are overcome. These defense mechanisms were reviewed earlier in this chapter. Bacterial adherence to epithelial cells then leads to successful colonization. Adherence involves specific binding between bacterial and epithelial surface molecules. Pili or fimbriae are the bacterial surface structures involved in adherence. The epithelial cell receptors are frequently simple carbohydrate moieties, which in turn are part of more complex membrane structures. For example, D-mannose on epithelial cells is thought to be the receptor for Klebsiella, Serratia, and Enterobacter species. Different sites in the respiratory tract favor localization of certain species. Ciliated sites in the nasal and tracheal mucosa seem to bind *Pseudomonas aeruginosa* more avidly than buccal epithelial cells.

The molecular basis for bacterial colonization is a complex process and involves structures in addition to the epithelial carbohydrate moieties. Fibronectin, a large molecular weight surface glycoprotein that is highly sensitive to trypsin, may serve as a receptor for the binding of Gram-positive bacteria. Under normal conditions, mucosal cells are coated with fibronectin, which in turn selects for adherence of Gram-positive cocci and prevents adherence of Gram-negative bacteria to cells. Increased protease content of saliva is associated with loss of fibronectin from buccal cell surfaces. Salivary protease activity has been measured to be greatly elevated in patients with respiratory failure who were colonized with Gram-negative rods. Protease activity is increased in postoperative patients. Polymorphonuclear leukocytes in airway secretions may be the source of this protease. During illness or postoperative stress, an increase in salivary protease activity may result in cleavage of cell-associated fibronectin, with exposure of sugar-containing attachment sites for Gram-negative bacteria.

Oral bacteria that are normally present in the oropharynx appear to be capable of inhibiting the growth of pathogenic Gram-negative bacteria. This mechanism has been called bacterial interference. *Streptococcus viridans* have been shown to be inhibitory to Gram-negative rods. Alteration of the normal flora by the use of antibiotics can create conditions under which pathogenic bacteria gain a foothold, and eventually lead to colonization.

The relationship between tracheobronchial colonization and subsequent development of nosocomial pneumonia is well established. In ICUs, 7% to 20% of patients develop pneumonia, with over 60% of cases due to aerobic Gram-negative bacilli. Pneumonia develops in the vast majority of cases as a consequence of aspiration of pathogenic organisms that have colonized the tracheobronchial tree. The lower pulmonary defenses are overwhelmed or previously compromised and cannot handle the bacterial challenge. Aspiration is commonplace in hospitalized patients and is facilitated through the frequent use of endotracheal tubes, tracheostomies, and nasogastric tubes. Hematogenous seeding of the lung is infrequently encountered.

It is imperative that a distinction be made between colonization and true infection. Antibiotics should not be administered for colonization because this only predisposes to superinfection with resistant pathogens. Making this distinction is problematic, particularly in the ICU patient. A detailed discussion about distinguishing colonization from infection is beyond the scope of this chapter. Sputum examination, quantitative microbiologic techniques, and a number of invasive diagnostic procedures have all been employed. Maneuvers to limit colonization have met with some success in decreasing the incidence of pneumonia. The importance of handwashing by hospital personnel, meticulous care of endotracheal tubes and tracheostomies, and frequent changes in ventilator circuits has been emphasized. Unnecessary use of histamine type-2 blockers and antacids should be minimized. Their use results in nonacidic gastric contents that become overgrown with Gram-negative rods, contributing to the common problem of microaspiration in these severely ill patients. Administration of sucralfate for stress ulcer prophylaxis avoids these problems by maintaining an acidic gastric pH.

SUMMARY

The human airway is continuously called on to defend itself and the lower respiratory tract from foreign invaders. It has a wide and varied arsenal available to perform this task. The nasopharyngeal passages carry out a vital filtration function. Intruders can be ejected via an explosive cough. The delicate and intricate "ciliary escalator" constantly sweeps the airway clean. Local production of IgA allows neutralization of viruses. Normal resident bacterial flora inhibit growth of pathogenic Gram-negative organisms.

Occasionally, airway defenses are overcome and infection or colonization occurs. The croup syndrome represents such an occurrence. Subglottic inflammation and obstruction results from a variety of viral agents, but predominantly from parainfluenza virus types 1 and 3. It is a self-limited illness of young children, managed by close observation and good supportive care. Children and adults are both susceptible to epiglottitis, a rapidly progressive, life-threatening infection of the upper airway caused mainly by *Haemophilus influenzae* type b. Inflammation of the epiglottis and supraglottic structures with normal subglottic region distinguishes this from the croup syndrome. Definitive control of the airway and antibacterial therapy are the critical components of management.

Numerous risk factors exist for bacterial colonization of the airway. Major risk factors include intubation, surgery, and critical illness. Colonization is strongly associated with infection of the lower respiratory tract. This generally occurs via aspiration into the lungs, rather than hematogenous seeding of the lungs. During airway colonization, bacterial pili bind to epithelial cell receptors. Mucosal fibronectin may modulate the ecology of this colonization by favoring adherence of Gram-positive cocci and preventing Gram-negative adherence.

References

1. Battista SP, Mione P, Lapey A, et al. Role of clotting factor(s) in the etiology of lung disease related to ciliostasis. Arch Environ Health 35(4):239–246, 1980.
2. Johanson WG, Pierce AK, Sanford JP. Nosocomial respiratory infections with Gram-negative bacilli: The significance of colonization of the respiratory tract. Ann Intern Med 77:701–706, 1972.
3. Craven DE, et al. Risk factors for pneumonia and fatality in patients receiving continuous mechanical ventilation. Am Rev Respir Dis 133:792–795, 1986.

Bibliography

Abraham SN, et al. Adherence of *Streptococcus pyogenes, Escherichia coli,* and *Pseudomonas aeruginosa* to fibronectin-coated and uncoated epithelial cells. Infect Immunol 41:1261–1268, 1983.

Burns JE, Hendley JO. Epiglottitis. In Mandell GL, Douglas RG Jr, Bennett JE (eds). Principles and Practice of Infectious Disease. New York: Wiley, 1990; pp. 514–516.

Craven DE, Steger KA. Nosocomial pneumonia in the intubated patient. Infect Dis Clin North Am 3:843–866, 1989.

Green GM, et al. Defense mechanisms of the respiratory membrane. Am Rev Respir Dis 115:479–496, 1977.

Hall CB. Acute laryngotracheobronchitis. In Mandell GL, Douglas RG Jr, Bennett JE (eds). Principles and Practice of Infectious Disease. New York: Wiley, 1990; pp. 499–504.

Murray JF. Defense mechanisms. In The Normal Lung. Philadelphia: W. B. Saunders, 1986; pp. 313–337.

Pennington JE. Nosocomial respiratory infection. In Mandell GL, Douglas RG Jr, Bennett JE (eds). Principles and Practice of Infectious Disease. New York: Wiley, 1990; pp. 2199–2204.

Reynolds HY. Host defense impairments that may lead to respiratory infections. Clin Chest Med 8:339–358, 1987.

Salata RA, Ellner JJ. Bacterial colonization of the tracheobronchial tree. Clin Chest Med 9:623–631, 1988.

Wanner A. Mucociliary clearance in the trachea. Clin Chest Med 7:247–257, 1986.

CHAPTER 33

Physical Factors in High-Frequency Ventilation

Jose G. Venegas, Ph.D., and Denise J. Strieder, M.D.

High-frequency ventilation (HFV) can support gas exchange with small tidal volumes and small pressure swings, and therefore with reduced barotrauma to the lungs. The success of HFV depends on two sets of physical phenomena: the mechanics of the respiratory system and the modalities of gas transport in the lungs. Much is known about respiratory mechanics, enough to predict the response of the respiratory system to HFV on the basis of realistic models of the airways, lungs, and chest wall. Much is also known about gas transport modalities applicable to HFV, although models are not yet quantitatively reliable. By combining the imperatives of respiratory mechanics and the empirically recognized relationship between ventilation and gas exchange, we can estimate the desirable setting of any respirator, whether in the conventional ventilation (CV) or in the HFV range.

A list of symbols is given in the Appendix. References to the literature are limited to articles whose results and conclusions are essential in supporting the validity of our rationale. Reviews of the literature are available elsewhere.[1–3]

RESPIRATORY MECHANICS

Models of respiratory mechanics can be laid out in terms of mechanical components[2] or in terms of equivalent electrical components.[4] A preference for electrical models has emerged through the years, together with the acceptance of sine waves as approximations of the respiratory waveform (Fig. 33–1). Therefore, we shall use electrical models. In so doing, we must remember that the usefulness of models depends on several attributes: a clear relationship to the physical system under study; an

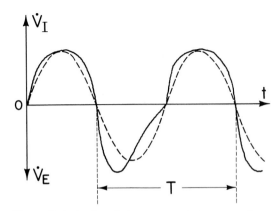

Figure 33–1. Analogy between a respiratory wave form, recorded with a pneumotachograph (*solid curve*), and a sine wave (*dashed curve*). Inspiratory flow, $\dot{V}_I$, is more closely similar to the sine wave than is expiratory flow, $\dot{V}_E$. The period, T, is the inverse of respiratory frequency, f.

Table 33–1. CORRESPONDENCE BETWEEN MECHANICAL AND ELECTRICAL SYSTEMS

Symbols	Mechanical Variables	Units*	Symbols	Electrical Variables	Units
$\dot{V}$	Flow	L/sec	i	Current	Ampere
P	Pressure	cm H_2O	v	Voltage	Volt
R	Resistance	cm H_2O/L·sec^{-1}	R	Resistance	Ohm
I	Inertance	cm H_2O/L·sec^{-2}	L	Inductance	Henry
C	Compliance	L/cm H_2O	C	Capacitance	Farad

*Unit of time may be changed to minutes or hour. Unit of pressure may be changed to mm Hg or Pascal.

optimal simplification that does not leave out essential characteristics of the system but reduces their complexity to a manageable set of components; and the use of measurable variables, so that the model may be amenable to experimental testing.

The RC Model

In 1956, Otis and associates[4] used the analogy between mechanical and electrical systems (Table 33–1) to analyze the mechanical behavior of the lungs. Once resistance (R) and compliance (C) in the lungs were modeled by a resistor and a capacitor (Fig. 33–2), the relationship between flow and pressure through the model could be predicted for the case in which flow and pressure had the form of a sine wave. Different breathing waveforms would complicate the details of the mathematical solutions, but would not change the generality of the conclusions.

The behavior of the single RC pathway in Figure 33–2 is dictated by the fact that the same flow, which passes through the resistance R, is stored in the compliance C, while the driving pressure P is the sum of the pressure differences across the resistance, P_R, and across the compliance, P_C. *Resistance* determines the energy dissipated by unit of flow. In

the case of laminar flow, resistance is a constant and the relationship between pressure and flow, $\dot{V}$, is given by Ohm's law, the equivalent in electricity of Poiseuille's law in fluid mechanics:

$$P_R = R\dot{V}$$

P_R differs from $\dot{V}$ in amplitude only: the two signals are in phase (Fig. 33–3).

Compliance reflects the elastic properties of the lungs. The greater the compliance, the less pressure is needed for the lungs to accept flow and store gas. Therefore, P_C is inversely proportional to lung compliance. Also, because P_C increases as the gas volume stored in the lung increases during inspiration, it is proportional to integrated flow. Thus, P_C reaches a maximum at the end of inspiration, when $P_C = V_T/C$, with V_T the tidal volume. In contrast, flow reaches a maximum at mid-inspiration; therefore, P_C and flow are out of phase: P_C lags flow by 1/4 of the period T, the inverse of the respiratory frequency. To express the relationship of P_C to flow in magnitude and time, we can write P_C as a vector $\vec{P}_C$, of magnitude V_T/C and phase angle -90 degrees $= -T/4$, related to flow by the expression

$$\vec{P}_C = \vec{X}_C \dot{V}$$

This equation is for a compliance the equivalent of Ohm's law for a resistance. The *reactance*, $\vec{X}_C$, is also a vector, characterized by a

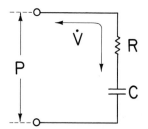
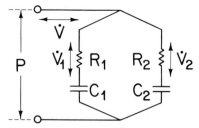

Figure 33–2. *Left,* Single RC pathway. The same flow $\dot{V}$ goes through the resistance R and the compliance C. The pressure P across the terminals is the sum of a pressure drop across the resistance and another across the compliance. *Right,* Two RC pathways in parallel are driven by the same pressure difference P, but the division of flow between the two branches is governed by their respective time constants, R_1C_1 and R_2C_2.

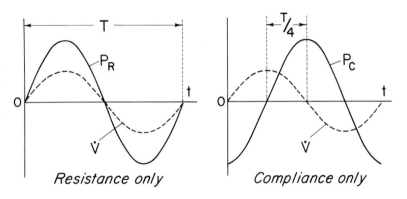

Figure 33–3. *Left,* The pressure difference across a resistance P_R and the flow $\dot{V}$ differ only in amplitude: pressure and flow are in phase. *Right,* The pressure difference across a compliance P_C is out of phase with flow. Pressure lags flow by a time equal to one quarter of the period T.

magnitude, $|\vec{X}_c| = 1/2\pi fC$, inversely proportional to compliance, and a phase angle $\varphi = +90$ degrees (see Fig. 33–7). In the case of Ohm's law for a resistance, the vectorial notation can also be used. Then resistance is a vector $\vec{R}$ in phase with flow (its phase angle is 0) and with magnitude: $|\vec{R}| = R$.

Returning to the single RC pathway, we can now appreciate that the pressure at the airway opening is the vector sum: $\vec{P}_R + \vec{P}_c = (R + \vec{X}_c)\dot{V}$. The term $R + \vec{X}_c$ measures the *impedance* $\vec{Z}$ of the pathway, so that the generalized Ohm's Law for an RC pathway can be written:

$$\vec{P} = \vec{Z}\dot{V}$$

$\vec{Z}$ is a vector whose magnitude is $\sqrt{R^2 + |\vec{X}|^2}$ (Fig. 33–4). The phase angle φ between $\vec{Z}$ (or $\vec{P}$) and $\dot{V}$ depends on the ratio of reactance to resistance: φ is the angle whose tangent equals $1/2\pi fRC$. The product RC, measured in units of time (Table 33–1) and called the *time constant* of the pathway,

together with f, determines the phase angle between pressure and flow for an RC pathway.

Leaving for a moment the sine wave analogy, let us recall that the rate of passive expiration is also determined by the time constant. At the onset of expiration, alveolar pressure is proportional to tidal volume and inversely proportional to compliance. Expiratory flow begins, driven by alveolar pressure V_T/C and opposed by resistance: the initial flow, V_T/RC, is also the maximal flow. As expiration progresses, lung volume, alveolar pressure and expiratory flow decrease exponentially (Fig. 33–5). For all three functions the argument of the exponential is $-t/RC$, where t is the expiratory time. During spontaneous breathing and in CV, expiratory durations $>3RC$ are needed for end-expiratory lung volume to approach the *static* functional residual capacity (FRC) and for the end-xpiratory alveolar pressure to approach zero (Table 33–2). With expiratory durations $<3RC$, lung volume increases with successive

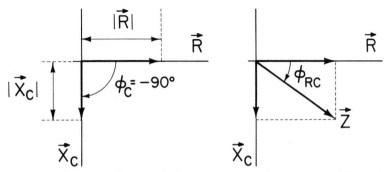

Figure 33–4. In vectorial coordinates, the horizontal axis represents zero phase angle, and the vertical axis represents phase angles of 90°, either positive or negative. *Left,* Resistance, which is in phase with flow, plots on the horizontal axis and compliant reactance, $\vec{X}_c$, plots on the vertical axis with a negative magnitude, $-1/2\pi fC$, and negative phase angle, $\varphi = -90°$. *Right,* Impedance $\vec{Z}$ is the vector sum of resistance and reactance, with magnitude $|\vec{Z}| = \sqrt{R^2 + |\vec{X}_c|^2}$ (Pythagorean theorem). The phase angle of impedance is that which has a tangent equal to $|\vec{X}_c|/R$: $= \tan^{-1}|\vec{X}_c|/R$.

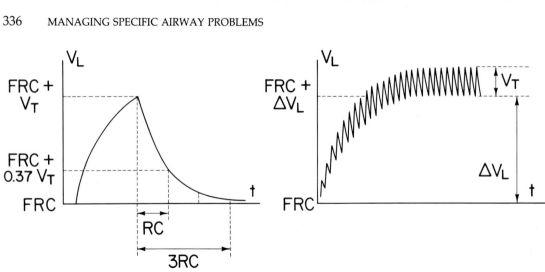

Figure 33–5. *Left,* Change in lung volume above FRC during a single breath in conventional ventilation with tidal volume, V_T. During expiration, alveolar pressure and lung volume fall exponentially, so that at least three times the time constant RC must be allowed for expiration, if the end-expiratory lung volume is to approximate FRC. *Right,* When expiratory time is shorter than three times the initial time constant, lung volume rises until the decreased compliance reduces the time constant, enough to allow the tidal volume V_T to be exhaled in the time allotted by the respirator. The end-expiratory lung volume is then dynamically determined and equal to FRC + ΔV.

breaths and consequently expiratory flow increases (Fig. 33–5): a new equilibrium is reached when expired tidal volume equals inspired tidal volume, but then FRC is *dynamically* determined. In HFV, expiratory times are small: unless RC is small also, as in the respiratory distress syndrome, a rise in lung volume will be needed to boost expiratory flow and again FRC will be dynamically determined.

The frequency dependence of impedance for an RC pathway is also governed by its time constant. The compliant reactance, of magnitude $1/2\pi fC$, falls with increasing frequency, and so does the magnitude of impedance, rapidly over the low-frequency range and slowly over the high-frequency range (Fig. 33–6). One can identify the frequency at which impedance changes from one to the other behavior as that for which reactance equals resistance, or *corner frequency*, which is inversely proportional to the time constant: $f_c = 1/2\pi RC$. For a constant ventilation, impedance falls markedly with increasing frequency up to f_c, because smaller tidal volumes require smaller P_C, while the resistance is constant. With frequencies greater than f_c, impedance continues to fall with increasing frequency, but slowly, because resistance has become the greater part of impedance (Fig. 33–6). In practice, ventilation must be increased when frequency is raised, but below f_c raising frequency is advantageous, because the fall of impedance is much steeper than the rise of ventilatory requirement. There is no advantage to raising frequency much above f_c.

To represent possible inhomogeneities among parallel pathways in the lung, the RC model can be modified to include two parallel pathways of impedance, $\vec{Z}_1$ and $\vec{Z}_2$ (see Fig. 33–2). In that case, the total impedance of the system is given by:

$$\frac{1}{\vec{Z}} = \frac{1}{\vec{Z}_1} + \frac{1}{\vec{Z}_2}$$

Using similar equations, Otis and associates[4] were able to draw the following conclusions, applicable to a model composed of two or more RC pathways mounted in parallel and to the low-frequency range pertaining to CV. Flow will be equally distributed to the pathways if these have equal resistance and compliance. Flow will be distributed in unequal but constant proportions between pathways if these have equal time constants, because in that case the variation of phase angle with

Table 33–2. FRACTION OF TIDAL VOLUME REMAINING IN THE LUNG, EXP ($-t/RC$), AT DIFFERENT TIMES (t) DURING PASSIVE EXPIRATION

Time from Onset of Expiration	exp ($-t/RC$)
0	1
1 RC	0.37
2 RC	0.14
3 RC	0.05
4 RC	0.02
5 RC	0.006

RC, resistance × compliance.

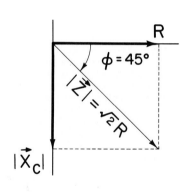
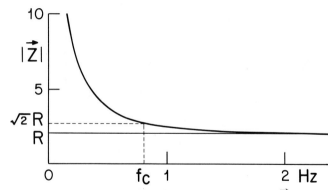

Figure 33–6. *Left,* For an RC pathway, the corner frequency, f_c, is that for which magnitude of reactance $|\vec{X}_C|$ equals resistance. At that frequency, the magnitude of impedance $|\vec{Z}|$ is $\sqrt{2}$ R and its phase angle is $-45°$. *Right,* Magnitude of impedance in cm H_2O/L·sec^{-1} as a function of frequency in Hz for a model of the respiratory system consisting of a single RC pathway. Compliance is 0.1 L/cm H_2O and resistance 2 cm H_2O/L·sec^{-1}. Corner frequency, f_c, is 0.8 Hz or 48/minute.

frequency will be the same for all pathways, regardless of the absolute values of R and C in each one. In all other cases, the distribution of flow between parallel pathways will vary with frequency, there will be intermittent flow back and forth between the compliances (asynchronous ventilation or Pendelluft), and the effective resistance and compliance of the system as a whole will be frequency-dependent. These conclusions, which have been experimentally confirmed, led to our current understanding of distribution of ventilation in the lungs at low breathing frequencies.

The RIC Model

Electrical models are equally useful in describing the flow–pressure relationships in HFV, but in that case the model needs to be altered to account for inertia. In HFV, tidal volumes are small but flow rates are large. The initiation of flow after each reversal requires acceleration, which is opposed by the *inertance* I of the respiratory system, mostly that of air in the airways. To produce acceleration, energy must be provided in the form of increased driving pressure at the airway opening. The magnitude of this pressure increment, P_I, depends on the acceleration, which in turn is proportional to the derivative of flow: $P_I = I\, d\dot{V}/dt$. For example, in a healthy adult, inertance has been measured[5] as 0.01 cm H_2O/L·sec^{-2}. In a typical HFV setting with f = 6 Hz and V_T = 120 mL, flow peaks at 2.4 L/sec and acceleration ($d\dot{V}/dt$) at 96 L·sec^{-2}: P_I = 1 cm H_2O. Because the pressure swings are small, the inertial component is never

negligible at high frequency. Therefore, to be applicable to HFV, a model of the respiratory system must include inertance as well as resistance and compliance.

If flow across an inertance is a sine wave, P_I is also a sine wave and, like P_C, it is displaced in time and reaches its maximum or minimum at points of no flow (Fig. 33–7). But P_I is proportional to the derivative of flow and runs 1/4 period ahead of flow, leading flow by an angle of +90 degrees. Again we can consider the vectors and write:

$$\vec{P}_I = \vec{X}_I\, \dot{V}$$

where $\vec{X}_I$, the *inertial reactance*, is a vector defined by its magnitude, $|\vec{X}_I|$ = I, and phase angle, φ = +90 degrees (Fig. 33–7).

In an RIC model (Fig. 33–8), the pressure across the system is the vector sum of the pressure drops across resistance, inertance, and compliance (RIC): $\vec{P} = P_R + \vec{P}_I + \vec{P}_C$. However, we can write Ohm's law for an RIC system as the simple expression:

$$\vec{P} = \vec{Z}\, \dot{V}$$

where the *impedance* $\vec{Z}$ is the vectorial sum of the resistance and the total reactance, $\vec{X} = \vec{X}_I + \vec{X}_C$. $\vec{X}$ has for magnitude the algebraic sum of $|\vec{X}_I|$ and $|\vec{X}_C|$ and for phase angle $\pm$ 90 degrees, the sign depending on which reactance has the largest magnitude. The magnitude of $\vec{Z}$ is $\sqrt{R^2 + |\vec{X}|^2}$ and its phase angle has a tangent equal to $|\vec{X}|/R$ (Fig. 33–8).

The magnitude of $\vec{X}_I$ increases with increasing frequency, whereas the magnitude of $\vec{X}_C$ decreases with increasing frequency, but $\vec{X}_I$ and $\vec{X}_C$ are opposite in direction. Therefore, there exists a frequency for which, as the magnitudes of $\vec{X}_I$ and $\vec{X}_C$ are equal, the two

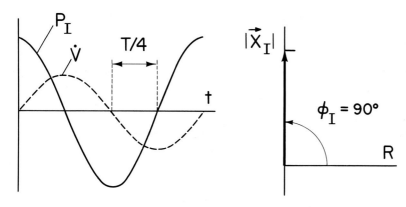

Figure 33–7. *Left,* The pressure difference across an inertance, P_I is out of phase with flow $\dot{V}$. Pressure leads flow by a time equal to one quarter of the period T, which is given a positive sign: the phase angle is $+90°$. *Right,* The inertial reactance is a vector defined by magnitude $2\pi fI$ and phase angle $+90°$.

vectors cancel each other out and $\vec{X} = 0$. This frequency, $f_o = 1/2\pi\sqrt{LC}$, is called the *resonant frequency*.

Pressure at the Airway Opening, in the Central Airways, and in the Alveoli

Resonant frequency is determined by the relative magnitudes of inertance and compliance. Because inertance is mostly linked to gas flow acceleration in the central airways,[5] inertance will be little affected by lung disease. In contrast, compliance can change by one order of magnitude in diseased lungs. Because the resonant frequency is proportional to the inverse of $\sqrt{C}$, the stiffer the lungs, the higher the resonant frequency (Table 33–3).

At the resonant frequency, $\vec{Z} = R$. At all other frequencies, $|\vec{Z}| > R$. At resonance, therefore, the pressure needed to drive the respiratory system for any given flow is mini-mized; we might hope that the barotrauma to the lungs could be minimized too. However, Fredberg and associates[6] have pointed out that ventilating at resonant frequency minimizes pressure swings at the airway opening, but not always in the alveoli. These authors reasoned from a model similar to that of Figure 33–9 applied to the case of excised lungs, so that pleural pressure, P_{pl}, is zero. Then the pressure at the airway opening P_{ao} is the driving pressure across the total impedance of the lungs and alveolar pressure $\vec{P}_A$ is the driving pressure across the compliant reactance of the lungs, with $|\vec{P}_A| = \dot{V}/2\pi fC$. At resonance, when $P_{ao} = R\dot{V}$, the ratio P_A/P_{ao} can be shown to equal the ratio of the corner frequency to the resonant frequency. This ratio is often referred to as the *quality factor* of the system, $Q = f_c/f_o$, or with f_o and f_c replaced by their actual values, $Q = \sqrt{I/C}/R$.

The quality factor governs the behavior of RIC systems on either side of resonant frequency. Systems with $Q < 1$ are said to be overdamped and show weak resonance. Sys-

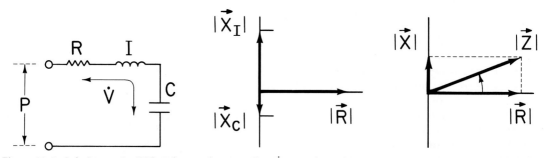

Figure 33–8. *Left,* In a series RIC pathway, the same flow $\dot{V}$ goes through resistance R, inertance I, and compliance C. The driving pressure P is the difference between pressures at the airway opening and either the pressure in the pleural space (lung model) or the pressure at the body surface (model of the respiratory system). R and I would be essentially the same in both models, but the compliance of the lung is greater than that of the respiratory system. *Center,* Three vectors representing inertial reactance, $\vec{X}_I$ ($\varphi = +90°$), compliant reactance, X_C ($\varphi = -90°$), and resistance, R ($\varphi = 0$). *Right,* The magnitude of total reactance $|\vec{X}|$ is the algebraic sum of $|\vec{X}_I|$ and $|\vec{X}_C|$. Impedance $\vec{Z}$ is the vectorial sum of R and $|\vec{X}|$ with phase angle equal to $\tan^{-1}|\vec{X}|/R$.

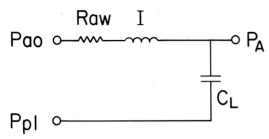

Figure 33–9. Three-terminal model of the lungs alone. The driving pressure across the lungs is the pressure at the airway opening P_{ao}, less the pleural pressure P_{pl}. R_{aw} is the airway resistance and I the inertance. A third terminal, on the right of the diagram, identifies alveolar pressure P_A, the driving pressure across the lung compliance C_L: P_A determines the barotrauma to distal airspaces.

Table 33–3. RESONANT FREQUENCY FOR ADULT LUNGS, AS PREDICTED FOR AN INVARIANT INERTANCE OF 0.01 cm $H_2O/L \cdot sec^{-2}$

Lung Compliance (C_L) L/cm H_2O	Resonant Frequency (f_o), Hz
0.2	3.2
0.1	5.1
0.05	7.2
0.02	10.6
0.01	16.0

airway pressure of 10 cm H_2O, Q was 1.26 only.[7]

In general, by knowing resistance, inertance, and compliance we can calculate the corner frequency, the resonant frequency, and the Q factor for any clinical situation (Table 33–4). For an adult patient with healthy lungs under general anesthesia, with a mean airway pressure of zero, Q = 0.32: the respiratory system is overdamped. Greater values of Q could be induced only by causing mean airway pressure, and therefore lung volume, to rise to the point where compliance falls appreciably. In adults with respiratory distress syndrome, Q is critically dependent on compliance. If the compliance of the respiratory system, C_{RS}, falls to 0.01, Q is 1 at resonance. For lower values of C_{RS}, Q > 1 near resonance. In premature infants with hyaline membrane disease, there is little risk of reaching Q > 1 because resistance is large as compared with $\sqrt{I/C}$ and f_c is

tems with Q > 1 are underdamped and develop strong resonance. In the respiratory system, when Q < 1, pressure swings are always smaller in the alveoli than at the airway opening. When Q > 1, pressure swings near the resonant frequency are greater in the alveoli than at the airway opening (Fig. 33–10). Such alveolar pressure amplification was observed by Fredberg and associates[6] in excised dog lungs. When mean airway pressure was increased from 5 to 25 cm H_2O, Q increased from 1.9 to 4.8 because lung compliance fell, whereas resistance and inertance showed little change. In live, anesthetized, vagotomized dogs, a similar, but more moderate behavior was observed at resonance and at a mean

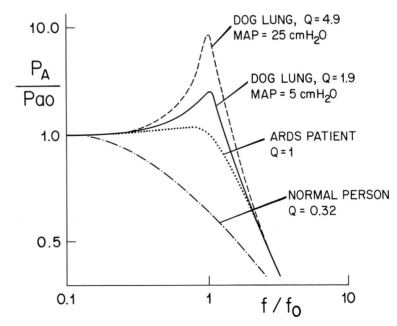

Figure 33–10. The ratio of alveolar pressure P_A to pressure at the airway opening P_{ao} is plotted as a function of frequency f divided by the resonant frequency f_o. The relationship is determined by the value of the quality factor, Q. Only in cases where Q>1, can alveolar pressure amplification take place near resonance (f/f_o near unity). MAP is the mean airway pressure.

Table 33-4. REPRESENTATIVE VALUES OF RESISTANCE (R), INERTANCE (L), COMPLIANCE OF THE RESPIRATORY SYSTEM (C_{RS}), CORNER FREQUENCY (f_c), RESONANT FREQUENCY (f_o), AND THE QUALITY FACTOR ($Q = f_c/f_o$) AT STATED MEAN AIRWAY PRESSURE (MAP) FOR DOGS AND FOR HUMANS: ADULTS WITH HEALTHY LUNGS, ADULTS WITH THE RESPIRATORY DISTRESS SYNDROME (RDS) OR CHRONIC OBSTRUCTIVE LUNG DISEASE (COPD), AND PREMATURE INFANTS WITH HYALINE MEMBRANE DISEASE (HMD). ONLY IN DOGS IS $f_c > f_o$ AND $Q > 1$

	MAP cm H_2O	R* cm $H_2O/L \cdot sec^{-1}$	L cm $H_2O/L \cdot sec^{-2}$	C_{RS} $L/cm\ H_2O$	f_c Hz	f_o Hz	Q
Dogs[7]	10	0.6	0.016	0.031	9	7	1.26
Humans							
Healthy adult	0	1	0.01	0.1	1.6	5	0.32
Adult RDS	10	1	0.01	0.02	5.7	11	0.52
Adult COPD	0	7.5	0.01	0.40	0.05	2.5	0.20
Infant HMD[13]	0	30	0.024	0.0004	13	50	0.26

*Measured from the tip of an endotracheal tube.

much smaller than f_o (Table 33-4): $Q = 0.26$ and the respiratory system should be markedly overdamped.

Because the lungs are a complex branching system, alveolar pressure swings, ΔP_A, can vary substantially between alveoli. High ΔP_A are most likely to be found in those alveoli that are governed by short bronchial pathways, but phase differences also can create differences in ΔP_A between alveolar regions. It is now thought that pressure gradients between adjacent regions could be as deleterious as the magnitude of alveolar pressure swings, a concept that invites limiting P_{ao} to the point of possibly compromising the efficacy of HFV. However, in HFV a sizeable portion of P_{ao} is dissipated by the resistance and inertance of the tracheal tube and the trachea. Therefore, the magnitude of pressure swings decreases rapidly as one moves the site of measurement from the airway opening to the carina. Minimizing pressure swings at the carina is an attractive option, one that sets a known upper bound to pressure swings in the alveoli and pressure gradients between neighboring regions.

The Airway Wall Shunt

Another important characteristic of the respiratory system is that airway walls are not rigid, but compliant. Part of each tidal volume is stored in the expanding airways during inspiration and released by the recoiling airways during expiration. In CV, the volume lost in distending the airway is a small fraction of tidal volume. In HFV, the loss can be considerable.[8] The compliance of the intrathoracic airway

walls, C_w, has been estimated[9] as 4 mL per cm H_2O of transmural pressure in the human adult. The presence of an intratracheal tube is unlikely to change this value by much.

Mead[9] considers the airways as a compliant pathway with negligible resistance to distention and therefore a negligibly small time constant. In that case, airway distention will be proportional to the static compliance of the airways. The distending pressure is the airway transmural pressure, which in a static condition equals or approximates the transpulmonary pressure, $P_{ao} - P_{pl}$. During flow, however, the airway transmural pressure becomes a complicated function of time within the breathing cycle and of distance along the airways: at time of maximal flow, distention affects the central more than the peripheral airways. At points of no flow, the static conditions are probably realized. Still, as a simplification, we can pose that $P_{ao} - P_{pl}$ is a working estimate of average airway distending pressure during the breathing cycle, although the accuracy of that estimate cannot be determined at present. We can then think of airway distention as a compliant shunt in parallel with lung impedance. For any pressure driving the model in Figure 33-11, the effective flow through the lung $\dot{V}_L$ is inversely proportional to the magnitude of lung impedance, $|\vec{Z}_L|$, and the flow lost to the shunt is inversely proportional to the magnitude of airway wall impedance, $|\vec{Z}_w| = 1/2\pi f C_w$. Therefore,

$$\dot{V}_w/\dot{V}_L = 2\pi f C_w |\vec{Z}_L|$$

In HFV, however, gas transport takes place partly in the airway, so that it becomes difficult to distinguish which fraction of $\dot{V}_w$ represents shunt ventilation and which contributes to effective ventilation, $\dot{V}_L$. To acknowledge this

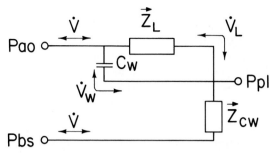

Figure 33–11. An electrical model of the respiratory system, applicable to HFV, includes lung impedance $\vec{Z}_L$, chest wall impedance $\vec{Z}_{cw}$, and the compliance of airway walls C_w. Ventilation is driven by the pressure at the airway opening P_{ao}, less the pressure at the body surface P_{bs}. A third terminal on the right of the diagram identifies pleural pressure, P_{pl}. Effective ventilation $\dot{V}_L$ is only a fraction of total ventilation $\dot{V}$, because some flow, $\dot{V}_w$, is lost to moving the airway wall (airway wall shunt).

uncertainty, we calculated the effect of the airway wall shunt not as a single value, but as a range between $2\pi f C_w \, |\vec{Z}_L|$ and $\pi f C_w \, |\vec{Z}_L|$, the latter expression implying that the shunt effect only involves one half of the airway volume (Fig. 33–12). Regardless of its exact magnitude, the airway wall shunt claims a fraction of the tidal volume, which increases with increasing frequency. At frequencies below 10 Hz, the calculated effect is modest for adults with healthy lungs or with respiratory distress syndrome, but quite large for a patient with chronic obstructive pulmonary disease (COPD) (Fig. 33–12). In practice, loss of tidal volume to the airway wall shunt has been considered a likely cause for limited effectiveness of HFV in ventilator-dependent patients thought to have small airway disease.[10]

Parallel RIC Pathways

The lungs contain not a single pathway but a variable number, depending on whether we consider as pathways two lungs, five lobes, 18 segments, etc., ending with some 300,000 primary lobules, all exhibiting resistance, inertance, and compliance in a complicated series-parallel network. From the electrical model we learn that if all pathways had identical resistance, inertance, and compliance, then the network would respond to a driving pressure in a manner identical to that of a single pathway.

From gross anatomy alone we can conclude that lung units are not equal. The length and number of bronchial branches vary from short

segments, such as the anterior segment of the right upper lobe, to long ones, such as the posterior segments of the lower lobes. Also, compliance is a function of transpulmonary pressure, and pleural pressure varies from the superior to the dependent regions of the lungs; therefore, regional compliance varies as well. Regional variations in inertance, although small, may be expected also, because of regional variability of airway length and branching. Severe regional variations occur as a result of lung disease, but even in healthy lungs the distribution of flow is uneven.

Measurements of dynamic compliance and effective resistance characterize the respiratory system as a single RC pathway, although it is known that neither resistance nor compliance are single-valued parameters. Because flow in the airways is predominantly non-Poiseuille, airway resistance, R_{aw}, is non-ohmic; rather, R_{aw} is flow dependent[11] and therefore greater in HFV than in CV. In addition, because of uneven distribution of flow, both R and C measurements preferentially register the behavior of well-ventilated regions, with the result that both resistance and dynamic compliance fall smoothly across the range of useful frequencies, as discussed by Otis and associates.[4] The airway wall shunt acts in the same way[9] and adds to the frequency dependence of

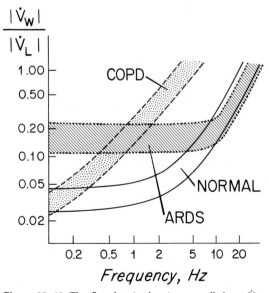

Figure 33–12. The flow lost in the airway wall shunt $\dot{V}_w$, expressed as a fraction of lung ventilation $\dot{V}_L$, increases with increasing frequency. The airway wall shunt is greatest in patients with increased airway resistance, such as chronic obstructive pulmonary disease (COPD) and asthma. ARDS, adult respiratory distress syndrome.

both resistance and dynamic compliance. The frequency dependence of inertance has received much less attention, but from theory and from actual reactance measurements it can be concluded that inertance rises with increasing frequency.

Methods now exist to measure the frequency spectra of impedance, reactance, compliance, resistance, and inertance in less than 30 seconds by oscillating the respiratory system with either a random noise[12] or with a frequency sweep.[13] Sometime in the future, these technologies are likely to be incorporated into smart respirators. At that time, it will become practical to acknowledge that R, I, and C are frequency-dependent parameters rather than constants. Models of the respiratory system that include parallel RIC pathways will then become useful, no matter how cumbersome the mathematical equations needed to describe the behavior of such systems.

For the present, it is reasonable to use the simple model of Figure 33–11, in which R, I, C_L, and C_w are taken as constants and given individual values that are representative of different clinical situations (Table 33–4). The usefulness of this model has been illustrated already by our discussion of resonant frequency and of the airway wall shunt.

GAS TRANSPORT MECHANISMS

We use the expression gas transport to designate the movement of distinct gas species, mainly O_2 and CO_2, in and out of the lungs. In contrast, ventilation only measures bulk flow, regardless of gas composition. Alveolar ventilation, $\dot{V}_A$, is a hybrid variable, defined as the ratio of CO_2 output, $\dot{V}_{CO_2}$, to the "ideal" alveolar CO_2 concentration, FA_{CO_2}, as calculated from the arterial P_{CO_2}.[14] The ratio $\dot{V}_A/\dot{V}$ measures the efficiency of gas transport, which for healthy lungs is 0.6 to 0.8 in CV and 0.02 to 0.2 in HFV[15]: this marked difference reflects the different importance, in CV and HFV, of various mechanisms of gas transport. In this section, we describe three major mechanisms: convection, diffusion, and convective dispersion.

Convection is another name for bulk flow, where volumes of fluid move en masse. In the case of a gas mixture, all molecular species travel the same average distance in the same time interval. The net transport of any species in the gas mixture is the product of the bulk flow, $\dot{V}$, by the fractional concentration, F_G, of the gas species. Convective transport is independent of molecular characteristics.

In contrast, transport by diffusion results from random molecular motion and depends on the molecular diffusivity of the gas, $DMOL_G$. Species transport by unit time, $\dot{V}_G$, is proportional to the cross-sectional area, A, across which diffusion takes place, and the concentration difference per unit distance (perpendicular to A), dC/dx, as stated by Fick's equation:

$$\dot{V}_G = A \, DMOL_G \, (dC/dx)$$

In the lungs, A and dC/dx are clearly defined at the alveolar–capillary interface, where A is the surface area of the alveolar walls (or rather the summed area of the fractions of wall surface apposed to capillaries) and dC/dx is the concentration difference between pulmonary capillary blood and alveolar air. Elsewhere in the lungs, where diffusion within the gas phase is to be considered, A is a function of airway geometry and dC/dx varies with distance from the alveolar wall, with different behaviors in CV and HFV.

Convective dispersion refers to the spreading of contiguous particles in a moving fluid, as produced by a non-uniform velocity profile. In the airways, dispersion is usually irreversible because the branching tree geometry and possibly molecular diffusion prohibit any gas molecule from retracing its path on successive inspirations and expirations. Irreversible dispersion results in a net transport of individual gas species across any plane of reference and is believed to play an important role in HFV.[16, 17]

Conventional Ventilation

Convection and diffusion are dominant mechanisms of gas transport in CV. Their relative roles are dictated by the structure of the airways. From the trachea downward, the summed cross-sectional area (CSA) of all airways increases.[18] By the 16th generation (mostly terminal bronchioles), total CSA for an adult is approximately 1000 cm². With an inspiratory flow of 500 cm³/sec, the forward bulk flow velocity of inspired air falls from 150 cm/sec in the trachea to 0.5 cm/sec in the terminal bronchioles. Beyond that, the forward velocity is so small and the total CSA so large that diffusion becomes the primary mechanism for transport of O_2 and CO_2 molecules down the existing concentration gradients; incoming gas takes on a composition similar to that of the resident gas: a large fraction of the inspired tidal volume becomes alveolar gas. This mixing of incoming and resident gas is facilitated by the motion of the heart.[19] Therefore, at the level of either the terminal or the respiratory bronchioles, a front of rapidly changing O_2 and CO_2 concentrations separates the incoming fresh air from the diffusion-mixed alveolar air.[20] At expiration, this front travels by convection up the airways to the mouth, where it can be observed with fast-responding gas analyzers.

By the time it reaches the mouth, the front of rapidly changing concentrations has lost some of its initial sharpness, in part because of uneven lengths of various bronchial pathways; it is still well enough defined to allow measurements of the volume of conducting airways or anatomic dead space, V_D. For the purpose of measuring anatomic dead space, the single-breath nitrogen test of Fowler[21] has become the method of reference, but the principles involved in the creation of an O_2–N_2 interface are identical to those involved with the O_2 and CO_2 concentration fronts.

During expiration in CV, alveolar gas flows through the airways, making up part of the expired air. Thus, the alveolar ventilation is breathed out in large aliquots (60% to 80% of tidal volume) and the concentration profiles along the airways are very much different during expiration and inspiration (Fig. 33–13). Although Fick's diffusion is clearly important in CV, the limiting mechanism for gas transport is convective bulk flow of inspired gas, which mixes with resident gas, and of alveolar air, which is breathed out.

High-Frequency Ventilation

In HFV, the tidal volumes are small and alveolar gas concentrations are never seen at the airway opening. Alveolar ventilation is still a real and measurable quantity, in so far as FA_{CO_2} can be estimated from arterial P_{CO_2} but it is no longer delivered to the outside in sizeable aliquots of alveolar gas: rather, each expiration contains some CO_2 at a concentration that rises during expiratory time from zero to a fraction of FA_{CO_2} (Fig. 33–14). One can still assess the efficiency of ventilation as the ratio of alveolar ventilation to total ventilation, $\dot{V}_A/\dot{V}$, which is always much smaller in HFV than in CV.[15] However, the focus of interest in HFV is not its low efficiency ratio, but the fact that it is efficient enough to sustain eucapnia with reduced alveolar pressure swings. Several mechanisms are thought to be responsible for gas transport in HFV.

First, mixing of resident gas by diffusion is as important in HFV as it is in CV. The oscillation that HFV imposes on all the resident gas adds to or even supplants the mixing action of the heart. Other mechanisms account for O_2 and CO_2 transport between well-mixed alveolar gas and ambient air at the airway opening. These mechanisms, which we will now examine, occur in varying degrees during CV as well. In CV, however, their effects are unimportant, because the first 100 mL or so of

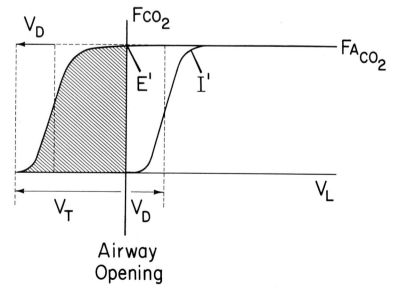

Figure 33–13. CO_2 concentration (F_{CO_2}) profiles in the lungs, from airway opening through the cumulative volume of airways toward the alveoli, and in the expired tidal volume, V_T. In CV the concentration profiles existing in the lungs at the end of inspiration (I′) and at the end of expiration (E′) are quite different. The shaded area highlights the CO_2-containing portion of expired tidal volume. The volume of the anatomic dead space can be derived from the rapidly changing CO_2 concentration in expired air as a function of tidal volume.

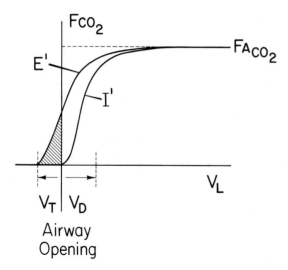

Figure 33–14. CO_2 concentration (F_{CO_2}) profiles in the lung from airway opening through the cumulative volume of airways toward the alveoli, and in the expired tidal volume, V_T, during HFV. End-inspiratory (I') and end-expiratory (E') profiles are schematic. The shaded area highlights the CO_2-containing portion of the tidal volume.

inspired air are forced further down into the lungs by the continuing inspiration and then mixed with resident gas to become alveolar air. In HFV, the small tidal volumes are immediately breathed out with increased CO_2 and decreased O_2 concentrations, showing that some gas transport has taken place.

Direct Alveolar Ventilation

Direct alveolar ventilation occurs whenever a fraction of the tidal volume, however small, actually reaches some of the distal air spaces, where it mixes with resident gas by diffusion. The observation that direct alveolar ventilation can occur without flushing the whole anatomic dead space goes back to Henderson,[22] Rohrer,[11] Briscoe,[23] and their coauthors. Several mechanisms are involved in this process alone. The existence of short pathways in the lung has been mentioned already. From anatomic measurement of the human lung, Rohrer[11] predicted that alveoli in the central regions would be directly ventilated with any tidal volume greater than 75% of dead space volume. From measurements of bronchial casts of dog lungs, Ross[24] estimated that direct alveolar ventilation would occur with tidal volumes greater than 54% of dead space. More recently, Kamm and associates[25] calculated that when tidal volume exceeds 80% of dead

space, most of the gas transport is due to direct alveolar ventilation. In these three studies it was assumed that regional tidal volumes, V_{Ti}, were evenly distributed, so that alveolar ventilation occured only where regional dead space, V_{Di}, was small.

Regardless of the absolute values of regional dead spaces, regional V_{Ti}/V_{Di} ratios greater than unity can occur in HFV as a result of uneven pathway impedances. Low-impedance pathways receive a larger fraction of tidal volume than would be expected from their alveolar volume and regional dead space. Other than pathway length and diameter, geometric characteristics such as branching angles affect pathway impedance. Indeed, in models of symmetric branching trees, Snyder and colleagues[26] observed a preferential distribution of flow to daughter branches that lay medial to the parent bifurcation. Asymmetric angles accentuate this type of uneven distribution, because inertia forces the inspired gas to flow preferentially into the straighter pathway. Pathologic changes in some airways also cause preferential distribution of inspired air to low-impedance pathways.[6]

In addition, inspiratory flow travels through the bronchi with non-uniform velocity profiles. In the well-known case of laminar flow in a straight tube and far from the entrance (Poiseuille flow), the fluid moves with a parabolic profile, whereby gas velocity in the center of the tube equals twice the average velocity of the flow. With this type of flow and in the absence of diffusion, some gas can reach the distal end of a tube without need for a complete flushing of the tube volume, a mechanism that has been considered to explain the observation of adequate alveolar ventilation with low tidal volumes.[11, 22, 23] However, inspiratory velocity profiles in the airways are by far more complex than Poiseuille flow. Direct measurements in branching tubes[3] and in a model of the human airways[27] showed skewed profiles with peak velocities near the medial wall of daughter branches. It is conceivable that inspired gas traveling along such velocity paths could reach alveoli with tidal volumes smaller than anatomic dead space.

Direct alveolar ventilation in HFV is favored by relatively large tidal volumes and is preferentially distributed to pathways that are shorter and straighter or have lower impedance than the rest of the lung (Fig. 33–15). Therefore, one would expect that increasing tidal volume in HFV might result in increasingly uneven distribution of ventilation, which indeed has been shown experimentally with ra-

PATH LENGTHS   IMPEDANCES   VELOCITY PROFILES

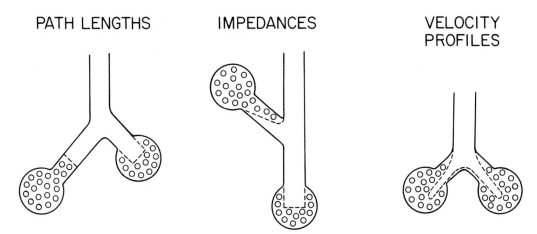

Figure 33–15. Direct alveolar ventilation in HFV can result from three distinct mechanisms: short path length, low path impedance, and asymmetrical velocity profiles.

dioactive gases. Using [133]xenon in dogs, Brusasco and associates[28] observed that ventilation was equally distributed to apical and basal regions lying in the same horizontal plane when tidal volume was less than 2/3 of V_D, but greater in the basal than in the apical region when tidal volume was greater than 2/3 of V_D. Using [13]nitrogen and constant ventilation, as measured by the product $V_T f$, also in dogs, one of us[29] observed that as tidal volume increased from 0.25 V_D to V_D, the ventilation to the basal regions of the lungs increased twofold, whereas that to the apical regions had only a slight increase. Using [13]nitrogen and constant $V_T f$ at varying frequencies, Yamada and colleagues[30] described a central region of the lungs in dogs, imaged by positron emission tomography (PET), which is preferentially ventilated as compared to the periphery. Using [133]xenon, Rehder and Didier[31] also found uneven distribution of ventilation in anesthetized and paralyzed human volunteers, but ventilation was delivered preferentially to the apical regions of the lungs; the effect of varying tidal volume was not examined. In these studies, however, all regions of the lungs received some ventilation, so that other mechanisms besides direct alveolar ventilation must come into play during HFV. These mechanisms may be referred to as irreversible dispersion.

Taylor Dispersion

Taylor[32] described the dispersion of an indicator substance injected into a unidirectional laminar flow in straight tubes. The relevance of this phenomenon to gas transport in HFV is a matter of controversy. However, Taylor's work is mentioned in articles concerned with HFV so often that some familiarity with this work is needed for a critical reading of the literature. Taylor's purpose was to refine existing techniques for measuring flow in water pipes by injecting brine at one site and calculating flow from changes in water conductivity at some other site downstream, a principle later applied to the measurement of cardiac output by the indicator dilution method. Although much of his work was concerned with the dispersion of a bolus, Taylor also considered the case in which a solution of constant indicator concentration enters a tube that initially contained pure solvent. The latter case may be considered as a simplified model of respiratory gas transport.

In laminar flow, because of the parabolic velocity profile, an initially sharp concentration front progressively takes the form of a paraboloid and creates a diffusion gradient at the interface between the advancing paraboloid and the surrounding fluid. The dispersion of the indicator "is due to the combined action of convection parallel to the axis and molecular diffusion in the radial direction."[32] At moderate rates of flow, when the convection is faster than radial diffusion, the cross-sectional average of indicator concentration falls linearly with the distance traveled down the tube. At low rates of flow, when radial diffusion is faster than longitudinal convection, the radial concentration gradients decay as soon as they are generated by the velocity profile. The overall result is a "strong tendency for molecular diffusion to prevent dispersion along the tube."[32] Accordingly, the zone of varying concentration remains narrower than that predicted for convection alone. Taylor's theoretical analysis showed that, in cases where the time needed for radial diffusion was much shorter than that needed for axial convection, the dispersion of a bolus could be treated as a diffusive process and would follow Fick's equation. This result was expressed quantitatively by an effective diffusion coefficient, K, such that

$$K = \frac{a^2 \ u^2}{48 \ \text{D}_{\text{MOL}}}$$

where a is the tube radius, u the *mean* velocity of the fluid, D_{MOL} the molecular diffusion coefficient of the indicator in the solvent, and 48 an integration constant. Because K is inversely proportional to D_{MOL}, poorly diffusive solutes undergo greater axial dispersion than highly diffusive ones. In a subsequent paper[33] Taylor showed that the above equation was valid only within a limited range of values of the dimensionless parameter, ua/D_{MOL}, similar to the better known Peclet number, $(\text{Pe}) = ud/\text{D}_{\text{MOL}}$ (d is the diameter of the tube), which measures the relative importance of axial convection velocity (u) and radial diffusive velocity (D_{MOL}/d). In a refinement of Taylor's analysis, Aris[34] showed that the correct expression for the effective diffusion coefficient of an indicator spreading through a moving fluid in laminar flow must include the axial dispersion due to molecular diffusion

$$D_{\text{eff}} = \text{D}_{\text{MOL}} + \frac{a^2 \ u^2}{48 \ \text{D}_{\text{MOL}}}$$

To emphasize the relationship between D_{eff} and the Peclet number, it is useful to rewrite the latter equation as a function of the tube diameter and reorder, which yields:

$$D_{\text{eff}}/\text{D}_{\text{MOL}} = 1 + \frac{(\text{Pe})^2}{192}$$

Taylor's analysis is strictly applicable only to steady laminar flow in long tubes. Nevertheless, the general conclusions from his work may be at least qualitatively relevant to gas transport in the distal airways. The lower the rate of flow, the more important the radial diffusion: the concentration front between inspired air and resident gas in the distal airways tends to be narrow. Conversely, for poorly diffusive indicators, convective dispersion is more important than radial diffusion. Smoke, for example, is a poorly diffusive aerosol, which at low rate of flow spreads through the whole length of a tube with a distinct leading spike, as observed by Henderson and associates.[22] Sulfur hexafluoride, added to inspired air, is carried deeper into the lungs than helium.[35]

In a five-generation branched model of the central airways, Scherer and colleagues[36] examined the dispersion of a bolus of benzene in air, for Reynolds numbers varying from 30 to 2000. These authors expressed their results as

$$D_{\text{eff}}/\text{D}_{\text{MOL}} = 1 + k(\text{Pe})$$

where (Pe) is the characteristic Peclet number for each individual branch and k is an experimental constant equal to 1.08 for inspiratory and 0.37 for expiratory flow. Scherer's equation can be rewritten as:

$$D_{\text{eff}} = \text{D}_{\text{MOL}} + k(ud)$$

which separates the invariant term for axial diffusion, D_{MOL}, from the variable term for dispersion due to convection. In the central airways, as a rule, D_{MOL} is very much smaller than k(ud), suggesting that dispersion is due to eddy formation at the bifurcations and not to the radial diffusion studied by Taylor.

The transition from laminar to turbulent flow for steady, unidirectional flow in a long straight tube takes place at Reynolds numbers close to 2200. In the airways, turbulence is found in the trachea because of high flow rates and because of flow disturbance at the laryngeal inlet. Once established, turbulence needs an adequate distance to die out and this process is slowed down by the branching structure of the airways. Hence, turbulence persists through several bronchial bifurcations, even though local Reynolds numbers fall rapidly.[37] The resulting flow profiles are complex[38] and quite different from those prevailing in straight tubes.

For turbulent flow, radial mixing is caused by swirls rather than molecular diffusion. The effective diffusion coefficient K′ calculated by Taylor[39] is a complex function of the Reynolds number, Re = du/v (v is the kinematic viscosity of the fluid), which with an acceptable approximation simplifies into

$$K' = \frac{10.1 \ a \ u}{5 \ \log \ (\text{Re})} = \frac{d \ u}{\log \ (\text{Re})}$$

Thus, dispersion is proportional to tube diameter and mean flow velocity for both turbulent flow in a straight tube and laminar flow in the branched model of Scherer. This observation further supports the concept that radial mixing in the central airways is primarily due to eddies and swirls (secondary flows), rather than molecular diffusion.

Dispersion in Oscillatory Flow

Velocity profiles for laminar oscillatory flow in straight tubes are parabolic at very low frequency and become increasingly blunt at higher frequencies, when inertia prevents the axial core of fluid from reaching a paraboloid profile in either direction.[40] However, in proximity to the tube wall (boundary layer), velocities and accelerations are comparatively small, inertia is unimportant, and the velocity profile is determined by viscosity alone. The thickness of the boundary layer is approximately $\sqrt{\nu/2\pi f}$ and the deviation from parabolic velocity profile is characterized by the ratio of the tube radius to the thickness of the boundary layer, known as the dimensionless Womersley parameter

$$\alpha = a/\sqrt{2\pi f/\nu}$$

For low values of α ($\alpha < 1$), oscillatory flow behaves like steady flow, develops parabolic velocity profiles at low rates of flow, and changes to turbulence for Reynolds numbers greater than 2200. With increasing values of α, the thickness of the boundary layer diminishes and the flow becomes progressively more blunt, approaching a flat velocity profile, often referred to as a plug flow or piston flow. At high values of α ($\alpha > 10$), the transition from laminar to turbulent flow in straight tubes does not occur at a given Reynolds number, but occurs when the ratio of Reynolds number to Womersley parameter, $(Re)/\alpha$, is in the range of 550 to 800, with the velocity in (Re) taken as the cross-sectional average velocity at the time of maximal flow.[41] Therefore, in oscillatory flow, the laminar conditions can prevail at high Reynolds numbers, which in steady flow would certainly cause turbulence.

In laminar oscillatory flow, the dispersion created in one half of the cycle will be exactly reversed in the second half, unless some radial mixing is present. Radial mixing renders the dispersion *irreversible* and therefore produces a net transport of fluid particles with each cycle. For the simple case of laminar oscillatory flow in straight tubes, an effective diffusion coefficient, theoretically determined[42] and experimentally validated[41] can be written as:

$$D_{eff}/D_{MOL} = 1 + f(\alpha)(Pe)^2$$

where the velocity in (Pe) is the temporal root mean square velocity, u_{rms}. This expression is similar to the Taylor-Aris equation expressed as a function of the Peclet number. However, $f(\alpha)$ is a complex function of the Womersley parameter between low- and high-frequency asymptotes. For low frequencies ($\alpha < 1$), $f = 1/192$, and D_{eff} takes the same value as for unidirectional flow. For high frequencies ($\alpha > 10$), $f(\alpha)$ is proportional to α^{-3} or $f^{-3/2}$: indicator dispersion decreases with increasing frequency because of the progressive blunting of velocity profiles.

Turbulent oscillatory flow in branched tubes has not been studied experimentally. Assuming that turbulent dispersion for oscillatory flow in the airways could be treated like dispersion for unidirectional flow, Fredberg[43] concluded that dispersion in HFV might be represented by:

$$D_{eff}/D_{MOL} = 1 + k\,(Pe)$$

the expression derived by Scherer and associates[36] for laminar flow in an airway model. Because u in (Pe) is proportional to the product $V_T f$, the equation proposed by Scherer and associates[36] and by Fredberg[43] implies that gas transport should be proportional to $V_T f$.

In this section and the previous one, we have reviewed theoretical work aimed at treating gas transport in HFV as a diffusion process, similar to the dispersion of a bolus studied by Taylor. These efforts have failed to provide a quantitatively useful model of gas transport in HFV. If the Taylor models were applicable, one would expect first that molecular diffusivity would strongly affect gas transport. To the contrary, experimental studies in HFV have found either no difference[44] or a small difference[45] between transport of tracer gases characterized by markedly different diffusivities. Second, one would expect gas transport to be proportional to $V_T f$, which does not fit experimental data.[25, 44, 46–49] One must conclude that Taylor diffusion at most could account for a small fraction of overall transport.

Asymmetric Velocity Profiles

Velocity profiles in branching systems such as the airways are markedly affected by the direction of flow. Divergent flow (inspiration) tends to stream along the medial walls of daughter branches after each bifurcation, whereas convergent flow (expiration) tends to have more uniform velocity profiles.[45] Haselton and Scherer[50] have pointed out that, whatever their shapes, different velocity profiles in opposite directions will result in net dispersion of a bolus after each cycle, even in the absence of radial diffusion (Fig. 33–16).

Haselton and Scherer[50] also studied the dispersion of nondiffusible beads in a mixture of glycerine and water, for Reynolds numbers ranging from 1 to 1000 (laminar flow). These authors demonstrated a net, irreversible dispersion of the beads into a five-generation model of the branching airways. The corresponding expression for gas transport becomes proportional to the square of the tidal volume:

$$\dot{V}_G \simeq V_T^2 f$$

the dispersion process being independent of diffusion. This result, confirmed by direct measurements in similar models of the branching airways and in animal experiments,[25, 44, 46–49] is consistent also with the empirical model of Permutt and associates.[51]

It can be concluded that, in contrast to the alveolar space, where gas transport is dominated by diffusion, mixing of respiratory gases in the airways is mainly dependent on nondiffusive dispersion due to eddies and swirls, and to the asymmetry of velocity profiles during inspiration and expiration.

TOWARD OPTIMIZING THE SELECTION OF FREQUENCY IN MECHANICAL VENTILATION

In spite of many theoretical and experimental studies of oscillatory flow characteristics, no model of gas transport in HFV has yet received widespread endorsement. Nevertheless, a consensus is emerging among authors who accept as experimentally validated the fact that gas transport in HFV is proportional not to ventilation, $V_T f$, but to the product $V_T^2 f$ or a slightly higher fractional power of V_T.

A General Gas Transport Relationship

We have found it helpful to represent gas transport in terms of dimensionless variables, yielding two general equations applicable to various mammalian species for CV and HFV, and allowing us to identify the transition frequency separating the CV and HFV domains.[15] The classical equation of Krogh and Lindhard:[52]

$$V_T f = \dot{V}_A + V_D f$$

in which, V_D is the volume of the conducting airways, describes gas transport in CV. Dividing both sides by $\dot{V}_A$ yields a dimensionless equation:

$$\underline{Q} = 1 + \underline{F}$$

where $\underline{Q} = V_T f / \dot{V}_A$ is the inverse of the efficiency of ventilation and $\underline{F} = f V_D / \dot{V}_A$ is the ratio of anatomic dead space to the alveolar ventilation per breath, $\dot{V}_A / f$. Regression analysis of published HFV data, obtained in animal models ranging from rat to horse, yields a dimensionless HFV equation:

$$\underline{Q} = \left(\frac{\underline{F}}{0.19} \right)^{0.54}$$

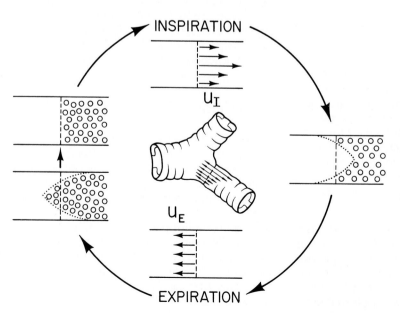

Figure 33–16. When flow profiles are laminar in one direction and flat in the reverse direction, oscillatory flow causes net transfer of an indicator across a plane of reference.

which is equivalent to $\dot{V}_A = (V_T/V_D)^{1.2}(V_Tf)$. This equation, therefore, supports the consensus that gas transport in HFV is approximately proportional to V_T^2f. Additionally, the equation predicts that $\dot{V}_A$ should be inversely proportional to V_D, which has been confirmed experimentally in dogs, by manipulating V_D through changes in mean lung volume.[53]

The intersection between the two equations (Fig. 33–17), which marks the transition from CV to HFV, is found at $\underline{F} = 5$ and corresponds to different transition frequencies in different species, because of variations in the value of $V_D/\dot{V}_A$. For all species, the eucapnic tidal volume at the transition frequency equals 1.2 V_D.

The combination of the CV and HFV equations makes it possible to preset a respirator to values of frequency and tidal volume that should approximate eucapnic ventilation in healthy subjects. One needs only to calculate $\dot{V}_A$, from measured or estimated metabolic CO_2 production and desired FA_{CO_2}, and to measure or estimate anatomic dead space. The preliminary settings will be as good as the estimated CO_2 production and dead space; that is, within 10% or 20% of eucapnic ventilation. Then a single measurement of arterial P_{CO_2} will suggest any needed corrections to the respirator settings.

Another practical advantage of the dimensionless CV and HFV equations is that they allow us to combine the gas transport requirements and the mechanical response of the lungs. By so doing, we can rationally select the ventilation modality best suited to any clinical situation.

Combining Mechanics and Gas Transport

From low frequencies to resonance, the magnitude of lung impedance decreases, but ventilatory requirements increase. It follows that there must exist an optimal frequency in mechanical ventilation, for which eucapnia is achieved with the smallest possible pressure swings imposed on the lungs. The alveolar pressure swings, which are most relevant, cannot be measured at the bedside. The second best variable of interest is the transpulmonary pressure, which is measurable, but with difficulties arising either from physiologic artifacts (esophageal pressure) or intermittent catheter obstruction (chest tube). Practically, one must rely on monitoring pressure at the airway opening, $P_{ao} = \dot{V}\,\vec{Z}_{RS}$, where $\vec{Z}_{RS}$ is the impedance of the respiratory system, or the pressure near the carina, P_c, which sees $\vec{Z}_{RS}$ minus the impedance of the tracheal tube. This is acceptable for two reasons. First, the chest wall impedance is usually little affected by disease. Second, the human respiratory system is generally overdamped, so that P_{ao} or P_c gives an estimate of the largest possible pressure swings anywhere in the lungs. Even if some underdamped regions exist in nonhomogeneous lungs, the resonant frequencies of such regions are likely to be much higher than the desirable ventilating frequency for the respiratory system as a whole. Any underdamped region will be ventilated far enough from its own resonant frequency to prohibit alveolar pressure amplification.

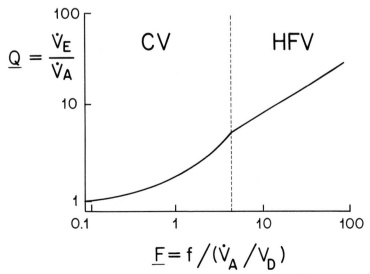

Figure 33–17. Relationship between the dimensionless variables $\underline{Q} = V_Tf/\dot{V}_A$ and $\underline{F} = fV_D/\dot{V}_A$, showing the transition from CV to HFV at $\underline{F} = 5$. (Modified from Venegas JG, Hales CA, Strieder DJ. A general dimensionless equation of gas transport during high frequency ventilation in dogs. J Appl Physiol 59:1539–1547, 1989; with permission.)

$$\underline{Q} = \frac{\dot{V}_E}{\dot{V}_A}$$

$$\underline{F} = f\,\big/\,(\dot{V}_A / V_D)$$

To combine mechanical and gas transport equations, we normalize $\dot{V}$ by $\dot{V}_A$ and $\vec{Z}$ by R. This yields the dimensionless variable:

$$\underline{P} = \frac{\dot{V}\,\vec{Z}}{\dot{V}_A\,R}$$

With increasing frequency below resonance, changes in $\underline{P}$ reflect the combination of a loss of ventilatory efficiency (as $\dot{V}/\dot{V}_A$ rises or $\dot{V}_A/\dot{V}$ falls) and a gain in mechanical efficiency (as $|\vec{Z}|/R$ falls). Whereas $|\vec{Z}|$ is minimum at resonant frequency, the combined variable $\underline{P}$ reaches its minimum at a lower frequency.

Because the human respiratory system is overdamped, the function relating $|\vec{Z}|$ to frequency is flat in the vicinity of f_o, particularly on the lower frequency side, which is illustrated by plotting $|\vec{Z}|/R$ as a function of $\underline{F}$ (Fig. 33–18). In contrast, the $\underline{Q}$ versus $\underline{F}$ relationship (Fig. 33–17) increases monotonically with frequency through the CV and HFV range. The combined variable $\underline{P}$ passes through a minimum when the negative slope of $|\vec{Z}|/R$ is equal in absolute value to the positive slope of $\underline{Q}$ versus $\underline{F}$. For overdamped systems, the corresponding frequency is always lower than f_o and close to f_c. The optimal frequency, for which eucapnia is achieved with minimal pressure swings at the airway opening, can be calculated; but, for practical purposes, a good approximation is given[48] by

optimal frequency in HFV = corner frequency

and

optimal frequency in CV = (corner frequency)$^{2/3}$

the appropriate selection depending on whether f_c falls in the CV or HFV range.

As an illustration, we calculated the function $\underline{P}$ versus $\underline{F}$ in representative cases (Fig. 33–19), using the mechanics data of Table 33–4 and standard estimates of anatomic dead space and alveolar ventilation. The curves show that the optimal frequency for mechanical ventilation is indeed found in the HFV range for healthy adults, adults with the respiratory distress syndrome, and infants with hyaline membrane disease. We also calculated the $\underline{P}$ versus $\underline{F}$ relationship for an adult with chronic obstructive pulmonary disease: in that case, the optimal frequency is found in the low-frequency region of conventional ventilation. A similar result will be obtained in all patients whose airway resistance is high, and for whom, therefore, the corner frequency is low.

This analysis has allowed us to identify the optimal frequency for mechanical ventilation and the ventilatory requirements at that frequency. To deliver that ventilation, however, the tidal volume dialed on the respirator must take into account the ventilation lost to the airway wall shunt, $\dot{V}_w$. The latter is never known exactly but can be estimated from Figure 33–11. In addition, any increase in lung volume increases anatomic dead space and therefore the ventilatory requirements in HFV.[53] Several mechanisms may lead to increased lung volume during mechanical ventilation. The role of long time constants already mentioned in the case of CV (see Fig. 33–5) can be important in HFV as well.[54] The difference between inspiratory and expiratory resistance[55] and even expiratory flow limi-

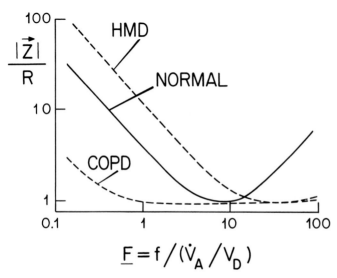

Figure 33–18. The normalized impedance $|\vec{Z}|/R$ plotted as a function of $\underline{F} = fV_D/\dot{V}_A$ for a healthy adult, for an adult with chronic obstructive pulmonary disease (COPD), and for an infant with hyaline membrane disease (HMD). In all instances, the function reaches its minimum, $|\vec{Z}|/R = 1$, at resonant frequency and is nearly flat on either side of that point.

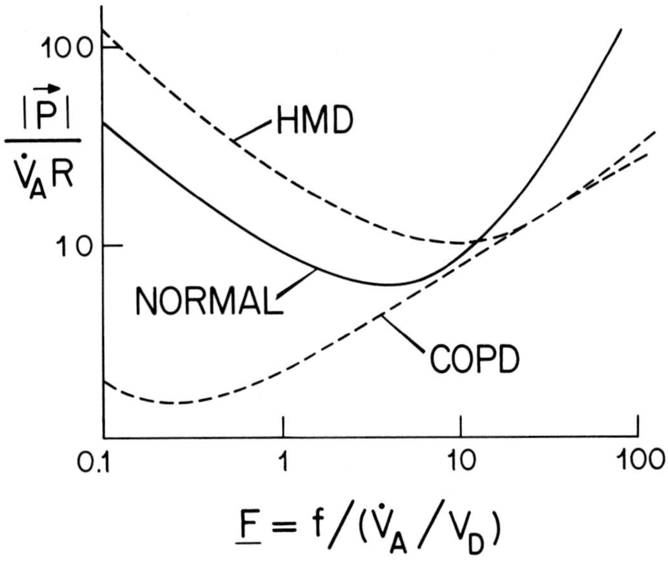

Figure 33–19. Normalized pressure requirements $\underline{P}$ for eucapnic ventilation as a function of $\underline{F} = fV_D/\dot{V}_A$. The optimal frequency for a healthy adult is 1.6 Hz; for a patient with chronic obstructive pulmonary disease (COPD), 0.1 Hz; and for an infant with hyaline membrane disease (HMD), 14 Hz.

tation[44] may also play a role in HFV. Often, however, increased lung volume results from the high end-expiratory pressure needed in some patients to optimize oxygenation.

CONCLUSION

Less than 15 years have passed since the effectiveness of HFV was demonstrated experimentally in animals.[56–58] In that short time, physiologists and physicists have made great progress toward understanding how HFV works and, therefore, when it works; that is, when the airway resistance is low and when both corner and resonant frequencies are high. In such cases, HFV can support gas transport with a marked reduction of the magnitude of pressure swings imposed on the lungs, even if mean airway pressure must be raised in order to ensure adequate oxygenation.

References

1. Chang HK. Mechanisms of gas transport during ventilation by high-frequency ventilation. J Appl Physiol 56:553–563, 1984.
2. Hoppin FG Jr, Hildebrandt J. Mechanical properties of the lung. In West JB (ed). Lung Biology in Health and Disease, vol. 3: Bioengineering Aspects of the Lung. New York: Marcel Dekker, 1977; pp. 118–162.
3. Pedley TJ, Schroter RC, Sudlow MF. Gas flow and mixing in the airways. In West JB (ed). Lung Biology in Health and Disease, vol. 3: Bioengineering Aspects of the Lung. New York: Marcel Dekker, 1977; pp. 163–265.
4. Otis AB, McKerrow CB, Bartlett RA, Mead J, Mc-
Ilroy MB, Selverstone NJ, Radford EP, Jr. Mechanical factors in distribution of pulmonary ventilation. J Appl Physiol 8:427–443, 1956.
5. Mead J. Measurement of inertia of the lungs at increased ambient pressure. J Appl Physiol 9:208–212, 1956.
6. Fredberg JJ, Keefe DH, Glass GM, Castile RG, Frantz ID, III. Alveolar pressure nonhomogeneity during small-amplitude high frequency oscillation. J Appl Physiol 57:788–800, 1984.
7. Fredberg JJ, Ingram RH Jr, Castile RG, et al. Nonhomogeneity of lung response to inhaled histamine assessed with alveolar capsules. J Appl Physiol 58:1914–1922, 1985.
8. Gavriely NJ, Solway J, Drazen JM, Slutzky AS, Brown R, Loring SH, Ingram RH, Jr. Radiographic visualization of airway wall movement during oscillatory flow in dogs. J Appl Physiol 58:645–652, 1985.
9. Mead J. Contribution of compliance of airways to frequency-dependent behavior of the lung. J Appl Physiol 26:670–673, 1969.
10. Rossing TH, Slutsky AS, Lehr J, Drinker PA, Kamm R, Drazen JM. Tidal volume and frequency dependence of carbon dioxide elimination in high-frequency ventilation. N Engl J Med 305:1375–1379, 1981.
11. Rohrer F. Der Stroemungswiderstand in den menschlichen Atemwegen und der Einfluss der unregelmaessigen Verzweigung des Bronkialsystems auf den Atmungsverlauf in verschiedenen Lungenbezirken. Pfluegers Arch 162:225–299, 1915.
12. Michaelson ED, Grassman ED, Peters WR. Pulmonary mechanics by spectral analysis of forced random noise. J Clin Invest 56:1210–1230, 1975.
13. Dorkin HL, Stark AR, Werthammer JW, Strieder DY, Fredberg JJ, Frantz ID, III. Respiratory system impedance from 4 to 40 Hz in paralyzed intubated infants with respiratory disease. J Clin Invest 72:903–910, 1983.
14. Riley RL, Cournand A. "Ideal" alveolar air and the analysis of ventilation/perfusion relationships in the lungs. J Appl Physiol 1:825–843; 846–847, 1949.
15. Venegas JG, Hales CA, Strieder DJ. A general dimensionless equation of gas transport by high frequency ventilation. J Appl Physiol 60:1025–1030, 1986.

16. Scherer PW, Haselton FR. Convective exchange in oscillatory flow through bronchial-tree models. J Appl Physiol 53:1023–1033, 1982.
17. Scherer PW, Haselton FR, Seybert JR. Gas transport in branched airways during high-frequency ventilation. Ann Biomed Eng 12:385–405, 1984.
18. Weibel ER. Morphometry of the Human Lung. New York: Academy Press, 1963.
19. Engel LA, Menkes H, Wood LDH, Utz G, Joubert J, Macklein PT. Gas mixing during breathholding studied by intrapulmonary gas sampling. J Appl Physiol 35:9–17, 1973.
20. Fahri LE. Diffusive and convective movement of gas in the lung. In Wolstenholme CEW, Knight J (eds). Circulatory and Respiratory Gas Transport. Boston: Little, Brown & Co., 1969, pp. 277–292.
21. Fowler WS. Lung function studies. II: The respiratory dead space. Am J Physiol 154:405–416, 1948.
22. Henderson Y, Chillingworth FP, Whitney JL. The respiratory dead space. Am J Physiol 38:1–19, 1915.
23. Briscoe WA, Forster RE, Comroe JH Jr. Alveolar ventilation at very low tidal volumes. J Appl Physiol 7:27–30, 1954.
24. Ross BB. Influence of bronchial tree structure on ventilation in the dog's lung, as inferred from measurements of a plastic cast. J Appl Physiol 10:1–14, 1957.
25. Kamm RD, Collins JM, Joshi CH, Greiner M, Shapiro AH. Axial dispersion of a passive contaminant in oscillatory flow. Proceedings of the American Conference on Engineering in Medicine and Biology 35:23, 1982.
26. Snyder B, Dantzer RD, Jaeger MJ. Flow partitioning in symmetric cascades of branches. J Appl Physiol 51:598–606, 1981.
27. Chang HK, El Masry OA. A model study of flow dynamics in human central airways. I: Axial velocity profiles. Respir Physiol 49:75–95, 1982.
28. Brusasco V, Knopp TJ, Rehder K. Gas transport during high-frequency ventilation. J Appl Physiol 55:472–478, 1983.
29. Venegas JG. Efficiency and regional distribution of high frequency ventilation. PhD thesis. Cambridge, MA: Massachusetts Institute of Technology, 1983.
30. Yamada J, Burnham C, Hales CA, Venegas JG. Regional mapping of gas transport during high-frequency and conventional ventilation. J Appl Physiol 66:1209–1218, 1989.
31. Rehder K, Didier EP. Gas transport and pulmonary perfusion during high-frequency ventilation in humans. J Appl Physiol 57:1231–1237, 1984.
32. Taylor G. Dispersion of soluble matter in solvent flowing slowly through a tube. Proc R Soc Lond [Biol] 219:186–203, 1953.
33. Taylor G. Conditions under which dispersion of a solute in a stream of solvent can be used to measure molecular diffusion. Proc R Soc Lond [Biol] 22:473–477, 1954.
34. Aris R. On the dispersion of a solute in a fluid moving through a tube. Proc R Soc Lond [Biol] 235:67–77, 1956.
35. Power GG. Gaseous diffusion between airways and alveoli in the human lung. J Appl Physiol 27:701–709, 1969.
36. Scherer PW, Schendalman LH, Greene NM, Bouhuys A. Measurement of axial diffusivities in a model of the the bronchial airways. J Appl Physiol 38:719–723, 1975.
37. Winter DC, Nerem RM. Turbulence in pulsatile flows. Ann Biomed Eng 12:357–369, 1984.
38. Olson DE, Iliff LD, Sudlow MF. Some aspects of the physics of flow in the central airways. Bull Physio-Pathol Respir 8:391–408, 1972.
39. Taylor G. The dispersion of matter in turbulent flow through a pipe. Proc R Soc Lond [Biol] 223:446–468, 1954.
40. Menon AS, Weber ME, Chang HK. Model study of flow dynamics in human central airways. III: Oscillatory velocity profiles. Respir Physiol 55:255–275, 1984.
41. Joshi CH, Kamm RD, Drazen JM, Slutsky AS. An experimental study of gas exchange in laminar oscillatory flow. Journal of Fluid Mechanics 133:245–254, 1983.
42. Watson EJ. Diffusion in oscillatory pipe flow. Journal of Fluid Mechanics 133:233–244, 1983.
43. Fredberg JJ. Augmented diffusion in the airways can support pulmonary gas exchange. J Appl Physiol 49:232–238, 1980.
44. Knopp TJ, Kaethner T, Meyer M, Rehder K, Scheid P. Gas mixing in the airways of dog lungs during high frequency ventilation. J Appl Physiol 55:1141–1146, 1983.
45. Van Der Kooij AM, Luijendijk SCM. Longitudinal dispersion of gases measured in a model of the bronchial airways. J Appl Physiol 59:1343–1349, 1985.
46. Jaeger MJ, Banner M, Gallagher J. Alveolar ventilation in high frequency studies [abstract]. Fed Proc 42:1351, 1983.
47. Venegas JG, Custer J, Kamm RD, Hales CA. A relationship for gas transport during high frequency ventilation in dogs. J Appl Physiol 59:1539–1547, 1985.
48. Venegas JG. A rationale for selecting respiratory frequency [abstract]. Am Rev Respir Dis 133:A346, 1986.
49. Weinmann GG, Mitzner W, Permutts S. Physiological dead space during high frequency ventilation. J Appl Physiol 57:881–887, 1984.
50. Haselton FR, Scherer PW. Bronchial bifurcations and respiratory gas transport. Science 208:69–71, 1980.
51. Permutt S, Mitzner W, Weinmann G. Model of gas transport during high-frequency ventilation. J Appl Physiol 58:1956–1970, 1985.
52. Krogh A, Lindhard J. The volume of the "dead space" in breathing. J Physiol (Lond) 47:30–43, 1913.
53. Yamada J, Venegas JG, Strieder DJ, Hales CA. Effect of mean airway pressure on gas transport during high-frequency ventilation in dogs. J Appl Physiol 61:1896–1902, 1986.
54. Saari AF, Rossing TH, Solway J, Drazen JM. Lung inflation during high-frequency ventilation. Am Rev Respir Dis 129:333–336, 1984.
55. Simon BA, Weinmann GG, Mitzner W. Mean airway pressure and alveolar pressure during high-frequency ventilation. J Appl Physiol 57:1069–1079, 1984.
56. Bohn DJ, Mijasakak, Marchak EB, Thompson WK, Froese AB, Bryan AC. Ventilation by high-frequency oscillation. J Appl Physiol 48:710–716, 1980.
57. Bunnell JB, Karlson KH, Shannon DC. High frequency positive pressure ventilation in dogs and rabbits [abstract]. Am Rev Respir Dis 119:226A, 1979.
58. Slutsky AS, Drazen JM, Ingram RH, Kamm RD, Shapiro AH, Fredberg JJ. Effective pulmonary ventilation with small-volume oscillations at high frequency. Science 209:609–611, 1980.

APPENDIX
Table of Symbols

Acromyms

CSA	Cross-sectional area
CV	Conventional ventilation
HFV	High-frequency ventilation
RC	Resistance–compliance
RIC	Resistance–inertance–compliance

Principal Symbols

a	Radius
A	Cross-sectional area
C	Compliance
C_L	Lung compliance
C_{RS}	Compliance of the respiratory system
C_w	Compliance of the airway wall
d	Diameter
D	Diffusion coefficient
f	Frequency
f_c	Corner frequency
f_o	Resonant frequency
F	Fractional concentration
$\underline{F}$	Dimensionless variable $f V_D / \dot{V}_A$
Hz	Hertz = cycles per second
I	Inertance
L	Liter or inductance
P	Pressure or partial pressure
$\underline{P}$	Dimensionless variable $\dot{V} \, | \, \vec{Z} \, | \, / \dot{V}_A R$
P_{ao}	Pressure at the airway opening
P_{bs}	Pressure at the body surface
P_{pl}	Pleural pressure
P_A	Alveolar pressure
P_C	Pressure across a compliance
P_I	Pressure across an inertance
P_R	Pressure across a resistance
Pe	Dimensionless Peclet number $u d / D_{MOL}$
Q	Dimensionless quality factor f_c / f_o
$\underline{Q}$	Dimensionless variable $V_T f / \dot{V}_A$
R	Resistance
R_{aw}	Airway resistance
Re	Dimensionless Reynolds number = $d u / \nu$
t	Time
T	Period = 1/f
u	Velocity
v	Voltage
V	Volume
V_D	Dead space volume
V_L	Lung volume
$\dot{V}$	Ventilation, flow or flux
$\dot{V}_w$	Flow lost to the airway wall shunt
$\dot{V}_A$	Alveolar ventilation
$\dot{V}_G$	Flux of a gas species, uptake or output
$\dot{V}_L$	Lung ventilation or flow to the lungs

$\vec{X}$	Reactance
$\vec{X}_c$	Compliant reactance
$\vec{X}_I$	Inertial reactance
$\vec{Z}$	Impedance
$\vec{Z}_L$	Lung impedance
$\vec{Z}_w$	Impedance of the airway wall
α	Dimensionless Womersley parameter $a/\sqrt{2\pi f/\nu}$
ν	Kinematic viscosity
π	3.14159
φ	Phase angle
Δ	Change or range of variability

Subscripts

ao	Airway opening
aw	Airway
bs	Body surface
c	Corner for corner frequency
	Carina for carinal pressure
cw	Chest wall
eff	Effective
i	1,2,3 . . . n
rms	Root mean square
A	Alveolar
G	Gas species
L	Lung
MOL	Molecular
RS	Respiratory system
T	Tidal
w	Airway wall

CHAPTER 34

Lasers and the Airway

Anne-Marie Cros, M.D.

In 1960, Mainman and Javan performed the first stimulated emission of laser light using ruby as activating material. In 1966, Yahr and Strully discovered that the carbon dioxide laser could cut tissue and be useful in medicine. Jako first used the CO_2 laser in the dog in 1971. Soon Jako, Strong, Vaughan, and Andrews used the CO_2 laser in otolaryngology, thanks to the development of micromanipulation that allowed the use of the CO_2 laser with a microscope. The neodymium-yttrium-aluminum-garnet (Nd:YAG) laser was introduced in medicine in 1975. Since then, surgeons have increasingly used lasers for precise, bloodless airway surgery. These techniques pose new problems. A good knowledge of the physiologic effects of lasers and their hazards is essential for progress in the future.

LASERS: PHYSICS AND PHYSIOLOGIC EFFECTS

Principles of Laser Technology

In 1960, Mainman developed the first ruby laser, based on Einstein's work on quantum theory and stimulated emission. Visible light is an electromagnetic radiation whose wavelengths are located between 4000 Å and 8000 Å. Each radiation is characterized by its wavelength. According to Bohr's theorem, the electrons of an atom circle the nucleus in different orbits. The orbits, populated by the electrons, determine the energy level of the atom. All atoms are able to increase their energy level when the electrons rise from a low to a higher orbit by absorbing a specific amount of radiation; the atom is said to be in an excited state. Conversely, an atom in an excited state tends to lose energy when the electrons are transferred to a lower orbit. Three possible radiative processes are involved in laser production (Fig. 34–1).

Spontaneous Emission. Any electron in an excited state tends to lose energy spontaneously by moving to a lower orbit, resulting in the emission of a photon or light wave. Each atom is characterized by a precise amount of energy and therefore by a precise wavelength related to the orbit to which it dropped.

Absorption. An electron can be raised to an excited energy state by the absorption of a photon of appropriate wavelength. It is the opposite process to emission.

Stimulated Emission. A photon produced from an electron in an excited state can interact with another electron in the same state, resulting in the emission of another photon of equal wavelength and in phase. The two photons are said to be coherent, coordinated in space and time.

The stimulation of a corpuscular population (atoms, molecules, and electrons at different

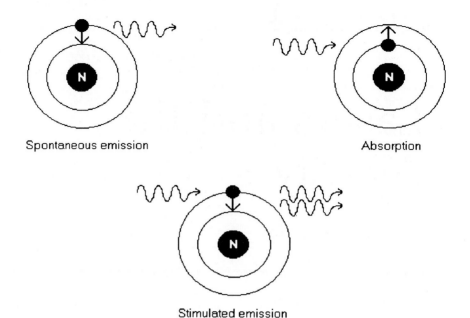

Figure 34–1. The three processes involved in laser beam production. N, nucleus.

energy levels) by a high electromagnetic field could result in a transfer of energy and in a *population inversion*. A population is said to be inversed when the higher energy levels of atoms or molecules are more populated than the lower ones. This state is unstable or transitional. The inversed population tends to return spontaneously to the normal state with emission of a noncoherent radiation. The laser effect is obtained by stimulating the return of an inversed population to a normal state, thus producing a coherent beam: the laser beam. The emission is of the same wavelength *(temporal coherence)*: all beams are parallel *(spatial coherence)*, resulting in a monochromatic, narrow, nondivergent, powerful beam.

The components of a laser system include (Fig. 34–2): (1) a quantitatively active population, the *lasing medium*, whose electrons create the photons; (2) an energy source that produces the population inversion, the process is called *pumping*, which may consist of a xenon flash lamp or an electric spark generator; and (3) a resonator that stimulates the return to the normal state. The lasing medium is placed between two mirrors that allow repeated passes of photons through the medium, thus stimulating the emission of additional photons. One mirror is completely reflective, and the other is partially transmissive for a determined wavelength, allowing the beam to escape.

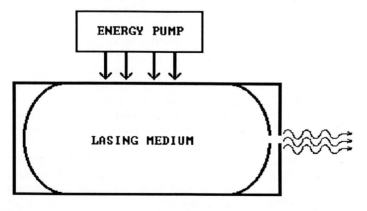

Figure 34–2. Components of a laser system: an optical cavity containing the lasing medium (eg, CO_2 or Nd:YAG); an energy source (eg, xenon flash or an electric spark generator); a pair of axial mirrors.

Characteristics of Lasers Used for Airway Surgery

The name of the laser refers to the type of material used as a lasing medium. The wavelength of the emitted radiation is determined by the lasing medium. Two types of laser are used for airway surgery. The carbon dioxide (CO_2) laser produces an invisible radiation located in the infrared region, with a wavelength of 10.6/μm.[1] Because the radiation of the CO_2 laser is invisible, a helium–neon laser of very low power is used to aim the beam. The two beams must be coaxial. The spot size of a laser beam depends on its wavelength. Thanks to its coherence, the power density of the laser beam can be increased by focusing the beam with appropriate lenses.[1] If the CO_2 laser is unfocused, its beam diameter is nearly 1 cm because of its long wavelength. If it is focused on a 1-mm spot size, the power density is increased by 100.[2] The depth of penetration is a function of the power density and the duration of firing. If the laser is used in the "continuous" wave mode, no time limit is set; but with a pulsed mode, the duration of firing is preset. The CO_2 laser beam cannot be transmitted through optical fibers. It is directed by a system of mirrors and prisms to reach the target. It may be used only when lesions are visible and superficial, as in laryngeal surgery. The beam may be deflected with the aid of a mirror or a mirror-like polished surface.[1]

The Nd:YAG laser produces a shorter wavelength in the near-infrared portion of the spectrum of 1.06 μm. It is invisible and the beam must be aimed like the CO_2 laser by using a visible, red beam of helium–neon laser, thus allowing precise alignment. It is more powerful than the CO_2 laser—50 to 100 W. The lasing medium is composed of a laser-passive material, a synthetic gem crystal (YAG) that contains ionic impurities known as dopants (neodymium), which is the lasing material. The Nd:YAG laser can be transmitted by flexible optic fibers, permitting surgical access for endoscopic resections of tumor or stenosis of the major airways. It is preferentially absorbed by pigmented tissues. The Nd:YAG laser can be used in a continuous or pulsative mode with an energy of up to 10^{10}Wem^{-2}.[3, 4]

Biologic Effects: Interaction With Tissues

The effects of the laser are due to the conversion of light energy into heat. The CO_2 laser, with its long infrared wavelength, is strongly absorbed by water and consequently by human tissues that contain approximately 80% water.[5] The laser beam can be focused on an extremely small spot. This, together with the high intensity of the laser beam, is responsible for an extremely high-power energy, almost completely transformed into caloric energy. The very strong heat emitted at the focused impact is capable of vaporizing any tissue.[2, 5] The water of the cells that absorb the laser beam is immediately heated up to 100°C and boils, resulting in cellular explosive vaporization.[2] The CO_2 laser is strongly absorbed within the first 200 μm of any tissue crossed and can damage all surface soft-tissue cells. Carbonization of proteins occurs at the edge, but the penetration results in minimal damage to underlying and surrounding tissues.[5] Postoperative edema formation is minimal because of immediate coagulation due to the heat generated.[2]

The Nd:YAG laser is preferentially absorbed by pigmented tissues. The cellular penetration is strong because it is much less absorbed by water than occurs with the CO_2 laser. Consequently, the Nd:YAG laser produces less vaporization and more thermal coagulation.[5] Unlike with the CO_2 laser, carbonization occurs over a large area. The extension length is 30 to 100 times longer and the volume of tissue that interacts with the laser beam is 100 to 900 times larger.[2] Van Der Spek and associates[2] compare the area affected by the Nd:YAG laser to an iceberg. Only the tip of this area is visible on the surface. Some of the effects, like edema or necrosis-induced perforation resulting from damage to the underlying tissue by the diffuse scattering of the Nd:YAG laser, may not be apparent for hours or even days after exposure.[4]

LASER HAZARDS

The use of lasers for airway surgery entails specific risks for the operating team, the operating room personnel, and the patient. There are three main types of hazard: hazards due to misdirection or reflection of the laser beam, endotracheal tube fire, and atmospheric contamination by smoke and fine particles that result from tissue vaporization. The primary concern is to ensure the safety of the patient and personnel, and the operating room should have a warning sign that a laser is in use, according to the American National Standard for the safe use of lasers in health care facilities (Z136.3. 1988) published by the American National Standards Institute (ANSI).[5]

Hazards Due to Misdirection or Reflection of Beam

Among the 21 injuries reported to the Food and Drug Administration (FDA) over a period of 18 months, eye injuries represented 19% and other burns 9%. A laser beam can be reflected from a mirror-like surface without its properties and energy being changed.[1] The beam can be misdirected in an unexpected direction. The eye is the most susceptible tissue; because the CO_2 beam is absorbed within the first 200 μm of tissue, it can cause corneal injury. The Nd:YAG laser is most likely to cause damage to the retina,[3, 5] although there is a significant deposition in the aqueous tissues of the cornea and lens.[3] To prevent hazards to the eye, all personnel in the operating room must wear appropriate protection, goggles or lenses that are specific for the wavelength emitted by the laser in use.[5] Eye protection should have side protectors to provide lateral protection from a reflected beam and should fit well around the forehead.[3] Because it is opaque to the CO_2 beam, any clear glass can be used for the CO_2 laser. Regular spectacles can be sufficient, but do not provide lateral protection,[5] and contact lenses do not afford sufficient protection.[2] The Nd:YAG laser requires special, green-tinted goggles, which may hinder observation of the patient, mainly his or her skin color.[5] Continuous monitoring of hemoglobin saturation must be used.[2] Clear lenses with a special coating opaque to near-infrared light are now available. The patient's eyes should also be protected, with the lids closed and covered with water-moistened eye pads,[1, 2] gauze,[3] or a metal shield.[5] Plastic or paper tapes must be avoided.[2] Absorption of a laser beam on the skin can cause a burn, mainly with the CO_2 laser. Damage to the skin of a team member is unlikely to happen because the energy density decreases rapidly beyond the focal point.[3] No skin protection is needed for the patient beyond the routine surgical drapes. Wet cloth towels must protect the surrounding surgical field. Paper or plastic-coated paper towels must be avoided because they wet poorly.[2] Accidental burns from laser-ignited combustion of flammable material such as surgical gloves in the direct vicinity of the surgical field could occur.[6] Normal tissue surrounding the operating field can be damaged, especially from a reflected beam, and may cause laryngotracheal tear and pneumothorax.[7] Tissue adjacent to the lesion can be protected by water-moistened gauze or swabs.[3] When the Nd:YAG laser is used, the depth of damage is impossible to judge and necrosis-induced perforation may occur several days later.[5] Proper maintenance of general anesthesia with neuromuscular blockade is necessary to prevent unexpected coughing or movement, because appropriate ventilation is essential for providing a quiet operating field.

Another means of protecting both patient and operating room personnel from a reflected beam is to disperse the laser energy by using a matte-finished, nonreflective, rough-surfaced instrument for laryngoscopy or suction.

Endotracheal Tube Fire

Fire danger and its prevention are of particular importance in airway surgery. The incidence of endotracheal tube ignition varies from 0.4% to 1.5% according to reports.[3] Airway fire represents 14% of laser injuries reported to the FDA.[5] All commercially available tracheal tubes made from rubber polyvinyl chloride (PVC) or silicone can be ignited either by a focused laser beam or by sparks and incandescent particles secondary to tissue combustion[5-8]; the risk is higher in 100% oxygen or in an oxygen-enriched atmosphere. Nitrous oxide allows combustion, as does oxygen. When a tracheal tube fire is induced in these circumstances, the tube becomes a blow torch because of the high oxygen percentage and the high gas flow caused by ventilation. Heat and toxic products from material combustion are blown down the airway and can cause widespread deposits of carbonaceous debris and ulceration of the trachea.[3-5]

In most cases, minimal damage or no harm to the airway occurs,[5, 6, 9, 10] but serious injuries are possible.[5, 11] Puncturing the tracheal cuff with the laser may lead to a high risk of airway fire if oxygen is used.[10] The likelihood of tracheal tube ignition depends, on the one hand, on the setting of the laser beam, duration of exposure, and power and, on the other hand, the material.[2] Two indices are used to compare the commercially available raw material (PVC, silicone, red rubber): ignitability; ie, the amount of energy needed to ignite a fuel in a given atmosphere, and flammability; ie, the ability to sustain a flame in a given atmosphere. Red rubber has the lowest ignitability and PVC the highest. However, PVC flammability is lower than that of silicone and red rubber[2, 12]; moreover, PVC self-extinguishes in air. In other words, PVC is more likely to be ignited but needs more oxygen to sustain the flame than silicone and red rubber.

In practice, raw materials do not have the same behavior with regard to the laser used. Red rubber is more resistant than PVC to the CO_2 laser beam.[2, 4, 5] Modern PVC strongly absorbs far-infrared light and consequently is very sensitive to CO_2 laser energy.[5] Conversely, because the Nd:YAG laser is absorbed by a dark color like purple or black, the red rubber tube is more likely to be burned. An unmarked, transparent PVC tube is more appropriate for Nd:YAG laser use,[13] except when the laser is used in the continuous mode, when serious damage and flame can happen. Areas of black lettering are at high risk of ignition.[13] The silicone tube is damaged by both CO_2 and Nd:YAG lasers. PVC produces more dense smoke and debris when it burns.[1, 2] A silicone fire results in abundant white silica ash.[5] Red rubber burns with little smoke.

The effects of an endotracheal tube fire on the airway depend mainly on the magnitude of the event. Most fires are located on the outside of the tube and can result in local thermal damage. If the tube is perforated by a laser beam or if the cuff is punctured, the oxygen-enriched gas and ventilation flow may act as a bellow; this can result in a blow torch flame and great devastation to the tracheobronchial tree.[5, 6, 8, 11, 14] Airway burn due to the thermal effect of explosion can be worsened by a chemical burn due to toxic fumes. When it burns, PVC produces HCl and chlorine vapor; silicone produces silica ash. The potential risk of silicosis is speculative.[14]

When a tracheal tube fire occurs, the first step is to disconnect the oxygen, stop ventilation, and remove the tube, then to carry out a rigid bronchoscopy to remove the foreign body and fumes and to lavage the tracheobronchial tree. A fiberoptic bronchoscope must be used for smaller airways. Antibiotics and steroids should be prescribed for several days. It is of great importance to provide a high-humidity environment to the airway. In some cases, patients should be intubated and ventilated.[1]

Several approaches have been developed to reduce the incidence of airway fire: reduce the flammability of the endotracheal tube, protect the tube with aluminum tape, or use a specially designed laser tube or jet ventilation.

Reducing Flammability of the Tracheal Tube

Reducing flammability of the tracheal tube is a permanent objective for the anesthetist. It has been suggested that helium can significantly reduce the flammability of an unmarked PVC tube.[10] In a study carried out in 523 cases of CO_2 laser surgery using 60% He in O_2, no fire occurred in spite of the fact that more than 50% of the tubes received laser impacts. In this study, the power was 10 W and the spot beam size was limited to 0.8 cm. However, another study from Simpson and colleagues[15] showed that O_2 diluted in He increases the delay until ignition, but the flammability is little altered. Moreover, He increases the intraluminal flame velocity. Because airway fire can be induced when potentially flammable material is used in an O_2-enriched atmosphere, the FIO_2 must be reduced below 30% even when the tube is protected. Volatile anesthetics are nonflammable and nonexplosive, but during an airway fire they may pyrolize to toxic compounds.[5] The ANSI Z136.3 standards advise anesthetists against their use during laser surgery.[5]

Protective Taping

The most popular method of producing a laser-protected tube is to wrap the tracheal tube with an aluminum or copper tape. Recent work[16] showed that only 3M tape #425 (St. Paul-Minneapolis, MN) and copper foil tape provided excellent protection of the endotracheal tube against a CO_2 laser beam. For protection against a Nd:YAG laser beam, 3M #433 aluminum foil tape and Venture copper foil tape (Rockland, MA) are safest. However, the anesthetist has to keep in mind that aluminum and copper tape do not protect against indirect combustion of the lumen from hot, carbonized fragments. The tube material must be chosen according to the laser used; ie, red rubber for CO_2 laser and clean PVC for Nd:YAG laser. For the same reason, FIO_2 ought to be lower than 30%. The tracheal cuff may not be protected by aluminum tape, so perforation of the cuff by the laser beam is a potential hazard.

Filling of the tracheal tube cuff with saline provides moderate protection during CO_2 laser surgery.[17] It has also been suggested to use dye as a control of cuff perforation. The most effective protection is obtained by placing wet pledgets above the cuff and keeping them moist throughout laser use.[17]

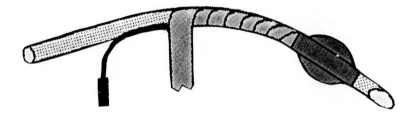

Figure 34–3. Endotracheal tube wrapped with aluminum tape. The tube has to be wrapped in a spiral manner from the tip of the cuff to the pilot balloon.

The tube has to be wrapped in a spiral manner from the tip of the cuff to the level of the uvula. The end should be cut to approximately 60 degrees.[5] A 30% overlap between layers is necessary to ensure perfect protection. Care needs to be taken to prevent wrinkles that could injure the tracheal mucosa. Tubes should not be wrapped longitudinally, in order to avoid kinking of the tube. Several complications from wrapped tubes have been published, such as injuries to tissue by rough edges, pieces of tape dropping into the airway, obstruction of a kinking tube, and tearing of the trachea by a reflecting beam. Most can be avoided by careful maneuvers (Fig. 34–3).

Muslin strips have been recommended to protect the tracheal tube. Muslin is soaked in saline before intubation and has to be kept wet during laser surgery. However, the real protection of muslin is not proven and fire can occur.[3] Another recent means of tube protection is the Merocel "Laser Guard" wrap (Mystic, CT), which has an adhesive metal foil with a synthetic sponge surface. It provides good protection against CO_2 and Nd:YAG lasers, but its main disadvantage is to increase the diameter of the endotracheal tube by 2 mm.[5]

Specially Designed Laser Tube

Several special tubes have been designed for laser surgery. An excellent review of these has been made by Rampil.[5] They are either metallic or made from material specially treated to improve resistance to fire. The Xomed laser shield tube (Xomed-Tleace, Jacksonville, FL) is made from silicone, with an outer layer made of silicone loaded with aluminum powder, which covers the tube and the cuff. This feature does not completely protect against ignition risk.[5] The Porges Milhaud tube (Sar Lat, France), also made of silicone with aluminum powder, uses nitrogen that flows above the vocal cords to cool the tube. It also has a protective shield made of the same material to protect the cuff.[2] The Norton tube (available from Baxter Healthcare Corp, Niles, IL) is

made of a stainless steel spiral coil that is not airtight and may make ventilation difficult.

The "Laser Flex" tube (Mallinckrodt, St. Louis, MO) is made of an airtight stainless steel spiral with two cuffs made from PVC. Because of the PVC cuff, it is not recommended for Nd:YAG laser use. The Bivona "foam cuff" laser tube (Gary, IN) is made of an aluminum spiral covered with silicone. It is approved for CO_2 laser use. The cuff is filled with polyurethane foam and ensures protection against airleaks, but can be ignited.

Jet Ventilation

The jet ventilation technique offers several advantages over conventional ventilation via an endotracheal tube. It produces optimal surgical conditions and patient safety. Good alveolar ventilation and oxygenation can be obtained without an endotracheal tube. Jet ventilation allows a free operating field and the avoidance of flammable material. It can be used either for laryngoscopy or bronchoscopy and with the CO_2 or Nd:YAG laser. The smoke is almost constantly blown out from the airway if a high frequency is used. Jet ventilation is particularly useful in infant and child surgery, allowing good gas exchange with a 1-mm inner dimension (ID) catheter and lower airway pressure than in conventional ventilation. It is the method of choice for airway laser surgery. Perfect knowledge of the technique is necessary before it is used, and contraindications ought to be known and respected. It is safer to use a jet ventilator, especially if high frequencies are used, with a driving pressure Ti/Ttot ratio and frequency setting, and airway pressure monitoring with an alarm, blocking insufflation if the airway pressure is too high. Manual systems with a pressure-reducing valve, like the Sanders jet oxygenator, can be used[2, 18] but do not offer the same safety, mainly with regard to pressure alarm. Moreover, manual systems should not be used for high-frequency jet ventilation. Various techniques for jet ventilation have been described and various materials have been used.[1, 18] The injection can be carried out in front of or below the glottis, or transtracheal. Many operating laryngoscopes have side channels that can be used to provide jet ventilation. The injector tube used is, in most cases, a long, stainless steel needle that is inserted coaxially into the lumen of the laryngoscope or through the special side channel. Supraglottic jet ventilation has the disadvantage of linking ventilation with the laryngoscope. Moreover, smoke and possibly some fragments of the tumor are blown into the airway, down to the tracheobronchial tree. Patients can be hypoventilated in case of partial upper airway obstruction by tumor, stenosis, or papilloma. In such cases, if jet ventilation is not contraindicated, it should be carried out under the stenosis.[19] A copper tube suction device and a suction PVC catheter protected by aluminum tape can be used. Because the tracheal part of the Carden tube cannot be protected, it can be ignited by the laser. Jet ventilation through the Norton tube has also been proposed for CO_2 laser surgery. Transtracheal jet ventilation can be performed with a needle (16 gauge for children and 14 gauge for adults). A specially designed percutaneous transtracheal catheter[20] introduced through the cricothyroid membrane is recommended for laryngeal papillomatosis and stenosis laser surgery, mainly in children.[20] During jet ventilation, a close relationship has been found between the tidal volume and the position of the catheter.[18, 21] When the catheter is not in the middle of the trachea but against the tracheal wall, the tidal volume can be decreased to 50%,[18] mainly because of a lack of entrainment and an inspiratory backflow. To improve entrainment, a catheter has been designed with a special device that can be opened in the trachea to center the catheter (Fig. 34–4). The Teflon catheter, which is nonflammable even in O_2, can be used for laser surgery. Unpublished preliminary results show that tidal volume is improved when the "centering device" of the catheter is opened, caused by an increase in entrainment and a lack of inspiratory backflow.

Jet ventilation is also carried out through the special channel of the rigid bronchoscope during Nd:YAG laser surgery of endobronchial tumors.[4, 22]

Atmospheric Contamination

Vaporization of tissues by the laser beam produces smoke with fine particles of 0.1 to 0.8 µm diameter[5] that can be blown down toward the alveoli by ventilatory gas flow. Experimentally in the rat, these laser smoke particles can be responsible for an interstitial pneumonia bronchiolitis, a decrease in mucociliary clearance, and inflammation.[5] No evidence of such injuries has been found in clinical practice,[4, 23, 24] but because of the potential risk of bronchospasm and alveolar edema, authors recommend alternative phasing of ventilation and vaporization with suction.[1, 18, 24] Airway tumor laser surgery has been suspected as being mutagenic and a vector for viral infection, but no tumor cells able to grow in culture have ever been found,[4, 5] and transmission of viral infection, eg, the papilloma virus, has not been demonstrated. No work has yet been published on the detection of human immunodeficiency virus (HIV) in laser smoke plumes. Laser smoke may contain viable bacterial spores.[2, 3, 5] As protection against the potential hazard of inhaling laser smoke, the surgeon and the people surrounding the patient must wear surgical masks, especially when jet ventilation is used. Smoke produced during laser resection of a tracheobronchial tumor does not increase the concentration of carboxyhemoglobin, as could be suspected.

ANESTHESIA MANAGEMENT

Laser microsurgery of the airway presents specific problems to the anesthetist. Because of the precarious medical state of certain patients (ie, patients with a life-threatening ob-

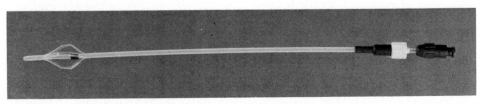

Figure 34–4. Teflon catheter specially designed for jet ventilation. It is composed of two tubes that slide one in the other, with the outer one opening like an umbrella to center the catheter.

struction of the airway), a close cooperation between anesthetist and surgeon is necessary. Methods of oxygenation and ventilation and drugs used for anesthesia need to be well understood. The first preoccupation of the anesthetist should be precise preoperative assessment of the patient.

Preoperative Evaluation of Patient

Patients must be evaluated for chronic lung disease, respiratory obstruction, and pulmonary infection. Most patients scheduled for Nd:YAG laser bronchial surgery are heavy smokers, and this results in a variable degree of chronic bronchitis and emphysema. Due to the partially obstructed airway, patients may have poor pulmonary toilet, with trapping of secretions and pulmonary infection. The quality of the voice, coughing, and the presence of dyspnea or stridor during normal respiration or deep breathing give important information on the degree of respiratory obstruction. Physical work-up should seek excess tracheobronchial secretions, localized hypoventilation, bronchospasm, and predictive factors of difficult intubation.

A chest radiograph, tomography of tracheal and main stem bronchi, and computed tomography (CT) scan provide information on anatomic changes and the involvement of extrabronchial structures. Flow–volume curves can determine the degree of obstruction, and pulmonary testing spirometry may indicate the degree of obstructive pathology. Central airway obstruction produces a plateau during forced exhalation, instead of the rise to and descent from peak flow.

Arterial blood gases provide information on the repercussion of the airway and lung pathologies on lung ventilatory function and gas exchange. Assessment of the tracheobronchial obstruction and its repercussions, like hypoxemia, makes it possible to anticipate problems that can occur during surgery. If respiratory distress requires emergency laser resection, only chest radiography and blood gases can be carried out. Other routine preoperative evaluation consists of an electrocardiogram (ECG) and a coagulation test.

Premedication

Premedication is important, particularly in children with papillomatosis that requires mul-

tiple surgical procedures. Appropriate premedication should be selected according to age and the degree of respiratory depression. An antisialagogue, like atropine or glycopyrrolate, reduces oral secretions, thus providing a dry field that facilitates the surgeon's task. It is particularly useful before CO_2 laser surgery, because saliva absorbs the energy of the beam and decreases its power. Moreover, the parasympatholytic effect of atropine is indicated to prevent laryngoscopy-induced bradycardia, particularly in children. Except for patients with severe obstruction and respiratory depression, a tranquilizing agent should be used. Benzodiazepines, which provide amnesia and sedation, are normally prescribed by anesthetists. Phenothiazine derivatives are reported to increase excitatory phenomena and should be avoided.[3] Drugs such as theophylline, steroids, or β_2-receptor agonists are not discontinued before the surgical procedure. Aminophylline can be used for prevention of bronchospasm in Nd:YAG laser bronchial surgery.[23]

Anesthesia

Anesthesia for direct laryngoscopy should be able to prevent the hypertensive catecholamine response that is a result of the stimulation of the pharyngolaryngeal structures. Fast recovery is desirable in order to avoid postoperative respiratory depression.

If there is no airway obstruction, standard intravenous techniques of induction can be used. In children, mask induction is more common, and rectal barbiturates may be useful, but intravenous access must be obtained before intubation. In patients with a compromised airway, intubation can be planned before or after the loss of consciousness. If severe airway obstruction is predicted, intubation over a 3-mm pediatric ventilating bronchoscope can be used. An awake intubation is recommended in adults; in children, the best technique is inhalation induction with spontaneous ventilation. In all cases, an anesthetist competent in fiberoptic intubation is required to perform intubation quickly. Before intubation, all equipment required for difficult intubation should be at hand: straight laryngoscope blades, a variety of endotracheal tubes of different sizes, bronchoscope, and equipment for performing percutaneous transtracheal ventilation. A surgeon experienced in performing tracheostomy should be in attendance. Once the airway is secure, the patient can be anesthetized with an intravenous agent. Volatile anesthetics are not recommended if a flammable material is used.[5] Moreover, they cannot be used with jet ventilation. Ketamine may lead to laryngospasm because it increases airway reflexes, and so it should be avoided.[3]

Immobilizing of the surgical field is mandatory, because coughing or swallowing can lead to misdirection of the laser beam and damage to normal tissues. Therefore, deep anesthesia and muscle relaxants are necessary. Succinylcholine infusion and intermediate-acting muscle relaxants like atracurium or vecuronium are the most suitable with the procedure. Sulfentanil citrate and alfentanil provide a deep level of narcotic anesthesia, a shorter duration of action than fentanyl, and cardiovascular stability. They provide a more rapid recovery rate than fentanyl at equipotent doses.[18] The gag reflex and the hypertensive response can be blunted by local anesthesia, and lidocaine is the most frequently used. Proper monitoring includes an ECG, a noninvasive blood pressure cuff, a pulse oximeter and, at best if jet ventilation is used, a neuromuscular blockade monitoring unit. It should be remembered that SpO_2 only monitors oxygenation and not alveolar ventilation or CO_2 elimination.

Airway Management for Laryngeal Laser Surgery

There are three main techniques for airway management. Anesthetists should take into account the patient's age and previous history, particularly the degree of airway obstruction and respiratory insufficiency, and his or her own experience and that of the surgeon.

No Tube in Airway

This technique provides moderately deep anesthesia with spontaneous ventilation. Topical anesthesia of the pharyngeal and laryngeal structures with lidocaine spray is carried out after induction. Local anesthesia can be affected by superior laryngeal nerve blockade and transtracheal injection. Patients may also receive 10 to 15 mL of 4% lidocaine via an ultrasonic nebulizer 15 minutes before induction. Anesthesia is maintained with insufflation of a volatile anesthetic via a nasal catheter[3] or via a needle through a side channel of the laryngoscope. Local anesthesia supplemented with sedation should be avoided for laser surgery. This technique offers a free operating field to the surgeon, and is more appropriate for infants, but is not innocuous. It is difficult to find the best level of anesthesia. Too deep an anesthesia may result in hypoventilation and hypercarbia or apnea; too light an anesthesia may lead to coughing and laryngospasm, so that the airway is not secured and the vocal cords are not immobile, thus increasing the risk of damage to normal tissue and making the surgeon's task difficult. Moreover, the expired gases pollute the surrounding environment. For all these reasons, several authors[25, 26] recommend *apneic anesthesia* in children. Following induction and neuromuscular blockade, the child is intubated with a suitable size of endotracheal tube, and suspension laryngoscopy is performed. The child is then hyperventilated to an end-tidal CO_2 of nearly 30 mm Hg with O_2 and a volatile anesthetic. The tube is removed and laser surgery is performed with an apneic technique until SpO_2 reaches 97%. Surgery is performed with successive periods of hyperventilation and apnea. The apnea should not exceed 90 seconds in children under 2 years of age and 3 minutes in older children.[25]

Laser-Proof Endotracheal Tube

The laser-proof tube should be smaller than usual in order to allow good visualization of the glottis. A 6-mm cuff tracheal tube is usually used for adults and a 3-mm uncuffed tracheal tube for children. Ventilation is maintained with air in oxygen ($FIO_2 \leq 30\%$) or helium in oxygen ($FIO_2 \leq 40\%$), with or without a volatile agent, by positive-pressure ventilation. The increased airway resistances due to the smaller tube and the inspiratory gas leak in children have to be taken into account for setting of ventilatory parameters. If the cuff is penetrated by the laser beam, the endotracheal tube should be changed to avoid severe hypoventilation due to a large inspiratory gas flow leak. In patients with tracheostomy, a nonfenestrated metal tracheostomy or a laser-proof tracheostomy tube is inserted through the stoma.

This simple technique can be used by all anesthetists and ensures protection of the airway, prevents aspiration of blood and debris, and allows ventilation without specialized material. Tracheal intubation is particularly adapted for anterior commissure laryngeal lesions, the tube providing a good opening of the glottis. However, the endotracheal tube partially obstructs the surgeon's view for surgery of the posterior commissure, and it risks being compressed by the laryngoscope if it is maintained in the anterior commissure. The main disadvantage of this technique is the risk of tube ignition.

Jet Ventilation

The use of jet ventilation requires close cooperation between anesthetist and surgeon. Video monitoring of the operating field is particularly useful. There is no need for an endotracheal tube, so there is no risk of airway fire; this gives a free operating field. Gas is injected through a narrow needle or catheter, 2- to 2.5-mm ID or 14 gauge in adults and 1- to 2-mm ID or 16 gauge in infants and children. The driving pressure is regulated according to chest expansion, airway pressure, and SpO_2. In adults, the recommended driving pressure is between 20 to 40 psi; in children, up to 20 psi; and in infants and neonates, 10 psi. The driving pressure is at first set at the lower pressure and is altered by 5 to 10 psi increments according to chest expansion and SpO_2. It is safer to use an actuated solenoid valve jet ventilator, mainly if high frequencies are used, with driving pressure Ti/Ttot ratio and frequency setting and airway pressure monitoring with an alarm device. Manual systems with a pressure-reducing valve like the Sanders jet oxygenator can be used,[3, 18] but do not offer the same safety, mainly with regard to the pressure alarm. Barotrauma is the most important complication of jet ventilation. The incidence can be decreased and nearly suppressed by using a pressure monitoring alarm and by respecting contraindications; eg, large tumor that can act as a ball valve, stenosis that reduces airway diameter up to 0.5 cm in adults and up to 50% in children,[19] patients with lung heterogeneity, or a high time constant. In such cases, jet ventilation with 60% He in O_2 can be used to increase alveolar gas exchange without increasing airway pressure,[2, 17] thereby allowing the use of a lower driving pressure. Moreover, because of its low density, helium facilitates gas flow past the airway obstruction[10] and decreases the expiratory pressure. Gastric distention[1, 5, 18] occurs only when jetting in front of the glottis. High-frequency jet ventilation (HFJV) has several advantages over jet ventilation. HFJV produces an immobile field because of low tidal volume and high frequency. The smoke is blown outside nearly constantly and lower tidal volumes of 150 to 200 mL are used, resulting in lower airway pressure for the same alveolar ventilation. Due to a slight

intrinsic positive end-expiratory pressure (PEEP) effect reducing the shunt fraction, oxygenation is improved. Pressure monitoring should be used, especially in children. Conversely, manual jet ventilation needs a simple, inexpensive device. It may be more suitable for surgical procedures if there is a need for alternate phasing of ventilation and vaporization with suction. It produces abnormal forced movement of the vocal cords due to higher tidal volume. Jet ventilation does not offer protection of the airway; slight bleeding is blown out,[20] but extensive bleeding should lead to conversion to intubation.

Airway Management for Tracheobronchial Laser Surgery

Anesthesia and airway management for tracheobronchial laser surgery problems are different from those of laryngeal surgery. The greatest problem is the difficulty of maintaining alveolar ventilation and oxygenation in the presence of a large tumor obstruction and distally high airway resistances.[1] The risk of fire is minimal, because metallic material is used in most cases. Several methods of anesthesia have been described[1, 2, 4, 5, 22] and are linked to surgical methods.

Spontaneous Ventilation

This is proposed with the use of a flexible bronchoscope in patients with a precarious medical state.[27] The anesthesia associates local anesthesia with sedation. It is proposed when the middle or lower tracheal lumen is decreased by more than 50%, in emergency situations with a high degree of obstruction, or when the lesion involves the trachea above the carina.[27] In such cases, the negative pressure created by spontaneous respiration may be the margin of safety necessary to maintain oxygenation and may prevent the tumor ball-valve effect that can occur with positive pressure ventilation.[27] However, it increases the respiratory workload, does not give sufficient control of the airway,[4] and could be complicated by severe hypoxia due to sedation and by asphyxiation from hemorrhage.[4] Moreover, the procedure can last more than 1 hour and coughing and restlessness can occur.

Ventilation Through an Endotracheal Tube

The flexible bronchoscope may be introduced through a rubber diaphragm within a large-diameter, laser-proof endotracheal tube, or into the trachea alongside a smaller diameter tube. This method is not recommended, because it does not suppress the risk of laser ignition.

Ventilation Through a Rigid Bronchoscope

A rigid bronchoscope should be used whenever possible.[1, 4, 27] It gives better access to lesions and an easier passage through the stenosis. Suction of blood, secretions, smoke, and tumor debris is easier. It allows the use of a fiberscope or a laser probe and the control of bleeding. The large diameter of the bronchoscope[7, 9] reduces ventilatory resistances and improves the operating field view.[27] A tracheoscope can also be used.[22] Two methods of ventilation are proposed. The anesthetic circuit is connected to the ventilation port of the bronchoscope and the patient is ventilated with bag ventilation with a gas mixture of 40% O_2 in air or in He.[27] A concentration of O_2 higher than 40% could allow combustion of organic material in theory,[4] and a high gas flow is needed to compensate for the inspiratory leak. Alternate periods of ventilation and suction prevent smoke pollution of the alveoli. Hypercapnia during bag ventilation has led to favoring jet ventilation. Although no comparative studies have been carried out to prove the better efficiency of jet ventilation in laser surgery, several studies have proved that jet ventilation and especially high-frequency jet ventilation provides good gas exchange and higher oxygenation.[1, 4, 22, 27] Jet ventilation can be performed either through the special ventilating port of the bronchoscope especially adapted for an Nd:YAG laser or CO_2 laser,[2] or through a metallic needle inserted into the bronchoscope,[4] the tracheoscope,[22] or through the suction port of the bronchoscope[1] (Fig. 34–5). Tidal volume and entrainment depend on the position of the tip of the jet.[2]

Whatever the technique, the main danger is hypoxemia and hypercarbia. SpO_2 is highly mandatory and transcutaneous Po_2 and Pco_2 can be useful especially in children. If hypoxemia occurs, the surgical procedure is stopped and the patient is ventilated with 100% O_2.

Postoperative Airway Complications

At the end of the surgical procedure, the patient is awakened and extubated in the op-

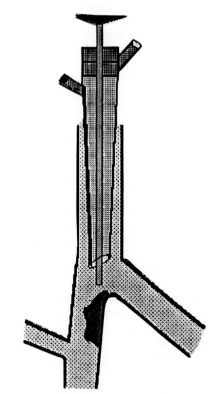

Figure 34–5. Schematic representation of use of Nd:YAG laser through a bronchoscope. Jet ventilation can be performed either through the suction or ventilating port, or with a metallic needle inserted into the bronchoscope.

erating room. The protected endotracheal tube has to be inspected; if tape is missing, laryngoscopy and bronchoscopy are performed. The patient should be monitored with SpO_2 and chest examination. Postoperative edema, laryngospasm, and bronchospasm can occur as indicated by inspiratory stridor, retraction, and a decrease in SpO_2. These must be prevented and treated as usual.[1, 2, 23] A high incidence of muscle weakness has been reported after laser resection of bronchial tumor under general anesthesia.[23] Pneumothorax should be suspected if there is a respiratory insufficiency, especially if jet ventilation has been performed.

SUMMARY

The use of lasers in airway surgery improves operating conditions, allowing bloodless surgery with a low risk of edema. However, it poses the problem of sharing the airway. Both anesthetist and surgeon should cooperate throughout the procedure. The best approach to the airway management of patients is to have excellent knowledge of the different techniques and to have several alternatives available before induction.

The laser principle is based on Einstein's quantum theory and stimulated emission. Three processes are involved in laser production: spontaneous emission, absorption and stimulated emission. The laser beam is characterized by its temporal and spatial coherence, resulting in a narrow, nondivergent powerful beam. Two types of lasers are used in airway surgery. The CO_2 laser, whose wavelength is located in the infrared region, and the Nd:YAG laser, which produces a wavelength in the near-infrared region. Unlike the CO_2 laser, the Nd:YAG laser can be transmitted by flexible optic fibers. The CO_2 laser beam is absorbed by water and vaporizes tissue. The Nd:YAG laser is absorbed by pigmented tissue and mainly produces a thermal coagulation.

Laser hazards can be grouped into three main categories. With misdirection or reflection of the beam, eye injuries are more likely to occur. The CO_2 laser can cause corneal injury, although the Nd:YAG laser may damage the retina. Glasses or goggles specially adapted to each laser should be worn by the operating room personnel. The patient's eyes and face should be protected by wet gauze and cloth. Endotracheal tube fire represents 14% of laser injuries. If O_2 exceeds 30%, the burning tube becomes a blow torch and can cause serious damage to the trachea and airway. Red rubber is more resistant to the CO_2 beam, whereas PVC is more resistant to the Nd:YAG beam. The flammability of the tracheal tube can be reduced by using He in 40% O_2 instead of nitrogen. Aluminum or copper tapes provide excellent protection for the endotracheal tube against the laser beam, but the cuff and the inside of the tube are not protected. Of the specially designed laser tubes, only the metallic tubes are nonflammable. Jet ventilation allows the use of nonflammable materials; eg, metallic needles or Teflon translaryngeal or transtracheal catheters. Moreover, with jet ventilation the operating field is free of the tube, providing an excellent view.

Although atmospheric contamination of the airway has never been proved in clinical practice, protection against exhaled laser smoke is highly recommended.

Close cooperation between anesthetist and surgeon is necessary for safe management of anesthesia. The main preoccupation of the anesthetist should be precise preoperative assessment of the patient, especially the reper-

cussion of the airway pathology on the respiratory system and possibly difficult intubation. Immobility of the surgical field is mandatory during anesthesia, because coughing or swallowing should be avoided. Therefore, deep anesthesia and muscle relaxants are required. Airway management is the main problem during CO_2 laser surgery. Spontaneous ventilation without an endotracheal tube is no longer used. Apneic anesthesia is proposed in children, but the best solution is intubation with a small, laser-proof endotracheal tube or jet ventilation. The FIO_2 should be up to 40% if nonflammable material is used. Jet ventilation can be performed with a manual system, but high-frequency jet ventilation (HFJV) ought to be used with a special device that combines airway pressure monitoring. HFJV produces an immobile field and improves oxygenation. Spontaneous ventilation has few indications in tracheobronchial laser surgery. Bag ventilation or, better still, jet ventilation should be used.

References

1. Paes ML. General anaesthesia for carbon dioxide laser surgery within the airway. Br J Anaesth 59:1610–1620, 1987.
2. Van Der Spek AF, Spargo PM, Norton ML. The physics of lasers and implications for their use during airway surgery. Br J Anaesth 60:709–729, 1988.
3. Hermens IM, Bennet MJ, Hirshman CA. Anaesthesia for laser surgery. Anesth Analg 62:218–229, 1983.
4. Blowquist S, Algotsson L, Karlsson SE. Anaesthesia for resection of tumours in the trachea and central bronchi using the Nd:YAG laser technique. Acta Anaesthesiol Scand 34:506–510, 1990.
5. Rampil IJ. Anaesthetic considerations for laser surgery. Anesth Analg 74:424–435, 1992.
6. Wegrzynowicz ES, Jensen NF, Pearson KS, Watchel RE, Scamman FL. Airway fire during jet ventilation for laser excision of vocal cord papillomata. Anesthesiology 76:468–469, 1992.
7. Gaufield RA, Chapin JW. Pneumothorax with upper airway laser surgery. Anesthesiology 56:398–399, 1982.
8. Hirshman CA, Smith I. Indirect ignition of the endotracheal tube during carbon dioxide laser surgery. Arch Otolaryngol 106:639–641, 1980.
9. Casey KR, Fairfay WR, Smith SJ, Dixon JA. Intratracheal fire ignited by the Nd:YAG laser during treatment of tracheal stenosis. Chest 84:295–296, 1983.
10. Pashayan AG, Gravenstein JS, Cassisi NJ, McLaughlin G. The helium protocol for laryngotracheal operations with CO_2 laser: A retrospective review of 523 cases. Anesthesiology 68:801–804, 1988.
11. Sosis MB. Airway fire during CO_2 laser surgery using a Xomed laser endotracheal tube. Anesthesiology 72:747–749, 1990.
12. Wolf GL, Sidebothan GW. Tracheal tube intraluminal flame spread in opposed flow oxidant: Helium versus nitrogen dilution. Anesth Analg 70:S438, 1990.

13. Geffin B, Shapsay SM, Bellack GS, Hobin K, Setzer SE. Flammability of endotracheal tubes during Nd YAG laser application in the airway. Anesthesiology 65:511–515, 1986.
14. Ossof RH, Duncarage JA, Eisenman TS, Karlan MS. Comparison of tracheal damage from laser-ignital endotracheal tube fires. Ann Otol Rhinol Laryngol 92:233–236, 1983.
15. Simpson JI, Schiff GA, Wolf GL. The effect of helium on endotracheal tube flammability. Anesthesiology 73:538–540, 1990.
16. Sosis MB. Evaluation of five metallic tapes for protection of endotracheal tubes during CO_2 laser surgery. Anesth Analg 69:392–393, 1989.
17. Sosis MB, Dillon FX. Saline-filled cuffs help prevent laser-induced polyvinylchloride endotracheal tube fires. Anesth Analg 72:187–189, 1991.
18. Shikowitz MJ, Abramson AL, Liberatore L. Endotracheal jet ventilation: A 10 year review. Laryngoscope 101:455–461, 1991.
19. Belaguid A, Ben Jebria A, Cros AM, Boudey C, Guenard H. High frequency jet ventilation and upper tracheal stenosis: A model study. Intensive Care Med 17:479–483, 1991.
20. Monnier PH, Ravussin P, Savary M. Percutaneous transtracheal ventilation for laser endoscopic treatment of laryngeal and subglottic lesions. Clin Otolaryngol 13:209–217, 1988.
21. Cros AM, Guenard H, Boudey C. High frequency jet ventilation with helium and oxygen versus nitrogen and oxygen. Anesthesiology 69:417–419, 1988.
22. Schneider M, Probst R. High-frequency jet ventilation via a tracheoscope for endobronchial laser surgery. Can J Anaesth 37:372–376, 1990.
23. Hanowell LH, Martin WR, Savelle JE, Foppiano LE. Complications of general anesthesia for Nd:YAG resection of endobronchial tumors. Chest 98:72–76, 1991.
24. Gussack GS, Evans RF, Tacchi EJ. Intravenous anesthesia and jet ventilation for laser microlaryngeal surgery. Ann Otol Rhinol Laryngol 96:29–33, 1987.
25. Cohen SR, Herbert WI, Thompson JW. Anesthesia management of microlaryngeal laser surgery in children: Apneic technique anesthesia. Laryngoscope 98:347–348, 1988.
26. Weisberger EC, Miner ID. Apneic anesthesia for improved endoscopic removal of laryngeal papillomata. Laryngoscope 98:693–697, 1988.
27. Rontal M, Rontal E, Wendkul ME, Elson L. Anesthetic management for tracheobronchial laser surgery. Ann Otol Laryngol 95:556–560, 1986.

Bibliography

Apfelberg DB. Evaluation and Installation of Surgical Laser Systems. New York: Springer Verlag, 1987.

Carlon GC. High frequency ventilation in intensive care and during surgery. In Howland WS (ed). Lung Biology in Health and Disease. New York: Marcel Dekker, 1985.

Lunkenheimer PP, Whemster WF, Sykes MK. High frequency ventilation: 20 years of endeavour reviewed. Acta Anaesthesiol Scand 33:suppl 90, 1989.

Wilson J, Hawkes JFB. Lasers: Principles and Applications. New York: Prentice-Hall, 1987.

CHAPTER 35

Congenital Airway Abnormalities

Charles J. Coté, M.D., Norbert Rolf, M.D., and I. David Todres, M.D.

In order to approach the management of children with congenital airway abnormalities in a logical and rational manner, it is helpful to have a basic understanding of the embryologic development of the airway, normal airway anatomy, and the differences between the pediatric and the adult airway.

EMBRYOLOGY

The lung bud develops from the alimentary component of the foregut at the fourth week of gestation, and is the precursor of the future larynx, trachea, bronchi, and alveoli. During the fourth week of gestation, the lateral ridges separate the alimentary and the respiratory portions of the foregut.[1-3] Failure of these ridges to develop or to fuse leads to various forms of tracheoesophageal fistulae or clefts; failure to separate results in laryngeal webs.

The paired bronchial arches and pharyngeal pouches form the facial and pharyngeal structures of the airway (nose, mouth, pharynx). Failure of these structures to fuse in the fifth week leads to microstomia and various cleft malformations of the oropharynx; these are among the most common developmental upper airway abnormalities. Hypoplasia of the second bronchial arch, which forms the mandible, results in microstomia abnormalities.[1] Devel-

opment of the nasal cavity is completed by the end of the seventh week of gestation. Choanal atresia or stenosis is the result of a partial or total persistence of the septum between the nose and the stomodeum.[4] The majority of congenital airway abnormalities are therefore the result of abnormal development during the first 12 weeks of gestation.

THE NORMAL PEDIATRIC AIRWAY

The airway of the infant differs from the adult in five ways:[5-7] (1) The infant tongue is relatively large in relation to the oropharygeal cavity and thus easily obstructs the upper airway, with loss of consciousness or neuromuscular relaxation. The relatively large tongue may make its control difficult with the laryngoscope blade. (2) The infant larynx is located higher in the neck (C3–4), compared with the adult larynx (C4–5) (Fig. 35–1). The infant larynx is usually characterized as being "anterior"; this is incorrect. The infant larynx is higher or more rostral in the neck than the adult, making direct visualization of laryngeal structures more difficult because the angulation between the base of the tongue and the glottic opening is more acute than in the adult. It is for this reason that straight laryngoscope

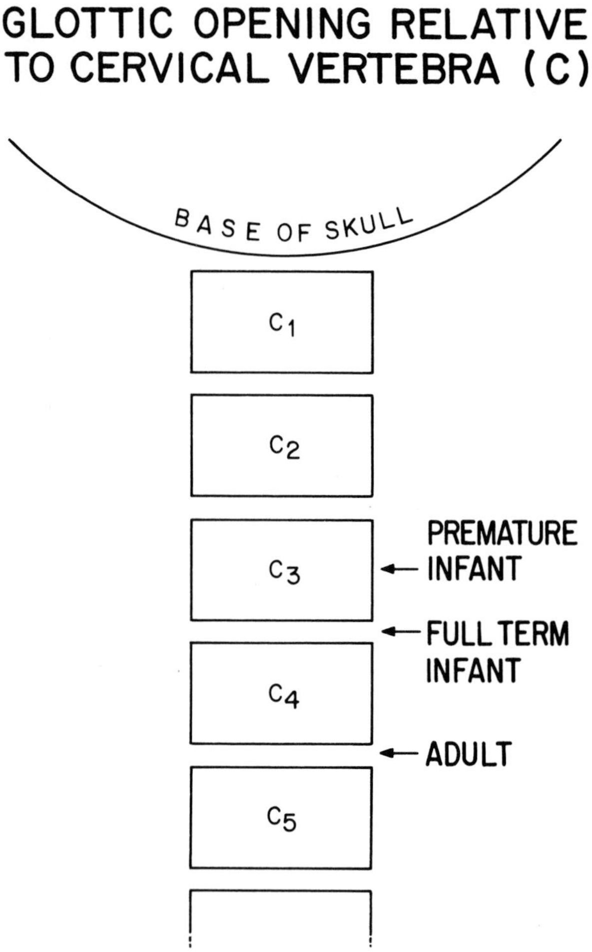

GLOTTIC OPENING RELATIVE TO CERVICAL VERTEBRA (C)

Figure 35–1. The premature infant larynx is located at the middle of the third cervical vertebra (C3), the full-term infant larynx is at the C3–4 interspace, whereas the adult larynx is at the C4–5 interspace. (Adapted from Negus VE. The comparative anatomy and physiology of the larynx. New York. Grune & Stratton, 1949; with permission. Coté CJ, Ryan JF, Todres ID, Goudsouzian NG (eds). A practice of anesthesia for infants and children, 2nd ed. Philadelphia, WB Saunders Co, 1993, p. 58.)

blades facilitate endotracheal intubation in infants. (3) The infant epiglottis is angled (45 degrees) from the axis of the trachea and therefore control (ie, lifting) of the epiglottis may be more difficult in the infant compared with the older child or adult, in whom the axis of the epiglottis is parallel to that of the trachea. (4) The vocal cords have a lower attachment anteriorly than posteriorly compared with the adult; this angulation may result in the endotracheal tube being caught at the anterior commissure with nasotracheal intubation. (5) An important difference between the child and adult larynx is that the narrowest portion of the infant larynx is the nondistensible ring of cricoid cartilage (Fig. 35–2), whereas in the adult it is the rima glottidis (ie, the laryngeal inlet). Thus, an endotracheal tube that readily passes through the glottic opening may not pass through the subglottic region or may fit too tightly in the young pediatric patient. By age 10 to 12 years, the larynx has undergone normal growth and de-

velopment and no longer has this subglottic narrowing. It is for this reason that a child may develop postintubation "croup" when a "snug" endotracheal tube is placed. The circular narrowing in the subglottic region allows the anesthesiologist to place uncuffed endotracheal tubes, allowing an acceptable leak around the tube while at the same time ensuring effective ventilation. If a cuffed endotracheal tube were passed, because of the space occupied by the cuff, a smaller internal diameter endotracheal tube would need to be placed in order to avoid excessive pressure to the mucosa in the subglottic region. Generally, we endeavor to have a leak at a peak inflation pressure of 20 to 30 cm H_2O with either an uncuffed endotracheal tube or a cuffed endotracheal tube with the cuff partially inflated.

FUNCTIONAL ANATOMY

The infant larynx does not achieve normal functional coordination until approximately 5

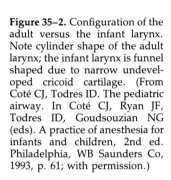

Figure 35–2. Configuration of the adult versus the infant larynx. Note cylinder shape of the adult larynx; the infant larynx is funnel shaped due to narrow undeveloped cricoid cartilage. (From Coté CJ, Todres ID. The pediatric airway. In Coté CJ, Ryan JF, Todres ID, Goudsouzian NG (eds). A practice of anesthesia for infants and children, 2nd ed. Philadelphia, WB Saunders Co, 1993, p. 61; with permission.)

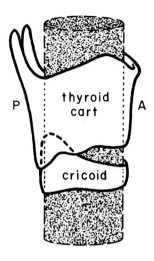

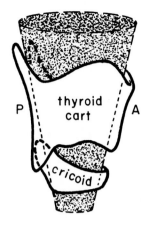

ADULT
(cylinder)

INFANT
(funnel)

months of age; ie, the infant has difficulty in coordinating swallowing and ventilation.[8, 9] The infant is frequently characterized as being an obligate nasal breather. This is a developmental process that occurs during the first 5 months following birth. Among infants of 31 weeks gestational age, only about 8% are able to overcome nasal obstruction and breathe through their mouths.[10, 11] About 40% of full-term newborns are able to overcome nasal airway obstruction and breathe through their mouths. By 5 months of age, nearly all infants are able to overcome nasal obstruction and breathe through their mouths. Maturational differences in laryngeal function account in part for why some infants are greatly affected by choanal atresia and others minimally so.

An important functional difference between the infant and adult airway results from the highly compliant nature of the laryngeal and tracheal structures in the infant.[12–14] The trachea is particularly susceptible to distending and compressive forces as a result of differences between intrathoracic and extrathoracic transluminal pressure.[15] When a child inspires, there is little dilatation of the intrathoracic airways and dynamic collapse of the extrathoracic trachea, particularly at the thoracic inlet, due to the pressure differential between atmosphere and intratracheal pressure. If a child develops upper airway obstruction (eg, epi-

glottitis, croup, or an extrathoracic intratracheal foreign body), there will be a much greater dynamic collapse of the trachea at the thoracic inlet when the child attempts to breathe against this obstructed airway. Dynamic collapse of the trachea is even further exaggerated when the child cries and becomes agitated (Fig. 35–3). For this reason, we attempt to keep children with obstructed airways as calm as possible. For the anesthesiologist, a knowledge of this aspect of functional anatomy leads to the rational application of positive end-expiratory pressure (PEEP) to "stent" the airway open and overcome transluminal pressure differentials. Laryngomalacia and tracheomalacia are examples of congenital airway anomalies that make the child more susceptible to the effects of dynamic airway collapse; ie, because these areas are less rigid than normal, there is greater dynamic extrathoracic airway collapse.[1] With laryngomalacia, the soft, redundant epiglottis and aryepiglottic folds are paradoxically pulled into apposition and into the laryngeal inlet during inspiration.

With lower airway obstruction (eg, bronchiolitis, pulmonary edema, an intrathoracic tracheal foreign body, or intrathoracic tracheomalacia), there will be obstruction during expiration.[16] When the child forcefully exhales against this obstruction, the intrathoracic pressure compresses the highly compliant intratho-

A = Atmospheric pressure
− = Negative to A
+ = Positive to A

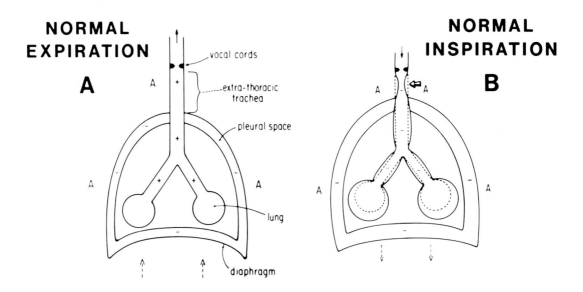

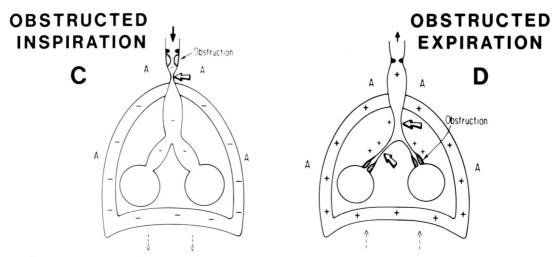

Figure 35–3. A, Normal expiration. The normal sequence of events at end-expiration is a slight negative intrapleural pressure stenting the airways open. In infants, the highly compliant chest does not provide the support required; thus, airway closure occurs with each breath. Intraluminal pressures are slightly positive in relation to atmospheric pressure, resulting in air being forced out of the lungs. With descent of the diaphragm and contraction of the intercostal muscles, a greater negative intrathoracic pressure relative to intraluminal and atmospheric pressure is developed. B, Normal inspiration. The net result is a stretching longitudinally of the larynx and trachea, dilatation of the intrathoracic trachea and bronchi, movement of air into the lungs, and some dynamic collapse of the extrathoracic trachea *(open arrow)*. The dynamic collapse is due to the highly compliant trachea and the negative intraluminal pressure in relation to atmospheric pressure. C, Obstructed inspiration. Note the severe dynamic collapse of the extrathoracic trachea below the level of obstruction. This collapse is greatest at the thoracic inlet where the largest pressure gradient exists between negative intratracheal pressure and atmospheric pressure *(open arrow)*. D, Obstructed expiration. Breathing against an obstructed lower airway (bronchiolitis, asthma) results in greater positive intrathoracic pressures, with dynamic collapse of the intrathoracic airways (prolonged expiration of wheezing *[open arrows]*). (From Coté CJ, Todres ID. The pediatric airway. In Coté CJ, Ryan JF, Todres ID, Goudsouzian NG (eds). A practice of anesthesia for infants and children, 2nd ed. Philadelphia, WB Saunders Co, 1993, p. 63; with permission.)

racic airways, thus creating small airway obstruction, which manifests as prolonged expiration (Fig. 35–3). This obstruction may be overcome with the application of PEEP. Therefore, upper airway obstruction primarily manifests with inspiratory stridor and lower airway obstruction with wheezing and prolonged expiration.[17]

The work of breathing is similar on a per kg basis in infants and adults.[18–20] Pathologic narrowing of the infant airway has much greater adverse effect on the work of breathing.[21–23] For example, resistance to air flow is inversely proportional to the radius of the lumen to the fourth power for *laminar* flow and inversely proportional to the radius of the lumen to the fifth power for *turbulent* flow.[24] Therefore, if a pediatric airway of 4 mm diameter developed 1 mm circumferential edema, this would result in a 75% reduction in cross-sectional area and 16-fold increase in resistance to airflow with marked increase in the work of breathing (Fig. 35–4).[5, 24] If the child cried and developed greater transluminal pressures, this would re-

sult in turbulent flow and therefore would increase the work of breathing 32 times! When compared with the adult airway (approximately 8 mm) and having 1 mm of edema, this would result in a 44% reduction in cross-sectional area and only a three-fold increase in the work of breathing.[5] Therefore, any pathology that causes intraluminal airway obstruction has much greater adverse effects in the infant compared with the adult.

Another difference in functional anatomy involves the respiratory muscles (intercostals, diaphragm), which have a lower proportion of type I muscle fibers; these allow for repetitive motion without fatigue.[25–27] The infant has a smaller content of type I muscle fibers, and thus fatigues more readily than the older child or adult. The diaphragm and intercostal muscles do not develop a normal proportion of type I muscle fibers until approximately 2 years of age.[26] Therefore, children under 2 years of age are more susceptible to respiratory failure as the work of breathing is increased.

EFFECTS OF AIRWAY EDEMA ON FLOW RESISTANCE AND CROSS-SECTIONAL AREA

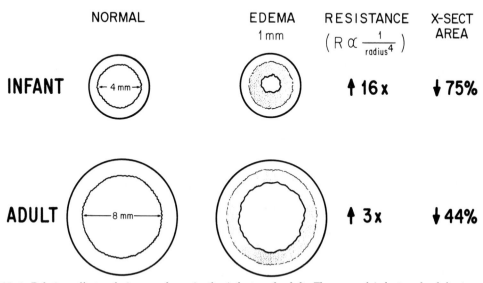

Figure 35–4. Relative effects of airway edema in the infant and adult. The normal infant and adult airways are presented on the left, edematous airways (1 mm circumferential) on the right. Note that resistance to flow is inversely proportional to radius of the lumen to the fourth power for laminar flow, and the radius of the lumen to the fifth power for turbulent flow. The net result in the infant is a 75% reduction in cross-sectional area, and a 16-fold increase in resistance, as compared with a 44% reduction in cross-sectional area and a threefold increase in resistance in the adult. (From Coté CJ, Todres ID. The pediatric airway. In Coté CJ, Ryan JF, Todres ID, Goudsouzian NG (eds). A practice of anesthesia for infants and children, 2nd ed. Philadelphia, WB Saunders Co, 1993, p. 62; with permission.)

SPECIFIC CONGENITAL MALFORMATIONS

General Concepts

When one plans the anesthesia of a pediatric patient, it is vital to perform a careful physical examination. *If there is one congenital malformation present, one must look for associated malformations.* In particular, if one sees an external ear deformity, this is often associated with mid-facial hypoplasia and renal developmental abnormalities.

The physical examination begins with an overall observation of the patient and how he or she is interacting with the parents. This interaction helps guide the approach to the anesthetic management (premedication, no premedication, mask versus intravenous induction). During this period of observation, one notes the color of the nail beds, respiratory rate, quality of the voice and the presence of normal or abnormal respiratory patterns (ie, stridor, retractions, cyanosis).

Once general observations have been carried out, one may proceed to a more careful physical examination. First ask the child to open his or her mouth, and note how large the tongue is in proportion to the oral pharynx, note how large the oral cavity is, and if there is a high arched palate, tonsillar hypertrophy, and missing or loose teeth. One then examines the ramus of the mandible to determine the distance between the mentum of the mandible and the upper border of the thyroid cartilage. For the teenager, one should be able to fit approximately three fingerbreadths between the mentum of the mandible and the thyroid cartilage. The younger the child, the smaller this distance. Performing this careful physical examination routinely in every pediatric patient, and then reviewing any difficulties encountered with the airway during the induction of anesthesia, the anesthesiologist gains experience, being able to predict those patients who might have simple as opposed to complex airway management problems with anesthesia.

One should then examine for mobility of the head and neck structures, looking for possible fusion of the cervical spine. Some syndromes are associated with instability of the cervical spine; eg, approximately 15% of Down's syndrome children have unstable atlantoaxial structures.[28, 29]

The physical examination then proceeds to the thorax, examining for stridor or signs of infection. On the basis of this interview and physical examination, the decision is made as to whether further evaluation of the airway for other associated medical conditions is required before the child comes to the operating room.[30–33] In addition, during this time one begins to formulate the "game plan" regarding the type of anesthetic induction and the need for a premedication.[34]

Macroglossia

If a child has a large tongue (macroglossia), one must consider a variety of syndromes, such as congenital hypothyroidism, Down's syndrome, mucopolysaccharidosis, glycogen storage diseases, and the Beckwith-Wiedemann syndrome.[35–37] The Beckwith-Wiedemann syndrome is associated with hyperviscosity, hypoglycemia, and organomegaly. The large tongue will present mechanical difficulty during laryngoscopy because the position of the large tongue may be difficult to control with a laryngoscope blade. In addition, the large tongue will more readily obstruct the oral pharynx when the child loses consciousness.

Mid-Facial Hypoplasia

Mid-facial hypoplasia syndromes present perhaps the most difficult airway management problems because, in addition to having a hypoplastic mandible, these children tend to have a narrow high-arched palate and a small mouth. The normal position of the larynx in relation to the base of the tongue is distorted, so that the angle between the base of the tongue and the laryngeal inlet is much more acute; ie, these children have a larynx located more posteriorly in the neck than the normal neonate. Examples of this include the Pierre Robin syndrome, Goldenhar's syndrome, and Treacher Collins syndrome.[38–44]

The Pierre Robin abnormality consists of mandibular hypoplasia, which can vary from mild to very severe hypoplasia (Fig. 35–5). These children are usually physiologically and developmentally normal except for the mandibular hypoplasia. The mandible eventually grows to near normal position and configuration by approximately 3 years of age in most children.[38, 40] Children with Treacher Collins syndrome (craniofacial dysostosis) have a triangular-shaped face, high arched palate, small mouth, hypoplastic mandible, and a larynx that is located more posteriorly. These children are

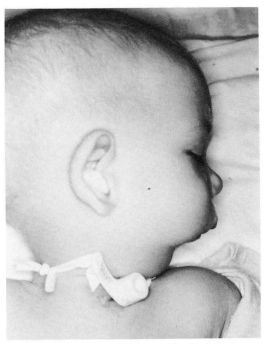

Figure 35–5. Pierre Robin anomaly. Note the near complete absence of the mandible in this extreme example. (Courtesy of Roland Eavey, MD.)

among the most difficult airway management problems because the posterior location of the larynx exaggerates the angulation between the base of the tongue and the laryngeal inlet (Fig. 35–6).[41, 42] They also have a high incidence of associated congenital heart disease. Goldenhar's syndrome (oculo-auriculo-vertebral syndrome) involves abnormalities of the eye and external ear. These children have a hypoplastic mandible that may be normal on one side, resulting in mandibular displacement to one side during mouth opening. Similar to Treacher Collins children, they have a high-arched palate, a small mouth, and the larynx is located more posteriorly than normal. They may also have fusion of the base of the skull with the cervical spine, limiting the ability to extend or flex the neck (Fig. 35–7).[43, 44] These children may have associated congenital heart disease.

Other common mid-facial hypoplasia syndromes include Apert's syndrome, Marfan's syndrome, Turner's syndrome, and achondroplasia.[45, 46] In all these children, the insertion of an oral airway soon after they lose consciousness frequently facilitates air exchange, because the tongue is relatively large and easily obstructs the airway. The majority of these patients do not present the same difficulty with

airway management as children with Pierre Robin, Treacher Collins, or Goldenhar syndromes because the angulation between the base of the tongue and the laryngeal inlet is not so acute; ie, the larynx does not have as much of a posterior location.

Clefting of the lip and palate is another common congenital malformation.[1] Generally, children with isolated clefting anomalies present with fairly normal laryngeal anatomy and do not present difficulty in airway management other than the technical problem of obtaining a good mask fit.[47] When one sees this malformation, seek other abnormalities. These children are more susceptible to ear infections, as well as aspiration pneumonia.

Malformations of the Larynx and Trachea

Laryngomalacia is the most common cause of congenital laryngeal stridor.[48, 49] This is the

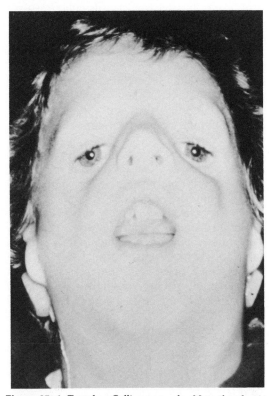

Figure 35–6. Treacher Collins anomaly. Note the classic triangular-shaped facies, small mouth, high-arched palate, mid-facial and mandibular hypoplasia, and external ear deformity. These children should also be evaluated for possible associated congenital heart disease. (Courtesy of Frederick Berry, MD.)

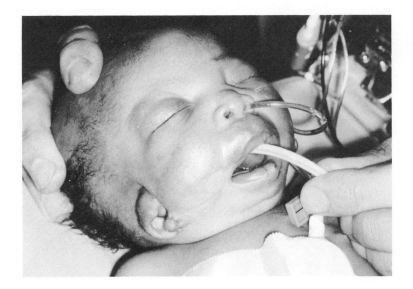

Figure 35–7. Goldenhar's anomaly. Note the marked mid-facial hypoplasia, hypoplastic mandible, and external ear deformity. Fusion of cervical vertebra with the base of the skull may limit flexion and extension.

result of soft laryngeal structures, especially the epiglottis and redundant aryepiglottic folds, allowing collapse of these structures on inspiration, resulting in glottic obstruction. This collapse is exaggerated during crying. The stridor of laryngomalacia usually resolves spontaneously as the child matures during the first 6 to 12 months of life.

Laryngeal webs may present with stridor in the delivery room and occasionally may present with a total obstruction of the airway; in this situation, the infant usually does not survive.[1, 2] Partial webs are compatible with life and require urgent treatment—dilation or tracheostomy.

Congenital subglottic stenosis is a more common abnormality. These children may have stridor at the time of delivery or, more commonly, manifest episodes of "croup" at a very young age. They may unknowingly present for a routine surgical procedure when the anesthesiologist discovers the inability to pass an "appropriate size" endotracheal tube. These patients may present for the first time with postintubation stridor ("postintubation croup") after a routine surgical procedure. This should be a red flag that there is probably an abnormality of the subglottic region.

MANAGEMENT OF CONGENITAL AIRWAY PROBLEMS

After completing a careful history, physical examination, and obtaining appropriate radiologic and laboratory evaluation of the patient, one must decide on a technique that allows the securing of the airway without presenting unnecessary danger to the patient. When formulating an anesthetic plan for patients with congenital airway problems, one must consider the need for a premedication and prophylaxis against acid aspiration syndrome.[34, 50] Although the incidence of pulmonary aspiration of gastric fluid is extremely rare in pediatric patients (10 per 10,000), there is a higher incidence of aspiration in children with difficult airways.[51–53] The most likely reason for an increased incidence of pulmonary aspiration is that mask ventilation prior to placement of the endotracheal tube often results in gaseous distention of the stomach, which then induces vomiting. It is for this reason that children in whom one anticipates a difficult airway might benefit from the full regimen of acid aspiration prophylaxis.[50] Histamine$_2$ blocking agents, metoclopramide, and clear antacids decrease gastric residual volume and increase gastric pH.

The subject of preoperative fasting has recently undergone considerable revision, so that infants 1 to 5 months of age may fast for 4 hours from milk and solids but have clear liquids up until 2 hours prior to anesthesia induction. Infants 6 to 36 months of age may fast from milk and solids for 6 hours and then receive clear liquids up to 3 hours prior to anesthetic induction; children more than 36 months of age may fast from milk and solids for 8 hours but receive clear liquids up to 3 hours prior to anesthetic induction.[54–61] This fasting regimen should be encouraged, because it results in a better hydrated patient compared

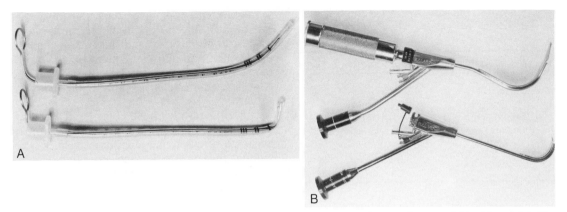

Figure 35–8. *A,* Endotracheal tubes may be inserted with greater assurity when made more rigid with a stylet. The upper endotracheal tube is shaped with the classic "hockey-stick" configuration for patients with a normal airway. The lower endotracheal tube has a 90-degree bend, which is required to allow passage in patients with mid-facial hypoplasia. *B,* The Bullard laryngoscope may be a useful aid to laryngoscopy in patients with mid-facial hypoplasia or cervical spine fracture. Note the 90-degree bend in the optics (similar to the endotracheal tube above), which permits direct visualization of the larynx.

with the traditional longer fasting periods and most likely reduces the incidence of anesthetic-induced hypotension secondary to relative hypovolemia.[50] This may be particularly advantageous for patients with difficult airways because of the need to provide a deep level of anesthesia while preserving spontaneous ventilation, because tracheal intubation is usually performed with inhalational agents only.

The anesthesiologist must have a clear understanding of the airway anatomy so that the "anesthetic game plan" may be appropriately designed; eg, if a child has a large tongue, one can anticipate airway obstruction due to this large tongue very early in the anesthetic induction. Therefore, one might consider applying a topical anesthetic agent to the surface of the tongue and coating the oral airway with local anesthetic paste prior to the induction of anesthesia. This then allows the relatively early insertion of the oral airway without stimulating laryngeal reflexes.

If the child has abnormal airway anatomy that will provide a technical challenge to endotracheal intubation, muscle relaxants are contraindicated because one does not want to lose control of the airway and the breath sounds may be used as a guide to the entrance of the larynx.[13, 14, 62, 63] Thus, one might plan a gaseous induction by mask and minimize the pre-induction use of sedatives or narcotics to provide the optimal ventilatory mechanics. A modified laryngoscope blade capable of delivering oxygen at the tip is most helpful in preventing desaturation in this situation.[64] Typically, the most difficult pediatric airways to

manage are those with mid-facial hypoplasia, such as Goldenhar's syndrome, Pierre Robin syndrome, Treacher Collins syndrome, and children with neck burn contracture or unstable cervical spine. All of these problems will likely prevent normal visualization of laryngeal structures. In these conditions, one may be limited to being able to visualize only the tip of the epiglottis during direct laryngoscopy. The anesthesiologist must therefore be prepared to insert the endotracheal tube either in a "blind" fashion or with the aid of special airway equipment. Our approach is to anesthetize children with anatomic airway problems using halothane in oxygen and avoiding the use of sedatives and narcotics so as to maintain spontaneous ventilation during laryngoscopy and intubation. One shapes the endotracheal tube with a *stylet* so that it has a near 90-degree bend at the tip (usually the distal 1 cm) (Fig. 35–8*A*). Understanding the normal laryngeal anatomy (the epiglottis is always at the *center* of the base of the tongue), one then inserts the laryngoscope blade down the *center* of the tongue, after the child is appropriately (usually deep level) anesthetized. When the tip of the epiglottis is visualized, one can move the larygoscope blade to the right (the traditional location) and sweep the tongue to the left, providing the best visualization of the laryngeal inlet. This avoids possible trauma to the larynx, because the blade is not first passed beyond the larynx into the esophagus and then withdrawn.

When the laryngeal inlet cannot be directly visualized, one can place the tip of the endo-

Table 35–1. INTERNAL DIAMETER (mm ID) OF ENDOTRACHEAL TUBES FOR INFANTS AND CHILDREN

Age	Size (ID)
Premature	
≤1000 g	2.5
>1000 g	3.0
Term to 6 months	3.0
6 months to 1 year	3.5–4.0
1–2 years	4.0–5.0
Older than 2 years	$\dfrac{\text{age (years)} + 16}{4}$

tracheal tube (with stylet) in the midline, just posterior to the epiglottis, and listen for breath sounds. When one hears air exchange coming through the 15-mm connector of the endotracheal tube, one can then pass the endotracheal tube over the stylet into the airway. With this maneuver, successful intubation occurs approximately 50% of the time. If the patient is breathing spontaneously and the endotracheal tube does not advance into the trachea but into the esophagus, this will become evident by the loss of breath sounds and inability to record expired carbon dioxide on the capnograph. At this point, no harm is done, provided that one has not grossly inflated the stomach with anesthetic agent and oxygen. One then simply removes the endotracheal tube, reinserts the oral airway, and deepens the level of anesthesia for the next attempt at intubation. If the stomach becomes distended, it should be decompressed with an orogastric tube prior to the next attempt at laryngoscopy.

AIDS TO PROVIDE DIRECT VISUALIZATION OF THE LARYNX

With many of the difficult anatomic problems, there is a need to visualize the laryngeal inlet around a near 90-degree turn at the base of the tongue. Special aids to laryngoscopy and intubation are directed at making this sharp turn so as to allow successful placement of an endotracheal tube. Hence the design of the Bullard laryngoscope, which has a fixed 90-degree bend and fiberoptics that allow direct visualization of laryngeal structures (Fig. 35–8B).[65] Another aid to intubation is the lighted malleable stylet ("light wand"). The ability to bend the light wand into the desired shape is extremely helpful.[66, 67] The fiberoptic laryngo-scope/bronchoscope is perhaps the most useful, because the tip of the fiberoptic laryngoscope can be directed and then advanced into the trachea; this allows the fiberoptic bronchoscope to function as a stylet over which the endotracheal tube is advanced into the trachea.[68–70]

One must always have considered an alternate plan should acute airway obstruction or an acute airway emergency arise. Before beginning the anesthetic, one must have all the normal monitoring equipment available for the management of such a patient. This includes a variety of endotracheal tubes, oral airways, and stylet and laryngoscope blades. Table 35–1 presents the appropriate-sized endotracheal tubes (internal diameter) for age; Table 35–2 presents the size of laryngoscope blades appropriate to patient age.

One must also have available special airway management equipment, such as a laryngoscope that provides for the delivery of oxygen at the tip of the blade (Oxyscope, Foregger, Langhorne, PA).[64] A fiberoptic laryngoscope/bronchoscope may be particularly helpful, as may a light wand and Bullard laryngoscope. Emergency equipment to perform a cricothyroid puncture to provide oxygen delivery via the cricothyroid membrane to the airway might be helpful should other methods to secure an airway fail.[71] In addition, a surgeon skilled in pediatric tracheostomy must also be immediately available in the room should an airway emergency result. Table 35–3 lists equipment helpful in these circumstances.

After successful endotracheal intubation, anesthesiologists must be concerned with safe extubation at the end of the procedure. Thus, the patient must be fully alert with airway reflexes intact and the stomach suctioned prior to extubation.

The Lighted Stylet

The lighted stylet (light wand) is a malleable stylet with a bright light at its tip.[66, 67] The

Table 35–2. LARYNGOSCOPE BLADES AND SIZES FOR INFANTS AND CHILDREN

Age	Blade Type:	Blade Size Miller	Blade Size Wis-Hippel	Blade Size Macintosh
Premature		0	—	—
Term		0	—	—
Neonate to 2 years		1	1	—
2–6 years		2	1.5	2
6–12 years		2	—	2–3
Older		2–3	—	3

Table 35–3. SUGGESTED EQUIPMENT FOR
THE DIFFICULT AIRWAY

Masks (multiple sizes and shapes)
Oral airways (multiple sizes)
Several laryngoscope handles
Laryngoscope blades (multiple sizes and shapes)
Suction catheters
Two functioning suction systems
Endotracheal tubes (multiple sizes, cuffed and
    uncuffed)
Stylets appropriate for endotracheal tube size
Lubricant
Topical anesthetic spray
Topical anesthetic paste
Pediatric fiberoptic bronchoscope
Light wand
Bullard laryngoscope
Equipment for pediatric tracheostomy
Tracheostomy tubes and connectors
Equipment for Seldinger technique
Equipment for percutaneous cricothyrotomy
5% carbon dioxide source
Doxapram hydrochloride

---

stylet is shaped into a bend resembling the direction an endotracheal tube would take to pass through the laryngeal inlet. The stylet is well lubricated, and an appropriate size endotracheal tube (without the 15-mm connector) is threaded over the stylet. After the patient is adequately anesthetized, the lighted stylet is passed into the mouth, keeping the tip in the midline of the tongue. The tip is advanced into the approximate location of the cricothyroid membrane. One then looks for a very bright point of light on the neck at the cricothyroid membrane, indicating the tip of the light wand is at the laryngeal inlet; if there is no sharp point of light, then the tip of the stylet is either not in the midline or not in the laryngeal inlet. The disadvantage of this technique is that it is not performed under direct vision, so that there is potential for trauma to the larynx and other structures unless one is particularly gentle. Also, the size of the light bulb at the end of the stylet may require the diameter of the endotracheal tube through which it can be passed to be 5.0 mm or larger.[66, 67] This technique is of greatest value in the larger pediatric patient; a fiberoptic light source, rather than a light bulb, may correct this limitation.

The Bullard Laryngoscope

Another useful instrument for managing congenital airway problems is the Bullard laryngoscope.[65] This is a fiberoptic laryngoscope with a built-in, fixed 90-degree bend at the tip (Fig. 35–8B). This configuration allows direct visualization of the laryngeal inlet in congenital airway abnormalities because its shape and fiberoptics allow one to "look" around the base of the tongue. This is particularly helpful in mid-facial hypoplasia syndromes and in patients with unstable cervical spines. The limitation of this technique is that the depth perspective provided is quite different from that usually observed with direct laryngoscopy. Additionally, one is not able to advance the instrument into the laryngeal inlet, as with a fiberoptic bronchoscope. Because the depth perspective is distorted, when one inserts the endotracheal tube, which is also configured with a 90-degree bend (Fig. 35–8A), one may lose sight of the laryngeal inlet; ie, the endotracheal tube obstructs the view. Therefore, this technique can be a "semi-blind" technique. This laryngoscope is made in only two sizes, so that there may be some patients for whom one size is too small, whereas the other is too large. A further limitation is that in patients with a small mouth, there may be a mechanical problem; ie, it is difficult to introduce both the laryngoscope blade and a styletted endotracheal tube simultaneously.

Fiberoptic Laryngoscopy/Bronchoscopy

The principles for performing successful fiberoptic laryngoscopy in the pediatric patient are similar to those for the adult patient and are well described elsewhere in this text. However, there are unique considerations for the pediatric patient.[68–75] The young pediatric patient obviously requires a smaller-sized bronchoscope; in the smaller fiberoptic bronchoscopes, however, there is no suction port. This is unfortunate, because the suction port can be used as a means of delivering oxygen to the spontaneously breathing patient. Delivery of oxygen into the pharynx and larynx is particularly valuable in the small patient who has a very high oxygen consumption and may rapidly desaturate.[76] We have found that using a plastic mask with a hole drilled through it that is large enough to fit both the flexible fiberoptic bronchoscope and the endotracheal tube allows the delivery of oxygen and maintains the depth of anesthesia during prolonged bronchoscopy. A second individual is required to observe heart rate, oxygen saturation, blood pressure, and to hold the mask securely in place while the first individual is performing the laryngoscopy.

Another difference between children and adults is that in the adult patient, the procedure is generally performed under sedation and topical anesthesia of the airway, whereas children frequently require general anesthesia.[77, 78] If laryngoscopy is prolonged, then the child may wake up, develop return of airway reflexes, and become prone to laryngospasm, gagging, and vomiting. The use of topical anesthesia may be helpful even in the presence of general anesthesia. It is critical to have the child adequately anesthetized so as to blunt laryngeal reflexes while not dangerously depressing the cardiovascular system. Therefore, maintaining spontaneous ventilation, having the child well hydrated, and administering atropine (to dry secretions and to maintain heart rate despite moderately deep levels of anesthesia) may be particularly helpful in avoiding some of these problems. Halothane has proved to be the best inhalation agent for the difficult pediatric airway.

One further concern in the child is the propensity toward adenoidal hypertrophy; this may result in nose bleeds or disruption of adenoidal tissue when the fiberoptic bronchoscope or the endotracheal tube is passed. Nevertheless, the nasal route is the easiest, because it maintains the tip of the fiberoptic bronchoscope in the midline, thus lining it up with the laryngeal inlet.

Other Techniques

Transtracheal retrograde passage of a flexible guidewire and the use of doxapram hydrochloride or carbon dioxide added to the inspired gases to increase tidal volume have been successfully used as adjuncts to managing the difficult airway.[77-84] Each of these techniques has associated problems, and the risks must outweigh the benefits. The single most important concept to be recalled is that hypercarbia is very well tolerated provided hypoxemia is avoided.[85] Therefore, whatever problem arises, one must maintain oxygenation, even in the face of inadequate ventilation.

A new method for airway management, the laryngeal mask airway, has recently been introduced.[86-88] This may provide an alternative means for maintaining a clear, unobstructed airway, but must not be a substitute for securing the airway with an endotracheal tube or a tracheostomy should that be required. Trans-

tracheal jet ventilation is an additional technique that has been successfully used.[89-91] However, this technique must be used with caution because of the danger of pneumothorax, pneumomediastinum, and massive subcutaneous emphysema.[92]

SUMMARY

With all special techniques for management of the difficult airway, the ability to insert an endotracheal tube is directly proportional to the experience of the person performing the technique; the patient with a difficult airway is not the patient on whom to learn rarely used techniques. Fiberoptic bronchoscopy techniques, use of the light wand, or the Bullard laryngoscope should first be learned on normal patients.[75] One should develop these skills in patients with normal airway anatomy so that when patients with an abnormal airway present, the anesthesiologist has the skills already developed to allow safe airway management.[93] Selected syndromes with potential airway problems and associated medical conditions have been reviewed. Much rarer syndromes have not been considered in this chapter, and the reader is referred to several excellent reviews for details.[94, 95]

References

1. Ogura JH, Mallen RW. Developmental anatomy of the larynx. In Ballenger JJ (ed). Diseases of the Nose, Throat and Ear. Philadelphia: Lea & Febiger, 1977.
2. O'Rahilly R, Tucker JA. The early development of the larynx in staged human embryos. I: Embryos of the first five weeks (to stage 15). Ann Otol Rhinol Laryngol 82:3–27, 1973.
3. Fink RB, Demarest RJ. Laryngeal Biomechanics. Cambridge, MA: Harvard University Press, 1978.
4. Hobolth N, Buchmann G, Sandberg LE. Congenital choanal atresia. Acta Paediatr Scand 56:286–294, 1967.
5. Eckenhoff JE. Some anatomic considerations of the infant larynx influencing endotracheal anesthesia. Anesthesiology 12:401–410, 1951.
6. Negus VE. The Comparative Anatomy and Physiology of the Larynx. New York: Grune & Stratton, 1949.
7. Wilson TG. Some observations on the anatomy of the infant larynx. Acta Otolaryngol 43:95–99, 1953.
8. Pressman JJ, Kelemen G. Physiology of the larynx. Physiol Rev 35:506–554, 1955.
9. Bosma JF. Introduction. In Bosma JF, Showacre J (eds). Symposium on Development of Upper Respiratory Anatomy and Function: Implications of Sudden Infant Death Syndrome. Washington, DC: U.S. Government Printing Office, 1974; pp. 5–49.
10. Miller MJ, Carlo WA, Strohl KP, Fanaroff AA, Martin

RJ. Effect of maturation on oral breathing in sleeping premature infants. J Pediatr 109:515–519, 1986.

11. Miller MJ, Martin RJ, Carlo WA, Fouke JM, Strohl KP, Fanaroff AA. Oral breathing in newborn infants. J Pediatr 107:465–469, 1985.

12. Wittenborg MH, Gyepes MT, Crocker D. Tracheal dynamics in infants with respiratory distress, stridor, and collapsing trachea. Radiology 88:653–662, 1967.

13. Wilson TG. Stridor in infancy. J Laryngol Otol 66:437–451, 1952.

14. Maze A, Bloch E. Stridor in pediatric patients. Anesthesiology 50:132–145, 1979.

15. Grunebaum M, Adler S, Varsano I. The paradoxical movement of the mediastinum: A diagnostic sign of foreign body aspiration during childhood. Pediatr Radiol 8:213–218, 1979.

16. Wohl MEB, Stigol LC, Mead J. Resistance of the total respiratory system in healthy infants and infants with bronchiolitis. Pediatrics 43:495–509, 1969.

17. Bhutani VK, Rubenstein D, Shaffer TH. Pressure-induced deformation in immature airways. Pediatr Res 15:829–832, 1981.

18. Briscoe WA, DuBois AB. The relationship between airway resistance, airway conductance, and lung volume in subjects of different age and body size. J Clin Invest 37:1279–1285, 1958.

19. Cook CD, Sutherland JM, Segal S, Mead CJ, McIlroy MB, Smith CA. Studies of respiratory physiology in the newborn infant. III: Measurements of mechanics of respiration. J Clin Invest 36:440–448, 1957.

20. Phelan PD, Williams HE. Ventilatory studies in healthy infants. Pediatr Res 3:425–432, 1969.

21. O'Brodorich HM, Haddad GG. The functional basis of respiratory pathology. In Kendig EL Jr (ed). Disorders of the Respiratory Tract in Children, 5th ed. Philadelphia: W. B. Saunders, 1990, pp. 3–46.

22. Thibeault DW, Clutario B, Auld PAM. The oxygen cost of breathing in the premature infant. Pediatrics 37:954–959, 1966.

23. Epstein RA, Hyman AI. Ventilatory requirements of critically ill neonates. Anesthesiology 53:379–384, 1980.

24. Macintosh R, Mushin WW, Epstein HG. Physics for the Anaesthetist, 2nd ed. Oxford: Blackwell Scientific, 1958; pp. 156–191.

25. Keens TG, Bryan AC, Levison H, Ianuzzo CD. Developmental pattern of muscle fiber types in human ventilatory muscles. J Appl Physiol 44:909–913, 1978.

26. Keens TG, Ianuzzo CD. Development of fatigue-resistant fibers in human ventilatory muscles. Am Rev Respir Dis 119:139–141, 1979.

27. Keens TG, Chen V, Patel P, O'Brien P, Levison H, Ianuzzo CD. Cellular adaptations of the ventilatory muscles to a chronic increased respiratory load. J Appl Physiol 44:905–908, 1978.

28. Williams JP, Somerville GM, Miner ME, Reilly D. Atlanto-axial subluxation and trisomy-21: Another perioperative complication. Anesthesiology 67:253–254, 1987.

29. Moore RA, McNichols KW, Warran SP. Atlantoaxial subluxation with symptomatic spinal cord compression in a child with Down's syndrome. Anesth Analg 66:89–90, 1987.

30. Kushner DC, Harris GB. Obstructing lesions of the larynx and trachea in infants and children. Radiol Clin North Am 16:181–194, 1978.

31. Doust BD, Ting YM. Xeroradiography of the larynx. Radiology 110:727–730, 1974.

32. Rosenfield NS, Peck DR, Lowman RM. Xeroradiography in the evaluation of acquired airway abnormalities in children. Am J Dis Child 132:1177–1180, 1978.

33. Slovis TL, Haller JO, Berdon WE, Baker DH, Joseph PM. Noninvasive visualization of the pediatric airway. Curr Probl Diagn Radiol 8:1–67, 1979.

34. Coté CJ. Induction techniques in pediatric anesthesia. Refresher Courses in Anesthesiology ASA 17:43–57, 1989.

35. Clark RW, Schmidt HS, Schuller DE. Sleep induced ventilatory dysfunction in Down's syndrome. Arch Intern Med 140:45–50, 1980.

36. Smith DF, Mihm FG, Flynn M. Chronic alveolar hypoventilation secondary to macroglossia in the Beckwith-Wiedemann syndrome. Pediatrics 70:695–697, 1982.

37. Sjogren P, Pedersen T, Steinmetz H: Mucopolysaccharidoses and anaesthetic risks. Acta Anaesthesiol Scand 31:214–218, 1987.

38. Fletcher MM, Blum SL, Blanchard CL. Pierre Robin syndrome, pathophysiology of obstructive episodes. Laryngoscope 79:547–560, 1969.

39. Hawkins DB, Simpson JV. Micrognathia and glossoptosis in the newborn. Surgical tacking of the tongue in small jaw syndromes. Clin Pediatr 13:1066–1073, 1974.

40. Lewis MB, Pashayan HM. Management of infants with Robin anomaly. Clin Pediatr (Phila) 19:519–521, 525–528; 1981.

41. MacLennan FM, Robertson GS. Ketamine for induction and intubation in Treacher-Collins syndrome. Anaesthesia 36:196–198, 1981.

42. Sklar GS, King BD. Endotracheal intubation and Treacher-Collins syndrome. Anesthesiology 44:247–249, 1976.

43. Scholtes JL, Veyckemans F, VanObbergh L, Verellen G, Gribomont BF. Neonatal anaesthetic management of a patient with Goldenhar's syndrome with hydrocephalus. Anaesth Intensive Care 15:338–340, 1987.

44. Madan R, Trikha A, Venkataraman RK, Batra R, Kalia P. Goldenhar's syndrome: An analysis of anaesthetic management—a retrospective study of seventeen cases. Anaesthesia 45:49–52, 1990.

45. Walts LF, Finerman G, Wyatt GM. Anaesthesia for dwarfs and other patients of pathological small stature. Can Anaesth Soc J 22:703–709, 1975.

46. Pauli RM, Gilbert EF. Upper cervical cord compression as cause of death in osteogenesis imperfecta type II. J Pediatr 108:579–581, 1986.

47. Morgan GAR, Steward DJ. Linear airway dimensions in children: Including those with cleft palate. Can Anaesth Soc J 29:1–8, 1982.

48. Holinger PH, Brown WT. Congenital webs, cysts, laryngocoeles and other anomalies of the larynx. Ann Otol Rhinol Laryngol 76:744–752, 1967.

49. Holinger PH, Johnston KC. Factors responsible for laryngeal obstruction in infants. JAMA 143:1229–1232, 1950.

50. Coté CJ. NPO after midnight for children—a reappraisal. Anesthesiology 72:589–592, 1990.

51. Borland LM, Saitz EW, Woelfel SK. Evaluation of pediatric anesthesia care. Presented at the Section on Anesthesiology, American Academy of Pediatrics, Orlando, FL, March, 1989.

52. Tiret L, Nivoche Y, Hatton F, Desmonts JM, Vourc'h G. Complications related to anaesthesia in infants and children: A prospective survey of 40240 anaesthetics. Br J Anaesth 61:263–269, 1988.

53. Olsson GL, Hallen B, Hambraeus-Jonzon K. Aspiration during anaesthesia: A computer-aided study of 185 358 anaesthetics. Acta Anaesthesiol Scand 30:84–92, 1986.

54. Schreiner MS, Triebwasser A, Keon TP. Oral fluids

compared to preoperative fasting in pediatric outpatients. Anesthesiology 72:593–597, 1990.

55. Sandhar BK, Goresky GV, Maltby JR, Shaffer EA. Effect of oral liquids and ranitidine on gastric fluid volume and pH in children undergoing outpatient surgery. Anesthesiology 71:327–330, 1989.

56. Splinter WM, Stewart JA, Muir JG. The effect of preoperative apple juice on gastric contents, thirst and hunger in children. Can J Anaesth 36:55–58, 1989.

57. Meakin G, Dingwall AE, Addison GM. Effects of fasting and oral premedication on the pH and volume of gastric aspirate in children. Br J Anaesth 59:678–682, 1987.

58. Splinter WM, Schaefer JD, Zunder IH. Clear fluids three hours before surgery do not affect the gastric fluid contents of children. Can J Anaesth 37:498–501, 1990.

59. Crawford M, Lerman J, Christensen S, Farrow-Gillespie A. Effects of duration of fasting on gastric fluid pH and volume in healthy children. Anesth Analg 71:400–403, 1990.

60. Splinter WM, Stewart JA, Muir JG. Large volumes of apple juice preoperatively do not affect gastric pH and volume in children. Can J Anaesth 37:36–39, 1990.

61. Splinter WM, Schaefer JD. Ingestion of clear fluids is safe for adolescents up to 3 H before anaesthesia. Br J Anaesth 66:48–52, 1991.

62. Salem MR, Mathrubhutham M, Bennet EJ. Current concepts: Difficult intubation. N Engl J Med 295:879–881, 1976.

63. Gordon RA. Anesthetic management of patients with airway problems. Int Anesthesiol Clin 10:37–59, 1972.

64. Todres ID, Crone RK. Experience with a modified laryngoscope in sick infants. Crit Care Med 9:544–545, 1981.

65. Borland LM, Casselbrant M. The Bullard laryngoscope: A new indirect oral laryngoscope (pediatric version). Anesth Analg 70:105–108, 1990.

66. Holzman RS, Nargozian CD, Florence FB. Lightwand intubation in children with abnormal upper airways. Anesthesiology 69:784–787, 1988.

67. Ellis DG, Jakymec A, Kaplan RM, Stewart RD, Freeman JA, Bleyaert A, Berkebile PE. Guided orotracheal intubation in the operating room using a lighted stylet: A comparison with direct laryngoscopic technique. Anesthesiology 64:823–826, 1986.

68. Fan LL, Flynn JW. Laryngoscopy in neonates and infants: Experience with the flexible fiberoptic bronchoscope. Laryngoscope 91:451–456, 1981.

69. Taylor PA, Towey RM. The broncho-fiberscope as an aid to endotracheal intubation. Br J Anaesth 44:611–612, 1972.

70. Katz RL, Berci G. The optical stylet—a new intubation technique for adults and children with specific reference to teaching. Anesthesiology 51:251–254, 1979.

71. Coté CJ, Eavey RD, Todres ID, Jones DE. Cricothyroid membrane puncture: Oxygenation and ventilation in a dog model using an intravenous catheter. Crit Care Med 16:615–619, 1988.

72. Wood RE, Sherman JM. Pediatric flexible bronchoscopy. Ann Otol Rhinol Laryngol 89:414–416, 1980.

73. Wood RE, Postma D. Endoscopy of the airway in infants and children. J Pediatr 112:1–6, 1988.

74. Berthelsen P, Prytz S, Jacobsen E. Two-stage fiberoptic nasotracheal intubation in infants: A new approach to difficult pediatric intubation. Anesthesiology 63:457–458, 1985.

75. Ovassapian A, Yelich SJ, Dykes MHM, Golman ME. Learning fibreoptic intubation: Use of simulators v. traditional teaching. Br J Anaesth 61:217–220, 1988.

76. Cross KW, Tizard JPM, Trythall DAH. The gaseous metabolism of the newborn infant. Acta Paediatr 46:265–285, 1957.

77. Gordon RA. Anesthetic management of patients with airway problems. Int Anesthesiol Clin 10:37–59, 1972.

78. Webster AC. Anesthesia for operations on the upper airway. Int Anesthesiol Clin 10:61–122, 1972.

79. Roberts KW. New use for Swan-Ganz introducer wire. Anesth Analg 60:67, 1981.

80. Cooper CMS, Murray-Wilson A. Retrograde intubation: Management of a 4.8-kg, 5-month infant. Anaesthesia 42:1197–1200, 1987.

81. Ledbetter JL, Rasch DK, Pollard TG, Helsel P, Smith RB. Reducing the risks of laryngoscopy in anaesthetized infants. Anaesthesia 43:151–153, 1988.

82. Borland LM, Swan DM, Leff S. Difficult pediatric intubation: A new approach to the retrograde technique. Anesthesiology 55:577–578, 1981.

83. Bourke D, Levesque PR. Modification of retrograde guide for endotracheal intubation. Anesth Analg 53:1013–1014, 1974.

84. Davies JAH. Blind nasal intubation using doxapram hydrochloride. Br J Anaesth 40:361–364, 1968.

85. Goldstein B, Shannon DC, Todres ID. Supercarbia in children: Clinical course and outcome. Crit Care Med 18:166–168, 1990.

86. Brain AIJ. The laryngeal mask—a new concept in airway management. Br J Anaesth 55:801–805, 1983.

87. Brain AIJ. Three cases of difficult intubation overcome by the laryngeal mask airway. Anaesthesia 40:353–355, 1985.

88. Grebenik CR, Ferguson C, White A. The laryngeal mask airway in pediatric radiotherapy. Anesthesiology 72:474–477, 1990.

89. Ravussin P, Bayer-Berger M, Monnier P, Savary M, Freeman J. Percutaneous transtracheal ventilation for laser endoscopic procedures in infants and small children with laryngeal obstruction: Report of two cases. Can J Anaesth 34:83–86, 1987.

90. Bedger RC Jr, Chang J-L. A jet-stylet endotracheal catheter for difficult airway management. Anesthesiology 66:221–223, 1987.

91. Schur MS, Maccioli GA, Azizkhan RG, Wood RE. High-frequency jet ventilation in the management of congenital tracheal stenosis. Anesthesiology 69:952–955, 1988.

92. Steward DJ. Percutaneous transtracheal ventilation for laser endoscopic procedures in infants and small children. Can J Anaesth 34:429–430, 1987.

93. Badgwell JM, McLeod ME, Friedberg J. Airway obstruction in infants and children. Can J Anaesth 34:90–98, 1987.

94. Smith DW. Recognizable Patterns of Human Malformation, 2nd ed. Philadelphia: W. B. Saunders, 1976.

95. Jones AEP, Pelton DA. An index of syndromes and their anesthetic implications. Can Anaesth Soc J 23:207–266, 1976.

CHAPTER 36

Critical Upper Airway Obstruction in Children

I. David Todres, M.D., and Praveen Khilnani, M.D.

Acute upper airway obstruction is a potentially life-threatening condition in the infant or child. The progression of airway obstruction may be rapid, therefore requiring astute recognition and anticipation of the problem. A basic knowledge of the embryologic development, anatomy, and physiology of the upper and lower airways is important to understand the pathology and management of airway obstruction.

DEVELOPMENTAL ANATOMY

The respiratory tract develops from the ventral surface of the foregut in the early embryonic period. A definable larynx is seen at 6 weeks of gestation, and by the 10th and 11th weeks of gestation, the major structures of the larynx have developed.[1, 2] Failure of the true cords to separate appropriately to form the primitive glottis results in a complete or partial laryngeal web. By 26 weeks of gestation, the larynx develops the important function of protecting the lower airway and phonation. Protection of the lower airway occurs through neurally controlled closure of the glottis during swallowing. Development of receptors that respond to irritant stimuli by inducing laryngo-spasm also takes place by 26 weeks of gestation.

In the trachea and major bronchi, C-shaped rings of cartilage support the airway structure. Cartilage is present in airways as small as 1 to 2 mm in diameter.[1] It maintains airway patency despite large changes in intrathoracic pressure with the phases of respiration.

Developmentally, there are several anatomic differences between the airway of the child and that of the adult. Infants have a cephalad larynx (C3–4, compared with adult larynx, C5–6) and a large epiglottis that constantly touches the soft palate, thereby preventing mouth breathing. By 4 to 5 months of age, as the larynx descends down, the epiglottis no longer touches the soft palate, thereby allowing mouth breathing.

The child's tongue is relatively large for the smaller oral cavity due to buccal fat pads and receded mandible. Increase in size of the tongue (eg, hemangioma, Down syndrome, Beckwith-Wiedemann syndrome) or markedly receded mandible (Pierre Robin, Treacher Collins syndromes) readily leads to airway obstruction.

In the child, the attachment of the vocal cords is lower at its anterior attachment than posteriorly (in the adult, the vocal cords are

383

on a horizontal plane) occasionally making endotracheal intubation more difficult in the child as a result of the tube being held up at the anterior commissures of the vocal folds.

The area within the cricoid cartilage, or subglottic region, is the narrowest part of the child's upper airway (Fig. 36–1), as opposed to the rima glottidis in the adult (Fig. 36–2). The relatively narrow subglottic area is predisposed to edema from croup or following endotracheal intubation or bronchoscopy. Swelling in this area in the child may cause stridor and respiratory distress. An equivalent amount of swelling in the adult would have minimal effects due to much larger diameter, resistance to flow being inversely proportional to the radius of the lumen of the airway.

Histologically, the mucosa of the mouth is continuous with that of the larynx and trachea. The mucosa is covered with squamous and pseudostratified ciliated epithelium and is tightly adherent to the vocal cords and tracheal surface of the epiglottis, but loosely adherent elsewhere. Inflammatory changes above the vocal cords are limited by the barrier formed by the tightly adherent mucosa at the vocal cords. Thus, supraglottitis (epiglottitis) is usually limited to the supraglottic area. Similarly, inflammation in the subglottic region leads to subglottic edema in the loosely adherent mucosa below the vocal cords, but does not usually spread above the level of the vocal cords.

PHYSIOLOGY

In the neonate, the nasal passages account for 25% of the total resistance to airflow, compared with 60% in the adult. The lower airway contributes the majority of airway resistance due to relatively small size of the airways and lack of supportive structures. Because of relatively soft cartilaginous support, the larynx, trachea, and bronchi in the infant are considerably more compliant than in the adult. Various distending and compressive forces have a significant effect on airway caliber. The *extra*thoracic trachea is subject to different stresses than the *intra*thoracic trachea. With normal inspiration, the negative pressure developed within the chest is transmitted to the large airways, including the intrathoracic trachea, tending to cause dilation. However, at the thoracic inlet, dynamic com-

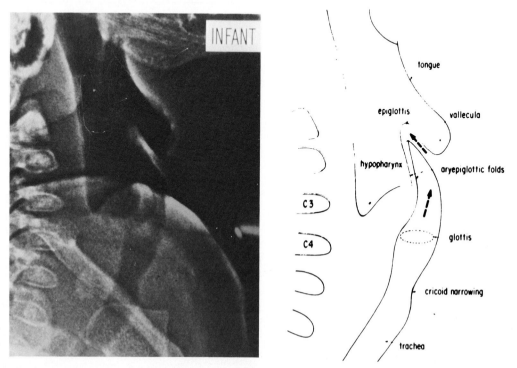

Figure 36–1. Note the narrow cricoid cartilage in the child, creating a funnel-shaped larynx. (From Coté CJ, Ryan JF, Todres ID, Goudsouzian NG (eds). A practice of anesthesia in infants and children, 2nd ed. Philadelphia: W.B. Saunders, 1993, p. 61; with permission.)

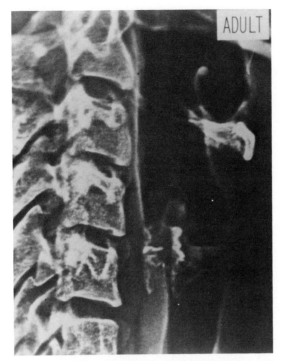
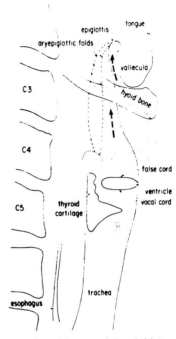

Figure 36–2. Note the adult larynx is cylindrical compared with the funnel-shaped larynx of the child (see Fig. 36–1). (From Coté CJ, Ryan JF, Todres ID, Goudsouzian NG (eds). A practice of anesthesia in infants and children, 2nd ed. Philadelphia: W.B. Saunders, 1993, p. 60; with permission.)

pression occurs as a result of the pressure differential between atmospheric pressure and the negative pressure within the *extra*thoracic trachea. With normal inspiration, this compression is relatively slight and patency of the airway is not compromised (Fig. 36–3*A*). Normal expiration is a passive process, driven by the elastic recoil of the lung. Transmural pressures are positive along the entire tracheobronchial tree. There are no significant changes in airway caliber. With obstruction of the extrathoracic airway (eg, laryngotracheobronchitis, supraglottitis, foreign body), inspiratory effort leads to increased negative pressure within the chest and airway. This leads to a greater difference between ambient pressure and the negative pressure within the extrathoracic trachea. As a result, significant dynamic inspiratory collapse of the extrathoracic trachea occurs, particularly at the thoracic inlet. Intrathoracic airway caliber is only minimally affected because inspiratory pressures within the airways and pleural pressure fall to a similar extent (Fig. 36–3*B*). Obstructed expiration is illustrated in Figure 36–3*C* and *D*.

The phenomenon of dynamic collapse of the airway has particular relevance in treating acute airway obstruction. Marked transmural pressure changes occur when the infant is agitated and crying. Thus, efforts to relieve anxiety and crying are crucial in minimizing dynamic collapse of the airway. In addition, applying continuous positive pressure via a face mask and adjustable pop-off valve in the severely obstructed child counteracts dynamic collapses of the airway and facilitates gas exchange.

HISTORY AND PHYSICAL EXAMINATION

In evaluating a child with airway obstruction, a history of the illness should not be overlooked. Careful recounting of the onset may suggest foreign body aspiration. Some illnesses progress more slowly (eg, laryngotracheobronchitis), as opposed to a more sudden and acute onset in a sicker child (eg, supraglottitis). The time of onset of the illness may suggest a congenital abnormality; that is, symptoms starting at birth or shortly after. An

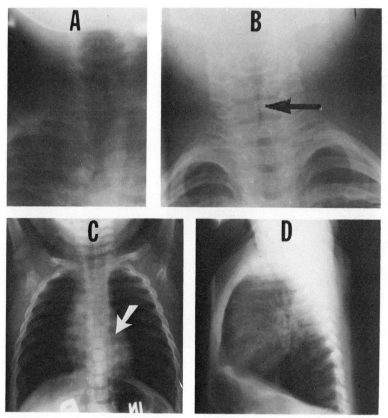

Figure 36–3. Roentgenograms of the upper and lower airways of the child. *A* illustrates the normal upper airway anatomy. Note buckling of the trachea, which is normally seen on expiration. *B* illustrates dynamic collapse of the upper airway *(arrow)* due to subglottic narrowing associated with croup. *C* illustrates dynamic collapse of the lower airway *(arrow)* due to bronchiolar obstruction associated with asthma. Note the hyperinflated chest and flattened diaphragm *(D)*. (Courtesy of Susan Connelly, M.D.)

infant presenting with "inspiratory stridor" at 1 month of age should not be diagnosed as croup; an alternate diagnosis (eg, subglottic hemangioma) or another condition must be considered.

An initial physical examination involves observing the child to assess how severe the airway obstruction is and whether immediate therapeutic intervention is necessary. Listening to the child provides clues to the approximate location of the obstruction. Inspiratory stridor is characteristic of upper airway obstruction (eg, croup, supraglottitis, vocal cord paralysis), whereas expiratory stridor has its origin in obstruction of the distal respiratory tract (foreign body, compression from a vascular ring).[3, 4] In severe situations, a to-and-fro stridor may exist.

Signs of acute distress are reflected by an increased respiratory rate, nasal flaring, retrac-

tions (suprasternal, sternal, intercostal, and subcostal), and cyanosis when breathing air. Cyanosis reflects severe hypoxemia. The child may be leaning forward with an open mouth and drooling (eg, supraglottitis). Drooling of secretions can occur because of an inability to swallow secretions. Dysphagia occurs with supraglottitis and esophageal foreign bodies. The agitated child is one who is hypoxemic. In a critical situation, aggressive therapy (eg, intubation) to secure a safe and adequate airway may be necessary.

In suspected cases of supraglottitis, direct examination of the throat is best avoided, because attempts at visualizing the pharynx with a tongue blade may precipitate acute airway obstruction. Pulse oximetry is a good, noninvasive measure of oxygen saturation in a child with stridor. Transcutaneous CO_2 monitoring has been shown to correlate with in-

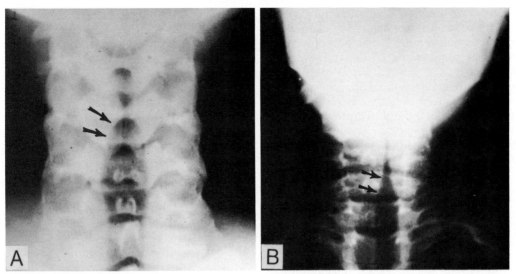

Figure 36–4. Roentgenogram (anteroposterior view) of the upper airway of the child. *A*, Normal; *B*, laryngotracheo-bronchitis—note the "tapered" subglottic area (steeple sign). (From Coté CJ, Ryan JF, Todres ID, Goudsouzian NG (eds). A practice of anesthesia in infants and children, 2nd ed. Philadelphia: W. B. Saunders, 1993, p. 254; with permission.)

creasing upper airway obstruction in laryngo-tracheobronchitis.[5]

SPECIAL INVESTIGATIONS

Roentgenograms

The need for radiographic studies must be carefully evaluated, because the manipulations

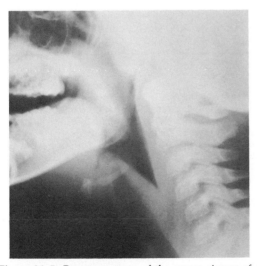

Figure 36–5. Roentgenogram of the upper airway of a child (lateral view) shows edema of the epiglottis and aryepiglottic folds. (From Coté CJ, Ryan JF, Todres ID, Goudsouzian NG (eds). A practice of anesthesia in infants and children. Philadelphia: W. B. Saunders, 1993, p. 252; with permission.)

of the procedure must not increase the risk of further airway obstruction. Anteroposterior and lateral views of the entire airway should be obtained. The procedure should be performed with the child in the upright position, because this is usually the most comfortable for the patient. Placing a child with supraglottitis in the supine position may precipitate acute and dangerous airway obstruction. On anteroposterior view of airway, subglottic narrowing is usually apparent in laryngotracheobronchitis (Fig. 36–4). Severe upper airway obstruction is associated with distention of the hypopharynx. Lateral view of airway may show a swollen epiglottis as the outline of the posterior part of the tongue is followed inferiorly to the level of the epiglottis (thumb sign) (Fig. 36–5). If epiglottitis is clinically suspected, a normal lateral view of the airway may not be enough to rule it out. A direct visualization in the operating room under general anesthesia is therefore necessary based on clinical suspicion alone.

Chest roentgenogram may also reveal the presence of acute pulmonary edema, seen occasionally with severe upper airway obstruction.[6–8] Pulmonary edema may manifest immediately following relief of airway obstruction with, for example, tracheal intubation. In long-standing upper airway obstruction, hypoxemia and pulmonary hypertension lead to cardiac failure, and evidence of this may be seen on radiographs. Fluoroscopy and computed tomography (CT) may be helpful when standard radiographs are unsatisfactory in defining the site and extent of airway obstruction. A barium swallow may be a helpful procedure in defining compression of the trachea by a vascular ring, eg, double aortic arch. It is important to keep in mind that stridor is a symptom produced by upper airway obstruction. A cause for stridor therefore must be looked for even if radiologic studies, including airway fluoroscopy and CT scan, of the airway are negative.

Endoscopy

Direct examination of the airway by laryngoscopy and bronchoscopy is necessary for making a diagnosis of the site of the obstruction, its extent, and the cause.[9] Flexible fiberoptic bronchoscopy is now being routinely used for evaluation of stridor in children. Instruments have been designed that have an outer diameter of 3.5 mm and a 1.2-mm suction channel. An ultrathin fiberoptic bronchoscope with an outer diameter of 2.2 mm is now available for airway evaluation of premature and younger infants. In the hands of the experienced physician, it is a safe and effective instrument for exploring the pediatric airway.[9-11] Performed under sedation and local anesthesia, it carries less risk than rigid bronchoscopy under general anesthesia. It is particularly advantageous in evaluating the cause of stridor, because there is less distortion of the child's airway anatomy; also, dynamic airway collapse during respiration is better appreciated than would be the case if the child was under general anesthesia. When rigid bronchoscopy is performed, the procedure must be carried out under appropriate conditions with skilled surgeons and anesthesiologists. The rigid Storz bronchoscope and Hopkins rod-lens systems are excellent devices for removal of a foreign body from the airway when compared with fiberoptic bronchoscopes. Passage of a fiberoptic bronchoscope through the rigid bronchoscope may be used to visualize smaller airways difficult to reach via rigid bronchoscopy. Airway obstruction may also be caused by a foreign body in the esophagus that compresses the trachea and requires esophagoscopy for its removal.

Physiologic Studies

Physiologic studies of airway resistance by measuring inspiratory and expiratory airflow produces flow–volume loops. These are sensitive indicators of airway obstruction when traditional clinical methods are unable to detect an obstruction. They may be diagnostic in identifying the site of obstruction.

SPECIFIC DISEASES

Various causes of upper airway obstruction in neonates and older children are listed in Table 36–1. The majority of conditions with stridor as a presenting symptom are due to causes at the level of larynx and above. Ten percent of all children presenting with stridor have an underlying cause below the level of the larynx. In neonates, the most common cause of stridor is laryngomalacia, followed by vocal cord paresis/paralysis as the second most common cause. Selected conditions that have airway obstruction as their primary pathology are reviewed in detail.

Supraglottitis (Epiglottitis)

Supraglottitis (epiglottitis) is a life-threatening infection that occurs predominantly in children between the ages of 9 months and 7 years, but may occasionally affect adolescents and adults.[12]

The acute inflammation involves the epiglottis and aryepiglottic folds, producing a su-

Table 36–1. CAUSES OF UPPER AIRWAY OBSTRUCTION

Neonate and Infant	Child
Laryngomalacia	Laryngotracheobronchitis
Vocal cord paralysis	Supraglottitis (epiglottitis)
Malformation of laryngeal cartilages	Bacterial tracheitis
Subglottic hemangioma	Acute tonsillitis
Laryngeal web	Diphtheria
Vascular ring	Retropharyngeal abscess
Neonatal tetany	Peritonsillar abscess
Cervical spine abnormality	Glossitis
Macroglossia	Ludwig's angina
Down syndrome	Subglottic edema
Beckwith-Wiedemann syndrome	Airway trauma
	Airway burns
Traumatic laryngeal edema	Laryngeal stenosis
Choanal atresia	Adenoid hypertrophy
Craniofacial deformities	Mediastinal tumors
Nasal encephalocele	Airway tumors
Cystic hygroma	Foreign body, airway and esophagus
Tracheoesophageal fistula	Vascular ring
	Tracheobronchomalacia

praglottitis. The infection may start within the aryepiglottic folds and cause obstruction before involving the epiglottis. The organism responsible is usually *Haemophilus influenzae* type B.[13]

Clinical Presentation

The child has high fever, drooling, with a preferred position of sitting with the head pushed forward to have a less obstructed airway. Inspiratory stridor is not as striking as that seen in laryngotracheobronchitis; it is softer and lower pitched. The voice and cry are muffled. Rapid and unpredictable progression of the disease may cause total acute airway obstruction.[14] It is this feature of the disease that makes this condition one that requires urgent evaluation and treatment.

Differential Diagnosis

Supraglottitis should be differentiated from other significant life-threatening causes of upper airway obstruction. Usually, the differentiation from laryngotracheobronchitis (croup) is fairly clear. However, it may be more difficult to differentiate from bacterial tracheitis (usually due to *Staphylococcus aureus*), in which inflammatory changes and thick, inspissated, mucopurulent secretions may cause life-threatening airway obstruction.[15, 16]

Foreign body aspiration should always be considered in any acute upper airway obstruction. The history, clinical examination, and radiographic findings provide clues to this diagnosis. A retropharyngeal abscess may present with acute upper airway obstruction. Occasionally, acute tonsillitis in severely hypertrophied tonsils may cause acute upper airway obstruction. Diphtheria, a rare but important bacterial infection occurring in the nonimmunized child, may be responsible for acute upper airway obstruction.

Management

A well-organized protocol is necessary for the management of the child with supraglottitis. Acute and total obstruction may be precipitated by crying and agitation in the child. The child should be allowed to assume the position of comfort and not be separated from the parent if being held in a comfortable position. Throat examination, arterial puncture for blood gas analysis, and placement of an intravenous line should be deferred until control of

the airway has been secured by placement of an endotracheal tube[17] or tracheostomy.[18] The unpredictable progression of this disease and the significant risks of morbidity and mortality make placement of an artificial airway the safest course. The choice of artificial airway, endotracheal tube or tracheostomy, depends on the experience of the physician and the site where this procedure is performed. In most intensive care settings today, the choice is endotracheal intubation.

Radiography of the upper airway may be helpful in making the diagnosis of supraglottitis (Fig. 36–5), and in differentiating it from laryngotracheobronchitis (Fig. 36–4) or a radiopaque foreign body. However, if the child is in acute distress, radiographic procedures may delay life-saving intervention. An appropriate management plan consists of transferring the child from the emergency room to the operating room where, under controlled conditions, general anesthesia is administered for placement of the endotracheal tube with a surgeon (pediatric surgeon or otolaryngologist) ready to perform an emergency tracheostomy should attempts at endotracheal intubation fail. In the procedure of tracheal intubation, prevention of hypoxemia and cardiovascular collapse is critical. Oxygen insufflation with laryngoscopy using a modified laryngoscope (Oxyscope) may be helpful.[19] Other centers perform endotracheal intubation in the pediatric intensive care unit (PICU). In skilled hands, the endotracheal tube may be placed nasotracheally with the aid of a flexible fiberoptic bronchoscope. Cultures of the blood and supraglottic structures are obtained once the artificial airway has been secured. Antibiotics (ampicillin and chloramphenicol or third-generation cephalosporins) are administered and are given for 10 days once organism sensitivity has been identified.

On occasion, it may not be possible to establish an artificial airway either with an endotracheal tube or tracheostomy to ventilate the child. In this desperate situation, percutaneous cricothyroid membrane puncture and oxygen insufflation may be life saving.[20, 21] Note, however, that the cricothyroid membrane is extremely small in the infant and that the procedure is more difficult to accomplish than in the adult. However, on rare occasions, one may have no choice. In most cases, endotracheal intubation can be successfully performed, and tracheostomy is rarely necessary. After endotracheal intubation is performed, the patient is transferred to the PICU. Extubation can usually be accomplished in 24 to 36 hours when the inflammation subsides, causing a leak around the endotracheal tube. Direct laryngoscopy may also be performed to visualize the epiglottis in order to make a decision to extubate.

Occasionally, pulmonary edema may be seen with supraglottitis, as with other severe forms of acute upper airway obstruction. Metastatic complications of the *H. influenzae* infection are serious and must be suspected when toxicity and fever do not resolve and when new symptoms appear. Metastatic infections lead to pneumonia, meningitis, pericarditis, and periarticular abscess.[22-26]

Prophylactic rifampin is administered to intimate contacts and to siblings under 8 years of age in order to abolish the nasopharyngeal carrier state and to minimize the risk of spreading the invasive *H. influenzae* disease.

Laryngotracheobronchitis

Laryngotracheobronchitis (croup) is a very common cause of acute upper airway obstruction in children from 6 months to 5 years of age. The parainfluenza virus group appears to cause the majority of cases. Influenza, adenovirus, and respiratory syncytial virus have also been incriminated in some cases. Inflammation and edema of the subglottic region cause an increase in resistance to breathing. The effect of narrowing the child's relatively small airway causes a disproportionate increase in airway resistance compared with the older child and adult. Laminar flow resistance at a given flow rate increases with the fourth power of the reduction in radius of the tube. This is described by the Hagen-Poiseuille equation

$$Q = \frac{Pr^4}{8ln}$$

where Q = flow, P = pressure drop across the tube, r = radius, l = length, and *n* = viscosity of gas.

Clinical Presentation

The onset of laryngotracheobronchitis is insidious, with a history of upper respiratory infection characterized by a "barking cough" that is followed by inspiratory stridor. Low-grade fever is common. The child is tachypneic with chest retractions. With progression of the disease, the child may develop cyanosis. This indicates severe hypoxemia due to ventilation–perfusion mismatching.[27] Increasing tachyp-

nea, tachycardia, increasingly more severe sternal and chest retractions, and deepening cyanosis may occur and signal life-threatening airway obstruction. Croup score has been used to objectively assess the severity of upper airway obstruction based on presence of inspiratory stridor, severity of retractions, air entry, cyanosis, and level of consciousness.[28] The score may be affected by interobserver variability.

Roentgenograms of the upper airway (particularly the anteroposterior view) that show subglottic narrowing may be helpful when the history and examination are atypical.

The differential diagnosis must consider other causes of a severe acute upper airway obstruction; namely, supraglottitis, bacterial tracheitis, a foreign body, subglottic hemangioma, and diphtheria.

Management

In the majority of cases, management includes allaying patient and family anxiety and providing oxygen therapy to treat hypoxemia. Humidified air therapy is widely used but lacks support in the scientific literature.[29] Antibiotics have no role in treatment of croup.

Inhalation of racemic epinephrine (0.5 mL in 3 mL saline) may benefit the child on a short-term basis. This form of treatment probably does not affect the duration or ultimate severity of the child's illness. The treatments may need to be repeated every 1 to 3 hours. Rebound airway swelling may result 45 minutes to 1 hour after racemic epinephrine treatment; therefore, close observation of the patient for airway obstruction and cardiovascular symptoms is necessary.[28, 30, 31]

There has been recent interest in the use of steroids for laryngotracheobronchitis.[32, 33] In one prospective randomized study, single-dose dexamethasone 0.6 mg/kg was used.[32] Overall, severity of moderate to severe acute laryngotracheitis was found to be decreased, requiring racemic epinephrine less frequently compared with control group; however, oxygen saturation, respiratory rates, and duration of hospitalization were no different. The role of corticosteroids in preventing the need for intubation in severe croup at present is at best controversial.

Increasing distress in the child, manifested by progressive tachycardia, tachypnea, stridor, and cyanosis, warrants more active measures to relieve potential life-threatening airway obstruction. With increasing airway obstruction and fatigue, the child may not generate vigorous respiratory efforts and therefore stridor may diminish. This may erroneously be interpreted as improvement in the child's condition. Depression of the level of consciousness and decreased muscle tone are important clinical signs of critical deterioration. Decision to perform endotracheal intubation is therefore based on clinical assessment that reveals worsening airway obstruction. Skilled personnel are essential when performing this maneuver. In some situations, progressive respiratory distress is compounded by the presence of thick, inspissated secretions that the child is unable to cough up. Tracheal intubation provides a means for suctioning the airway and maintaining patency. The endotracheal tube should have a 0.5-mm to 1.0-mm internal diameter, smaller than would normally be used, in order to avoid ischemic necrosis in the subglottic area with potential subsequent stenosis. Nasotracheal intubation has been extensively used.[34] Based on our experience, when required, endotracheal intubation via the oral route can be used as successfully as nasotracheal intubation, and tracheostomy is rarely necessary.

Extubation is carried out in the PICU after 3 to 5 days, or earlier if an air leak develops around the endotracheal tube.[35]

The use of helium–oxygen mixtures in the management of acute upper airway obstruction due to croup was practiced many years ago. There has been a recent renewal of interest in this method of treatment.[36, 37] Although endotracheal intubation or tracheostomy remains the definitive treatment for life-threatening airway obstruction, this technique may be helpful in guiding the child through a crisis so that definitive therapy may be carried out under more optimally controlled conditions. A limitation of this technique to be kept in mind is that the fractional concentration of oxygen in "heliox" is only 30% to 40%, therefore limiting its use in severely hypoxemic conditions requiring higher FIO_2.

Bacterial Tracheitis

Bacterial tracheitis is also referred to as pseudomembranous croup and membranous croup.[16, 38–41] It is considered a primary infection that is most commonly due to *S. aureus*. Occasionally, *H. influenzae*, streptococcus, and *Branhamella catarrhalis* have been identified. Severe subglottic edema with tracheal mucosal sloughing occurs. This is associated with copious mucopurulent secretions and inadequate mucociliary clearance, and may rapidly lead to serious and potentially life-threatening airway obstruction.

Clinical Presentation

The disease affects infants and children until early adolescence. It usually starts with an upper respiratory infection that rapidly progresses over hours with the child becoming acutely toxic and severely distressed. High fever, hoarseness, stridor, and cough are prominent, and airway obstruction may lead to hypoxemia and death. The child may have pulmonary infiltrates on chest roentgenogram and becomes rapidly exhausted and unable to clear the airway. Establishment of an artificial airway by tracheal intubation is usually necessary. Bronchoscopy may be helpful in clarifying the diagnosis and clearing the airway of sloughing debris. Intensive airway care is essential in order to prevent obstruction of the child's own airway, as well as obstruction of the endotracheal tube. A combination of intravenous nafcillin and a third-generation cephalosporin is usually adequate. Bacterial tracheitis should be considered in the differential diagnosis if the child does not respond to conventional therapy for croup.

Foreign Bodies

Foreign body aspiration may cause acute, life-threatening airway obstruction or, if initially undetected, may result in severe lung damage.[42–46] Children in the first 2 to 3 years of life are particularly prone to aspirating a wide array of foreign objects. Eighty percent of cases occur under 4 years of age, and aspiration occurs twice as commonly in males. Sixty-five percent of food asphyxial deaths occurred in infants younger than 2 years of age.[47]

Peanuts, hot dogs, candy, and grapes are among the most common offenders. Most lodge in a main or stem bronchus; the right bronchus is obstructed more often than the left. Sharp foreign bodies include plastic, egg shells, and pins; they can impact in the larynx and produce symptoms of acute laryngeal edema. One should also suspect that a foreign body aspiration may involve multiple foreign bodies. Foreign bodies are also subject to movement from their original position. Foreign body aspiration of a balloon has been reported in a 3-month-old infant.[48] Therefore, foreign body aspiration must be considered in all cases of sudden respiratory distress, regardless of age.

Clinical Presentation

In two thirds of children, the diagnosis is made within the first few days. In a significant number, however, there are no symptoms. Thus, the clinical picture is modified by the interval that has elapsed from the time of foreign body aspiration. There may be a history of violent coughing, gagging, and severe respiratory distress with cyanosis. Wheezing may be present. However, the diagnostic triad of wheezing, coughing, and decreased breath sounds over the affected side are more commonly encountered in the late diagnosed case. The diagnostic triad is incomplete in 61% of aspirating patients.[49] Cough and wheezing may persist without respiratory distress. These patients frequently may be diagnosed as having chronic asthma.

Chest roentgenograms and fluoroscopy are important diagnostic procedures. It should be appreciated that the majority of aspirated foreign bodies are *not* radiopaque. Atelectasis or obstructive emphysema may be seen on the obstructed side. Hyperinflation may be enhanced by forced expiration. In some situations, the movement of the foreign body and its breaking up into fragments may produce atelectasis followed by hyperinflation.

Recurrent, persistent localized pneumonitis that does not respond to standard medical therapy requires investigation for an underlying foreign body. More than half of the patients with aspirated foreign bodies are diagnosed late, even when there is evidence of significant airway obstruction from the history of choking.

Foreign bodies impacting in the esophagus, especially at sites of anatomic constriction (namely, the postcricoid region and at the level of the aortic arch), may produce compression of the trachea and serious airway obstruction.

Management

The physician should be familiar with emergency measures to dislodge a foreign body that is producing a life-threatening crisis.[50] Debate continues over the various maneuvers. The Academy of Pediatrics (Section of Accident and Poison Prevention) recommends back blows followed by abdominal thrusts. Back blows have been blamed by some investigators for causing further distal impaction of the foreign body. Abdominal thrusts (Heimlich maneuver) have been known to be effective. In infants, liver trauma is possible with abdominal thrusts; hence, chest thrusts are recommended. Blind finger sweeps to remove the foreign body from the pharynx are not recommended.

The Storz pediatric bronchoscope with the Hopkins rod lens telescope provides excellent visualization of the foreign body and allows introduction of a forceps to remove the foreign body.[51-54]

On occasion, a Fogarty embolectomy balloon catheter has been used to dislodge an impacted foreign body.[55] The catheter is pulled back together with the bronchoscope to the pharynx, from which the foreign body is removed. Rarely, the foreign body, if deeply lodged in the bronchus, may have to be removed via a thoracotomy and bronchotomy. Extraction may be difficult with foreign bodies that tend to crumble; eg, peanuts.

Following removal of the foreign body, the child may still have symptoms due to the presence of residual foreign bodies. Flexible fiberoptic bronchoscopy appears to be a useful technique in this situation to screen for residual foreign body fragments.[56]

Following a difficult removal of a foreign body, the child may have residual glottic and airway edema and may require steroid therapy and racemic epinephrine inhalations. The value of steroids, although frequently advocated, remains uncertain.

Tracheal Stenosis

Tracheal stenosis in infants and children may be congenital or acquired.[57]

Congenital Tracheal Stenosis

Congenital tracheal stenosis is a rare, life-threatening condition.[58] Pathologically, the luminal narrowing is due to the presence of complete tracheal rings, as opposed to C-shaped cartilaginous rings. In 50% of cases, congenital tracheal stenosis is associated with pulmonary artery sling, where compression and narrowing of the posterior tracheal wall is due to the anomalous origin of the left pulmonary artery from the right pulmonary artery. The anomalous left pulmonary artery passes behind the trachea to supply the left lung. Surgical correction of the vascular anomaly leaves the child with tracheal stenosis because of the underlying tracheal defect. In other vascular anomalies, compression of the trachea may also occur; eg, double aortic arch. Here, correction of the vascular anomaly largely improves the airway problem. However, this is variable and some infants continue to have respiratory difficulty for prolonged periods. In some cases, the ligamentum arteriosum is responsible for the compression and remains unsuspected because it cannot be visualized on an angiogram. Innominate artery compression of the trachea may be severe enough in some children to cause significant narrowing of the airway lumen. Aortopexy in this situation relieves the airway occlusion.

Acquired Tracheal Stenosis

Acquired tracheal stenosis occurs in a number of different circumstances:[59] (1) postintubation (endotracheal tube or tracheostomy), (2) post-trauma, (3) thermal and chemical burns, and (4) primary tumors (rare). Tracheal stenosis is relatively uncommon in neonates, being more frequently encountered in older children. Tracheal pressure necrosis from the endotracheal or tracheostomy tube leads to mucosal injury, the formation of granulation tissue, perichondritis and, finally, scar formation with stricture. Symptoms of obstruction are delayed following the removal of the tube.

Clinical Presentation

Congenital tracheal stenosis must be considered in any infant who has episodes of stridor, cyanosis, wheezing, recurrent pneumonias, or sudden respiratory arrest. Symptoms may appear at birth or shortly thereafter as the stenosed airway becomes inadequate for the growing child's greater ventilatory needs. Following upper respiratory infection, mucus plugs and inflammatory reaction may acutely precipitate respiratory failure. Respiratory distress, stridor, and retractions increase with agitation and crying in the child as a result of dynamic collapse of the airway associated with increased respiratory efforts. Airway obstruction is aggravated by the inability to clear mucus.

Depending on the site of tracheal obstruction, wheezing may be heard and may be misdiagnosed as "allergic asthma." Thus, a thorough history is necessary and a suspicion of this complication should exist if there is a history of recent tracheal intubation or tracheostomy and, particularly, if a diagnosis of asthma has been made that has not responded to standard therapeutic maneuvers. Examination of the child should include a search for other anatomic anomalies, especially vascular ones. This includes barium swallow, echocardiography and, in selected cases, angiography.

Roentgenograms of the anteroposterior and lateral cervical and chest views provide visualization of the location and extent of the tracheal pathology. Airway fluoroscopy demonstrates the dynamic movements of the airway with respiration and any associated degree of tracheomalacia. Tracheobronchography is potentially dangerous because of possible reaction to the contrast material, causing further obstruction of the airway. CT scans can delineate tracheal dimensions, the extent of the stenosis, and also mediastinal and vascular pathology. Patients undergoing these studies who have an endotracheal tube in place may be at grave risk if extubated for the radiologic study. A physician skilled in airway control should be in attendance at the radiographic facility, in order to replace the child's endotracheal tube if necessary.

Management

Bronchoscopy is performed for the definitive diagnosis, and the trachea may then be dilated.[60] Airway bleeding and edema may occur, leading to increasing respiratory difficulty after the dilatation. This should be anticipated. The child should be observed in the intensive care unit following the procedure. Inhalation of racemic epinephrine may alleviate some obstruction due to edema. However, progressively increasing distress from obstruction may necessitate tracheal intubation. Prior to intubation, if this is required, positive pressure with a face mask, 100% oxygen, and an adjustable pop-off positive end-expiratory pressure (PEEP) valve can force oxygen into the lungs by counteracting the dynamic airway collapse that occurs with increasing respiratory efforts.

The child should remain in an intensive care unit where airway compromise may be carefully monitored and treated should deterioration occur. With significant airway obstruction, narcotics and sedatives should *not* be given, because they may cause central respiratory depression and precipitate acute respiratory failure. In selected cases, clinical, radiologic, and endoscopic evaluation may be all that is required in assessing the need for conservative management or surgical correction. If the child is relatively stable, then conservative management is preferred, delaying surgical resection until the child is at an age when tracheal resection would be considered a safer procedure.[61, 62]

A variety of techniques have been used before tracheal resection is undertaken in selected cases. These include dilatations, steroid injections, resecting with diathermy, cryosurgery, and laser therapy. These techniques may be helpful while granulation tissue is present or while the scar is still in the early stages. Once the scar tissue becomes hard and fibrous, then resection would appear to offer the best chances for success. Resection of tracheal stenosis is possible even in small infants.[63, 64]

As much as 50% of the trachea may be resected and a primary anastomosis performed.[62] However, with extensive tracheal stenosis, newer techniques such as the use of cartilage grafts, pericardial patch, and stents made of a flexible steel spring coated with silicone rubber have been employed.[58, 65–68]

It is usually possible to extubate the child at the conclusion of surgery. This is preferred, because the presence of the tube (a foreign body) in the trachea may predispose to breakdown of the anastomosis. However, should the child have to remain intubated, endotracheal tube positioning is critical, because the infant's shortened trachea and flexed head may predispose to accidental main stem bronchial intubation or extubation with minimal movement.

Tracheomalacia

Tracheomalacia is a condition of abnormal flaccidity of the tracheal wall that leads to tracheal collapse during respiration. Congenital tracheomalacia as a primary defect is uncommon. The use of flexible fiberoptic bronchoscopy has allowed the visualization of the airway dynamics in the child with respiratory distress and has revealed a more frequent occurrence of tracheomalacia than previously suspected. In this situation, there is a congenital malformation of the tracheobronchial cartilages such that they provide inadequate support and allow expiratory collapse. The condition may be associated with tracheoesophageal fistula, where there is deficiency of tracheal cartilage, or when extrinsic compression occurs with vascular anomalies and mediastinal masses. It may occur with systemic diseases affecting cartilage and connective tis-

sue; namely, Ehlers-Danlos syndrome. Acquired tracheomalacia follows tracheostomy and prolonged tracheal intubation, especially with cuffed endotracheal tubes.

Clinical Presentation

In primary tracheomalacia, the symptoms of respiratory distress manifested by stridor and cyanosis appear after the first few weeks of life, aggravated by infections and agitation. Spontaneous resolution takes at least 2 years.[69]

The clinical history of previous intubation or tracheostomy may suggest this diagnosis in a child who has symptoms of airway obstruction that is aggravated by stress, crying, and agitation.

Airway fluoroscopy defines the dynamic aspects of tracheomalacia; that is, constriction and dilatation of the tracheal wall related to phases of respiration. Bronchoscopy at *light* levels of anesthesia confirms the radiologic findings. Fiberoptic bronchoscopy with sedation and local anesthesia provides the best indication of the child's airway dynamics under normal conditions.

Management

The natural tendency for the trachea is to stiffen with time, usually by 2 years of age, and thus surgery is rarely indicated. However, underlying causes for secondary tracheomalacia should be identified and treated. Occasionally, tracheostomy may be required until the trachea has firmed and stabilized. Those children requiring tracheostomy to maintain a safe, clear airway appear to take longer to stabilize their airways. In selected cases, vascular suspension of the aorta or innominate artery relieves the problem. Long-term (approximately 24 months) PEEP of 8 to 10 cm H_2O via a tracheostomy tube has been effective in stabilizing the upper airway until the tracheal wall has become firm and less compliant.[70, 71] Tracheomalacia may extend into the main stem bronchi (bronchomalacia). Surgical treatment with an implanted synthetic graft has been successfully carried out, apparently without compromising airway growth.[72]

Mediastinal Masses

Mediastinal masses occur in the anterior, middle, and posterior mediastinum. Common mediastinal masses according to location are

(a) anterior mediastinum: lymphoma, teratoma, cystic hygroma, pericardial cyst, diaphragmatic hernia (via foramen of Morgagni); (b) middle mediastinum: lymphoma, tuberculous lymphadenopathy; and (c) posterior mediastinum: neurogenic tumor (neuroblastoma, ganglioneuroma, neurofibroma), esophageal duplication, bronchogenic cyst, diaphragmatic hernia (via foramen of Bochdalek). Of concern is the effect of mediastinal masses on the airways, lungs, and cardiovascular system. Anesthesia, bronchoscopy and surgery in these patients are potentially hazardous; therefore, thorough investigation and preparation are mandatory.[73, 74]

Anterior Mediastinum

Anterior mediastinal masses may produce severe respiratory and cardiovascular complications.[73, 74] Obstruction of major airways, cardiac compression that produces tamponade, and superior vena caval obstruction may occur. Malignant lymphoma may surround the heart with infiltration of the pericardium, producing pericardial tamponade.[75]

Most anterior mediastinal masses are lymphoid in origin (Hodgkin's and non-Hodgkin's lymphoma). It is important to appreciate that cervical masses (eg, cystic hygroma) may extend into the mediastinum.

Posterior Mediastinum

Posterior mediastinal masses (eg, esophageal duplication cyst) may cause respiratory distress through pressure on the adjacent lung. In addition, compression of the esophagus can lead to dysphagia and, possibly, reflux and aspiration.

Symptoms may be incorrectly attributed to benign and chronic conditions. For example, a child with "asthma" unresponsive to treatment with bronchodilators was shown to have a large mediastinal mass (neurogenic tumor) obstructing the airway.

Anesthetic Implications

Preoperative preparation of the child with a mediastinal mass includes evaluation of the degree of airway obstruction and any possible cardiovascular compromise. In addition to clinical evaluation of airway patency and hemodynamic stability, other special studies are carried out. Roentgenograms of the airway might include tomography and fluoroscopy.

CT scans of the airway provide better definition of obstruction. Pulmonary flow–volume loop studies, both in the upright and supine positions, are sensitive indicators of obstructive lesions of the major airways. Peak flow rate may show a significant decrease, even when the CT scan has revealed no airway obstruction.

In evaluating hemodynamic stability, the possibility of cardiac tamponade must be considered;[75] thus, it is important to examine for pulsus paradoxus. Echocardiography and barium swallow examinations are performed in selected cases.

In some cases, especially in Hodgkin's disease, in which compression of the trachea and bronchi by the mediastinal mass is perceived as life-threatening, irradiation of the tumor prior to anesthesia may ameliorate the degree of airway obstruction and provide a safer induction. General anesthesia and, especially, the use of muscle relaxants in these patients may be extremely hazardous. In the absence of spontaneous respiration, they may be extremely difficult to ventilate even with an endotracheal tube in place. Local anesthesia in preference to general anesthesia should be used for the biopsy procedure, if suitable. In rare situations, standby cardiopulmonary bypass is necessary. Irradiation of the tumor distorts the cellular picture and interferes with making a clear histologic diagnosis. Hence, a practice of general anesthesia prior to irradiation of anterior mediastinal masses has been proposed, even in the presence of respiratory or cardiovascular symptoms.[76] Thoracotomy is usually necessary to make the specific diagnosis. Excision of the entire mediastinal mass is undertaken if possible.

References

1. Tucker JA, O'Rahilly R. Observations on the embryology of the human larynx. Ann Otol Rhinol Laryngol 81:520, 1972.
2. Tucker JA, Tucker GF. Some aspects of fetal laryngeal development. Ann Otol Rhinol Laryngol 84:49, 1975.
3. Maze A, Bloch E. Stridor in pediatric patients. Anesthesiology 50:132, 1979.
4. Holinger LD. Etiology of stridor in the neonate, infant and child. Ann Otol Rhinol Laryngol 89:397, 1980.
5. Fanconi S, Burger R, Maurer H, Uehlinger J, Ghelfi D, Muhlemann C. Transcutaneous carbon dioxide pressure for monitoring patients with severe croup. J Pediatr 117:701–705, 1990.
6. Travis KW, Todres ID, Shannon DC. Pulmonary edema associated with croup and epiglottitis. Pediatrics 50:695, 1977.

7. Oswalt CE, Gates GA, Holmstrom FMG. Pulmonary edema as a complication of acute airway obstruction. JAMA 238:1833, 1977.

8. Kanter RK, Watchko JF. Pulmonary edema associated with upper airway obstruction. Am J Dis Child 138:356, 1984.

9. Benjamin B. Endoscopy in congenital tracheal anomalies. J Pediatr Surg 15:164, 1980.

10. Wood RE. Spelunking in the pediatric airways: Explorations with the flexible fiberoptic bronchoscope. Pediatr Clin North Am 31:785, 1986.

11. Noviski N, Todres ID. Fiberoptic bronchoscopy in the pediatric patient. Anesthesiol Clin North Am 9:163–174, 1991.

12. MayoSmith MF, Hirsch PJ, Wodzinski SF, Schiffman FJ. Acute epiglottitis in adults: An eight year experience in the state of Rhode Island. N Engl J Med 314:1133, 1986.

13. Baker AS, Eavey RD. Adult supraglottitis (epiglottitis). N Engl J Med 314:1185, 1986.

14. Faden HS. Toxicity of Hemophilus influenzae type B epiglottitis. Pediatrics 63:402, 1979.

15. Kilham H, Gillis J, Benjamin B. Severe upper airway obstruction. Pediatr Clin North Am 34:1, 1987.

16. Jones R, Santos JI, Overall JB. Bacterial tracheitis. JAMA 242:721, 1979.

17. Rapkin RH. Nasotracheal intubation in epiglottitis. Pediatrics 56:110, 1975.

18. Cohen SR, Chai J. Epiglottitis, 20 year study with tracheostomy. Ann Otol Rhinol Laryngol 87:1, 1978.

19. Todres ID, Crone RK. Experience with a modified laryngoscope in sick infants. Crit Care Med 9:544, 1981.

20. Slutsky AS, Watson J, Leith DE, Brown R. Tracheal insufflation of O_2 at low flow rates sustains life for several hours. Anesthesiology 63:278, 1985.

21. Coté CJ, Eavey RD, Todres ID, Jones DE. Cricothyroid membrane puncture. Oxygen ventilation in a dog model using an intravenous catheter. Crit Care Med 16:615, 1988.

22. Molteni RA. Epiglottitis: Incidence of extra-epiglottic infection: Report of 72 cases and review of the literature. Pediatrics 58:526, 1976.

23. Dajani AS, Asmar BI, Thirumoorthi MC. Systemic hemophilus influenzae disease: An overview. J Pediatr 94:355, 1979.

24. Walker SH. Influenza b epiglottitis and meningitis. Pediatrics 67:581, 1981.

25. Friedman EM, Damion J, Healy GB, McGill TJ. Supraglottitis and concurrent hemophilus meningitis. Ann Otol Rhinol Laryngol 94:470, 1985.

26. Kresch MJ. Pericarditis complicating hemophilus epiglottitis. Pediatr Infect Dis 4:559, 1985.

27. Newth CJL, Levison H, Bryan HC. The respiratory status of children with croup. J Pediatr 81:1068, 1972.

28. Westley CR, Cotton EK, Brooks JG. Nebulized racemic epinephrine by IPPB for the treatment of croup. Am J Dis Child 132:484, 1978.

29. Henry R. Moist air in the treatment of laryngotracheitis. Arch Dis Child 58:572, 1983.

30. Taussig LM, Castro O, Beaudry PH, Fox WW, Bureau M. Treatment of laryngotracheobronchitis (croup): Use of intermittent positive pressure breathing and racemic epinephrine. Am J Dis Child 129:790, 1975.

31. Fogel JM, Berg IJ, Gerber MA, Sherter CB. Racemic epinephrine in the treatment of croup: Nebulization alone versus nebulization with intermittent positive pressure breathing. J Pediatr 101:1028, 1982.

32. Kairys SW, Olmstead EM, O'Connor GT. Steroid treatment of laryngotracheitis: A meta analysis of the evidence from randomized trials. Pediatrics 83:683–693, 1989.

33. Super DM, Cartelli NA, Brooks LJ, Lembo RM, Kumar ML. A prospective randomized double blind study to evaluate the effect of dexamethasone in acute laryngotracheitis. J Pediatr 115:323–329, 1989.

34. McEniery J, Gillis J, Kilham H, Benjamin B. Review of intubation in severe laryngotracheobronchitis. Pediatrics 87:847–853, 1991.

35. Adderly RJ, Mullins GC. When to extubate the croup patient: The 'Leak' test. Can J Anaesth 34:304–306, 1987.

36. Duncan PG. Efficacy of helium–oxygen mixtures in the management of severe viral and post-intubation croup. Can Anaesth Soc J 26:206, 1979.

37. Skrinkas GJ, Hyland RH, Hutcheon MA. Using helium–oxygen mixtures in the management of acute upper airway obstruction. Can Med Assoc J 128:555, 1983.

38. Han BK, Dunbar JS, Striker TW. Membranous laryngotracheobronchitis (membranous croup). AJR 133:53, 1979.

39. Listen S, Gehrz R, Jaris C. Bacterial tracheitis. Arch Otolaryngol 107:561, 1981.

40. Denneny JC, Handler SD. Membranous laryngotracheobronchitis. Pediatrics 70:705, 1982.

41. Friedman EM, Jorgensen K, Healy GB, McGill TJ. Bacterial tracheitis: Two-year experience. Laryngoscope 95:9, 1985.

42. Strome M. Tracheobronchial foreign bodies: An updated approach. Ann Otol Rhinol Laryngol 86:649, 1977.

43. Rothmann BF, Boeckman CR. Foreign bodies in the larynx and tracheobronchial tree in children. Ann Otol Rhinol Laryngol 89:434, 1980.

44. Blazer S, Navelo Y, Friedman A. Foreign body in the airway. Am J Dis Child 134:68, 1980.

45. Cotton E, Yasuda K. Foreign body aspiration. Pediatr Clin North Am 31:937, 1984.

46. Aytac A, Yurdakul Y, Ikizler C, Olga R, Saylam A. Inhalation of foreign bodies in children: Report of 500 cases. J Thorac Cardiovasc Surg 74:145, 1977.

47. Harris CS, Baker SP, Smith GA, Harris RM. Childhood asphyxiation by food. JAMA 251:2231, 1984.

48. Anas NG, Perkin MD. Aspiration of a balloon by a 3 month old. JAMA 250:285, 1983.

49. Wiseman NE. The diagnosis of foreign body aspiration in childhood. J Pediatr Surg 19:531, 1984.

50. Abman SH, Fan LL, Colton EK. Emergency treatment of foreign body obstruction of the upper airway in children. J Emerg Med 2:7, 1984.

51. Cohen SR, Herbert WI, Lewis GB Jr, Geller KA. Foreign bodies in the airway: Five year retrospective study with special reference to management. Ann Otol Rhinol Laryngol 89:437, 1980.

52. Hight EW, Phillipart AI, Hertzler JH. The treatment of retained foreign bodies in the pediatric airway. J Pediatr Surg 16:694, 1981.

53. Kosloske AM. Bronchoscopic extraction of aspirated foreign bodies in children. Am J Dis Child 136:924, 1982.

54. Black RE, Choi KJ, Syme WC, Johnson DG, Matlak ME. Bronchoscopic removal of aspirated foreign bodies in children. Am J Surg 14:77, 1984.

55. Hunsicker RC, Gartner WS. Fogarty catheter technique for removal of endobronchial foreign body. Arch Otolaryngol 103:103, 1977.

56. Wood RE, Gauderer MW. Flexible fiberoptic bronchoscopy in the management of tracheobronchial foreign bodies in children: The value of a combined

approach with open tube bronchoscopy. J Pediatr Surg 19:693, 1984.

57. Cotton RT. Pediatric laryngotracheal stenosis. J Pediatr Surg 19:699, 1984.

58. Loeff DC, Filler RM, Vinograd I, Ein SH, Williams WG, Smith CR, Bahoric A. Congenital tracheal stenosis: A review of 22 patients from 1965 to 1987. J Pediatr Surg 23:744, 1988.

59. O'Neill JA Jr. Experience with iatrogenic laryngeal and tracheal stenosis. J Pediatr Surg 19:235, 1984.

60. Benjamin B. Endoscopy in congenital tracheal abnormalities. J Pediatr Surg 15:164, 1980.

61. Benjamin B, Pitkin J, Cohen D. Congenital tracheal stenosis. Ann Otol Rhinol Laryngol 90:364, 1981.

62. Grillo HC, Zannini P. Management of obstructive tracheal disease in children. J Pediatr Surg 19:414, 1984.

63. Akl BF, Yahek SM, Berman W Jr. Total tracheal reconstruction in a three month old infant. J Thorac Cardiovasc Surg 87:543, 1984.

64. Sorensen HR, Holsteen V. Resection of congenital stenosis of the trachea in an infant. Acta Paediatr Scand 73:141, 1984.

65. Majeski JA, Schreiber JT, Cotton R, MacMillan BG. Tracheoplasty for tracheal stenosis in the pediatric burned patient. J Trauma 20:81, 1980.

66. Filler RM, Buck JR, Bahoric A, Steward DJ. Treatment of segmental tracheomalacia and bronchomalacia by implantation of an airway splint. J Pediatr Surg 17:597, 1982.

67. Idriss FS, DeLeon SY, Ilbawi MN, Gerson CR, Tucker GF, Holinger L. Tracheoplasty with pericardial patch for extensive tracheal stenosis in infants and children. J Thorac Cardiovasc Surg 19:527, 1984.

68. Saad SA, Falla S. Management of intractable and extensive tracheal stenosis by implantation of cartilage graft. J Pediatr Surg 18:472, 1983.

69. Cogbill TH, Moore FA, Accurso FJ, Lilly JR. Primary tracheomalacia. Ann Thoracic Surg 35:538, 1983.

70. Wiseman NE, Duncan PG, Camberon CB. Management of tracheobronchomalacia with continuous positive airway pressure. J Pediatr Surg 20:489, 1985.

71. Sotomayor JL, Godinez RI, Borden S, Wilmott RW. Large-airway collapse due to acquired tracheobronchomalacia in infancy. Am J Dis Child 140:367, 1986.

72. Vinograd I, Filler RM, Bahoric A. Long-term functional results of prosthetic airway splinting in tracheomalacia and bronchomalacia. J Pediatr Surg 22:38, 1987.

73. Piro AH, Weiss DR, Hellman S. Mediastinal Hodgkin's disease: A possible danger from intubation anesthesia. Int J Radiat Oncol Biol Phys 1:415, 1976.

74. Todres ID, Reppert G, Walker PF, Grillo HC. Management of critical airway obstruction in a child with a mediastinal tumor. Anesthesiology 45:100, 1976.

75. Keon TP. Death on induction of anesthesia for cervical node biopsy. Anesthesiology 55:471, 1981.

76. Ferrari LR, Bedford RF. General anesthesia prior to treatment of anterior mediastinal masses in pediatric cancer patients. Anesthesiology 72:991, 1990.

CHAPTER 37

Anesthetic Considerations for Maxillofacial Trauma

Alexander W. Gotta, M.D., and
Colleen A. Sullivan, M.B.Ch.B.

The average anesthesiologist deals with severe maxillofacial trauma only occasionally. This lack of familiarity with the consequences of injury-induced alterations in the soft tissue and bony and cartilaginous components of the upper airway can lead to serious errors in assessment and clinical management. The practitioner should have some awareness of the anatomy of the facial skeleton; common fractures of the face; preoperative evaluation of the traumatized patient; airway assessment; and choice of anesthetic agent and technique, to include airway management.

ANATOMY

The facial skeleton is conventionally divided into thirds. The lowest third consists of the mandible, extending from the symphysis anteriorly, to the ramus, with the condyle and coronoid process posteriorly. The middle third is formed by the maxillae, zygomata, nasal bone, and orbits, whereas the upper third contains the frontal bones.

A series of bony arches protect the facial structures from the effects of blows, and a series of buttresses serve to limit motion and displacement of the facial and cranial skeletons. Thus, a protective arch is formed by the zygomatic process of the temporal bone and its union with the zygoma. Another arch stretches between condyle and coronoid process of the mandible.

Horizontal posterior displacement of the face in relation to the skull is prevented by the zygomatic process of the temporal bone. Oblique posterior displacement is limited by the pterygoid process of the sphenoid bone, and vertical posterior displacement by the greater wing of the sphenoid.

Upward displacement of the facial skeleton is limited by the zygomatic process of the frontal bone, the nasal part of the frontal bone, and the roof of the mandibular fossa.

The arches and buttresses create a vector of force dispersion and redistribution, helping to protect the facial and cranial skeletons from the effects of the great forces developed within the oral cavity during mastication and from the effects of blows to the face (Fig. 37–1). Thus, a blow to the mandible may fracture this bone, but very rarely will this fracture extend into the skull. Concurrent fractures of both mandible and skull are, of course, possible,

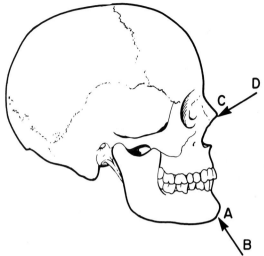

Figure 37–1. Although the mandible may be fractured by the force of a blow delivered along vector AB, the series of arches and buttresses within the cranial and facial skeletons redistribute the force so that a fracture of the skull will usually not result from the same blow. However, a blow to the midface along the vector CD will generate an abnormal shearing force, tending to tear apart the cranial and facial skeletons and extend a fracture line from the midface into the base of the skull. (From Gotta AW. Maxillofacial trauma: Anesthetic considerations. ASA Refresher Courses in Anesthesiology 15:39–50, 1985; with permission.)

but usually result from a series of blows to the face and skull or simultaneous trauma to both areas, as might occur when someone is buffeted about in a closed container, such as an overturning automobile. However, a blow to the midface, especially from in front and above, does not follow a normal vector of force dispersion, and such a blow may generate an abnormal shearing force, which tends to tear the facial and cranial skeletons apart or extend a mid-facial fracture into the base of the skull.

FACIAL FRACTURES

The mandible is a tubular bone, and as such derives its strength from the cortex. The jaw bone thus is strongest and most resistant to fracture where the cortex is thickest; ie, at its anteroinferior border.[1] The cortex thins as the mandible extends posteriorly and is most vulnerable in the ramus. The ramus is the most frequently fractured part of the mandible.[2–5] A fracture of the condyle at the temporomandibular joint may imperil function of this joint, limiting mobility of the jaw, and making endotracheal intubation under direct vision impossible.

The second most common point of fracture of the mandible is at the level of the first or second molar.[4] A bimandibular fracture at this point may cause the anterior fracture segment to be pulled posteriorly by the digastric, mylohyoid, and genioglossus muscles, thus impacting the fracture segment together with the tongue and paraglottic soft tissues into the upper airway, and causing total airway closure.[6] This type of fracture is usually recognized by the foreshortened mandible, and is known as an "Andy Gump fracture" after a chinless comic book character popular many years ago. This type of break is most likely to occur in an elderly, edentulous patient who does not wear his or her dentures and thus has had extensive decalcification of the mandible. The force of the blow is usually from below, as being struck by an "uppercut" or by falling forward and striking the unprotected jaw against a countertop. The Andy Gump fracture may occur in an automobile accident when the face is thrown violently forward and strikes the steering wheel.

Almost 100 years ago, LeFort of France subjected cadaver skulls to a series of maneuvers in an attempt to discover the common lines of fracture of the face.[7] At the same time, he discovered that the extent of facial skeletal trauma cannot be assessed by external (ie, soft tissue) trauma, and severe facial fracture may exist with little obvious soft-tissue disruption. The converse is also true—severe soft-tissue injury does not necessarily mean severe or even any bony deformity. His studies led to the commonly used LeFort classification of midface fractures (Fig. 37–2).

LeFort I

The LeFort I fracture is a horizontal fracture of the maxilla, passing above the floor of the nose. The lower third of the nasal septum is involved, and the palate, maxillary alveolar process, and the lower third of the pterygoid plates and parts of the palatine bones are mobilized. The fracture segment may be displaced posteriorly or laterally, rotated about a vertical axis, or a combination of any of these. Oral or nasal intubation may be carried out, and the airway can usually be secured without difficulty.

LeFort II

The LeFort II fracture is a pyramidal fracture, beginning at the junction of the thick

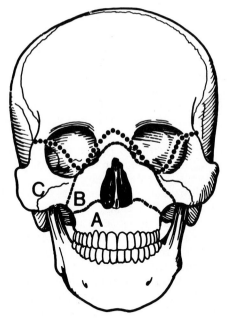

Figure 37–2. The lines of fracture for LeFort I (A), LeFort II (B), and LeFort III (C). (From Gotta AW. Maxillofacial trauma: Anesthetic considerations. ASA Refresher Courses in Anesthesiology, 15:39–50, 1985; with permission.)

upper part of the nasal bone and the thinner portion that forms the upper margin of the anterior nasal aperture. The fracture line crosses the medial orbital wall, the lacrimal bone, beneath the zygomaticomaxillary suture, across the lateral wall of the antrum, and posteriorly through the pterygoid plates. The mobile segment may be displaced posteriorly or rotated about an axis. A concomitant fracture of the base of the skull must always be considered in the presence of a LeFort II fracture.

LeFort III

In a LeFort III fracture, the line of fracture runs parallel to the base of the skull, separating the midface from the cranial base. The fracture extends through the base of the nose and the ethmoid in depth, through the orbital plates and near the cribriform plate, which may also be fractured. The fracture line crosses the lesser wing of the sphenoid, then downward to the pterygomaxillary fissure and sphenopalatine fossa. From the base of the inferior orbital fissue, the fracture line extends laterally and upward to the frontozygomatic suture and downward and posteriorly to the root of the

pterygoid plates. The zygomatic arch is also fractured.

Because the ethmoid is involved in the fracture line, there may be a fracture of the base of the skull, with access to the subarachnoid space. Attempted nasotracheal intubation may lead to introduction of the tube into the cranium, with consequent direct brain trauma. Cerebrospinal fluid rhinorrhea is an absolute indication of basal skull fracture and an absolute contraindication to nasal tracheal intubation. Even ventilation by mask risks the introduction of foreign matter into the subarachnoid space and the development of meningitis.[8]

With a LeFort III fracture, the midface is mobile and often pushed posteriorly. A concavity replaces the normal facial convexity, giving the patient a characteristic "dish-face" deformity.

Incidence of Maxillofacial Injury

In 1984, 145,012 people died in the United States as a result of trauma. Care for victims of trauma costs 6.9% of total health care expenditure and 2.3% of the gross national product of the United States. Despite the importance of trauma and the resultant morbidity and mortality there are great deficiencies in our knowledge of the mechanisms of injury and their consequences. The Committee on Trauma Research of the National Research Council Commission on Life Sciences points out that meaningful data on fractures of the smaller facial bones are not available; nor is there adequate assessment technology. Indeed, the mechanics of injury to the head and neck and resultant functional alteration are also poorly understood. Basic data are missing, including the incidence of various facial fractures.

Preoperative Evaluation

The patient who has sustained severe injury to his or her face often presents so dramatic a picture of obvious injury to the readily visible portion of his or her anatomy that the evaluating physician may disregard even more serious trauma to other parts of the body. An adequate history is mandatory, as is a complete physical examination. A traumatized patient admitted to the dental or oral surgical service of a hospital may be seen by no physician other than the anesthesiologist. The preanesthetic evaluation thus assumes even greater importance.

The history must determine, as much as possible, the nature of the blow; the possibility of multiple blows to the face, head, and other parts of the body; and the possibility of loss of consciousness. Significant prior illness must be sought, as well as use of drugs, both legitimate and illegitimate. Very often the traumatized patient is a substance abuser, and this abuse may have played a significant role in the cause of the injuries.

The face and oral cavity must be carefully examined for mobility, loose teeth, bone fragments, or any obstruction to respiration or hindrance to intubation. The patient must be able both to flex and extend the head and point the chin at either shoulder. Inability to do so warrants investigation as to the cause. The larynx or trachea may be compressed, deviated, or distorted by an increasing volume of blood trapped within the fixed and relatively immobile fascial planes of the neck, thus obstructing the free flow of respiratory air and making endotracheal intubation difficult or impossible.

Signs of respiratory obstruction may be evident—flaring of the alae nasi, obvious effort on inspiration and even expiration, and noisy stridor. Airway obstruction is usually dynamic and rapidly changing, and an acceptable airway quickly can become completely obstructed.

The physician must examine the chest for evidence of trauma. In an acceleration–deceleration type of injury, as in an automobile accident where the patient is thrown forcibly against the steering wheel or dashboard, ribs may be fractured, or the heart may be trapped between the sternum anteriorly and the vertebral column posteriorly, with resultant myocardial contusion or pericardial tamponade.

Broken ribs may be palpated or may evidence themselves with hematoma or tenderness. Subcutaneous emphysema indicates puncture of the lung and pneumothorax. Pneumothoraces, which may be small and apparently insignificant when the patient is first seen, may become very significant indeed on institution of positive-pressure ventilation, especially if nitrous oxide is used. Auscultation of the lungs must be performed carefully, looking for the decreased breath sounds of pneumothorax or lung contusion.

Beck's triad of hypotension, increased venous pressure, and a silent heart may indicate cardiac tamponade. Be especially wary of profound hypotension with little evidence of blood loss; this often indicates cardiac dysfunction secondary to entrapment within a pericardial sac with an expanding volume of blood, or heart failure caused by myocardial contusion.

The anesthesiologist should not hesitate to examine the abdomen for tenderness, signs of peritoneal sensitivity, and an increasing girth that is indicative of intra-abdominal hemorrhage. A neurologic examination is always in order to establish the baseline and to evaluate the possibility of concurrent central or peripheral nervous system damage.

Laboratory data should include hemoglobin or hematocrit as a rough indicator of blood loss and urinalysis as a marker for trauma elsewhere than the face and head. If alcoholism is suspected, liver function tests and clotting profile will probably prove helpful. Trauma to the chest warrants an electrocardiogram and a chest radiograph. Pneumothorax may be very difficult to see when early. Even fractured ribs may be difficult to visualize if the fractures are not displaced and the ribs are well apposed. It should be remembered that a fracture through the cartilaginous part of the rib may create cartilaginous spicules that may also penetrate the lung and cause pneumothorax. This type of fracture is not readily evident on radiographs.

As part of the preoperative evaluation, the physician must consider common concurrent medical and surgical problems. Common medical problems that may influence anesthetic management include (1) acute alcoholic intoxication, (2) chronic alcoholism, (3) drug intoxication, (4) chronic drug abuse, (5) myocardial infarct, and (6) stroke.

Alcoholism, both acute alcoholic intoxication and chronic abuse, is frequently associated with injury. It may be very difficult to obtain an adequate history, perform an appropriate physical examination, and secure the airway in an intoxicated, contentious, or violent patient. Acute intoxication always suggests chronic abuse, and the physician must consider the alterations in liver and myocardial function and the blood clotting mechanisms. Liver function tests and coagulation are especially important in this group of patients.

Similarly, acute drug intoxication and chronic abuse syndromes other than alcohol are frequently associated with trauma. The marked increase in the use of free-base cocaine ("crack") has been associated with great increases in the incidence of personal injury among those who use this potent psychotropic drug.

The acutely intoxicated crack user may be

psychotic, with hallucinations, illusions, delusions, paranoia, and usually is extremely difficult to manage. Other drugs of abuse, although fading in popularity before crack's onslaught, present their own problems. It must be remembered that it is rare for only one drug to be used to excess, and that the drug abuser is almost always a multiple substance abuser. Thus, the narcotic addict is almost invariably an alcoholic.[9] The converse need not be true; ie, the alcoholic is not usually a narcotic user. The polypharmacy of the abuser demands an inquiring in-depth history. Withdrawal from narcotics is unpleasant, but rarely deadly. Withdrawal from alcohol can be very unpleasant and, in its extreme manifestation, often fatal, whereas withdrawal from crack can create an acute psychotic state. The physician must be aware of the drug history and the possibility of withdrawal from one or many substances of abuse.

One must also consider myocardial infarct and stroke as preliminary events in the development of injury. The elderly gentleman admitted after an automobile accident and with obvious maxillofacial injury may have lost control of his car because he lost consciousness after myocardial infarct or stroke. It may take great diagnostic skill to determine whether the post-injury neurologic deficit is a result of trauma to the nervous system, or whether a nervous system deficit preceded the trauma.

Concurrent surgical problems in patients with maxillofacial trauma may include (1) fracture of the skull, (2) intracranial hemorrhage, (3) subdural hematoma, (4) fracture of the cervical spine, (5) fat embolism, (6) pneumothorax, (7) flail chest, (8) cardiac tamponade, (9) cardiac hematoma, and (10) ruptured spleen or liver.

The skull may be fractured along with the facial skeleton by repeated blows to the face and head. Although a mandibular fracture rarely extends into the skull, fractures of the base of the skull are not uncommon with severe maxillary injury, especially a LeFort III fracture.

Intracranial hemorrhage or subdural hematoma may occur with the application of any force sufficient to injure the facial skeleton. Protean manifestations of such central nervous system injury can make adequate evaluation of an ever-changing clinical picture quite difficult.

Fracture of the cervical spine must be considered in injuries to the neck and may demand radiologic evaluation. The technique of endotracheal intubation is often altered, or even determined outright, by the presence of cervical fractures.

Fat embolism may develop with any significant injury and is especially prone to develop after concurrent long-bone fracture. The central nervous system manifestations of fat embolism may be confusing in the presence of possible central nervous system trauma.

Pneumothorax may occur after lung penetration by a fractured rib, and flail chest with multiple fractures is likely to result from a steering wheel injury. Cardiac tamponade and cardiac hematoma may occur with any forceful blow to the chest. An intra-abdominal organ may also rupture when great force is directed to the abdomen, and must be considered whenever hypotension is not accompanied by visible blood loss.

Airway Assessment

The patient who has sustained serious maxillofacial injury may have upper airway obstruction secondary to the presence of foreign matter in the airway, edema, or obstruction due to compression of the larynx or trachea by active bleeding contained within the closed fascial planes of the neck. Flaring of the alae nasi, use of the accessory muscles of respiration, obvious effort during respiration, or stridor should alert the anesthesiologist to the presence of an obstructed airway.

The mouth must be examined, and broken teeth, clotted blood, or vomitus removed manually if necessary. The presence of an "Andy Gump" fracture is manifested by an apparent shortening of the mandible, or maxillary protusion, with obvious difficulty in breathing. It may be possible to reduce this type of fracture and restore a troubled airway by gentle yet forceful anterior traction on the mandible. The neck must be examined for laryngeal injury, or turgor within the neck, possibly exerting pressure on the airway.

The patient with severe mandibular trauma, with section of the muscles of the floor of the mouth, may find it necessary to lean forward constantly so that gravity will pull his or her loosened tongue and paraglottic soft tissue forward and out of their impaction into the oropharynx. If this patient is made to lie back, complete airway occlusion may occur.

In order to effect endotracheal intubation under direct vision, at a minimum the patient must be able to open his or her mouth and extend his or her tongue between the incisors.

Inability to open the mouth sufficiently may be due to (1) trismus, (2) edema, (3) pain, (4) fractures through the temporomandibular joint, and (5) fracture of the zygomatic process of the temporal bone.

Trismus is masseter spasm secondary to trauma or infection, and may be overcome by anesthesia and muscle relaxants. Similarly, oral closure due to pain is overcome by anesthesia and relaxant. Edema alone is rarely so severe as to make visualized endotracheal intubation impossible. However, a fracture through the temporomandibular joint may cause enough mechanical impairment of this joint to make visualization of the larynx impossible.

The zygomatic process of the temporal bone is enveloped in the tough temporal fascia, and is thus fractured only with the direct application of great force. However, should the fascia be ruptured and a fracture of this process ensue, then the fracture segments may be driven inferoposteriorly, impacting on the coronoid process of the temporomandibular joint. It thus may be impossible to open the mouth and visualize the larynx. The advice of the surgeon as to the cause of jaw immobility should be sought. But if in doubt, awake intubation is mandatory.

Endotracheal Intubation

Securing the airway in the patient with maxillofacial injury is often a serious challenge to the clinical skills of the anesthesiologist. Midface fractures, with anatomic distortion and the possibility of basal skull fracture, often mandate oral intubation or tracheostomy. Mandibular fractures, with mechanical impairment of the temporomandibular joint or with the jaw already wired shut, mandate awake intubation. This is facilitated by the use of the fiberoptic laryngoscope or bronchoscope, but can often be performed quite simply as a blind intubation.

The first step in nasotracheal intubation is to evaluate the nasal airway. The posterior nares offer the smallest diameter of the upper airway, but cannot be seen and thus cannot be evaluated. Air flow can be assessed, however, merely by closing one nostril at a time and feeling the air flow through the patent nostril. Intubation should be effected through the nostril with the best air flow.

Nasotracheal intubation involves placing a rather formidable piece of plastic or rubber into a very resistant airway that has powerful reflexes designed primarily to prevent the entry of any foreign body. These reflexes may be overcome and intubation facilitated by anesthetizing the airway from nose to carina.

Lidocaine, 2% to 4%, dripped into the nose, anesthetizes the mucosa quite well. The addition of several drops of 0.25% to 0.50% phenylephrine causes vasoconstriction in the mucosa, thus increasing the airway's patency and minimizing the risk of epistaxis. Cocaine may be used, but offers little advantage over the combination of lidocaine and phenylephrine, and adds the risk of serious cardiac arrhythmias and the problems of storing a drug with great street value. The mouth, even if wired closed, may be anesthetized by spraying lidocaine onto the tongue and base of the oropharynx.

The interior of the larynx, from the base of the tongue to the vocal cords, may be anesthetized by blocking the internal branch of the superior laryngeal nerve. The superior laryngeal nerve is a branch of the vagus arising from the nodose ganglion. The nerve travels with the main vagal trunk to the level of the larynx, then springs forward and terminates in an internal (sensory) branch and an external (motor) branch that penetrates and innervates the cricothyroid muscle.[10] This muscle is a tensor of the vocal cords, and its blockade causes no serious dysfunction of the laryngeal musculature. The internal branch of the superior laryngeal nerve penetrates the thyrohyoid membrane and ramifies immediately in a closed space bounded laterally by the thyrohyoid membrane, medially by the laryngeal mucosa, superiorly by the inferior border of the hyoid bone, and inferiorly by the superior border of the thyroid cartilage. The terminal ramifications of the nerve provide sensory innervation from the base of the tongue to the vocal cords. Within the closed space, the nerve may be blocked by introducing the tip of a needle and injecting a local anesthetic.[11, 12] Thus, the landmarks for a superior laryngeal nerve block are the hyoid bone, the thyroid cartilage, and the thyrohyoid membrane that links the two. The hyoid is usually easily identified as a freely movable bone in the upper neck. The thyroid cartilage is the largest component of the larynx, and the thyreohyoid membrane may be appreciated as a shallow depression between bone and cartilage.

In order to perform the block, the patient, lying supine, must extend his or her head. A 22-gauge needle, attached to a syringe containing 2 mL of 2% lidocaine, is aimed directly at the hyoid in its posterior third. The approach is lateral, not anterior. When the needle strikes the hyoid, the characteristic "gritty" feeling of needle on bone is appreciated (similar to an intercostal block, when the needle strikes the rib). The needle is then walked caudad until it just slips off the bone, and then advanced 2 to 3 mm. A suddenly yielding resistance may signal penetration of the membrane, and entrance into the closed space containing the nerve's ramifications. Aspiration should produce nothing; neither air (indicative of penetrance of the larynx), nor blood (indicative of penetrance of a blood vessel). It should be noted that the carotid sheath is directly posterior to the point of needle entry, and its puncture could lead to injection of the local anesthetic into either the carotid artery or internal jugular vein. If there is no aspirate, then the local anesthetic should be injected, and the block repeated on the other side.

Contraindications to a superior laryngeal nerve block are relative, not absolute, and include a full stomach, because of the possibility of aspiration after ablation of the protective laryngeal reflexes. Tumor or infection at the site of block would also be a contraindication because of the possibility of dissemination of either infection or tumor. Complications include direct intravascular injection of local anesthetic or hematoma after vessel injury.

Sensory innervation to the trachea is provided by the recurrent laryngeal branch of the vagus. Because it is the major innervator of the laryngeal muscles, it is imprudent to block the nerve directly. However, sensory block can be obtained by topical application of local anesthetic via translaryngeal puncture through the cricothyroid membrane and direct instillation of the anesthetic. A 22-gauge needle attached to a syringe containing 4 mL of 4% lidocaine is inserted through the membrane in the midline. The bevel of the needle is directed caudad and the patient is directed to exhale maximally. The lidocaine is then injected as rapidly as possible and the needle removed. The local anesthetic that strikes the carina initiates a vigorous cough, which sprays the local anesthetic on the trachea walls. Thus, the airway is anesthetized from nose to carina by topical anesthetic applied directly to nose and mouth, and via translaryngeal puncture to the trachea. This topical application, coupled with blockade of the internal branch of the superior laryngeal nerve, produces optimal conditions for acceptance of the endotracheal tube.

Nasotracheal intubation is facilitated by placing the patient's head on a folded sheet and into the "sniffing" position. It is best to avoid manipulating the injured face by allowing the patient to extend his or her head. The tube should be gently inserted parallel to the hard palate and advanced only as long as no significant resistance is felt. The bronchscope may be manipulated to enter the larynx, and the endotracheal tube is then slipped off the bronchoscope and into the trachea. If the airway has been properly anesthetized, the patient will offer no resistance and will not cough or strain.

If blind awake intubation is elected, then the tube should be inserted and maneuvered as close to the larynx as possible, while listening for quality and intensity of breath sounds. If the patient is made to hyperventilate, the tube can usually be inserted quickly and easily at the beginning of inspiration. Occasionally, it is necessary to flex the patient's head in order to facilitate entry of the tube into the trachea.

Tracheostomy may be necessary with unrelieved airway obstruction because of massive trauma and blood, bone, or teeth occluding the airway. An "Andy Gump" fracture may cause airway occlusion which, if it cannot be relieved, constitutes an emergency that necessitates immediate tracheostomy.

Anesthetic Agent and Technique

Minor surgical procedures may be carried out using local anesthesia, but only if the anesthesiologist is assured of the adequacy of the patient's ventilation and the ability to monitor the patient.

Intravenous anesthetics are suitable, but it may be difficult to determine an appropriate dose in the addicted patient. Ketamine should be used cautiously, if at all, because of its respiratory depressant effect[13] and its ability to alter cerebral metabolism[14, 15] and increase intracranial pressure[16] in the patient with an intracranial injury.

Inhalation anesthetics are excellent for providing adequate anesthesia, analgesia, and operative conditions. However, the halogenated ethers (either enflurane or isoflurane) are preferable to the alkane halothane, because of the higher incidence of serious cardiac arrhythmias when halothane is used in dental or maxillofacial surgery,[17] and because of the relative contraindication to the use of epinephrine in the presence of halothane.

SUMMARY

Adequate management of maxillofacial trauma demands a knowledge of normal facial anatomy, common fracture sites, and their implications. The anesthesiologist must be well versed in assessing and securing the airway, even when serious anatomic alteration has occurred.

References

1. Haskell R. Applied surgical anatomy. In Rowe NL, Williams JL (eds). Maxillo Facial Injuries. Edinburgh: Churchill Livingstone, 1985; pp. 3–4.
2. Huelke DF. Mechanics in the production of mandibular fractures: A study of the "stresscoat" technique. I: Symphyseal impacts. J Dent Res 40:1042–1056, 1961.
3. Huelke DF, Patrick LM. Mechanics in the production of mandibular fractures: Strain-gauge measurements of impacts to the chin. J Dent Res 43:437–446, 1964.
4. Halazonetis JA. The "weak" regions of the mandible. Br J Oral Surg 6:37–48, 1968.
5. Nahum AM. The biomechanics of facial bone fracture. Laryngoscope 85:140–156, 1975.
6. Seshul MB, Sinn DP, Gerlock AJ. The Andy Gump fracture of the mandible: A cause of respiratory obstruction or distress. J Trauma 18:611–612, 1978.
7. LeFort R. Etude experimentale sur les fractures de la machoire superieure. Rev Chir 23:208–227, 360–379, 479–507; 1901.
8. Kitahata LM, Collins WF. Meningitis as a complication of anesthesia in a patient with basal skull fracture. Anesthesiology 32:282–283, 1970.
9. Stimmel B, Vernace S, Tobias H. Hepatic dysfunction in heroin addicts: The role of alcohol. JAMA 222:811–812, 1972.
10. Durham CF, Harrison TS. The surgical anatomy of the superior laryngeal nerve. Surg Gynecol Obstet 118:38–44, 1964.
11. Gotta AW, Sullivan CA. Superior laryngeal nerve block: An aid to intubating the patient with fractured mandible. J Trauma 24:83–85, 1984.
12. Gotta AW, Sullivan CA. Anaesthesia of the upper airway using topical anaesthetic and superior laryngeal nerve block. Br J Anaesth 53:1055–1058, 1981.
13. Zsigmand EK, Matsuki A, Kothafy SP. Arterial hypoxemia caused by intravenous ketamine. Anesth Analg 55:311–314, 1976.
14. Takeshita H, Okuda Y, Sari A. The effects of ketamine on cerebral circulation and metabolism in man. Anesthesiology 36:69–75, 1972.
15. Crosby G, Crane AM, Sokoloff L. Local changes in cerebral glucose utilization during ketamine anesthesia. Anesthesiology 56:437–443, 1982.
16. Gardner AE, Olson BE, Lichtiger M. Cerebrospinal-fluid pressure during dissociative anesthesia with ketamine. Anesthesiology 35:226–228, 1971.
17. Gotta AW, Sullivan CA, Pelkofski J, Kangwalklai R, Kozam R. Aberrant conduction as a precursor to cardiac arrhythmias during anesthesia for oral surgery. J Oral Surg 34:421–427, 1976.

CHAPTER 38

Inhalational Injury: Management of the Burned Airway

William T. Denman, M.B.Ch.B., F.R.C. Anaes., and
Nishan G. Goudsouzian, M.D., M.S.

BURNS TO THE AIRWAY

Burns cause two million injuries per year in the United States.[1] Of these, 20,000 are admitted to specialist burn centers. In the 4000 to 8000 deaths per year from burns, inhalational injuries are one of the commonest causes of death; 55% to 80% of these are due to smoke inhalation.[2] In general, 20% to 30% of the patients admitted to burn centers have an inhalational injury.[3] The mortality associated with inhalational injury alone is of the order of 5% to 10%, but when combined with a large cutaneous injury, the mortality soars to 25% to 35%.[4]

MECHANISMS OF THERMAL INJURY

Inhalational injuries are usually associated with burns occurring in closed spaces, where toxic irritating gases accumulate. Blasts and explosions also cause such injuries in open spaces.[5] In either case, the damage to the respiratory system may be extensive, especially when impaired consciousness in the victim

causes a loss of protective reflexes and the subsequent inhalation of toxic fumes.

The upper airways may be injured in three discrete ways.

Inhalation of Hot, Dry Gases

Hot, dry air mainly causes lesions of the face, mouth, nasopharynx, oropharynx, and larynx. This is due to the fact that the respiratory mucosa has a large heat-exchanging capacity and the low heat-carrying capacity of dry air. Also, the larynx of an awake person closes immediately in response to hot gases. This helps to restrict injury to the area above the cords.[6, 7]

Smoke Inhalation

The inhalation of smoke causes chemical damage to the airway, the extent of which depends on the composition of the smoke. Toxic gases emitted during fires include carbon monoxide (CO), cyanide, acrolein, hydrogen chloride, phosgene, and ammonia.[8]

Acrolein is present when cellulosic materials burn. It is extremely irritating and denatures protein. Pulmonary edema may appear with levels as low as 10 ppm. Hydrogen chloride (HCl) is liberated in large quantities when polyvinyl chloride burns, because 40% of the gases released are HCl. This strong acid causes intense mucosal burns of the respiratory tract.[9] The toxins and acids may also be absorbed onto carbon particles and be carried peripherally as far as the alveoli. The smoke released by burning plastic is very much more dense than wood smoke and is released at lower temperatures.

Cyanide poisoning must also be considered in inhalational injuries. The polyurethanes emit cyanates, isocyanates, and hydrogen cyanide (HCN). These fumes produce a sensation of choking, dizziness, a loss of balance, and eventually loss of consciousness. Cyanide poisoning should be suspected in all victims with inhalational injuries.[10]

Steam Inhalation

Inhalational injury due to pure steam is uncommon. These types of accidents may occur in industrial injuries. Due to the very high heat-carrying capacity of steam (4000 times that of hot air), steam can cause severe damage to the entire respiratory system.

Combustion in a closed space consumes oxygen, causing the percentage of oxygen in the area to decrease from 21% and even to 10% to 15%.[12] The presence of toxic fumes and carbon monoxide also contributes to the victim's hypoxia. Of the deaths due to smoke inhalation, up to 80% may actually be the result of asphyxia or carbon monoxide poisoning.

It is convenient to attempt to isolate the type of injury. In reality, however, the trauma patient often has cutaneous thermal injuries, poisoning from toxic fumes, and may have other injuries, including fractures.[13] All aspects of resuscitation must be attended to if the victim is to receive optimal care.

PATHOPHYSIOLOGY

The pathologic changes seen in the respiratory tract after an inhalational injury depend on the products of combustion, the heat of the fire, and the duration of exposure. A general pattern is common to most.

Initially, the problem of asphyxia is encountered. The ensuing hypoxemia results in hyperventilation, further drawing products of combustion into the lungs. Thus, hypoxia is compounded by exposure to CO, HCl, HCN, and other toxins.

Edema is the body's acute response to a burn. Initially, the edema is confined to the area exposed to the thermal injury. In large cutaneous burns, however, the edema may extend away from the site of injury and include the respiratory tract.[14] If inhalational injury is present, marked edema and airway narrowing may occur, leading to respiratory obstruction. Within minutes of exposure to smoke and toxic fumes the cilia cease functioning, leading to impaired mucus and debris clearance.[15] Bronchial congestion and edema are early phenomena that result in airway obstruction. Bronchospasm often complicates smoke inhalation injuries and appears to have features indistinguishable from asthma. It has been shown that there is a strong correlation between exposure, carboxyhemoglobin levels, and initial airways conductance.[16]

At first, the mucosal lesions are the result of the heat from the burns. Mucosal hemorrhage, ulceration, and sloughing appear, adding to the problems of obstruction. The chemical effects of the injury progress more slowly, initially giving a mild but diffuse edema with submucosal edema. A mucopurulent membrane develops over the mucosa, and bronchorrhea is present. After 48 to 72 hours following severe injury, tracheal sloughing is established and casts may be expectorated.[17]

Lower airway obstruction results in airway trapping and demonstrable ventilation–perfusion ($\dot{V}/\dot{Q}$) mismatch. Intense bronchial congestion increases shunting of blood, further exacerbating $\dot{V}/\dot{Q}$ abnormalities. The surfactant in the alveoli is inactivated immediately, and atelectasis quickly supervenes.[18] Pulmonary capillary permeability increases, leading to both alveolar and interstitial edema.[19] This edema leads to an increase in the alveolar capillary gradient. The decrease in pulmonary compliance that accompanies the injury increases the work of breathing, leading to further pulmonary compromise.[20]

Toxic fume poisoning often accompanies inhalational injuries. These can be broadly classified as irritants,[21] chemical asphyxiants, and metals or metallic compounds.

The chemical asphyxiants CO and cyanide (CN) must be borne in mind with every burn victim.[22] These substances disrupt cellular metabolism by blocking oxygen usage.

CO intoxication is frequently the cause of death in fire victims. It occurs where the fire is in enclosed spaces and incomplete combustion is present. CO has an affinity of 200 times that of oxygen for hemoglobin; therefore, the oxygen-carrying capacity of the blood is greatly reduced. CO also shifts the oxyhemoglobin curve to the left, further reducing the oxygen available for the tissues. The signs and symptoms of CO intoxication initially correlate well with blood levels[12] (Table 38–1).

Treatment depends on recognition. Any burn victim brought to an emergency room from a fire in a closed space should be treated as if he or she has been exposed to CO. The cherry-red color may not be obvious due to soot and burns, and cyanosis may be a more overriding observation if respiration is markedly depressed; therefore, a more reliable test is to obtain CO blood levels. CN should be suspected when a patient presents with loss of consciousness and the carboxyhemoglobin levels are not elevated. The victim may present with gasping respirations and a profound metabolic acidosis.

Children are at greater risk from respiratory obstruction because of the smaller diameter of their airways. Resistance to flow is inversely proportional to the fourth power of the radius of the tube. Therefore, reducing the radius by one half increases resistance to flow 16 times.[23]

Cutaneous burns of the face and neck may affect the airway within hours. Edema of the face and neck impedes mouth opening, whereas burns of the neck and upper chest may obstruct lymphatic drainage, causing pharyngeal edema to worsen.[24]

Deep circumferential burns of the chest and abdomen may restrict respiratory excursion sufficiently to precipitate respiratory failure. The underlying edema and eschar formation act in tandem to severely restrict ventilation. Diaphragmatic excursion is diminished by the ileus that accompanies major trauma. In these patients, escharotomy may be necessary to allow respiratory excursion, which is performed by cutting the burned tissue vertically.[25] Often, this procedure does not require anesthesia and may be performed at the bedside.

Cutaneous burns alone do not generally affect lung function directly.[26] However, complications may arise during the post-burn period as a result of treatment. Initially, the pulmonary vascular resistance is moderately elevated (3 to 5 days).[27] This is thought to protect the lungs from pulmonary edema in spite of the large amounts of fluid used in resuscitation. However, over the next period (4 to 7 days post-burn), the pulmonary vascular resistance decreases toward normal and pulmonary edema may appear.[28]

CLINICAL ASSESSMENT

The assessment of a severe burn is a challenging and daunting prospect. The clinical picture is constantly changing, and a hard and fast diagnosis may be elusive. The burn victim is usually in pain, may be so disfigured as to frighten a young physician, and is at any stage in the continuum of an evolving process. The patient may appear stable, only to deteriorate as one watches; therefore, speed and thoroughness are of the essence.

Often, the patient is unconscious; therefore, the history must be obtained from the rescue workers, family, or other witnesses. It is also important to remain cognizant of the fact that the patient may be suffering from other injuries. There may be fractures or other traumatic injuries,[13] and the past medical history may be pertinent and must not be forgotten.

A systematic approach is necessary, and each organ system must be examined for evidence of both thermal and other insult. During the examination, particular care must be directed toward the likelihood of an inhalational injury.

The head and neck should be assessed for the presence of singed nasal hairs, soot in the mouth and pharynx, carbonaceous sputum, and burns of the face and oropharynx.[15, 17, 25] The examination of the respiratory system must look for tachypnea, dyspnea, accessory muscle recruitment, hoarseness, stridor, wheezing, and added breath sounds. An early sign of inhalational injury may be a bronchospastic response due to the intense irritation.[16, 29] The cardiovascular system may be affected in several ways. Arrhythmias occur due to hypoxia and catecholamine release; angina may occur

Table 38–1. CARBOXYHEMOGLOBIN

Level (%)	Symptoms
0–20	None
20–30	Headache, nausea, vomiting
30–50	Visual and cognitive disturbance
50–60	Loss of consciousness, permanent central nervous system damage
70–80	Death

in susceptible patients.[13] Hypertension or hypotension may be present, depending on pain, fluid status, or presence of poisoning. If poisoning figures largely, then myocardial depression is possible.[30]

The investigations available to evaluate an inhalational injury are:[31]

Pulse Oximetry. Pulse oximetry should be used in all inhalational injuries. A normal saturation may be erroneous in the presence of significant CO poisoning.[32]

Arterial Blood Gases (ABG). Oxygen tensions are usually lower in inhalational injuries. It must be remembered that the sample is taken with a patient on oxygen and hyperventilating. Therefore, a "normal" ABG may not actually be abnormal.[33, 26]

Carboxyhemoglobin. Blood samples should be taken for CO levels. However, if clinically necessary, treatment should not await this result.[30]

Chest Radiograph. Chest radiographs are a coarse method of determining inhalational damage early in the course of the injury.[34] However, a chest radiograph is necessary in trauma to provide a baseline and to identify other intrathoracic problems.[13]

Electrocardiogram (ECG). An ECG is important in assessing ischemia, conduction defects, and especially in the presence of chest pain.[35]

Pulmonary Function Tests. Spirometry is a sensitive indicator of inhalational injury to the lower tracheobronchial tree.[36] Alterations in FEV_1 and FVC occur early in the injury. This is so sensitive that normal spirometry is very unlikely in a case of significant lower respiratory tract injury.[37]

[133]Xenon Ventilation/Perfusion Lung Scan. This test is extremely sensitive in detecting areas of gas trapping due to bronchospasm or bronchial obstruction.[38] However, it is rarely available in emergency treatment settings.

Fiberoptic Bronchoscopy. Fiberoptic bronchoscopy is now accepted as the most easily performed and reliable diagnostic modality.[39, 40] It allows examination of the supraglottic and infraglottic region to assess both inflammatory changes and mucosal damage. The classical signs of respiratory burns consist of mucosal erythema, edema, ulceration, hemorrhagic necrosis, and carbon particles present in the respiratory tract.[41] In a hypotensive and inadequately resuscitated patient, erythema and edema may not have developed.[42] In mild cases of inhalational injury, the lumen of the airway is not compromised. If the injury is severe enough, the vocal cords may not be visible due to the prolapse of the false cords into the lumen of the larynx.[26] Once the false cords meet in the midline, respiratory obstruction becomes complete.

With experienced operators bronchoscopy is a procedure that carries minimal risk. It is diagnostic in delineating the extent and severity of the burn; also it gives information as to the imminence of airway obstruction and, if needed, it allows tracheal intubation to be carried out.[43] Bronchoscopy is also a beneficial therapeutic maneuver as a means of clearing debris and inspissated secretions.

As bronchscopes have improved, they have been used in pediatric practice to evaluate airways.[44] It may prove difficult to perform a bronchoscopy on a child who is awake, but the laryngeal mask airway (LMA) may be used to facilitate the procedure.[45]

Bronchoscopy can be carried out with topical anesthesia of the mucosa and judicious use of systemic analgesia and sedation.[46] Local anesthesia of the nose may be accomplished with cocaine or with a mixture of lignocaine and phenylephrine. Incremental doses of intravenous sedation/analgesia should be titrated to effect. It is imperative that supplemental oxygen be given during the bronchoscopy and pulse oximetry used to monitor the patient. The possibility of aspiration must be entertained as the patient is sedated and topical anesthesia is applied to the pharynx and larynx. If the trachea is not anesthetized, the cough reflex is maintained if foreign bodies are inhaled. During bronchoscopy, all resuscitative equipment must be readily available, along with skilled personnel. A gentle and speedy technique is necessary to avoid worsening the airway edema from manipulation.

PATIENT MANAGEMENT

Immediately following a burn, patients are often hypoxic, hypercapnic, and acidotic. The first therapy is the administration of a high concentration of oxygen and clinical resuscitation. As patient assessment continues, the extent of the inhalational injury is determined and, if present, treatment is begun immediately. If the injury is mild and there are no signs or symptoms of respiratory obstruction, then an approach of careful observation may be employed.[47] Fluid resuscitation is continued and humidified, oxygen-enriched air is given. Patients with moderate airway injury with minimal signs of airway narrowing may also be managed conservatively. However, these patients must be watched very closely, and the ability to secure their airways rapidly must be readily available. Nebulized racemic epinephrine 0.5%, 0.5 mL in 2 mL normal saline, may be a useful adjunct in treating mucosal edema. It must be stressed that if there is any doubt about the ability to maintain a patent airway, early tracheal intubation should be performed.[48]

Fiberoptic assessment of the airway is now becoming commonplace in the early management of inhalational injury. The use of the bronchoscope serves a dual role. In diagnostic procedures, the presence of erythema, ulceration, and luminal narrowing is distinctly documented. If intubation is necessary, then the trachea can be intubated at the same time.[43]

The patient with a severe airway burn or inhalational injury must be dealt with rapidly and thoroughly. Respiratory failure may rapidly overtake the victim due to increasing airflow resistance from edema (of the airway, face, chest wall, etc) or bronchospasm. If stridor, severe dyspnea, excessive tachypnea, or impending respiratory failure is imminent, the trachea should be intubated. In these circumstances or whenever there is doubt as to the severity of the injury, it is prudent to intubate the trachea. This is also true in cases of extensive facial burns. Prophylactic intubation virtually eliminates fatal obstructions of the upper airway in the 72 hours following an injury.[48]

Fluid Resuscitation

Burns cause capillary leaks that can lead to the profound hypovolemia seen when the burned area is greater than 20%.[49] Children are at risk with burns as small as 10%.[50] This fluid shift causes a decrease in cardiac output, a decrease in organ perfusion, and initially an increase in blood viscosity. Fluid replacement is now relatively well understood in burn therapy; as a result, the major problem is edema formation. Edema formation may decrease perfusion in burned areas, resulting in a diminution of blood flow. This can result in the death of cells that would have been viable if the only damage had been thermal injury. Unfortunately, airway edema is often made worse with aggressive fluid therapy.[51]

The aim of fluid resuscitation is to provide adequate circulating volume while minimizing edema formation.[52] These aims are proving increasingly important, because early operative intervention is now common. It has been shown that fluid retention greater than 4500 mL/m² total body surface area (TBSA)/48 h is an accurate predictor of mortality.[53] The development of edema varies depending on the damage to tissue. Immediately following the burn, blood flow is decreased to the tissues; therefore, significant edema does not develop until adequate fluid resuscitation has begun. During the period of resuscitation, edema gradually reaches a peak over 8 to 12 hours, providing that resuscitation is adequate. Also, fluid retention occurs in uninjured tissue as a result of a reduced oncotic pressure secondary to hypoproteinemia and capillary leak.[42, 52] Fluid resuscitation therapies using both crystalloid and colloid solutions are used. The amounts of fluid used are determined by the weight of the patient and the percent of the body surface burned.

Formulae to Guide Fluid Resuscitation

Several formulae are available to guide clinicians in managing patients with extensive burns; the most commonly used are:

Brooke: 1.5 mL crystalloid/kg/% burn/24 h
0.5 mL colloid/kg/% burn/24 h
2000 mL 5% dextrose 24 h
Parkland: 4 mL crystalloid/kg/% burn/24 h
Hypertonic lactated saline: This fluid is used in patients admitted in shock to restore volume and perfusion rapidly. The volume infused is adjusted to promote a urine flow of 0.5 ml/h with a solution containing 300 mEq/L sodium, 200 mEq/L lactate, and 100 mEq/L chloride.[25]

The aim of fluid resuscitation is to restore adequate organ perfusion. Due to a generalized capillary leak, it is believed by some that the administration of colloid-containing solutions is not beneficial, because the albumin would be lost to the interstitial space. It must be understood that these formulae are only guidelines. The most important aspect is that the patient be monitored closely and perfusion of tissues, urine output, hemodynamic stability, and edema formation be constantly monitored.[54]

Evaporative losses are greatly increased in burn patients and may be estimated by evaporative loss (mL/h) = (25 + % TBSA burn × TBSA) where TBSA = total body surface area. In a 70-kg patient with a 50% burn, this would lead to a loss of 125 mL/h.

In an effort to restrict the amount of fluid needed in resuscitation and therefore reduce edema, hypertonic and colloidal-based formulae have been used. When using the hypertonic solution in the elderly, hemodynamic stability and reasonable urine output were maintained.[55] Using this regimen, a reduced amount of fluid is necessary to resuscitate the patient and the time taken is less. Albumin can also be added to the solution to decrease the sodium load.[56] The serum sodium and osmolality must be monitored; if they rise above 160 mEq/L or 340 mOsm/L, respectively, lactated Ringer's solution should be substituted.

In some patients, the fluid requirements greatly exceed the volumes predicted by the formula. These patients have a poor prognosis.[57] Controversy surrounds the ideal fluid regimen, and some data show that burn victims who receive a combination of crystalloid and albumin in their resuscitation exhibit greater hemodynamic stability.[58] Therefore, centers often use a mixture of crystalloid and colloid solutions in their practice.

Endotracheal Intubation

In determining whether a patient needs tracheal intubation, many factors must be considered. Is respiratory failure imminent? Is there a worry that developing edema will lead to airway obstruction?[59] Also, associated injuries such as a head injury, flail chest, or the need to proceed to the operating room may determine the need for tracheal intubation.[13] However, in the burned patient, one must expect deterioration because it may occur rapidly, over the course of a few hours. Therefore, it is wiser to err on the side of caution and intubate when conditions are more amenable to success, rather than face an emergency later.[48] The most important aspects of the procedure are that an experienced person perform the intubation and that as thorough preparations are made as time allows. Intubation may be performed traditionally or by using a fiberoptic bronchoscope. The choice between fiberoptic and laryngoscopic intubation depends on the experience of the attending physician. If he or she is familiar with a fiberoptic bronchoscope, that would be the route of choice, because it provides diagnostic information. However, if he or she is not experienced with the fiberscope or if respiratory obstruction is imminent, then direct laryngoscopy and intubation is preferable.

Regardless of the route, certain equipment and preparations must be present to prepare for the worst possible scenario.[60]

Face Masks. Sterile face masks of various sizes must be readily available. The soft, transparent type provides the best seal to a swollen face. A transparent mask may also allow earlier detection of vomiting.

Laryngoscopes. A variety of types and sizes of laryngoscopes are necessary. A Macintosh type is the most popular blade for most clinicians. However, exposure is often better with a straight (Miller) blade. A straight blade is also commonly used in children due to the seemingly more anterior position of the larynx and floppy epiglottis. The choice depends on the operator, although it is prudent to have both types available.

Endotracheal Tubes. Tubes of several size must be immediately available. Often, the presence of edema has already narrowed the lumen of the airway. This makes the passage of the normal-sized tube impossible. Often, it is necessary to use a cuffed tube, even in children, because high inflation pressures may be needed. If the inflation pressures needed for ventilation are not raised, then the cuff can be deflated. Another advantage of a cuffed tube is greater protection from aspiration. In small children under 2 years of age, an adequate seal is usually possible without a cuffed tube. A stylet may make the intubation easier.

Oral and Nasal Airways. Sterile airways should always be available.

Positive Pressure Ventilation and a High Concentration of Oxygen. Optimally, this is provided via an anesthetic machine. However, if this is not available, an Ambu bag with an extension and oxygen is acceptable for emergencies. The provision of high inspiratory pressures may be difficult.

Suction. Suction apparatus and catheters must be readily available. Secretions are increased following inhalational injuries and aspiration is an ever-present threat in trauma situations.

Other Instruments/Materials. Other instruments and materials to have available include Magill forceps, nasogastric tubes, and stylet/gum elastic bougies.

Drugs. Antisialagogues are strongly recommended whether fiberoptic or traditional intubation is attempted. Airway manipulation increases the already profuse secretions in the burned patient.

Short-acting intravenous induction agents such as propofol, thiopental sodium, or methohexital are used to provide anesthesia, if required.

Muscle Relaxation. The use of suxamethonium (succinylcholine) during the first 24 hours following a burn is not known to cause hyper-kalemia.[61] However, most clinicians use the intermediate-acting relaxants atracurium or vecuronium.[62]

Before tracheal intubation is performed, the patient should be in optimum condition. Obviously, if the need for airway securement is urgent, intubation must proceed as an emergency. Ideally, cardiovascular stability must be assured before intubation is attempted. Resuscitation must be underway and adequate intravenous access is imperative. Monitoring should be in place before starting. If hydration is well established and hemodynamic perturbations due to hypovolemia are not present, patient care is much easier.

During intubation or bronchoscopy, hypoxia must be avoided. Prior to airway manipulation, 100% oxygen should be administered.[41] This allows for the largest margin of safety once the procedure begins. A pulse oximeter is invaluable as part of the monitoring of a patient's oxygenation. This allows a constant reference to the patient's oxygen saturation and assists in providing an early warning if the saturation begins to fall.

Analgesia is often necessary for burned patients. Sedation also is probably needed if bronchoscopy is to be performed. While the patient is breathing 100% oxygen, incremental doses of morphine can be judicially given. A starting dose of 0.1 mg/kg is usually used, with an increasing dose up to 0.5 mg/kg. It is also prudent to include an antisialogogue as part of the premedication prior to intubation (atropine 0.01 mg/kg or glycopyrrolate 0.005 mg/kg). If further sedation is needed, small doses of midazolam (0.05 mg/kg) or diazepam (0.1 mg/kg) may be used.

After sedation, it is useful to ascertain whether ventilation is possible with a tight-fitting face mask and the administration of positive pressure. If so, it makes the administration of anesthesia and the use of muscle relaxants much less worrisome.

A short-acting anesthetic may be given intravenously as ventilation is assessed. If doubt exists as to the ability to ventilate the patient, then a gaseous induction or an awake fiberoptic intubation should be considered. Suctioning the airway at this time gives an indication as to the patient's anesthetic level; if the patient coughs, swallows, or exhibits a sympathetic response, either further intravenous agents may be given or a volatile agent may be added. If the ventilation can be assumed by the anesthetist, muscular relaxation can be achieved. It is our practice to use relatively large doses of atracurium (0.6 mg/kg) or vecuronium (0.12 mg/kg).[62, 63]

The burned patient is as likely as any trauma patient to have a full stomach. Regurgitation and aspiration are both likely; therefore, cricoid pressure should be applied throughout the intubation procedure. Laryngoscopy is carried out in the burn patient as in the normal patient; however, attention to detail and position is paramount, because edema, facial trauma, and the risk of desaturation and aspiration may make the task more difficult. The task must be accomplished rapidly but without further injury to already damaged tissue. Edematous tissue may require slightly more pressure than usual, and again a stylet in the tube may be useful. Laryngeal manipulation via external pressure may be helpful.

Once the tracheal tube is in position, its placement should be checked by auscultation and, if possible, by the presence of CO_2 on exhalation.[64] A chest radiograph should also be performed following intubation. The tube must be secured properly to avoid accidental extubation. It is a tragedy to obtain an airway only to lose it when the edema is at its peak. Adhesive tape is inadequate; a soft tape (Harrington) is tied around the tube and then at the back of the head. The tape must be well padded and the tension checked regularly as the edema progresses; as the swelling occurs, the tape may cut into the face of the patient.

At this point, a stomach tube can be passed, usually via the nasal route. The stomach is emptied and abdominal distention secondary to an ileus is ameliorated.

Once the airway is secure, routine physiotherapy must begin.[65] Sloughing of the mucosa leads to obstruction of the bronchi and atelectasis. This must be avoided, and chest physiotherapy must be aggressive. Patients with alveolar injury are at risk of developing noncardiac pulmonary edema. This is due to a disruption of the alveolar–capillary membrane. The edema may form within minutes of intubation due to loss of natural positive end-expiratory pressure (PEEP) provided by the glottic structures. Resolution is usually obtained by providing continuous positive airway pressure (CPAP) or PEEP.[66]

Fiberoptic Bronchoscopy

Bronchoscopy is employed in the treatment of respiratory burns as a diagnostic procedure and as a means of performing intubation of the trachea. Repeated follow-up examination of the airway using flexible bronchoscopy may avoid intubation in some patients.[29]

Fiberoptic bronchoscopy does need good preparation. The patient must be calm, and the mucosa lining the route chosen for endoscopy must be adequately anesthetized. Many endoscopists prefer to have the patient sitting up and facing the operator. If the patient's condition will tolerate it, sedation and analgesia are used.

The more patent nostril is anesthetized with a mixture of lignocaine 4% and phenylephrine. This solution is applied to pledgets and gradually inserted into the nares. This provides local anesthesia and vasoconstriction of the mucosa.

A Guedel airway coated with lignocaine jelly 5% is given to the patient to suck and, as the tongue and palate become anesthetized, the airway can be advanced into the oropharynx and onto the posterior aspect of the tongue. A nebulizer mask with lignocaine 4% solution is given to the patient to breathe during this time. This provides a means of anesthetizing the respiratory mucosa down to the level of the vocal cords. Once adequate surface analgesia is complete, a gentle examination is conducted. Extreme care is called for, because the mucosa may be friable. An endotracheal tube should be in position on the bronchoscope should intubation be necessary. The mucosa is examined for hyperemia, bearing in mind that if resuscitation is in the early stages, the mucosa may still be vasoconstricted. Sloughing, soot particles, and hemorrhagic areas are all documented. If an area of the respiratory tract is not adequately anesthetized, particularly the cords or trachea, then lignocaine may be injected down the bronchoscope. Throughout the examination, oxygen should be given both through the bronchoscope channel and, if necessary, via nasal cannulae. Monitoring should continue, with particular care being paid to the pulse oximeter. When performing a bronchoscopy on an injured patient, there must always be trained personnel with the endoscopists to continue treating and evaluating the patient. If during the examination significant airway edema, necrosis, or other damage is seen, it is prudent to prophylactically intubate the trachea,[48] because respiratory causes of death are rare in intubated patients in the first 72 hours.

If the fiberoptic assessment shows minimal mucosal damage and if this is coupled with minimal flow–volume abnormalities, then a conservative approach may be taken.[37] How-ever, vigilance must be maintained, because deterioration may be precipitous.

Route for Tracheal Intubation

Tracheal intubation is usually easier to perform via the oral route, as opposed to the nasal route. The oral route is more common and, as such, the practitioner is usually more skilled in this approach. There is more room for manipulation of the tube in an oral approach. Swelling of the oral and nasal mucosa may limit the airway passages and make intubation, either orally or nasally, more difficult. Nasal intubation has several obvious drawbacks: bleeding is more likely from the nasal mucosa; it is often a technically more challenging procedure; and if swelling or anatomic conditions are unfavorable, it may not be possible. However, if intubation is expected to be prolonged or the conditions for nasal intubation are met, then there are several advantages. The presence of a nasal tube appears to be more easily tolerated by the patient, tube fixation is better, and the tube is not chewed on by the patient. Also, less laryngeal complications are seen following nasal intubation. Ulcerations of the laryngeal cartilage and posterior tracheal wall with incomplete laryngeal closing are seen following tube removal; this is thought to be due to tube movement. Because nasal intubation decreases tube movement, the incidence is diminished.[67, 68]

The usual order is to perform tracheal intubation via the oral route first, and change to a nasal route electively. If the initial intubation was difficult or swelling is problematic, then a tube change should wait until the patient is stable, the edema has subsided, or maybe not at all. Once a patient has been intubated, it is of paramount importance to maintain an adequate degree of sedation and analgesia for both comfort and tolerance of the tube. If orotracheal intubation has proven to be difficult and the tube needs to be changed to a nasal one, then extreme care must be taken not to jeopardize the patient while effecting the change.

In changing the tracheal tube, a fiberoptic technique is probably the most appropriate in the modern hospital setting.[43] The change may be necessary due to a damaged cuff, a tube that is small and becoming continuously obstructed, or a size that does not allow bronchoscopy through it. However, the most common reason for changing an oral tube to a nasal one is for long-term ventilation.

The conscious patient has the procedure explained to him or her, and then appropriate sedation is given to suppress the pharyngeal and laryngeal reflexes. The larger and more patent nostril should be prepared with either cocaine or a mixture of lignocaine and phenylephrine. Once the nostril is prepared, the tracheal tube is gently advanced into the pharynx. The fiberoptic bronchoscope is lubricated and advanced through the nasal tube. At our institution, we administer oxygen through the suction channel of the bronchoscope. This serves two functions: it allows for passive oxygenation during the time when the tube exchange is occurring, and secretions are blown away from the tip of the scope. The oral tube is lying in the posterior aspect of the larynx, thus leaving the anterior aspect of the glottic area open. The bronchoscope is manipulated to enter the trachea through the gap in the anterior aspect. In the awake patient, topical anesthesia may be applied to the larynx before entering the trachea. The fiberscope is then advanced into the trachea, anterior to the tube in place, and the cuff of the oral tube is deflated as the bronchoscope is advanced until the bifurcation of the trachea is identified. At this point, the orotracheal tube is removed and the nasal tube is threaded over the fiberoptic bronchoscope.

The advantages of changing the tube in this manner are that sedation requirements are less than needed for a conventional laryngoscopy and intubation, ventilation is interrupted for a only a short time, and tube placement may be confirmed.

Difficult Intubation

The keys to successful intubation are familiarity with the necessary equipment and assiduous preparation of the patient.[69] In most burn victims, this is sufficient to ensure a successful outcome. Occasionally, however, the edema and other injuries may be such as to make direct tracheal intubation practically impossible to perform. The patient may also have a preexisting condition (eg, ankylosing spondylitis) that makes intubation difficult. When faced a with a patient where difficulties with intubation are anticipated, a methodical approach must be taken and no maneuver performed that is irrevocable.

Difficult intubations may be the result of head and neck positioning; limited mouth opening; and in burns, swelling and edema of the upper airway passages. Presently, the most appropriate technique in experienced hands is fiberoptic intubation. The route of choice is via the nose, with the tracheal tube inserted into a prepared nostril and the fiberoptic bronchoscope advanced through the tube into the trachea. Once the trachea is entered, the tube is slid into the trachea.

Direct laryngoscopy can be as successful as fiberoptic intubation when experienced personnel are present. A variety of laryngoscope blades should be available and positioning of the patient must be optimal. Often, a difficult visualization may be overcome with a straight blade or repositioning. Stylets are useful for maintaining a curve on the tube and for aiding in gently maneuvering a tube through edematous tissue.

Blind nasal intubation is employed in cases where limited mouth opening and poor visualization is a problem. In these situations, maintaining spontaneous ventilation greatly increases the success; it is often helpful to lift the mandible forward.

The lightwand (Tube Stat, Concept Corporation, Clearwater, FL) is a battery-operated lighted stylet that can be used to aid intubation. The tube is placed over the lightwand and the distal end of the stylet is hooked. The lightwand is switched on and the lighted stylet is placed into the trachea after anesthesia is induced. A transilluminated glow is seen through the skin over the cricothyroid region as the light enters the trachea. The tube is then threaded into the trachea.[69]

The laryngeal mask airway (LMA) has been used in several occasions for both anticipated and unexpected difficult airways.[70–73] It is inserted after the induction of general anesthesia or adequate topical anesthesia to the upper airway. Once an adequate airway is established, the LMA is used as a route to facilitate tracheal intubation. The LMA is not sufficient as an airway alone, because laryngeal and vocal cord edema may lead to obstruction.

Retrograde translaryngeal guide wire intubation may be used. Following percutaneous needle puncture of the cricothyroid membrane, a flexible introducer wire is threaded cranially and grasped in the oropharynx.[74] A tracheal tube is then advanced over the wire as it is held under tension. Alternatively, the wire can be used as a guide for a fiberoptic bronchoscope.

If the intubation fails unexpectedly, every effort must be made to ensure adequate oxygenation during and between attempts of intubation.

Emergency criocothyroidotomy or tracheostomy is usually a last resort. A 12- to 14-gauge cannula can be inserted through the cricothyroid membrane and oxygen insufflated through it. The barrel of a 3-mL syringe is attached to the cannula and an 8-mm endotracheal tube adaptor can be inserted into the syringe.[75] There are now commercially available kits that are used for this purpose.

It must be emphasized that emergency tracheostomy or cricothyroid punctures are less than optimal; frequently, what unfortunately becomes a failed intubation may not have been if a more experienced operator had been available. If this awful scenario arises, then at least transtracheal insufflation should be employed until a surgical attempt at tracheostomy is attempted.

COMPLICATIONS OF PROLONGED INTUBATION

Complications considered to be of minor consequence in other patients may have devastating results in a patient with thermal injury.

Trauma resulting from intubation may be immediate or may result from the prolonged presence of a foreign body. During intubation, complications may arise concerning the cervical spine, direct trauma to the pharynx and larynx, nosebleeds, tracheal or bronchial rupture, and tooth damage.[76]

Some of the complications of prolonged nasotracheal intubation follow.

Obstruction of the Tube. This may occur due to external pressure or internal obstruction. Kinking may be present, or the patient may be biting or chewing on the tube. Internal causes are secretions, blood, or possibly foreign bodies.[77]

Erosion of the Nasal Arches or the Septum. This type of complication can be avoided by using smaller sized tubes made of softer material.[78] Sloughing of the nasal bridge can be prevented by careful positioning and by avoiding pressure on the nasal structures. Alternating the nares is helpful, if possible.

Sinusitis. Sinusitis can be the cause of unexplained fever in patients with a nasotracheal intubation.[79] If ultrasound is used, it can be shown that within 3 days 30% of patients nasally intubated developed a sinus effusion.[80]

Blocking of the Auditory Tube. Because the auditory (eustachian) tube opens into the nasal cavity, its blockade can lead to middle ear infection.

Erosion of Pharyngeal and Laryngeal Structures. The avoidance of these complications is extremely difficult in a patient with severe respiratory burns. Every effort needs to be made to avoid trauma, guard against infection, and use tubes that are designed to conform to respiratory tract anatomy.[81]

Incidence of Pneumonia. Intubation and mechanical ventilation can predispose to nosocomial pneumonia via several mechanisms. These include reduced local defenses, airway injury, direct organism entry into the lung, mucociliary dysfunction, and others.[82]

Tracheo-esophageal Fistula. This is a dreadful complication, the most probable cause of which is high inflation pressure in the cuff of the endotracheal tube. Ideally, the cuff should be inflated with the minimum amount of air to allow ventilation. The pulmonary status of the patient may, however, require high inflation pressures, and high pressures may be needed to allow ventilation. A contributory factor in the development of tracheo-esophageal fistula is the presence of a nasogastric tube; the soft swollen tissues compressed between this and an endotracheal tube are liable to necrosis and sloughing. The use of soft (Silastic) nasogastric tubes may help to avoid this complication.[77]

Once this condition is established, it becomes extremely difficult to treat. A gastrostomy precludes the need for a nasogastric tube; if the communication is high, a tracheotomy might be indicated. Alternatively, high-frequency ventilation can be used. The complete repair of this complication is deferred until all the wounds are healed.[83]

Erosion of Vascular Structures. This is a rare and catastrophic complication following prolonged endotracheal intubation. Erosion of the tracheal wall by the end of the tube may perforate the innominate artery, leading to exsanguination. Death is usually the outcome.[84]

PROLONGED NASOTRACHEAL INTUBATION OR TRACHEOTOMY

Even as recently as 10 to 15 years ago, tracheostomy was performed whenever the need for endotracheal intubation was expected to persist for more than 2 days.[85] Tracheostomy was originally used to obtain an airway in an emergency; however, now it is primarily used for control of secretions and where long-term ventilation is envisioned.[83] The availability of less irritating endotracheal tube materials and improved tube/cuff designs have since allowed progressively longer periods of translaryngeal intubation. Nowadays, 3 weeks or more would not be considered an unusually long period of intubation.[86]

Each route carries its own complications. Follow-up studies on patients with nonthermal prolonged intubation have shown a higher incidence of tracheal stenosis after tracheotomy[87]; it is actually three times higher than in patients treated with endotracheal intubation alone. The presence of tracheal dilation and subsequent tracheomalacia may be an early sign of impending problems of stenosis. The injuries reported from endotracheal intubation are due mostly to high cuff pressures,[68] whereas the stenosis following tracheotomies is mostly cicatricial, with the stenosis occurring at the site of surgery. Cuff pressure injuries are also seen with tracheostomies.[83] In general, the use of high-volume, low-pressure cuffs with low tracheal loading forces decreases but does not abolish the incidence of cuff-related injuries.[88, 77] In small children, uncuffed tubes with larger internal diameters can be usefully employed beyond the nondistensible cricoid cartilage, the result being less airway resistance.[26] In the severely burned child, however, cuffed tubes are more frequently used because of the need for higher airway pressures.

Glottic stenosis can follow endotracheal intubation, even after an interval as short as 24 hours. In burned patients, complications are more frequent and severe with tracheotomy than with translaryngeal intubation.[89, 90] Several factors contribute to this. Tracheotomy performed rapidly in emergency situations is liable to be complicated. Tracheostomy is ideally performed in a controlled situation, because there are complications arising from the surgery itself. Hemorrhage occurs in 1% to 37% of cases, and even minor bleeding may be life threatening if it interferes with tracheal identification. Pneumothorax, tracheoesophageal fistula, recurrent laryngeal nerve damage, and severe wound infections have all been documented. In an emergency, the procedure is likely to be done quickly, in the face of aggravating, even uncontrollable circumstances. When performed through burned skin or a damaged tracheal wall, the incision may easily become contaminated and necrosis may develop. Bronchial-based pulmonary sepsis is also very prevalent, particularly if the procedure is performed through the burn eschar.[82] Because of these deleterious and possibly fatal complications, tracheotomy is avoided as much

as possible in burned patients. It is much more preferable to maintain translaryngeal intubation as long as possible. If tracheotomy has to be performed, it should be delayed until burns at and near the site have healed. Late complications of tracheostomy include tracheal stenosis, tracheo-esophageal strictures, vascular erosion, and tracheocutaneous fistula.[83]

Extubation

The optimum time for extubation trachea is a matter of clinical judgment. Several criteria should be taken into account before proceeding to extubation.

1. The general condition of the patient should be carefully assessed. Mental status, cardiovascular stability, and lack of sepsis should be investigated.
2. Respiratory status must be carefully assessed.
3. Edema should have resolved. Extubation in the presence of facial, neck, or laryngeal edema is not advised.
4. Air leak around the endotracheal tube: on cuff deflation, if an air leak is present, the implication is that tracheal edema is subsiding.
5. Secretions: if purulent, excessive, or sooty secretions are present, a delay of extubation is wise. Pulmonary toilet may be better accomplished with an endotracheal tube.[82]
6. Clearing of pulmonary infiltrates: although an absolutely clear lung is not to be expected, prominent infiltrates are a contraindication to extubation.
7. Weaning: the advent of newer ventilators allows the transition of fully controlled ventilation to assisted ventilation to be achieved gradually, eventually with the patient on pressure support and then reduced to CPAP immediately prior to extubation.
8. Liaison: extubation is unnecessary if the patient is going to the operating room the next day.

MANAGEMENT OF BURN INJURIES IN THE RECONSTRUCTIVE STAGES

During healing, scar tissue is formed. Scars eventually contract, causing contracture deformities. In some areas of the body, the deformities result in either functional disability or cosmetically unacceptable scars; in the head and neck, the scars may be so severe as to compromise the airway. A special challenge is thus presented to the anesthesiologist.

Preoperative Evaluation

A thorough examination should be made, as in any patient presenting for surgery; however, the airway and sequelae resulting from burn injuries must be addressed.

The history pertaining to the airway needs to be obtained in detail. The presence of snoring needs to be elicited and whether episodes of periodic breathing occur. Obviously, this information is obtained from parents, spouses, or friends. Snoring may be an indicator of obstructive sleep apnea.[91] Chronic peripheral airway disease, although uncommon in these patients, is occasionally encountered with marked obstructive lung disease or bronchiolitis obliterans.[92]

The mouth opening must carefully evaluated. This gives an indication of type of laryngoscope blade to use and may be a portent to difficulty of intubation. Dentition should be noted, and the presence of caps and crowns documented.

The nares should be examined for patency. If a nasotracheal tube or a nasal airway needs to be inserted, the wider and more patent nostril is used.

A fixed, contracted neck makes intubation difficult, because extension of the head is not possible. The contractures may make mouth opening possible during neck flexion, but not during extension. A guide to difficulty is the thyroid mental distance. If the space is less than two finger breadths, expect difficulty.

Radiographs, scans, and occasionally tomograms or MRI of the trachea help to visualize stenosis or deviation.[83]

Preoperative Medication

Induction of anesthesia in patients where a difficult airway is expected is usually by an inhalation technique. Narcotics are avoided or used in a very careful manner. Anxiolytics, such as benzodiazepines, are often used. Often, H_2 receptor blockers such as cimetidine or ranitidine are used to decrease stomach acidity. Aspiration may occur during a difficult intubation due to the frequent need for positive pressure ventilation with a face mask and the almost inevitable gastric distention. Adequate hydration is important, particularly if a gaseous induction of anesthesia is planned. An intravenous line placed preoperatively allows adequate hydration and the opportunity to titrate sedation to the needs of the patient.

Anesthetic Management

There is no place in the preparation of the patient with a potentially difficult airway for lack of planning. Understanding of the planned procedure and availability of surgical colleagues should surgical intervention be necessary is mandatory.

Gaseous Induction. An inhalation induction allows constant assessment of the airway and, should obstruction occur, the patient is allowed to wake up.

Antisialagogue. Burn patients often have excessive secretions. A drying agent is useful in that it diminishes these secretions and diminishes the irritation of the airways during induction.

Adequate Depth of Anesthesia. It is imperative not to attempt manipulation of the airway until an adequate anesthetic level has been reached. Premature attempts at laryngoscopy or airway insertion may provoke coughing, breath holding, or laryngospasm.

Oxygenation. Hypoxia must be assiduously avoided. Throughout induction and airway manipulation, oxygenation should be monitored with a pulse oximeter.

Manipulation of the Tongue. In patients with severe contractures around the mouth, the tongue may cause obstruction and thus limit one's ability to manipulate the laryngoscope. Pulling the tongue out with gauze or even using a tongue stitch might prove very useful.

Stylet. Shaping the stylet after a preliminary look is often the best approach.

Fiberoptic Laryngoscope.[69] In experienced hands, this is an extremely valuable instrument. It is important to remember, however, that in some patients previous scarring may make it difficult to discern anatomic features.

Laryngeal Mask Airway.[70] The LMA is a useful device in patients where limited mouth opening or neck extension is present. The LMA is inserted without visualization blindly into the hypopharynx using local anesthesia, or under general anesthesia following a gaseous induction or an induction with propofol. Once the airway is established, the case may proceed or intubation through the mask may be performed in a controlled fashion.[93, 94]

Assistance from Surgeons. If contractures and scarring are severe, it is reasonable to start the anesthesia with a face mask; once a satisfactory anesthetic level is established, the surgeon can incise the neck and partially release the contracture. Endotracheal intubation can then be attempted.

Fixation of the Endotracheal Tube. In some situations, securing the endotracheal tube by a stainless steel wire to one of the teeth or suturing the tube is extremely helpful.

Extubation. Extubation should be performed once the patient is awake and able to protect his or her own airway.

Some surgical procedures do not need intubation. In those patients where this is true, yet the airway is thought to be difficult, ketamine can be useful,[95] or the LMA might be employed.

References

1. Accident Facts. Chicago: National Safety Council, 1988.
2. Coleman DL. Smoke inhalation. West J Med 1981;135:300.
3. Cahalane M, Demling RH. Early respiratory abnormalities from smoke inhalation. JAMA 251:771–773, 1984.
4. Crapo RO. Smoke inhalation injuries. JAMA 246:1694–1696, 1981.
5. Agee RN, Long JM, Hunt JL, Petroff PA, Lull RJ, Mason AD Jr, Pruitt BA Jr. Use of 133 Xenon in early diagnosis of inhalation injury. J Trauma 16:218–224, 1976.
6. Peters WJ. Inhalation injury caused by the products of combustion. Can Med Assoc J 125:249–252, 1981.
7. Cohen MA, Guzzardi LJ. Inhalation of products of combustion. Ann Emerg Med 12:628–632, 1983.
8. Terrill JB, Montgomery RR, Reinhardt CF. Toxic gases from fires. Science 200:1343–1347, 1978.
9. Dyer RF, Esch VH. Polyvinyl chloride toxicity in fires: Hydrogen chloride toxicity in fire fighters. JAMA 235:393–397, 1976.
10. Baud FJ, Barriot P, Toffis V, Riou B, Vicaut E, Lacarpentier Y, Bourdon R, Astier A, Bismuth C. Elevated blood cyanide concentrations in victims of smoke inhalation. N Engl J Med 325:1761–1802, 1991.
11. Püschel K, Mätzsch T, Brinkmann B. Clinical course and morphological findings after inhalation scalding. Unfallheikunde 83:592–598, 1980.
12. Davies JWL. Challenges for the future in burn research and burn care. The 1990 A. B. Wallace Memorial Lecture. Burns 17:25–32, 1991.
13. Grande CM, Stene JK, Bernhard WN. Airway management: Considerations in the trauma patient. Crit Care Clin 6:37–59, 1990.
14. Zellner PR. The 1990 Everett Idris Evans Memorial Lecture: The inhalation injury. J Burn Care Rehabil 11:487–495, 1990.
15. Formosa PJ, Waxman K. Inhalation injuries in burn patients. Hospital Physician July:69–82, 1986.
16. Kinsella J, Carter R, Reid W, Campbell D, Clark CJ. Increased airways reactivity after smoke inhalation. Lancet 337:595–596, 1991.
17. Pruitt BA, Cioffi WG, Shimazu T, Ikeuchi H, Mason AD. Evaluation and management of patients with inhalation injury. J Trauma 30:S63–S68, 1990.
18. Trunkey DD. Inhalation injury. Surg Clin North Am 58:1133–1140, 1978.
19. Barrow RE, Morris SE, Basadre JE, Herndon DN. Selective permeability changes in the lungs and airways of sheep after toxic smoke inhalation. J Appl Physiol 68:2165–2170, 1990.
20. Clarke WR, Bonaventura M, Myers W, Kellman R. Smoke inhalation and airway management at a regional burn unit: 1974 to 1983. II: Airway management. J Burn Care Rehabil 11:121–134, 1990.
21. Heidemann SM, Goetting MG. Treatment of acute hypoxemic respiratory failure caused by chlorine exposure. Pediatr Emerg Care 7:87–88, 1991.
22. Mayes RW. The toxicological examination of the victims of the British Air Tours Boeing 737 accident at Manchester in 1985. J Forensic Sci 36:179–184, 1991.
23. Coté CJ, Todres ID. The pediatric airway. In Ryan JF, Todres ID, Coté CJ, Goudsouzian NG (eds). A Practice of Anesthesia for Infants and Children. Orlando: Grune & Stratton, 1985; p. 35.
24. Haponik EF, Munster AM, Wise RA, Smith PL, Meyers DA, Britt EJ, Bleeker ER. Upper airway function in burn patients. Correlation of flow–volume curves and nasopharyngoscopy. Am Rev Resp Dis 129:251–257, 1984.
25. Welch GW. Care of the patient with thermal injury. In Capan LM, Miller SM, Turndorf H (eds). Trauma Anesthesia and Intensive Care. Philadelphia: J. B. Lippincott, 1991; pp. 629–648.
26. Madden MR, Finkelstein JL, Goodwin CW. Respiratory care of the burn patient. Clin Plast Surg 13:29–38, 1986.
27. Asch MD, Messerol PM, Mason AD Jr, Pruitt BA. Regional blood flow in the burned anaesthetized dog. Surg Forum 22:55–56, 1971.
28. Goodwin CW, Dorethy J, Lam V, Pruitt BA Jr. Randomized trial of efficacy of crystalloid and colloid resuscitation on hemodynamic response and lung water following thermal injury. Ann Surg 197:520–529, 1983.
29. Moylan JA. Smoke inhalation and burn injury. Surg Clin North Am 60:1533–1540, 1980.
30. Genovesi M. Transient hypoxemia in firemen following inhalation of smoke. Chest 71:41–44, 1977.
31. Heimbach DM, Waeckerle JF. Inhalation injuries. Ann Emerg Med 17:1316–1320, 1988.
32. Barker SJ, Tremper KK. The effect of carbon monoxide inhalation on pulse oximetry and transcutaneous PO_2. Anesthesiology 66:677–679, 1987.
33. Demling RH, LaLonde C. Moderate smoke inhalation produces decreased oxygen delivery, increased oxygen demands, and systemic but not lung parenchymal lipid peroxidation. Surgery 108:544–552, 1990.
34. Clark WR, Bonaventura M, Myers W. Smoke inhalation and airway management at a regional burn unit: 1974–1983. I: Diagnosis and consequences of smoke inhalation. J Burn Care Rehabil 10:52–62, 1989.
35. Holliman CJ, Saffle JR, Kravitz M, Warden GD. Early surgical decompression in the management of electrical injuries. Am J Surg 144:733, 1982.

36. Whitener DR, Whitener LM, Robertson KF, Baxter CR, Pierce AK. Pulmonary function measurements in patients with thermal injury and smoke inhalation. Ann Rev Resp Dis 122:731–739, 1980.

37. Haponik EF, Meyers DA, Munster AM, Smith PL, Britt EJ, Wise RA, Bleeker ER. Acute upper airway injury in burn patients. Serial changes of flow–volume curves and nasopharyngoscopy. Am Rev Respir Dis 135:360–366, 1987.

38. Moylan JA Jr, Wilmore DW, Mouton DE, Pruitt BA Jr. Early diagnosis of inhalation injury using [133]xenon lung scan. Ann Surg 176:477, 1972.

39. Brough MD. The King's Cross fire. I: The physical injuries. Burns 17:6–9, 1991.

40. Lukan J, Sandor L, Szabo M. The importance of fiberbronchoscopy in respiratory burns. Acta Chir Plast 32:107–113, 1990.

41. Clark CJ, Reid WH, Telfer BM, Campbell D. Respiratory injury in the burned patient. The role of flexible bronchoscopy. Anaesthesia 38:35–39, 1983.

42. Kramer GC, Herdon DN, Linares HA, Traber DL. Effects of inhalation injury on airway blood flow and edema formation. J Burn Care Rehabil 10:45–51, 1989.

43. Ovassapian A. Fiberoptic airway endoscopy in critical care. In Ovassapian A (ed). Fiberoptic Airway Endoscopy in Anesthesia and Critical Care. New York: Raven Press, 1990; p. 107.

44. Noviski N, Todres D. Fiberoptic bronchoscopy in the pediatric patient. Anesth Clin North Am 9:163–174, 1991.

45. Maekawa N, Mikawa K, Tanaka O, Goto R, Obara H. The laryngeal mask may be a useful device for fiberoptic airway endoscopy in pediatric anesthesia. Anesthesiology 75:169–170, 1991.

46. Tan WC, Lee ST, Lee CN, Wong S. The role of fiberoptic bronchoscopy in the management of respiratory burns. Ann Acad Med 14:430–434, 1985.

47. Ramon PH, Wallaert B, Galizzia JP, Gesterman X, Voisin C. Tracheo-bronchial endoscopy in burns to the face. Rev Mal Resp 2:97–101, 1985.

48. Venus B, Matsuda T, Copiozo JB, Mathru M. Prophylactic intubation and continuous positive airway pressure in the management of inhalation injury in burn victims. Crit Care Med 9:519–523, 1981.

49. Anderson G. Pathophysiology of the burn wound. Ann Clin Gynecol 69:178, 1980.

50. Merrell SW, Saffle JR, Sullivan JJ, Navar PD, Kravitz M, Warden LA. Fluid resuscitation in thermally injured children. Am J Surg 152:664, 1986.

51. Haberal M. Electrical burns: A five year experience—1985 Evans Lecture. J Trauma 26:103–109, 1986.

52. Demling RH. Fluid replacement in burned patients. Surg Clin North Am 67:15–30, 1987.

53. Carlson RG, Miller SF, Finley RK Jr, Billett JM, Fegelman E, Jones LM, Alkire S. Fluid retention and burn survival. J Trauma 27:127–135, 1987.

54. Matsuda T, Clark N, Hariyani GD, Bryant RS, Hanumadass ML, Kagan RJ. The effect of burn wound size on resting energy expenditure. J Trauma 27:115–118, 1987.

55. Bowser-Wallace BH, Cone JB, Caldwell FT Jr. Hypertonic lactated saline resuscitation of severely burned patients over 60 years of age. J Trauma 25:22–26, 1985.

56. Jelenko C 3rd, Williams J, Wheeler ML, Callaway BD, Fackler VK, Albers CA, Barger AA. Studies in shock and resuscitation. I: Use of hypertonic, albumin containing fluid demand regimen (HALFD) in resuscitation. Crit Care Med 7:157–167, 1979.

57. Rosenthal SR, Hawley PL, Hakim AA. Purified burn toxin and its composition. Surgery 71:527–536, 1972.

58. Dorethy JF, Welch G, Treat RC, Mason AD, Pruitt BA. Army Institute of Surgical Report. Progress report, 1977.

59. Wald P, Balmes J. Respiratory effects of short-term, high-intensity toxic inhalations: Smoke, gases, and fumes. J Intensive Care Med 2:260–278, 1987.

60. Goudsouzian N, Szyfelbein SK. Management of upper airway following burns. In Martyn JAJ (ed). Acute Management of the Burned Patient. Philadelphia: W.B. Saunders, 1990; pp. 46–65.

61. Martyn JAJ, Goldhill DR, Goudsouzian NG. Clinical pharmacology of muscle relaxants in patients with burns. J Clin Pharm 26:680–685, 1986.

62. Goudsouzian N, Young ET, Moss J, Liu L. Histamine release during the administration of atracurium and vecuronium in children. Br J Anaesth 58:1229–1233, 1986.

63. Dwersteg JF, Pavlin EC, Haschke R, Heimbach DM, Macintyre PE. High dose atracurium does not produce hypotension in the burned patient. Anesthesiology 65:A293, 1986.

64. Denman WT, Hayes M, Higgins D, Wilkinson DJ. The Fenem CO_2 detector device. An apparatus to prevent un-noticed oesophageal intubation. Anaesthesia 45:465–467, 1990.

65. Brown JM. Respiratory complications in burned patients. Physiotherapy 63:151–153, 1977.

66. Mathru M, Venus B, Rao TLK, et al. Noncardiac pulmonary edema precipitated by tracheal intubation in patients with inhalation injury. Crit Care Med 11:804–806, 1983.

67. Dubick MN, Wright BD. Comparison of laryngeal pathology following long-term oral and nasal endotracheal intubation. Anesth Analg 57:663–668, 1978.

68. Streitz JM, Shapshay SM. Airway injury after tracheotomy and endotracheal intubation. Surg Clin North Am 71:1211–1229, 1991.

69. Ovassapian A. The difficult intubation. In Ovassapian A (ed). Fiberoptic Airway Endoscopy in Anesthesia and Critical Care. New York: Raven Press, 1990, pp. 135–151.

70. Thomson KD, Ordman AJ, Parkhouse N, Morgan BDG. Use of the Brain laryngeal mask airway in anticipation of difficult tracheal intubation. Br J Plast Surg 42:478–480, 1989.

71. Laryngeal mask airway. Lancet 338:1046–1047, 1991.

72. Russell R, Judkins KC. The laryngeal mask airway and facial burns. Anaesthesia 45:894, 1990.

73. Allison A, McCrory J. Tracheal placement of a gum elastic bougie using the laryngeal mask airway. Anaesthesia 45:419–420, 1990.

74. Tobias R. Increased success with retrograde guide for endotracheal intubation. Anesth Analg 62:366–367, 1983.

75. Stinson TW III. A simple connector for transtracheal ventilation. Anesthesiology 47:232, 1977.

76. McCulloch TM, Bishop MJ. Complications of translaryngeal intubation. Clin Chest Med 12:507–521, 1991.

77. Stone DJ, Bogdonoff DL. Airway considerations in the management of patients requiring long-term endotracheal intubation. Anesth Analg 74:276–287, 1992.

78. Zwillich C, Pierson DJ. Nasal necrosis a complication of nasotracheal intubation. Chest 64:376–379, 1973.

79. Knodell AR, Beekman JF. Unexplained fever in patients with nasotracheal intubation. JAMA 248:868–870, 1982.

80. Bowers BL, Purdue GF, Hunt JL. Paranasal sinusitis in burn patients following nasotracheal intubation. Arch Surg 126:1411–1412, 1991.
81. Eckerbom B, Lindholm CE, Alexopoulos C. Airway lesions caused by prolonged intubation with standard and with anatomically shaped tracheal tubes. A post mortem study. Acta Anaesthesiol Scand 30:366–373, 1986.
82. Levine SA, Niederman MS. The impact of tracheal intubation on host defenses and risks for nosocomial pneumonia. Clin Chest Med 12:523–540, 1991.
83. Wood DE, Mathisen DJ. Late complications of tracheotomy. Clin Chest Med 12:597–609, 1991.
84. Myers EN, Carrau MRL. Early complications of tracheotomy incidence and management. Clin Chest Med 12:589–595, 1991.
85. Bendixen HH, Egbert LD, Hedley-Whyte J, Laver MB, Pontoppidan H. Respiratory Care. St. Louis: C. V. Mosby, 1965; pp. 114–137.
86. Berlauk JF. Prolonged endotracheal intubation vs tracheostomy. Crit Care Med 14:742–745, 1986.
87. Grillo HC, Cooper JD, Geffin LB, Pontoppidan H. A low pressure cuff for tracheostomy tubes to minimize tracheal injury. A comparative clinical trial. J Thorac Cardiovasc Surg 62:898–907, 1971.
88. Stauffer JL, Olson DE, Petty TL. Complications and consequences of endotracheal intubation and tracheostomy. Am J Med 70:65–76, 1981.
89. Lund T, Goodwin CW, McManus WF, Shirani KZ, Stallings RJ, Mason AD Jr, Pruitt BA Jr. Upper airway sequelae in burn patients requiring endotracheal intubation or tracheostomy. Ann Surg 201:374–382, 1985.
90. Eckhauser FE, Billote J, Burke JF, Quinby WC. Tracheostomy complicating massive burn injuries. A plea for conservatism. Am J Surg 127:418–423, 1974.
91. Robertson CF, Zuker R, Dabrowski B, Levison H. Obstructive sleep apnea: A complication of burn to the head and neck in children. J Burn Care Rehabil 6:353–357, 1985.
92. Jaspar N, Bracamonte M, Sergysels R. Severe peripheral airway obstruction after inhalation burn. Intensive Care Med 8:105–106, 1982.
93. Benumof JL. Use of the laryngeal mask airway to facilitate fiberscope-aided tracheal intubation. Anesth Analg 74:313–315, 1992.
94. Heath ML, Allagain J. Intubation through the laryngeal mask. A technique for unexpected difficult intubation. Anaesthesia 46:545–548, 1991.
95. Jacobacci S, Towy RM. Anaesthesia for severe burn contractures of the neck. A case report. East Afr Med J 55:543–545, 1978.

CHAPTER 39

The Airway in the Obstetric Patient

Mark Weiner, D.O., Michael C. Lawlor, D.O., M.S., and Calvin Johnson, M.D.

Airway management of the parturient has serious implications for the anesthesiologist. Anesthesia-related causes, particularly an inability to accomplish endotracheal intubation, remain a significant factor in maternal morbidity and mortality.[1-3] Davies and associates[4] report a composite incidence of failed intubation in parturients to be 1 in 500, whereas Lyons[5] experienced one for every 300 general anesthetics given. This problem is frequent enough that many anesthesiologists will, at some time in their career, be confronted with this frightening situation. Thus, all anesthesiologists must be familiar with the special anesthetic and airway needs of the pregnant woman and have a planned, thought-out management scheme ready to implement in the event of a failed intubation.

ANATOMIC AND PHYSIOLOGIC CHANGES IN THE PARTURIENT

Management of the obstetric airway necessitates full knowledge of the physiologic and anatomic demands placed on the mother by the fetus. These changes have a profound impact on the safe clinical management of the parturient.

Anatomic alterations of the respiratory system are an important consequence of pregnancy. Capillary engorgement of the respiratory tree, including the nasopharynx, larynx, and vocal cords, results in mucosa that is commonly edematous and friable.[6] The edema is accentuated in parturients with pregnancy-induced hypertension (PIH) or who have had a prolonged, strenuous second stage of labor.[7-9] Cephalad displacement of the diaphragm by the expanding uterus produces a compensatory increase in anterior-posterior and transverse diameter of the chest, resulting in an overall expansion of the thoracic cage circumference of 5 to 7 cm. Diaphragmatic breathing remains unaffected. The substernal angle is broadened from 70 degrees (first trimester) to 105 degrees (term). Radiographs of the lungs exhibit increased pulmonary markings that may simulate mild congestive heart failure.

Weight gain associated with pregnancy may further exaggerate anatomic changes that interfere with airway management. This is particularly evident in the obese parturient, whose propensity for large, pendulous breasts, fat shoulders, thick neck, large chest, and limited neck extension presents an additional challenge to the anesthesiologist.[10]

Respiratory physiology is altered dramatically during pregnancy (Table 39-1, Fig. 39-1).[10] Increases in tidal volume and minute volume are due to elevated progesterone levels

Table 39–1. CHANGES IN THE RESPIRATORY SYSTEM AT TERM

Variable	Direction of Change	Average Change
Minute ventilation	↑	+50%
Alveolar ventilation	↑	+70%
Tidal volume	↑	+40%
Respiratory rate	↑	+15%
Arterial P_{O_2}	↑	+10 torr
Inspiratory lung capacity	↑	+5%
Oxygen consumption	↑	+20%
Dead space	No change	
Lung compliance (alone)	No change	
Arterial pH	No change	
Vital capacity	No change	
Closing volume	No change or ↓	
Airway resistance	↓	−36%
Total pulmonary resistance	↓	−50%
Total compliance	↓	−30%
Chest wall compliance (alone)	↓	−45%
Arterial P_{CO_2}	↓	−10 torr
Serum bicarbonate	↓	−4 mEq/L
Total lung capacity	↓	−0 to 5%
Functional residual capacity	↓	−20%
Expiratory reserve volume	↓	−20%
Residual volume	↓	−20%

From Cheek TG, Gutsche BB. Maternal physiologic alterations during pregnancy. In Shnider SM, Levinson G (eds). Anesthesia for Obstetrics, pp. 3–13; © 1987, the Williams & Wilkins Co., Baltimore.

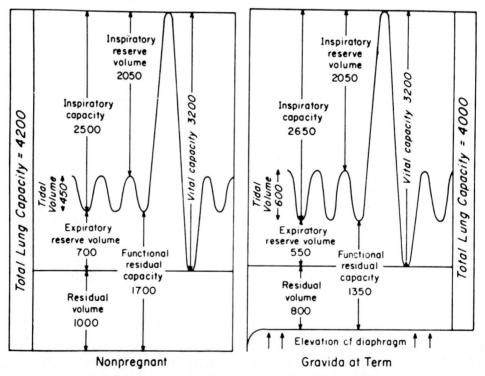

Figure 39–1. Pulmonary volumes and capacities during pregnancy, labor, and postpartum period. (From Cheek TG, Gutsche BB. Maternal physiologic alterations during pregnancy. In Shnider SM, Levinson G (eds). Anesthesia for obstetrics, pp. 3–13; © 1987, the Williams & Wilkins Co., Baltimore.)

and carbon dioxide production associated with pregnancy.[11, 12] The decrease in residual volume (RV), expiratory reserve volume (ERV), and functional residual capacity (FRC) are secondary to cephalad displacement of the diaphragm from the gravid uterus. Due to the decrease in ERV, closing volume (CV) may approximate FRC, creating the potential for regional ventilation–perfusion mismatching and hypoxia. Supine and, even worse, Trendelenburg positioning may further distort the relationship between CV and FRC. Up to one third of parturients may experience early airway closure during normal respiration in the supine position with PaO_2 values of less than 90 mm Hg.[13, 14] Preexisting conditions such as scoliosis, tobacco abuse, and obesity further exacerbate premature airway closure and associated hypoxemia in parturients of advanced gestation.[15]

The metabolic demands of the fetus and the additional energy expended during maternal respiration increase the parturient's oxygen consumption by 20%.[10] In preoxygenated patients undergoing caesarean section with general anesthesia, PaO_2 values decreased an average 139 mm Hg/min ± 13 mm Hg, as opposed to 58 mm Hg/min ± 8 mm Hg in nonpregnant patients during 1 minute of apnea.[16]

Gastrointestinal changes place the parturient at increased risk for regurgitation and aspiration. Elevated progesterone levels decrease gastric motility, food absorption, and lower esophageal sphincter tone.[17] Placental gastrin increases gastric volume and acid production. As many as 49% of parturients presenting for elective caesarean section after an overnight fast were found to have gastric volumes greater than 25 mL and a gastric pH less than 2.5, placing them at a high risk for aspiration pneumonitis.[10] The gravid uterus also produces upward displacement and rotation of the stomach with elevated intragastric pressure, delayed gastric emptying, and distortion of the gastroesophageal angle.[12]

CLINICAL IMPLICATIONS FOR THE ANESTHESIOLOGIST

All patients presenting for emergent or elective caesarean section should be considered to have full stomachs, and measures should be taken for rapid intubation of the trachea. Prior to induction, a nonparticulate antacid is administered orally and, if time permits, meto-

clopramide is administered to increase lower esophageal sphincter tone and gastric mobility and an H_2 antagonist is administered to increase gastric pH. Metoclopramide and cimetidine appear to be free of adverse effects in regard to the fetus.[12, 18] Properly applied cricoid pressure as a part of a rapid sequence induction technique is recommended in order to minimize risk of regurgitation and pulmonary aspiration.[19]

The combination of increased oxygen consumption and decreased pulmonary reserve render the parturient particularly susceptible to hypoxia after the induction of general anesthesia.[17] Preoxygenation for 3 to 5 minutes is an important step, although four deep breaths of 100% oxygen prior to induction may be sufficient in an emergency.[20, 21]

Edematous, friable mucosa within the respiratory tree make it imperative to avoid multiple traumatic attempts at tracheal intubation, which may cause a complete loss of airway due to hemorrhage and edema. Likewise, nasal intubation and nasogastric tubes are relatively contraindicated due to the risk of bleeding. Small-diameter endotracheal tubes may be necessary and therefore should be readily available. Postextubation obstruction due to upper airway edema may occur and requires constant observation in the immediate postoperative period.

The airway of the obese parturient can be unpredictable. Because 6% to 10% of pregnant patients may be considered obese[22] and at an increased risk for anesthesia-related morbidity and mortality,[1] the anesthesiologist must be particularly meticulous in the management of the patient's airway. A short-handled laryngoscope may be helpful when pendulous breasts or limited neck extension complicates laryngoscopy. Alternatively, one may insert the laryngoscope blade orally prior to attaching the handle. Elevation of the head and shoulders with blankets may alleviate many problems by favorably realigning the orolaryngeal axis and facilitating laryngoscopy.[10]

AIRWAY MANAGEMENT

Equipment for Airway Management

Proper equipment is essential for the management of the airway in the obstetric patient. Table 39–2 suggests basic equipment that should be readily available in the anesthetic

Table 39–2. BASIC AIRWAY EQUIPMENT

Laryngoscope
Curved blades #3, #4
Straight blades #2, #3
Malleable stylet
Endotracheal tubes: 6.5-, 7.0-, 7.5-mm inner diameter
Face masks: adult small, medium, large
Oropharyngeal airways: adult small, medium, large
Nasopharyngeal airways: various sizes (22-34 French)
Headstrap
Lubricating jelly
Suctioning equipment
Percutaneous transtracheal jet ventilation kit

work area of the operating room. A laryngo-scope with a variety of blades, endotracheal tubes, and a stylet should be all that is necessary for the routine and the somewhat more difficult intubation. If intubation proves to be very difficult, a selection of airways should be readily accessible to help provide for assisted ventilation while an assistant obtains the equipment reserved for difficult airways (Table 39–3). A difficult airway cart or box should be placed in a convenient location within the operating room suite. Specialty items, such as a short-handled laryngoscope, polio blade, bougie stylet, and a fiberoptic scope, may prove invaluable in a difficult intubation. It is recommended that a percutaneous transtracheal jet ventilation (PTJV) kit be readily available either in each operating room or in the difficult airway cart. Depending on the anesthesiologist's experience with a particular device, one may wish to stock a laryngeal mask airway, esophageal gastric tube airway, percutaneous cricothyrotomy or tracheostomy kit, and surgical cricothyrotomy kit. Anesthesiologists are encouraged to familiarize themselves with a variety of airway devices in order to be better prepared in the event of a difficult airway.

Techniques for Airway Management

Percutaneous Transtracheal Jet Ventilation

In the desperate situation when the parturient cannot be intubated or ventilated, PTJV is an effective and relatively safe method to temporarily establish oxygenation and remove carbon dioxide. Its use and efficacy is well documented in laboratory animals and humans,[23–28] but experience with this technique

in obstetrics is limited.[29, 30] Despite this, PTJV is an integral part of most obstetric protocols after failed intubation.[31–33]

Benumof and Scheller[23] recently described three acceptable systems for transtracheal ventilation. They preferred a jet injection powered by regulated wall or oxygen tank pressure. Unregulated wall or tank oxygen pressure with a jet injector was an acceptable alternative. The simplest and least expensive system consisted of oxygen supply tubing, a 15-mm endotracheal tube adaptor for a 4-mm inner diameter (ID) endotracheal tube, a 1/4-inch hose barb male Luer-Lok or cut-off 1 mL syringe, and a 14-g or 16-g intravenous catheter.

The technical aspects of establishing PTJV should be familiar to all anesthesiologists. With one hand on the cricothyroid membrane, a 14-g or 16-g intravenous catheter and needle with a syringe attached is advanced in the midline at a slightly caudad angle through the cricothyroid membrane. Using negative pressure, the trachea is identified by the aspiration of air into the attached syringe. The plastic intravenous catheter is advanced into the trachea, the needle is removed, and the position again is verified by the aspiration of air. With the catheter stabilized, the Luer-Lok or cut-off 1-mL syringe is affixed to the catheter hub while the 15-mm endotracheal tube adaptor is attached to the fresh gas outlet of the anesthesia machine (or to wall/tank oxygen if the jet injector device is used). The oxygen flush valve or jet ventilation apparatus is used to administer 40 to 50 breaths per minute.

This method of ventilation is capable of establishing normocarbia or hypocarbia and hyperoxia, but is considered a temporary device until the airway is secured by other means (ie, surgical cricothyrotomy or tracheostomy, fiberoptic intubation) or the patient resumes spontaneous ventilation.

Complications arising from PTJV occur in

Table 39–3. DIFFICULT AIRWAY EQUIPMENT

Laryngoscope: short handled
Specialty blades: polio blade, Bellhouse blade with
    prism
Endotracheal tubes: 5.0-, 5.5-, 6.0-mm inner diameter
Gum-elastic bougie stylet
Fiberoptic scope
Laryngeal mask airway
Esophageal gastric tube airway
Percutaneous cricothyrotomy/tracheostomy kit
Surgical cricothyrotomy kit
Retrograde tracheal intubation kit

up to 29% of cases and include subcutaneous emphysema (7.1%), mediastinal emphysema (3.6%), arterial perforation (3.6%), and difficulty with exhalation (14.3%).[27] The potential for laryngeal damage has led some to suggest that the puncture site be below the cricoid cartilage.[25] The anesthesiologist must be highly suspicious of any hypotension, tachycardia, or bradycardia that occurs during use of PTJV because of the possibility of barotrauma and pneumothorax.[34–39] The likelihood of barotrauma increases when a total upper airway obstruction causes an inability to exhale injected gas. This situation requires a surgical cricothyrotomy or tracheostomy as soon as is feasible.

Esophageal Gastric Tube Airway

Intubation of the esophagus, either deliberately or inadvertently, has been used as a means of establishing an airway in obstetric airway disasters.[28, 29, 31, 40–44] While using the esophageal tube as an obturator to prevent the passage of gastric contents from the esophagus into the trachea, it was discovered that the ability to ventilate was actually improved. It is believed that the cuffed tube helps to displace the larynx anteriorly away from the posterior pharyngeal wall, thus creating an open air passage from the pharynx to the trachea.

The esophageal gastric tube airway (EGTA) is a modification of the esophageal obturator airway first used for cardiopulmonary resuscitation by personnel untrained in tracheal intubation. The EGTA consists of an esophageal or endotracheal tube that passes through a holder in a special face mask, which allows for aspiration of gastric contents and also for a breathing circuit to be attached to a second aperture. Typically, the EGTA is placed in a paralyzed or anesthetized patient and the patient is subsequently allowed to breathe spontaneously while receiving general anesthesia. Potential risks include esophageal trauma, mediastinal perforation, and vomiting upon its withdrawal. In our practice, we do not initially consider the use of the EGTA in a difficult airway scenario, but if the esophagus is inadvertently intubated and emesis flows up through the tube, we will consider leaving it in the esophagus with the cuff inflated. The stomach is suctioned through the tube and an attempt to establish ventilation by mask is made. If ventilation is successful and further attempts to intubate are abandoned, we allow the patient to breathe spontaneously while maintaining general anesthesia. At the end of surgery, the patient is awakened and the stomach is suctioned again prior to removing the esophageal tube.

Laryngeal Mask Airway

A laryngeal mask airway has been reported in several instances to be a valuable tool in the very difficult airway. Experience with its use in obstetric anesthesia is limited[45, 46] but offers another viable alternative when intubation is unsuccessful. Cricoid pressure should be maintained after its insertion in order to reduce the risk of regurgitation and aspiration. It appears to be best suited to the patient who is spontaneously ventilating, although it has been used in conjunction with assisted ventilation until breathing resumes.[46] General anesthesia may be continued, if indicated, using the laryngeal mask airway and allowing the patient to breathe spontaneously. The airway is removed only when the patient is awake and able to protect her airway.

Percutaneous Tracheostomy/Cricothyrotomy

The desire to achieve a functional tracheal airway in an expedient fashion while avoiding surgical dissection has led to the development of several percutaneous tracheostomy and cricothyrotomy kits. Devices such as Nu-trake cricothyrotomy kit, Pertrach Emergency Percutaneous Airway, Rapitrac tracheostomy kit, and Melker Transcricothyrotomy Catheter were developed for this purpose. Each device follows a similar concept; that is, the insertion of a needle into the trachea and dilation of the puncture site to facilitate placement of a functional airway.[47, 48] Its advantages over surgical dissection include less bleeding and that it is easier to learn and faster to insert. Clinical experience in 100 patients revealed a complication rate of 14%, of which 6% was due to false passage of the device paratracheally rather than intratracheally.[47] One death was directly related to airway insertion in an obese woman in whom the tube was too short. The airway was lost, resulting in hypoxia and cardiac arrest. A longer length tube was subsequently developed. Use of this device in obstetrics has not been tested and cannot be recommended unless the anesthesiologist is familiar with its use.

Other Techniques of Airway Management

In the very difficult airway, one may wish to be familiar with as many techniques as possible in order to successfully ventilate the patient. One such technique involves the use of a long, lubricated, malleable gum-elastic bougie that has been flexed into a J shape.[49] The tip is extended approximately 6 cm beyond the end of a endotracheal tube, gently passed behind the epiglottis, and directed anteriorly toward the vocal cords. When the bougie is assumed to be in the trachea, the endotracheal tube is advanced over the bougie into the trachea. Alternatively, an endotracheal tube with an anterior bevel is used with the stylet placed through the eyelet.

A malleable illuminating stylet follows a similar premise to the bougie.[50] TUBE-STAT or Flexi-lum are illuminated stylets that, when placed in the trachea, are readily observed externally, particularly if the room is darkened. The stylet is lubricated, inserted into an endotracheal tube until the bulb just emerges from the distal tip, and then flexed into a J shape. After proper preparation, the awake patient is asked to protrude her tongue, and the stylet is inserted. With the anesthetized patient, the tongue is grasped with gauze and pulled forward. The illuminated stylet with endotracheal tube is placed in the oropharynx and advanced toward the larynx. As the tube is advanced into the trachea, a transilluminated glow from within the trachea is visible in the anterior neck at the level of the larynx. Light seen in the lateral neck suggests placement in the vallecula, whereas a dull, diffused light indicates esophageal placement. When successfully placed intratracheally, the endotracheal tube may then be advanced and the usual steps to confirm proper placement undertaken. In the obese patient or the patient with a thick neck, the light may be dimmer than expected when in the trachea and thus may be misleading to the anesthesiologist. Conversely, in the thin patient, the light may be bright despite being in the esophagus.

However efficient this method is in routine and difficult intubations, very little experience in obstetrics is available. It may be useful as an alternative intubation technique when direct laryngoscopy has failed, but only if the anesthesiologist is familiar with this method and cricoid pressure is maintained throughout intubation.

The Bullard laryngoscope is a rigid, hockey stick-shaped blade that contains a fiberoptic bundle along the posterior surface of the device, allowing the anesthesiologist excellent visualization of the larynx.[51, 52] Because use of this laryngoscope requires little or no manipulation of the neck, it has been recommended for patients with unstable cervical spine injuries.[52] An intubating stylet has been added as an integral part of the blade and appears to facilitate endotracheal tube placement. Although use of this new device may require some time and effort to master, it could be a useful addition to the anesthesiologist's armamentarium. It would seem particularly helpful in the patient with cervical spine disease or injury and in the parturient with a known or anticipated difficult airway who presents for elective caesarean section under general anesthesia. As with any fiberoptic device, excessive oral secretions or bleeding may interfere with visualization. Therefore, this may be a difficult device to use in the patient who is unable to be intubated after multiple attempts and has copious secretions, although the suction port provided may help somewhat. Another problem exists in patients with long necks. It has been reported that patients with significantly longer than normal necks, such as those who would require a #4 Macintosh or #3 Miller blade, cannot be successfully intubated due to the inadequate length of the Bullard laryngoscope.[52]

Other laryngoscope blades used in difficult airway management incorporate either one or two angles to take advantage of the features offered by both the straight and curved blades. The Belscope is a modified straight blade with a 45-degree bend at the midpoint. A prism can be added to further facilitate the line of vision anteriorly.[53] Another blade has two incremental curves of 20 degrees and 30 degrees along a wide, flat blade shaft.[54] By eliminating the flange, there is more room for manipulation of the endotracheal tube than with a standard straight blade. Jellicoe and Harris[55] have reported their modification of a standard Macintosh blade where the angle between the blade and the handle is increased to facilitate the introduction of the blade into the mouth, but is not obtuse enough to produce the difficulty associated with the polio blade. More experience with these new laryngoscope blades is necessary before their routine use in obstetrics can be recommended.

Although typically not recommended in obstetric patients, blind nasotracheal intubation has been performed successfully.[56, 57] In two cases, the intubation was accomplished in an awake patient, one of whom was a failed intubation who had been allowed to awaken. Topical nasopharyngeal anesthesia is considered essential to shrink the nasal mucosa and reduce its vascularity. Still, the passage of a nasal tube in this population must be considered dangerous in view of the potential for upper airway hemorrhage.

Surgical cricothyrotomy/tracheotomy should only be undertaken by an individual, preferably a surgeon, experienced with this procedure. The reader is referred to surgical texts for a review of the anatomy and technique.

Airway Management Scenarios

The initial step in airway management is to assess the patient's airway to, it is hoped, identify those patients at risk. In an ideal setting, the anesthesiologist would thoroughly evaluate the parturient's airway and devise an appropriate course of action prior to surgery. Unless the anesthesiologist is solely responsible for the obstetric ward and has the time to visit each patient early in her labor, the more likely first assessment will be on the way to the operating room for an emergency caesarean section.

Certainly, some difficult airways are easily recognized when a patient has obvious trauma or deformities of the face, upper airway, or cervical spine, or relates a history of difficult intubation. Difficult airways in other patients are much less obvious and it is for these patients that various criteria for estimating the probability of difficult intubation have been developed. One such simple maneuver is to evaluate the oropharyngeal structures in the seated patient with the mouth widely open and the tongue maximally protruded. First described by Mallampati and colleagues[58] and later modified by Samsoon and Young,[59] this technique found a significant correlation between visibility (or lack of visibility) of faucial pillars, soft palate and uvula, and exposure of glottis by direct laryngoscopy. Common errors include assessment in the supine position and having the patient phonate "ah," both of which were not part of the original studies and may distort the test's reliability.

Head extension is another important consideration in airway evaluation. Atlanto-occipital extension is assessed by visually estimating the angle traversed by the occlusal surface of the maxillary teeth when the head is extended from the neutral position.[60] Thirty-five degrees of extension is normal at the atlanto-occipital joint. Reduction of this angle by one third or

more predicts difficulty with intubation. A receding lower jaw reduces the space anterior to the larynx and diminishes the line of vision along the orolaryngeal axis when the head is extended. Described as the mandibular space by Bellhouse and Dore,[60] this is estimated by viewing the patient from the side with the mouth open and head extended. An imaginary line is drawn from the upper central incisor to a point 1.5 cm behind the laryngeal prominence of the thyroid cartilage. The observer then estimates the perpendicular distance to the mandibular genial tubercle in front of the line. A distance of less than 2.5 cm was associated with difficulty during laryngoscopy. Similarly, one may assess the thyromental distance by the number of fingerbreadths or with a ruler when the patient's head is extended. A distance of less than three fingerbreadths or 6 cm may suggest problems.

Besides these bedside evaluations, classic teachings emphasize visual assessment of physical characteristics that may pose problems.[61, 62] Beware of patients with a short muscular neck and a full set of teeth; a high, arched palate associated with a long, narrow mouth; poor mobility of the mandible; as well as a receding mandible, as previously mentioned.

The clinical evaluations of the airway as described are all relatively simple and quick to perform. Although these investigations were not performed in an obstetric population, the investigators using the three predictors (head extension, mandibular space, visualization of oropharyngeal structures) report 100% accuracy in identifying difficult intubations.[60] Although some clinicians suggest airway assessment of the parturient in the recumbent position,[4, 61] this would potentially negate the accuracy of these valuable predictors. In an emergency situation, we prefer to quickly assess body habitus and then evaluate the other three predictors in the sitting position. This can be done conveniently as the patient moves over the operating table or sits up to drink the required nonparticulate antacid. Such evaluation should take only seconds to perform and may impact profoundly on decision making during preparation for induction. If the situation precludes the patient sitting up, one should do the best assessment possible in the supine position while obtaining the patient's history.

Elective or Nonemergency Cesarean Section

In this situation, the anesthesiologist should have adequate time to assess the patient, her airway, and to administer a nonparticulate antacid (Fig. 39–2). A patient with a known difficult airway can be safely managed with awake or fiberoptic intubation. Regional anesthesia is an alternative, but one must always be prepared for the possibility of a high block, requiring respiratory support. A carefully placed epidural catheter may allow a more controlled dermatomal level of anesthesia than a single-shot spinal anesthetic. A slightly more difficult decision faces the anesthesiologist when a parturient's airway assessment is suspect. Again, regional anesthesia is a viable option. One may consider performing an awake laryngoscopy (after topical anesthesia is applied) to grade the visualization of the larynx prior to embarking on the anesthetic. Poor visualization of the larynx should encourage the anesthesiologist to either proceed with fiberoptic intubation or a cautious regional technique.

The most stressful scenario involves the unanticipated difficult airway. Should repeated attempts to intubate, including techniques using the flexible bougie or lightwand, fail, the anesthesiologist must make a critical decision to either wake the patient or proceed with another method of ventilation. If Doppler probe assessment of fetal heart tones indicates fetal stability, one should attempt to awaken the patient. However, if fetal status is tenuous and mask ventilation is possible, one may consider proceeding with the cesarean section. In all cases, the parturient's life takes priority and should be the prime concern of the anesthesiologist. If the patient cannot be ventilated by mask, the patient must be awakened. Often, the patient will not awaken in this situation and must be ventilated by other means. PTJV, laryngeal mask, EGTA, percutaneous or surgical cricothyrotomy are all viable options at this point, and the anesthesiologist should institute the technique most familiar to him or her. After the airway is secured, surgery may proceed. When the patient has been wakened but fetal status is precarious, consult with the surgeon regarding the delivery of the child under local anesthesia. Following delivery and hemostasis, the airway may be secured with awake or fiberoptic intubation.

Emergency Cesarean Section

The same caveats for nonemergency cesarean section apply to the emergency situation. Patient assessment, airway evaluation, and aspiration prophylaxis are performed, albeit more quickly (Fig. 39–3). Parturients with a known difficult airway should be considered for awake intubation or regional anesthesia (if not contraindicated). Time constraints make spinal anesthesia preferable to epidural anesthesia in this situation. If awake intubation is unsuccessful and regional anesthesia undesirable, local anesthesia may be used for delivery and hemostasis. The airway then can be secured and surgery completed.

If one suspects a probable difficult airway, these concerns should be conveyed immediately to the surgeon and patient; then proceed with awake laryngoscopy and intubation, if possible. Consider regional anesthesia (spinal) if awake laryngoscopy confirms these suspicions, or deliver the baby under local anesthesia.

When difficult intubation is not anticipated and cannot be achieved, the parturient's life is again the primary concern of the anesthesiologist. If mask ventilation is possible, the decision to proceed with surgery should be considered. When the patient cannot be ventilated by mask and shows no signs of awakening, institute other means of ventilation. The baby may be delivered once the airway is secured.

A few additional comments need to be mentioned regarding airway disasters. When problems arise, call for help. Extra experienced hands can be invaluable. The successful use of mask ventilation precludes further attempts at intubation unless one is reasonably assured of tracheal intubation. It is better to continue with a successful technique than to risk losing the airway due to trauma and excessive secretions from repeated laryngoscopy. Cricoid pressure needs to be maintained until the airway is secured. The only exception would be if the esophagus is intubated. Occasionally, misapplied cricoid pressure may interfere with intubation/ventilation and may be cautiously released to evaluate its effects. Some anesthesiologists recommend placing the patient in left lateral decubitis and head down position while maintaining mask ventilation.[31] This position may be difficult for many anesthesiologists. Typically, we keep the patient supine when using mask ventilation. However, if the patient has vomited, we immediately place the head down and tilt the patient to the left.

Use of muscle relaxants with mask ventilation is controversial.[31, 32, 63] When using mask ventilation, we prefer to allow the patient to resume spontaneous respiration while titrating doses of inhalation agent, narcotic, and midazolam. If we suspect difficult ventilation may

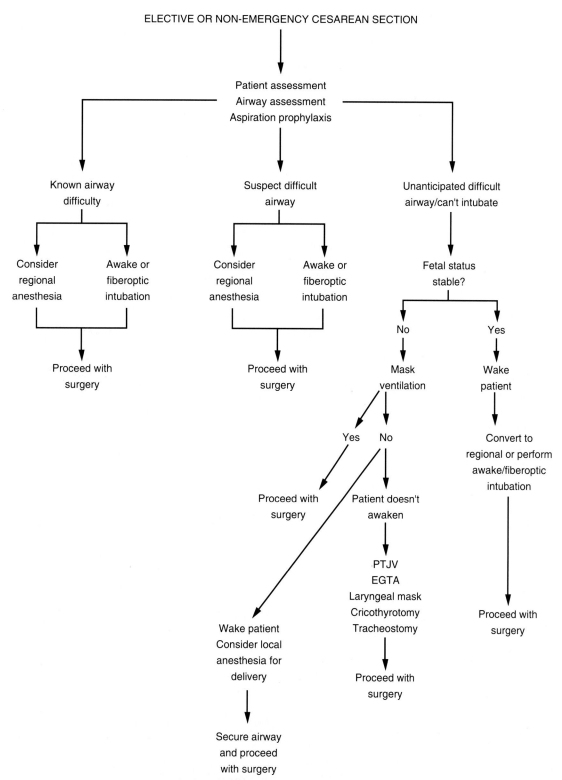

Figure 39–2. Airway management flowchart for elective or nonemergency cesarean section. PTJV, percutaneous transtracheal jet ventilation; EGTA esophageal gastric tube airway.

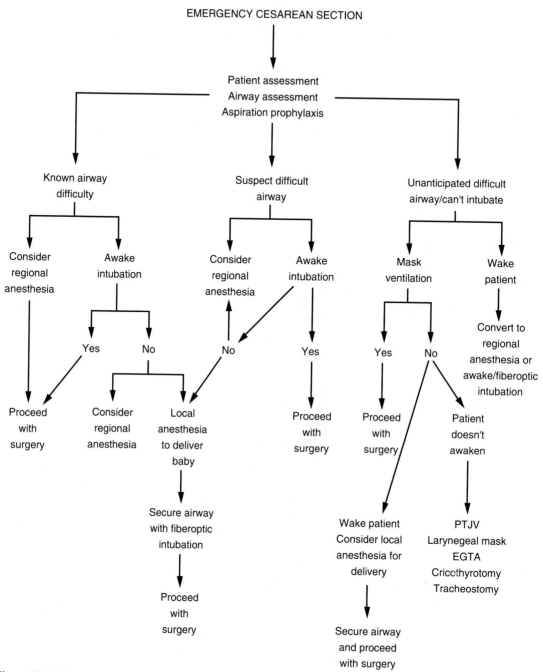

Figure 39–3. Airway management flowchart for emergency cesarean section. PTJV, percutaneous transtracheal jet ventilation; EGTA, esophageal gastric tube airway.

be improved with muscle relaxation, small incremental doses of succinylcholine may be cautiously administered.

Lastly, the patient who has proven to be difficult or impossible to intubate must be counseled regarding this problem postoperatively. Provide the patient with a letter that she can present to other anesthesiologists or suggest she wear a medical alert bracelet identifying her as a difficult airway patient.

References

1. Endler GC, Mariona FG, Sokol RJ, Stevenson LB. Anesthesia related maternal mortality in Michigan,

1972 to 1984. Am J Obstet Gynecol 159:187–193, 1988.

2. Turnbull AC, Tindall VR, Robson G, Dawson MP, Cloake EP, Ashley JS. Report on confidential inquiries into maternal deaths in England and Wales 1979–81. London: Her Majesty's Stationary Office, 1986.

3. Marx GF, Finster MD. Difficulty in endotracheal intubation associated with obstetric anaesthesia. Anesthesiology 51:364–365, 1979.

4. Davies JM, Weets S, Crone LA, Paulin E. Difficult intubation in the parturient. Can J Anaesth 36:668–674, 1989.

5. Lyons G. Failed intubation. Anaesthesia. 40:759–762, 1985.

6. Bonica JJ. Maternal respiratory changes during pregnancy. In Marx GF (ed). Parturition and Perinatology. Philadelphia: F. A. Davis, 1973; pp. 1–19.

7. MacKenzie AI. Laryngeal oedema complicating obstetric anaesthesia. Anaesthesia 33:271, 1978.

8. Jouppila R, Jouppila P, Hollmen A. Laryngeal oedema as an obstetric complication: Case reports. Acta Anaesth Scand 24:97–98, 1980.

9. Heller PJ, Scheider EP, Marx GF. Pharyngolaryngeal edema as a presenting symptom in preeclampsia. Obstet Gynecol 62:523–524, 1983.

10. Cheek TG, Gutsche BB. Maternal physiologic alterations during pregnancy. In Shnider SM, Levinson G (eds). Anesthesia for Obstetrics. Baltimore: Williams & Wilkins, 1987; pp. 3–13.

11. Gibbs CP. Maternal physiology. Clin Obstet Gynecol 24:533–538, 1981.

12. Conklin KA. Maternal physiological adaptations during gestation, labor and the puerperium. Seminars in Anesthesia 4:221–234, 1991.

13. Bevan DR, Holdcroft A, Loh L, MacGregor WG, O'Sullivan JC, Sykes MK. Closing volume and pregnancy. Br Med J 1:13–15, 1974.

14. Awe RJ, Nicotra MB, Newsom TD, Viles R. Arterial oxygenation and alveolar–arterial gradients in term pregnancy. Obstet Gynecol 53:182–186, 1979.

15. Leontie EA. Respiratory disease in pregnancy. Med Clin North Am 62:111, 1974.

16. Archer GW, Marx GF. Arterial oxygen tension during apnoea in parturient women. Br J Anaesth 45:358, 1974.

17. Camann WR, Ostheimer GW. Understanding the mother: Physiologic adaptations during pregnancy. In Ostheimer GW (eds). Manual of Obstetric Anesthesia, 2nd ed. New York: Churchill Livingstone, 1992; pp. 1–12.

18. Johnston JR, Moore J, McCaughey W, Dundee JW, Howard PJ, Toner W, McClean E. Use of cimetidine as an oral antacid in obstetric anesthesia. Anesth Analg 62:720–726, 1983.

19. Sellick BA. Cricoid pressure to control regurgitation of stomach contents during induction of anesthesia. Lancet 2:404, 1961.

20. Norris MC, Dewan DM. Preoxygenation for cesarean section: A comparison of two techniques. Anesthesiology 62:827–829, 1985.

21. Gambee AM, Hertzka RE, Fisher DM. Preoxygenation techniques: Comparison of three minutes and four breaths. Anesth Analg 66:468–470, 1987.

22. Dewan MD. Anesthesia for the morbidly obese parturient. Problems in Anesthesia 3:56, 1989.

23. Benumof JL, Scheller MS. The importance of transtracheal jet ventilation in the management of the difficult airway. Anesthesiology 71:769–778, 1989.

24. Scuderi PE, McLeskey CH, Comer PB. Emergency percutaneous transtracheal ventilation during anesthe-

sia using readily available equipment. Anesth Analg 61:867–870, 1982.

25. Spoerel WE, Narayanan PS, Singh NP. Transtracheal ventilation. Br J Anaesth 43:932–938, 1971.

26. Jacobs HB. Emergency percutaneous transtracheal catheter and ventilator. J Trauma 12:50–55, 1972.

27. Smith RB, Babinski M, Klain M, Pfaaffle H. Percutaneous transtracheal ventilation. J Am Coll Emer Phys 5:765–770, 1976.

28. Weymuller EA, Paugh D, Paulin EG, Cummings CW. Management of difficult airway problems with percutaneous transtracheal ventilation. Ann Otol Rhinol Laryngol 96:34–37, 1987.

29. Bready CL, Swartzman S, Adcock DC. Failed intubation—transtracheal ventilation. Br J Anaesth 55:1040, 1983.

30. Campbell WI. Failed intubation in obstetric anaesthesia. Br J Anaesth 55:1040, 1983.

31. Turnstall ME, Sheikh A. Failed intubation protocol: Oxygenation without aspiration. Clin Anaesth 4:171–187, 1986.

32. Davies JM, Weeks S, Crone LA, Paulin E. Difficult intubation in the parturient. Can J Anaesth 36:668–674, 1989.

33. Latto IP, Rosen M. Difficulties in Tracheal Intubation. London: Bailliere Tindall, 1984; pp. 152–155.

34. Weymuller EA, Paugh D, Pavlin EG, Cummings CW. Management of difficult airway problems with percutaneous transtracheal ventilation. Ann Otol Rhinol Laryngol 96:34–37, 1987.

35. Egol A, Culpepper JA, Synder JV. Barotrauma and hypotension resulting from jet ventilation in critically ill patients. Chest 88:98–102, 1985.

36. O'Sullivan TJ, Healy GB. Complications of venturi jet ventilation during microlaryngeal surgery. Arch Otolaryngol 111:127–131, 1985.

37. Oliverio R, Ruder CB, Fermon C, Curd A. Report on pneumothorax secondary to ball-valve obstruction during jet ventilation. Anesthesiology 51:255–256, 1979.

38. Smith RB, Schaer WB, Pfaeffle H. Percutaneous transtracheal ventilation for anesthesia: A review and report of complications. Can Anaesth Soc J 22:607–612, 1975.

39. Coté CJ, Eavey RD, Todres D, Jones DE. Cricothyroid membrane puncture: Oxygenation and ventilation in a dog model using an intravenous catheter. Crit Care Med 16:615–619, 1988.

40. Boys JE. Failed intubation in obstetric anaesthesia. Br J Anaesth 55:187–188, 1983.

41. Parker EO. Airway management in the parturient. Anesthesiology 60:167–168, 1984.

42. Brock-Utne JG, Rait C, Moodley J, Mayat N. Influence of preoperative gastric aspiration on the volume of pH of gastric contents in obstetric patients undergoing cesarean section. Br J Anaesth 62:397–401, 1989.

43. Swareswaren N, McGuinness JJ. Modified mask for failed intubation at emergency caesarean section. Anaesth Intensive Care 12:279–280, 1984.

44. Tunstall ME, Geddes C. "Failed intubation" in obstetric anesthesia. Br J Anaesth 56:659–661, 1984.

45. Chadwick IS, Vohra A. Anaesthesia for emergency cesarean section using the brain laryngeal airway. Anaesthesia 44:261–262, 1989.

46. McClune S, Regan M, Moore J. Laryngeal mask airway for cesarean section. Anaesthesia 45:227–228, 1990.

47. Toye FJ, Weinstein JD. Clinical experience with percutaneous tracheostomy and cricothyrotomy in 100 patients. J Trauma 26:1034–1040, 1986.

48. Toye FJ, Weinstein JD. A percutaneous tracheostomy device. Surgery 65:384–389, 1969.

49. Cormack RS, Lehane J. Difficult tracheal intubation in obstetrics. Anaesthesia 39:1105–1111, 1984.

50. Ellis DG, Jakymec A, Kaplan RM, Stewart RD, Freeman JA, Bleyaert A, Berkebile PE. Guided orotracheal intubation in the operating room using a lighted stylet: A comparison with direct laryngoscopic technique. Anesthesiology 69:784–787, 1989.

51. Benumof JL. Management of the difficult adult airway. Anesthesiology 75:1087–1110, 1991.

52. Gorback MS. Management of the challenging airway with the Bullard laryngoscope. J Clin Anesth 3:473–477, 1991.

53. Bellhouse CP. An angulated laryngoscope for routine and difficult tracheal intubation. Anesthesiology 69:126–129, 1988.

54. Choi JJ. A new double-angled blade for direct laryngoscopy [letter]. Anesthesiology 72:576, 1990.

55. Jellicoe JA, Harris NR. A modification of a standard laryngoscope for difficult tracheal intubation in obstetric cases. Anaesthesia 39:800–802, 1984.

56. Mokriski BK, Malinow AM, Gray WC, McGuinn WJ. Topical nasopharyngeal anaesthesia with vasoconstriction in preeclampsia-eclampsia. Can J Anaesth 35:641–643, 1988.

57. Edwards RM, Hunt TL. Blind nasal intubation in an awake patient for cesarean section. Anaesth Intensive Care 2:131–133, 1982.

58. Mallampati SR, Gatt SP, Gugimo LD, Desai SP, Waraksa B, Freiberger D, Liu PL. A clinical sign to predict difficult tracheal intubation: A prospective study. Can Anaesth Soc J 32:429–434, 1985.

59. Samsoon GLT, Young JRB. Difficult tracheal intubation: A retrospective study. Anaesthesia 42:487–490, 1987.

60. Bellhouse CP, Doré C. Criteria for estimating likelihood of difficulty of endotracheal intubation with the Macintosh laryngoscope. Anaesth Intensive Care 16:329–337, 1988.

61. McIntyre JWR. The difficult tracheal intubation. Can J Anaesth 34:204–213, 1987.

62. Cass NM, James NR, Lines V. Difficult direct laryngoscopy complicating intubation for anaesthesia. Br Med J 1:488–489, 1956.

63. Hewett E, Livingstone P. Management of failed endotracheal intubation at cesarean section. Anaesth Intensive Care 18:330–335, 1990.

CHAPTER 40

Airway Management in the Cardiac Patient

Lawrence Mason, M.D., and Calvin Johnson, M.D.

Endotracheal intubation is fraught with possible complications. Induction of general anesthesia in the cardiac patient is particularly associated with a variety of hemodynamic changes.[1]

Early clinicians noted the reflex cardiovascular disturbances when "light" general anesthesia was employed. Deep general anesthesia attenuated these responses.[2] With the advent of intraoperative electrocardiography (ECG) and continuous blood pressure monitoring in the 1950s, it was appreciated that these changes commenced with laryngeal stimulation prior to intubation.[3] Both systolic and diastolic hypertension occurred. Heart rate increased and dysrhythmias were noted. Dysrhythmias are associated more with intubation than with laryngoscopy. The cardiovascular response to intubation is transient, occurring seconds after laryngoscopy, reaching a peak in 1 to 2 minutes, and returning to baseline values in approximately 5 minutes.[4]

The reported incidence of dysrhythmias with general anesthesia ranges from 0 to 90%.[5] This emphasizes the importance of anesthetic technique and the medical condition of the patients, and also the recognition and recording of dysrhythmias.

The clinical significance of these cardiovascular changes is in most cases inconsequential; however, a subset of patients is at risk. These patients have increased intracranial pressure, aneurysms (both cerebral and aortic), hypertension, and ischemic heart disease.[1]

The hypertensive patient has an exaggerated cardiovascular response to laryngoscopy and intubation. It is imperative to continue the patient's antihypertensive regimen preoperatively in order to attenuate the response.[6] Failure to continue a patient's antihypertensive medication in the preoperative period may lead to withdrawal, which manifests itself as tachycardia, hypertension, and myocardial ischemia. Many investigators have reported ECG evidence of ischemia at laryngoscopy and intubation.[7] This has also been documented by the appearance of segmental wall motion abnormalities (SWMA) via echocardiographic techniques. Perioperative myocardial ischemia is associated with a significant increase in morbidity and mortality.[8]

Patients with ischemic heart disease are at risk because there is a critical balance between oxygen supply and demand. The two primary determinants of myocardial oxygen consumption are tachycardia and hypertension; both are known to occur during laryngoscopy and intubation. Tachycardia and hypertension can elevate myocardial oxygen demand and cause myocardial ischemia, ventricular dysfunction, and myocardial infarction. Myocardial reinfarction has a greater possibility of increase in patients who have had previous myocardial infarction, and mortality approaches 50% in some studies. Early institution of measures to prevent aberrations of the cardiovascular response results in improved outcome.[9]

Patients who have hypertension and ischemic heart disease are at even a higher risk for an untoward event. Preoperative evaluation should include a review of previous myocardial infarctions.[10] It is important to point out that patients who have long-standing hypertension and underlying myocardial disease may not have the myocardial reserve to generate a significant pressure response to an acute rise in systemic vascular resistance, and this could lead to ischemia or myocardial infarction. These patients with ischemic heart disease and long-standing hypertension have diastolic dysfunction. The increased ventricular mass not only requires more oxygen consumption per contraction, but one must remember that diastolic relaxation is an energy-requiring process and not a passive process. The clinical scenario that could arise with an acute rise in blood pressure with laryngoscopy and intubation is one of ventricular dilatation due to the decreased diastolic function. With the decrease in ventricular compliance, ejection fraction decreases, end-diastolic volume decreases, and left ventricular (LV) filling pressures increase, leading to pulmonary congestion. The preoperative history should emphasize whether the patient has a history of atrial enlargement; namely, atrial fibrillation, dyspnea, fatigue, and angina. This subset of patients should be addressed aggressively as far as blood pressure control is concerned during laryngoscopy and intubation. Decreased systolic function is also detrimental and is a sequela of long-standing hypertension.

The upper airway, larynx, and trachea are highly innervated with both sensory nerve endings and motor afferents. The afferent pathway for both the cardiovascular response and the laryngospastic reflex are mediated by the glossopharyngeal and vagus nerves. The sensory and anatomic distribution of the glossopharyngeal is superior to the vocal cords and includes the anterior surface of the epiglottis. The posterior aspect of the epiglottis and larynx is innervated primarily by the vagus nerve. The mucous membranes of the larynx are innervated by branches of the vagus; namely, the superior laryngeal and the recurrent laryngeal. The internal laryngeal nerve is predominantly sensory, except for a few motor fibers to the arytenoid muscles. The external branch is a motor branch of the cricothyroid. The recurrent laryngeal innervates all intrinsic muscles

of the larynx, except the cricothyroid and the arytenoids.

The cardiovascular response is mediated by both the sympathetic and parasympathetic nervous system. Reid and Brace in 1940 ascribed the ECG changes to a "vago-vagal" and postulated an afferent pathway mediated by the vagus nerve.[2] Later, other investigators could not reproduce ablation of the pressor response with 3 mg atropine, which is sufficient to block vagal action.[2, 11] In 1950, Burnstein ascribed the cardiovascular changes during laryngoscopy and intubation to be mediated via cardioaccelerator nerves, the reflex being potentiated by hypoxia.[12]

Current theory, as described by King and associates, believes the reflex to be less specific in character.[4] The reflex is thought to be polysynaptic, the afferent limb being the vagus with the efferent either due to increased sympathico-adrenal response or decreased parasympathetic response.[4] Impulses traverse brainstem and spinal cord through diffuse polysynaptic pathways. There is increased activity of the cardioaccelerator nerves, release of norepinephrine from vascular beds, and release of epinephrine from the adrenal medulla.[12] Also, there is evidence of activation of the renin-angiotensin system. As mentioned previously, the neuroendocrine response to tracheal intubation can lead to a number of complications in patients with cardiac or cerebrovascular disease.

Induction of general anesthesia in the cardiac patient is associated with a variety of hemodynamic changes. Some of these changes can be attributed to a heightened baroreceptor reflex, lack of appropriate baroreceptor response, and decreased cardiac reserve.

The peri-induction period is, therefore, a precarious time, and institution of timely and appropriate pharmacotherapy and technical skills are paramount.

Various pharmacologic regimens have been proposed; none, however, is without possible pitfalls. Historically, appreciation of depth of anesthesia was recognized early. The lighter the plane of anesthesia upon induction, the greater the changes in hemodynamics are appreciated. Various techniques and pharmacologic agents have been employed (Table 40–1).

CARDIAC ANESTHESIA

The state of anesthesia is composed of four basic components: amnesia, analgesia, muscle

Table 40–1. METHODS OF ATTENUATING CARDIOVASCULAR EFFECTS OF LARYNGOSCOPY AND INTUBATION

Deep anesthesia
  Inhalation
  Intravenous narcotics
    Sufentanil
    Fentanyl
    Alfentanil
  Topical anesthesia
    Direct spraying of larynx and trachea
    Transtracheal spraying
    Nebulization of the upper airway
Regional anesthesia
  Superior laryngeal nerve block
  Glossopharyngeal nerve block
Pharmacologic methods
  Vasodilators
  Calcium channel blockers
  Adrenergic blockers (beta-blockers, alpha-blockers)
  ACE inhibitors
  Intravenous and intratracheal lidocaine
  Prostaglandins
  α_2 agonists
  Hybrid antihypertensives
Techniques
  Nasal
  Lightwand
  Fiberoptic
  Retrograde

relaxation, and ablation of autonomic reflexes to surgery.[13] Induction of anesthesia and endotracheal intubation are generally accomplished by using a combination of intravenous anesthetic agents: volatile anesthetic agents, muscle relaxants, beta-blockers, calcium channel blockers, vasodilator agents, and other adjunctive antihypertensive agents.

Opioids

Opioids are very popular in cardiac anesthesia. These agents, in addition to supplying analgesia, are useful in attenuating the hemodynamic response to intubation, therefore reducing the requirement of potent volatile anesthetic agents. The upper airway and trachea are innervated by the ninth and tenth cranial nerves. As mentioned previously, the cardiac vascular response probably involves these nerves. In animal models, opiate receptors have been found to exist in these nerves and the closely associated solitary nucleus.[14] Opioids that are most useful in this application are the phenylperidine synthetic derivatives; notably, fentanyl, alfentanil, and sufentanil. Advantages over "old world" or first-generation narcotics (meperidine, morphine) are less

myocardial depression, histamine release, greater attenuation of the sympathetic nervous system, and less fluid retention. Fentanyl is used for induction of anesthesia and as the sole primary agent in doses anywhere from 25 to 100 µg/kg. When fentanyl is used as an adjunctive agent for attenuating the cardiovascular response during laryngoscopy and intubation, 8 µg/kg has been recommended. Sufentanil has been recommended as the sole anesthetic agent in the dose range of 10 to 20 µg/kg. Opioids, except for meperidine, usually produce a moderate to profound bradycardia.[15] Meperidine produces tachycardia, probably due to its structural similarity with atropine. Hypertension and tachycardia during laryngoscopy are not uncommon findings, even at higher doses. There is evidence that sufentanil may suppress the hypertensive response to a greater degree than fentanyl.[16–17] Sufentanil has been employed successfully at a dose of 1 µg/kg and has attenuated the cardiovascular response with a duration of action of 15 minutes. However, it must be emphasized that these agents are rarely sufficient in and of themselves for attenuation of the hyperdynamic response to intubation. Alfentanil may offer an advantage in the cardiac patient undergoing noncardiac surgery because of its pharmacokinetic properties; its rapid onset of action, short-elimination half-life, and small volume of distribution makes it a good agent for short surgeries. In one report, alfentanil 30 µg/kg suppressed hemodynamic response to laryngoscopy and intubation, with a duration of action lasting 12 minutes.[18] Other agents may have to be used in conjunction with opiates in order to attenuate the cardiovascular response. The ability of opioids to suppress the cardiovascular response may lie in their actions at this site.

Volatile Anesthetics

The volatile anesthetics (ie, halothane, enflurane, isoflurane) have been used with and without opioids in the cardiac patient. These agents are complete anesthetics but may not be tolerated by the patient with decreased myocardial reserve, because the concentration required to suppress the autonomic nervous system may have deleterious effects. During induction of anesthesia, laryngoscopy, and intubation, these agents are generally used in an adjunctive fashion. All volatile agents are myocardial depressants. Halothane and enflurane are the most potent myocardial depressants; isoflurane and enflurane are also potent vasodilators. Isoflurane is probably the most preferred volatile anesthetic for attenuating the response to laryngoscopy and intubation; it is the least myocardial depressant, maintains heart rate, provides systemic vasodilation, and has the highest threshold for generation of arrhythmias. Isoflurane is a potent coronary vasodilator. Areas of ischemic myocardium may be put at risk, because vasodilation can produce ischemia by causing an adverse redistribution of coronary blood flow. High concentrations of isoflurane should be avoided, because this may clinically produce coronary steal.[19, 20] If myocardial perfusion pressure is maintained, coronary steal clinically is not a problem; however, this concept remains controversial.[21]

Adrenergic Blockers

Adrenergic blockers have been employed extensively in cardiac anesthesia. A great number of patients may be on these agents preoperatively, and it is paramount that they not be withdrawn. Severe hypertensive episodes have been reported after beta-blocker and calcium channel blocker withdrawal. Adrenergic blockers work primarily by competitive inhibition of various receptor sites, resulting in the loss of sympathetic tone. Several different agents have been employed in the peri-induction period. Both alpha- and beta-receptor blockers have been used. Beta-blockers have a wide range of potency, efficacy, elimination kinetics, vascular effects, and cross-reactivity with β-$_2$ receptors.

Esmolol is a particularly useful agent in the peri-induction period. It has a rapid onset, a short clinical half-life, and a high selectivity for the β_1 receptor. Esmolol has a duration of action in minutes due to its rapid biotransformation by red cell esterases;[22] this pharmacokinetic property allows for its use as an infusion. Esmolol has been used in bolus doses of 150 mg 2 minutes prior to laryngoscopy and intubation. Labetalol is a unique agent that has both alpha- and beta-blocking properties. It produces a nonselective beta-blockade with the alpha- and beta-blocking properties. Labetalol produces a nonselective beta-blockade with the β/α ratio of 3:1 to 7:1 following oral or intravenous administration, respectively. It also may cause vasodilation via β_2 receptor stimulation. Labetalol has been advocated for

use in attenuating the cardiovascular response in the rapid-sequence induction of general anesthesia in the severely preeclamptic or eclamptic patient. The administration of beta-blockers to patients with a compromised myocardium or bronchospastic disease should be done with caution.[23]

Vasodilators

As with other classes of agents, there are a host of choices among vasodilators. Agents that are popular with anesthesiologists for control of blood pressure in the cardiac patient have a rapid onset, rapid elimination, and titrability.

Nitroglycerin is a very popular agent for use in the peri-induction period because it possesses all the aforementioned criteria. It produces relaxation of vascular smooth muscle, primarily on venous (capacitance) vessels and, to a lesser degree, reduction in arteriolar (resistance) vessel tone, resulting in a decrease in systemic blood pressure and pulmonary resistance. The higher blood levels required for arteriolar dilation are easily achieved by intravenous administration. Because of the decrease in preload and afterload, myocardial oxygen consumption is reduced. In addition, nitroglycerin has the added advantage of redistribution or increased blood flow to collateral myocardial vessels, which may increase perfusion to the ischemic myocardium. Nitroglycerin may be administered via the chest wall, sublingually, intravenously, or intranasally.[24–26]

Nitroprusside is a potent, rapid-acting peripheral vasodilator with direct smooth muscle effects on both venous (capacitance) and arterial vessels, thereby reducing preload and afterload. The hemodynamic effects of nitroprusside are titrable and can be interrupted abruptly by cessation of the infusion. Reflex tachycardia can occur and may limit its usefulness. Nitroprusside may cause an intracoronary steal by coronary arteriolar vasodilation that diverts blood from ischemic areas of myocardium. Also, a reduction of diastolic blood pressure may produce myocardial ischemia.[27, 28]

ACE Inhibitors

One of the proposed mechanisms of the cardiovascular response is thought to involve the renin-angiotensin system. Due to inhibition of the renin-angiotensin system with angiotensin-converting enzyme (ACE) inhibitors, these agents are attractive choices. Enalapril 6.5 mg orally has been shown to attenuate the responses; intravenous enalapril also has been used. ACE inhibitors cause vasodilation in the arteriolar vascular bed and, to a lesser degree, also in the capacitance vessels.[29]

Calcium Channel Blockers

Calcium channel blockers have been employed to prevent the cardiovascular reflex. These drugs should be continued through the preoperative period if the patient takes these medications on a chronic basis.

Calcium channel blockers are selective inhibitors of the influx of calcium ions from the extracellular space in to the cell, via the specific calcium channels in the sarcolemma. Calcium channel blockers exert their effect on myocardial muscle, vascular smooth muscle and, to a lesser extent, skeletal muscle. Calcium channel blockers produced decreased heart rate, decreased myocardial contractility, and vasodilation. A depressant action on cardiac tissues—reflected by decreased myocardial contraction, heart rate, and atrioventricular conduction—is limited to verapamil, diltiazem, and related drugs. Arterial vasodilation and its resultant antihypertensive action are common properties of all calcium channel antagonists. The dihydropyridines, of which nifedipine is the prototype, cause arterial vasodilation without action at the atrioventricular node. Therefore, nifedipine does not produce decrease in heart rate or atrioventricular conduction. Nifedipine causes a mild baroreceptor medial tachycardia. Nifedipine 10 mg sublingually has been shown to attenuate the cardiovascular response. Nifedipine action on the atrioventricular node is minimal, and tachycardia may be a problem.[30] Nicardipine, verapamil, and diltiazem all have been used to attenuate the cardiovascular response to laryngoscopy and intubation. Caution must be exercised when these drugs are used in a patient with decreased ventricular function, because they may cause myocardial depression and decreased cardiac output.[31]

Lidocaine

Lidocaine is a local anesthetic that has gained popularity among anesthesiologists for attenuation of the cardiovascular response. Authorities have demonstrated that either topical or intravenous lidocaine attenuates the cardiovascular response to laryngoscopy and intubation.[32, 33] The mechanism of action is unclear, but it seems that part of the action is caused by an increased depth of general anesthesia, because it causes a decrease of volatile anesthetic agents in dogs. The intravenous route is more efficacious. Topical lidocaine is less effective, probably for a number of reasons. Topical anesthesia is administered after laryngoscopy, and laryngoscopy itself may be associated with heightened cardiovascular response. Also, instillation of topical anesthetic solution due to initial stimulation by a foreign body may cause hypertension and tachycardia before the local anesthetic effect. Studies show that absorption of lidocaine topically sprayed in the pharynx does not reach effective levels until approximately 5 to 10 minutes later; therefore, most intubations occur before an effective concentration has been reached. Peak plasma concentration of local anesthesia occurs in 15 minutes after topical administration. Tracheal intubation proceeding 5 minutes after tracheal spraying is associated with a diminished cardiovascular response.[35] However, lidocaine 1.5 to 2 mg/kg intravenously attenuates the response after 1 minute and is probably the preferred method.[36]

Other Drugs

Other pharmacologic modalities on the horizon include prostaglandins, α_2 agonists, serotonin inhibitors, and hybrid drugs with mixed properties. Prostaglandin E_1 3 to 6 μg/kg has been advocated as a safe method for attenuation of the cardiovascular response. Ketanserin, a serotonin inhibitor, was found to have obtunding effects to the cardiovascular response at 0.5 mg/kg intravenously 5 minutes prior to induction. Urapidil, a selective alpha-blocker, has been used to blunt the cardiovascular response.[37–39]

Endotracheal intubation is facilitated by the use of muscle relaxants, but they also are not without untoward cardiovascular effects. Pancuronium is noted for the not-so-uncommon associated tachycardia, increased blood pressure over baseline.

D-tubocurare lowers blood pressure secondary to its ganglionic blocking properties. Many anesthesiologists use this drug alone or in combination with other muscle relaxants to attenuate the heightened response of hypertension to laryngoscopy. This effect is not predictable, because investigators find that this does not attenuate the hyperdynamic response to intubation.

Physical Manipulation

Alternative approaches to minimizing the cardiovascular response include avoiding excessive stimulation and stretching of tissues of the laryngopharynx and epipharynx. One of the earliest attempts was in laryngoscope design: the Macintosh blade was believed to be less stimulating because it avoids the vagus nerve directly. Macintosh blades fit into the vallecula, which is innervated by the glossopharyngeal nerve. No study has confirmed this theoretic advantage. Blind nasal intubation is controversial; the literature is divided as to its effectiveness. Recent information suggests that nasal intubation is associated with higher oxygen consumption, and this could present a problem in the patient with myocardial ischemia or ventricular dysfunction.[41] Fiberoptic intubation is also controversial, because there are conflicting reports as to its being less stimulating.[40] It may be that skill of the endoscopist, the technique employed, and the physical condition of the patient are the more important components in these physical maneuvers.

The peri-induction period of the cardiac patient is a time frame in which wide swings in blood pressure and pulse can occur. Dysrhythmia, with its potential for hemodynamic embarrassment, may also occur. The cardiac patient may have limited reserve. Potent inhalation anesthetic agents and intravenous agents may not allow for sufficient attenuation of the cardiovascular response to laryngoscopy and intubation. After endotracheal intubation, hypotension may ensue due to efforts to control this sympathoadrenal response. Via attempts to control this transient response, various other factors may complicate the picture. Positive-pressure ventilation decreases venous return by increasing intrathoracic pressure; this effect is magnified in patients with hypovolemia or ventricular dysfunction. Inadequate muscle paralysis with lack of ventilator synchronization may also lead to deterioration of the cardiac patient.

There are many methods to minimize the changes, but none is without potential pitfalls. Generally, one would want to increase the depth of anesthesia without depressing the cardiovascular system; some of these techniques have been discussed previously. Because ablation of the cardiovascular response requires a greater level of anesthesia than the baseline anesthetic, this presents a challenge. One must anticipate the early onset and transitory nature of the response and have strategies ready to circumvent the possible complications. The key again is anticipation, preparedness, adequate monitoring, and flexibility in handling this situation. Also, on extubation many of these changes may occur and require the same rationale in management.

VASCULAR ANOMALIES AND AIRWAY OBSTRUCTION

Extrinsic compression of the airway can result in significant morbidity and potential mortality. Airway obstruction can result from tracheobronchial compression by a vascular ring, a left pulmonary artery sling, or an anomalous innominate artery. Patients usually present with stridor, airway obstruction, or apnea in early childhood.[44] Reflex apnea occurs in many children secondary to respiratory arrest initiated by irritation of the area of compression of the trachea by the vascular anomaly. Reflex apnea is an indication for surgical correction.[45–47]

True vascular rings are a double aortic arch and a right aortic arch associated with a left-sided ligamentum arteriosum. These anomalies form a continuous circle around the trachea and esophagus and compress them.[49] Symptoms result from compression of the tracheobronchial tree or esophagus. The diagnosis is confirmed via chest computed tomography (CT) scan, barium swallow (a barium-filled esophagus is indented posteriorly by the vascular structure), and fiberoptic bronchoscopy demonstrating the flattened and obstructed trachea just above the carina. Surgical correction is performed via a left thoracotomy, and the vascular ring is divided at the appropriate point.

Surgical correction of the pulmonary artery sling may require cardiopulmonary bypass. The left pulmonary artery passes to the right of the trachea just before crossing back posteriorly to the left lung. As a result, this "sling" pulls on and compresses the trachea and right mainstream bronchus at the carina. The repair requires division of the left pulmonary artery, and removal of the left pulmonary artery from behind the trachea, and reanastomosis to the

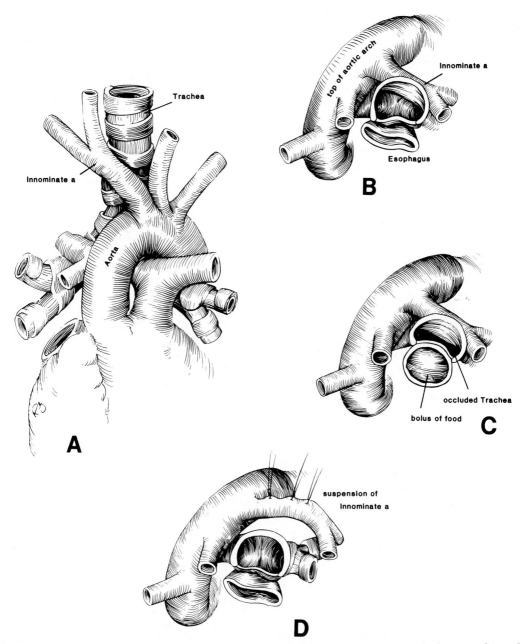

Figure 40–1. *A.* Depiction of the normal aorta, showing the innominate artery crossing the lower trachea, which produces compression of the trachea and buckling of the cartilages. *B.* Endoscopic view showing the buckled arch impinging on the lumen of the distal trachea. *C.* A bolus of food in the esophagus forces the posterior membranous portion of the trachea into the tracheal lumen, causing almost complete airway obliteration by the anterior compression and the posterior bulge. *D.* Suspension of the aorta and the innominate artery to eliminate the anterior compression and buckling of the tracheal rings, thereby increasing the cross-sectional diameter of the trachea. (From Fiston HC, Ferguson T, Oldham H. Airway obstruction by vascular anomalies. Ann Surg 205:541–548, 1987; with permission.)

main pulmonary artery just distal to the pulmonary valve.

Fiberoptic endoscopy is essential for diagnosis and intraoperative management for all vascular compression syndromes, particularly innominate artery syndrome.[48] Repair of innominate artery syndrome requires only that the innominate artery be pulled forward, away from the trachea that is being compressed (Fig. 40–1). The artery is then sutured to the posterior periosteum of the sternum to hold it away from the trachea. The results of the procedure are quite favorable in most cases.

MEDIASTINAL TUMORS AND AIRWAY OBSTRUCTION

Airway obstruction is the most common complication during anesthesia for mediastinal tumors. The majority of tumors in adults originate from involvement of the hilar lymph nodes with bronchial carcinoma or lymphoma; in children, the masses are often benign bronchial cysts, esophageal duplication, or teratoma. Tumors in the mediastinum can not only compress the tracheobronchial tree, but the pulmonary artery, atria, and superior vena cava as well.

The majority of mediastinal masses that cause obstruction of the airway are lymphomatous in origin. This usually requires a tissue diagnosis, resulting in the need for anesthesia for a diagnostic procedure (cervical or scalene node biopsy, staging laparotomy for Hodgkin's disease). Not all patients who develop severe intraoperative respiratory problems have respiratory symptoms and signs preoperatively. Loss of muscle tone secondary to general anesthesia can result in complete airway closure that cannot be relieved with placement of a standard endotracheal tube. As a result, a rigid bronchoscope should be readily available and set up, so that the airway can be ventilated below the level of collapse. This can be a life-saving maneuver.

The airway management of these patients is based on two overriding considerations.[50-52] First, loss of spontaneous ventilation seems to precipitate airway obstruction secondary to loss of chest wall tone. Also, intubation of a distorted or compressed trachea may cause complete obstruction if the orifice of the tube impinges on the tracheal wall. Second, lymphomatous tumors normally respond dramatically to radiation or chemotherapy. Thus, the treating physician should use radiation or chemotherapy before general anesthesia is employed.

General guidelines for managing mediastinal masses are listed in Table 40–2. If the patient is symptomatic (dyspnea or intolerance of the supine position), then local anesthesia should be used for all biopsy procedures. If the patient is asymptomatic, then a CT scan, flow–volume loop, and echocardiogram should be performed to evaluate the anatomic functional position of the tumor. Should a positive result of any of these tests occur, then local anesthesia should be used for biopsy.

If general anesthesia is required, fiberoptic bronchoscopy of the airway with topical anesthesia should be performed prior to general anesthesia. An armored endotracheal tube should be used for fiberoptic intubation. The patient should be placed in the semi-Fowler's position during induction of general anesthesia. Muscle relaxants should be avoided. The operating room team should be prepared to change the patient to the lateral or prone position to relieve airway complete obstruction. A rigid ventilating bronchoscope should be available to pass distal to the tracheal or carinal obstruction. The appropriate personnel and equipment for cardiopulmonary bypass should also be available.

Table 40–2. GUIDELINES FOR MANAGING MEDIASTINAL MASSES

1. If possible, use local anesthesia for all procedures.
2. If possible, perform radiation or chemotherapy before general anesthesia.
3. Inspect the tracheobronchial tree with fiberoptic bronchoscopy and intubate awake if general anesthesia is required.
4. Maintain spontaneous ventilation whenever general anesthesia is performed.

References

1. Fox EJ, Sklar GS, Hill CH, Villanueva R, King BD. Complications related to the pressor response to endotracheal intubation. Anesthesiology 47:524–525, 1977.
2. Reid LC, Brace DE. Irritation of respiratory tract and its reflex effect on heart rate. Surg Gynecol Obstet 70:157, 1940.
3. Siedlecki J. Disturbances in the function of cardiovascular system in patients following endotracheal intubation and attempts of their prevention by pharmacological blockade of the sympathetic system. Anaesthesia, Resuscitation, and Intensive Therapy 3:107–123, 1975.
4. King BD, Harris LC, Greifenstein FE, Elden JD, Dripps RD. Reflex circulatory responses to direct laryngoscopy and tracheal intubation performed during general anesthesia. Anesthesiology 12:556, 1951.
5. Katz RL, Bigger JT. Cardiac arrhythmias during anesthesia and operation. Anesthesiology 33:193, 1970.
6. Pyrs-Roberts C, Greene LT, Meloche R, Foer P. Studies of anesthesia in relation to hypertension: Hemodynamic consequences of induction and endotracheal intubation in normotensive man. Br J Anaesth 42:618, 1971.
7. Bedford F, Feinstein B. Hospital admission blood pressure: A predictor of hypertension following endotracheal intubation. Anesth Analg 59:367, 1980.

8. Rao TLK, Jacobs KLT, El-Etr AA. Reinfarction following anesthesia in patients with myocardial infarction. Anesthesiology 59:499, 1983.

9. Slogoff S, Keats A. Does perioperative myocardial ischemia lead to postoperative myocardial infarction? Anesthesiology 55:212–2i7, 1981.

10. Goldman L, Caldera DL. Risks of general anesthesia and elective operation in the hypertensive patient. Anesthesiology 50:285, 1979.

11. DeVault M, Greifenstein FE, Harris LC. Circulatory responses to endotracheal intubation in light general anesthesia—the effect of atropine and phentolamine. Anesthesiology 21:360, 1960.

12. Burnstein CL, Wotoshin G, Newman W. Electrocardiographic studies during endotracheal intubation. II: Effects during general anaesthesia and intravenous procaine. Anesthesiology 11:229, 1950.

13. Woodbridge PD. Changing concepts concerning depth of anesthesia. Anesthesiology 18:536–550, 1957.

14. Atweh SF, Kuhar MJ. Autoradiographic localization of opiate receptors in rat brains. I: Spinal cord and lower medulla. Brain Res 124:53–67, 1947.

15. Martin DE, Rosenberg H, Autberg SJ, Bartkowski RR, Edwards MW Jr, Greenhow DE, Klineberg PI. Low-dose fentanyl blunts response to tracheal intubation. Anesth Analg 61:680–684, 1982.

16. Hecker BR, Lake CL, DiFazio CA, et al. The decrease of the minimum alveolar anesthetic concentration produced by sufentanil in rats. Anesth Analg 62:987–990, 1983.

17. Althaus JS, Miller ED Jr, Mosciki JC, Hecker BR, DiFazio CA. Analgesic contribution of sufentanil during halothane anesthesia: A mechanism involving serotonin. Anesth Anal 64:857–863, 1985.

18. Black TE, Kay B, Healy TEJ. Reducing the hemodynamic responses to laryngoscopy and intubation. Anaesthesia 39:883–887, 1984.

19. Gallagher KP, Osakada G, Matsuzaki M, Kemper WS, Ross J Jr. Myocardial blood flow and function with critical coronary stenosis in exercising dogs. Am J Physiol 243(5):H698–707, 1982.

20. Reiz S, Balfors E, Sorensen MB, Anrola S, Friedmon A, Truedsson H. Isoflurane: A powerful coronary vasodilator in patients with coronary artery disease. Anesthesiology 59:91–97, 1983.

21. Wilton N, Knight P, Ullrich K, Martin B, Gallagher K. Transmural redistribution of myocardial blood flow during isoflurane anesthesia and its effects on regional myocardial function in a canine model of fixed coronary stenosis. Anesthesiology 78:510–523, 1993.

22. Sheppard S, Eagle CJ, Strumin L. A bolus dose of esmolol attenuates tachycardia and hypertension after tracheal intubation. Can J Anaesth 37:202–205, 1990.

23. Bernstein JS, Ebert TJ, Stowe DF, Schmeling WT, Nelson MA, Woods MP. Partial attenuation of hemodynamic responses to rapid sequence induction and intubation with labetalol. J Clin Anesth 1:444–450, 1989.

24. Grover VK, Sharma S, Mahajan RP, Singh H. Effect of intravenous nitroglycerine on circulatory responses to laryngoscopy and endotracheal intubation. Indian J Med Res 86:629–634, 1987.

25. Grover VK, Sharma S, Muhajan RP. Intranasal nitroglycerine attenuates pressor response to tracheal intubation in beta-blocker treated hypertensive patients. Anaesthesia 42:886–887, 1987.

26. Hood DD, Dewan DM, James F, Floyd H, Bogand T. The use of nitroglycerine in preventing the hypertensive response to tracheal intubation in severe preeclampsia. Anesthesiology 63:329–332, 1985.

27. Tinker JH, Mickenfelder JD. Sodium nitroprusside, pharmacology, toxicology and therapeutics. Anesthesiology 45:340–354, 1976.

28. Flaherty JT, Magee PA, Gardner TL, Potter A, MacAllister NP. Comparison of intravenous nitroglycerine and sodium nitroprusside for treatment of acute hypertension developing after coronary artery surgery. Circulation 65:1072–1077, 1982.

29. Yates AP, Hunter DN. Anaesthesia and angiotensin-converting enzyme inhibitors. The effect of enalapril on perioperative cardiovascular stability. Anaesthesia 43:935–938, 1988.

30. Puri G, Batra Y. Effect of nifedine on cardiovascular responses to laryngoscopy and intubation. Br J Anaesth 60:579–581, 1988.

31. Omote K, Kirita A, Namoki A, Iwasuki H. Effects of nifedipine on the circulatory responses to tracheal intubation in normotensive and hypertensive patients. Anaesthesia 47:24–27, 1992.

32. Denlinger JK, Ellison N, Ominsky AJ. Effects of intratracheal lidocaine on circulatory responses to tracheal intubation. Anesthesiology 41:409–412, 1974.

33. Abou-Madi MN, Keszler H, Yacoub JM. Cardiovascular reactions to laryngoscopy and tracheal intubation following small and large doses of lidocaine. Can Anaesth Soc J 24:12–19, 1977.

34. Himes DS, DiFazio CA, Burney RG. Effects of lidocaine on the anesthetic requirements for nitrous oxide and halothane. Anesthesiology 47:437–440, 1977.

35. Derbyshire D, Smith G, Achola K. Effect of topical lignocaine on the sympathoadrenal response to tracheal intubation. Br J Anaesth 59:300–304, 1987.

36. Hamill J, Bedford R, Weaver D, Colohan A. Lidocaine before endotracheal intubation: Intravenous or laryngotracheal? Anesthesiology 55:578–581, 1981.

37. Mikawa K, Ikegaki J, Maekawa N, Hoshina H, Tanaka O, Goto R, Obara H. Effects of prostaglandin E1 on the cardiovascular response to tracheal intubation. J Clin Anesth 2:420–424, 1990.

38. Murphy JD, Vaughn RS, Rosen M. Intravenous enalaprilat and autonic reflexes: The effects of enalaprilat on the cardiovascular responses to postural changes and tracheal intubation. Anaesthesia 44:816–821, 1989.

39. Murray W, Daniel C. Ketanserin and the cardiovascular response to intubation: A preliminary report. Eur J Anaesthesiol 4:401–409, 1987.

40. Smith E. Heart rate and arterial pressure changes during fiberoptic tracheal intubation under general anaesthesia. Anaesthesia 43:629–632, 1985.

41. Fassoddaki A, Andreopoulou K, Salah M, Kitharitz D. Metabolic and cardiovascular responses following oral and nasal intubation of the trachea. Acta Anaesthesiol Belg 41:281–286, 1990.

42. Rovenstine EA, Papper EM. Glossopharyngeal nerve block. Am J Surg 75:713–715, 1948.

43. Wu T, Luu KC. Suppression at hemodynamic changes before extubation—lidocaine through modified endotracheal tube. Ma Tsui Hsueh Tsa Chi 28:121–126, 1990.

44. Fearon B, Shortreed R. Tracheobronchial compression by congenital cardiovascular anomalies in children: Syndrome of apnea. Ann Otol Rhinol Laryngol 72:949–969, 1963.

45. Mustard WT, Bayliss CE, Fearon B, Pelton D, Trusler GA. Tracheal compression by the innominate artery in children. Ann Thorac Surg 8:312–319, 1969.

46. Moes CAF, Izukawa T, Trusler GA. Innominate artery compression of the trachea. Arch Otolaryngol 101:733–738, 1975.

47. Ardito JM, Ossoff RH, Tucker GF Jr, DeLeon SY. Innominate artery compression of the trachea in infants with reflex apnea. Ann Otol Rhinol Laryngol 89:401–405, 1980.
48. Fiston HC, Ferguson T, Oldham H. Airway obstruction by vascular anomalies. Ann Surg 205:541–548, 1987.
49. Benumof JL. Anesthesia for pediatric thoracic surgery. In Benumof JL (ed). Anesthesia for Thoracic Surgery. Philadelphia: W. B. Saunders, 1987; p. 21.
50. Benumof JL. Anesthesia for special elective therapeutic procedures. In Benumof JL (ed). Anesthesia for Thoracic Surgery. Philadelphia: W. B. Saunders, 1987; p. 343.
51. Mackie AM, Watson CB. Anaesthesia and mediastinal masses: A case report and review of the literature. Anaesthesia 39:899, 1984.
52. Neuman GG, Weingarten AE, Abramowitz RM, Kushins LG, Abramson AL, Ladner W. The anesthetic management of the patient with an anterior mediastinal mass. Anesthesiology 60:144, 1984.

CHAPTER 41

Airway Problems in the Postanesthesia Care Unit

George G. Collee, M.B.Ch.B., F.F.A.R.C.S. (Eng.), and
David J. Cullen, M.D., M.S.

Acute airway obstruction and aspiration remain significant causes of postoperative morbidity and mortality.[1] The postanesthesia care unit (PACU) provides an ideal environment for prevention, monitoring, and prompt treatment of circumstances that compromise the airway before adequate recovery of pharyngeal and laryngeal protective reflexes occurs. Specific anatomic abnormalities contributing to airway difficulties are discussed elsewhere in this book. This chapter is concerned with the multiple surgical and anesthetic sequelae contributing to airway difficulties in the immediate postoperative period (Table 41–1). Most of these factors are unavoidable consequences of general anesthesia, although their severity can be minimized by meticulous attention to detail during the perioperative period, so that few patients should require acute interventions.[2]

Many of the postoperative airway difficulties severe enough to require specific therapy result from preexisting airway abnormalities or from identifiable intraoperative events. It is therefore crucial to ensure good communication of such concerns from the anesthesiologist to the PACU staff. For example, multiple attempts at intubation may result in laryngeal edema, requiring intervention. Or if an attempted blind nasal intubation ruptured the pharyngeal mucosa, a prolonged period of observation in the PACU may be appropriate. Any concerns of intraoperative mishaps (such as aspiration of vomitus, pneumothorax) should be investigated and treated in the PACU. Similarly, specific surgical procedures may carry implications of which the PACU staff must be informed (eg, recurrent laryngeal nerve palsy following thyroid surgery). Early detection and prompt institution of appropriate therapy is key to the prevention of acute airway obstruction.

ROUTINE POSTOPERATIVE AIRWAY MANAGEMENT

All patients recovering from general anesthesia have some degree of decreased level of consciousness, depressed respiratory drive, decreased muscle tone, respiratory muscle weakness, and obtundation of pharyngeal and laryngeal reflexes. Nausea and vomiting are frequent sequelae of surgery and general anesthesia; decreased lower esophageal sphincter tone secondary to the use of vagolytic drugs[3]

Table 41–1. FACTORS CONTRIBUTING TO POSTOPERATIVE AIRWAY OBSTRUCTION

Decreased level of consciousness and respiratory drive
Decreased muscle tone and respiratory muscle
  weakness
Obtunded pharyngeal and laryngeal reflexes
Upper airway edema secondary to trauma/position/
  venous engorgement/allergy
Depressed mucociliary clearance
Presence of dry, inspissated secretions
Danger of malposition of existing endotracheal tubes

enhances the risk of passive regurgitation. Mucociliary clearance is depressed,[4] coughing may be weak due to posture, sedation, pain, or residual neuromuscular blockade, and secretions may be more viscid following long periods of ventilation with dry anesthetic gases. Together, these factors put every patient at risk of airway obstruction and aspiration during emergence from general anesthesia. This is especially true in those patients who are extubated while still deeply anesthetized. Other patients (eg, those with "difficult airways" or those considered at high risk of regurgitating stomach contents) are extubated when awake enough to be coughing on the endotracheal tube. Although these patients may superficially seem capable of maintaining a clear airway, protective reflexes may still be compromised by residual anesthetic.[5]

Silent aspiration may occur around the inflated cuff of an endotracheal tube.[6] Intubated patients require several hours following extubation to recover full vocal cord function in terms of preventing aspiration.[7] Elderly patients are particularly susceptible to aspiration because of the progressive loss of protective reflexes that occurs with aging.[8] In the immediate postoperative period, patients may therefore enter a worsening spiral of aspiration, atelectasis, hypoxia, drowsiness, and respiratory obstruction.

The optimal position for observation—with the patient lying supine—is suboptimal for prevention of obstruction or aspiration, goals better served by the lateral position. Surgical requirements may also impose restraints on patient posture, and postural hypotension may prevent sitting the patient up. In the supine patient, airway obstruction often results from soft tissues, particularly the tongue, infringing on the upper airway due to decreased tone of the genioglossus muscle and pharyngeal muscles, especially if the head is flexed.[10] A large tongue or epiglottis predisposes a patient to

airway obstruction when optimal positioning to maintain a patent airway is not possible.

The signs of upper airway obstruction are listed in Table 41–2, but it must always be remembered that a heavily sedated or narcotized patient may show no evidence of respiratory distress, despite a completely obstructed airway and total apnea. In less sedated patients, physical examination reveals obvious distress with vigorous contraction of the accessory muscles of respiration evidenced by intercostal retraction, tracheal tug (retraction at the suprasternal notch), and flaring of the nasal alae. Movement of the anterior chest wall may be minimal, or there may be paradoxical depression of the chest wall and simultaneous abdominal distension due to diaphragmatic contractions. Auscultation reveals poor air entry bilaterally, with inspiratory or expiratory stridor. Breath sounds may be high or low pitched or, in complete obstruction, totally absent. In partial or intermittent obstruction, the respiratory pattern may be irregular, periods of apnea interspersed with episodes of awakening and coughing, or the patient may be tachycardic and restless. Cyanosis and the associated cardiovascular effects of hypoxia and hypercarbia are late signs of respiratory obstruction with significant hypoventilation.

Postoperative airway obstruction may develop acutely or may be gradual in onset, requiring sequential assessment and prolonged observation. In such circumstances, the degree of airway obstruction may be objectively assessed using a scoring system such as that developed by Downes and Godinez for pediatric patients.[10] Such systems minimize interobserver variability in detecting whether or not a patient's situation is deteriorating.

Upper airway obstruction by the soft tissues of the oropharynx can usually be alleviated by manipulating the patient's head and neck. When the patient is supine, flexion of the neck and extension of the head (into the "sniffing" position) may relieve airway obstruction. If

Table 41–2. SIGNS OF UPPER AIRWAY OBSTRUCTION

Dyspnea ± cyanosis and tachycardia
Inspiratory or expiratory stridor
Decreased air entry
Activity of accessory muscles of inspiration with
  "Tracheal tug"
  Flaring of nares
  Intercostal indrawing
Altered sensorium

obstruction persists, anterior displacement of the mandible will pull the tongue forward off the posterior pharyngeal wall. This can be done by curling both index fingers around the rami of the mandible or pressing anteriorly at the angle of the jaw. At the same time, both thumbs should oppose each other on the mandibular symphysis, pushing the chin caudad and posteriorly to open the mouth (Fig. 41–1).

Drowsy patients who require more prolonged help to relieve soft tissue upper airway obstruction may benefit from the insertion of an oropharyngeal or nasopharyngeal airway; however, injudicious use of these devices may cause additional airway problems. The pharyngeal stimulation of airway placement may induce vomiting, or too long an airway may stimulate the larynx, causing reflex laryngospasm. Loose teeth may be dislodged during placement of an oropharyngeal airway, and caps or crowns may be damaged if a sedated patient bites down on the reinforced part of the airway. Nasopharyngeal airways may cause troublesome epistaxis during placement, but usually provide a clear airway for patients with upper airway obstruction secondary to masseter spasm. These devices are therefore helpful adjuncts to clinical skills but must be used with caution and good judgment.

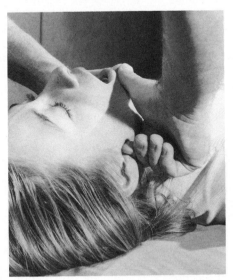

Figure 41–1. Clearing the airway. Curling both index fingers around the rami of the mandible and placing both thumbs on the mandibular symphysis, push the chin caudad and posteriorly to open the mouth while lifting the mandibular rami to pull the tongue off the posterior pharyngeal wall. (From Cullen DJ, Collee GC. Recovery from anesthesia. Care of the Critically Ill Patient, 2nd ed. In Tinher J, Zapol WM. London: Springer-Verlag, 1992, p. 392; with permission.)

Placing a patient in the lateral position lets the tongue fall forward naturally, making airway obstruction less likely. The left lateral position is preferred if direct laryngoscopy is being considered, because this lets the tongue fall away from the light of the laryngoscope blade. The prone position makes observation of the patient difficult, so that obstruction may go unnoticed.

In extreme situations where a patent airway cannot be obtained in a severely obstructed patient whose jaws have not clenched tightly, a ring forceps or towel clip may be used to pull the tongue forward, thereby clearing the pharynx of soft tissue obstruction.

When the airway cannot be secured by more conservative means, reintubation of a heavily obtunded patient with a difficult airway may be appropriate—a situation most frequently encountered with markedly obese patients, who may be slow to waken following general anesthesia.

Airway Access

Any surgical apparatus that prevents easy access to the patient's airway (eg, a halo device for immobilization following cervical fusion, wired jaws, traction devices) may make airway management difficult or impossible. The PACU staff must therefore be familiar with methods to remove such devices, and have the necessary tools available for use in an emergency. In extreme situations (such as cervical fusion with traumatic quadriplegia) where airway access is limited and problems anticipated, it is safer to leave the patient intubated until full assessment of secretions and respiratory function can be made.

Upper Airway Edema

The introduction of high-volume, low-pressure cuffs on endotracheal tubes has reduced the incidence and severity of mucosal damage secondary to endotracheal anesthesia. Nevertheless, edema of the upper airways may cause considerable obstruction in the postoperative period, especially in children.[11] It may result from traumatic or prolonged intubation, from generalized allergic reactions or local contact reactions to a particular type of endotracheal tube or anesthetic jelly, from prolonged Trendelenburg position intraoperatively, or from impairment of venous drainage secondary to surgical traction or arterial bleeding into the neck. Meticulous attention to detail during intubation is necessary to minimize the laryngeal and tracheal edema secondary to endotracheal tube placement. Tubes should be of the appropriate size to allow a low-pressure seal in adults. A small air leak should be present during ventilation when using cuffless tubes in children. After placement, manipulation of the tube and movement of the patient's head should be kept to a minimum.

Edema of the upper airway may present as a sore throat and hoarseness progressing to respiratory stridor and dyspnea, but significant edema may be present in the absence of symptoms.[12] Respiratory distress therefore may be present immediately after extubation or may develop gradually over the ensuing hours.

Subjective improvement is often achieved by sitting the patient up and by administering humidified oxygen by face mask. If there is difficulty in swallowing saliva, the patient should be encouraged to spit out accumulated oral secretions or be provided with a tonsil-tipped sucker. Edema secondary to trauma, infection, or allergy may respond rapidly to aerosolized racemic epinephrine—0.5 mL of 2.25% racemic epinephrine in 2 to 3 mL of normal saline. Only rarely are more than one or two treatments necessary. The administration of corticosteroids in the treatment of upper airway inflammation is controversial; objective clinical evidence of their benefit is limited to a few case reports in children.[13] A controlled trial in adults failed to demonstrate significant benefit of a single dose of betamethasone given immediately after intubation.[14] However, in a primate model in which investigators deliberately induced laryngeal edema with a large-bore endotracheal tube, the efficacy of a single dose of dexamethasone given immediately after extubation or 1 hour later was apparent.[15] A single intravenous dose of 10 mg of dexamethasone may therefore be justifiable on the grounds that it has few, if any, adverse effects. Similarly, mild degrees of laryngeal edema related to intraoperative Trendelenburg position may be empirically treated by inducing a diuresis with furosemide. Maintaining upright posture, avoiding the high intrathoracic pressures of persistent coughing, and therefore ensuring free venous drainage are probably more important mainstays of therapy. Intubation is performed only if increasing laryngeal edema makes air exchange progressively more difficult. Urgent tracheostomy is reserved for those patients in whom oral or nasotracheal intubation is impossible,

usually in conjunction with rare and bizarre causes of upper airway obstruction such as massive laryngeal or pharyngeal trauma or unrelenting tissue obstruction of the upper airway resulting from extensive edema, hemorrhage, or tumor. In acute cases of complete airway obstruction, an emergency cricothyroidotomy may be necessary. As a temporary life-saving maneuver, a 12- or 14-gauge cannula may be inserted through the cricothyroid membrane and connected to a syringe into which an endotracheal tube connector can be fixed. This assembly, first described by Stinson,[16] can provide a means of ventilating the patient until skilled help arrives to perform a more formal tracheostomy. Techniques for cricothyroidotomy and tracheostomy are fully discussed in Chapter 10.

Management of airway edema secondary to obstruction of venous drainage by tense cervical hematoma is primarily surgical. These patients may present extremely difficult airway management problems. There is some controversy as to whether the obstruction results from laryngeal edema or direct laryngotracheal compression by the expanding hematoma.[12, 17] Whatever the cause, its severity must not be underestimated; several deaths have been reported due to loss of the airway during anesthesia for evacuation of the hematoma. The problem may be encountered following any cervical dissection, but carotid endarterectomy, thyroidectomy, and anterior cervical fusion are most commonly associated. Early evacuation of the hematoma is the treatment of choice, using local anesthesia if circumstances permit. Alternatively, general anesthesia must be undertaken only after full preparation for possible problems in securing endotracheal intubation.

Obstruction following anterior cervical fusion or following a failed attempt at blind nasal intubation may result from accumulation of a large retropharyngeal hematoma. This is particularly difficult to manage, because decompression cannot be achieved without bleeding into the oropharynx. Attempts to intubate the patient may rupture the distended retropharyngeal mucous membrane, causing acute bleeding and complete obstruction. Patients in whom retropharyngeal swelling is suspected should be taken to the operating room and induced by an inhalational technique only after full preparation for an emergency tracheostomy has been arranged. Alternatively, the airway can be secured prior to induction by awake visual intubation under local anesthesia with or without the use of an intubating bronchoscope.

Laryngospasm

Laryngospasm, an acute tonic adduction of the vocal cords, is identified by the sudden onset of respiratory obstruction. It produces a characteristic high-pitched stridor in both inspiration and expiration, or may cause total obstruction to air flow. Frequently, its onset is heralded by a brief period of coughing or wheezing in response to laryngeal irritation by secretions, suctioning, airway manipulation, or insertion of oral or nasopharyngeal airways during emergence from extubation. Children are particularly prone to developing laryngospasm during both induction and emergence from anesthesia. The structural and functional basis of laryngospasm, and a discussion of the nerve pathways involved, has been reviewed in detail by Rex.[18] The degree of obstruction is often severe, requiring immediate intervention. The patient should be administered 100% oxygen by face mask, and the airway optimized by forward displacement of the mandible. Alternatively, one may use a resuscitation bag and mask to deliver pure oxygen with positive pressure, but the danger of distending the stomach with this approach must not be overlooked. Usually, laryngospasm lessens within a few seconds following either of these maneuvers. Rarely, it is necessary to cautiously administer intravenous sedation (eg, a small dose of midazolam or thiopental) or even to "break" the laryngospasm with succinylcholine. These maneuvers risk abolishing the respiratory efforts in a patient whose airway may be difficult to establish, but provide a more useful solution than the grim reassurance that the cords will ultimately relax when the patient becomes hypoxic enough. He or she may well suffer a cardiac arrest before that point is reached, so active intervention is essential. When laryngospasm occurs following cervical surgery, one must also consider the less common possible causes of hypocalcemia (eg, secondary to parathyroidectomy) and recurrent laryngeal nerve palsy (secondary to traction or section of those nerves). Hypocalcemia responds rapidly to the administration of intravenous calcium chloride. Recurrent laryngeal nerve palsy rarely produces complete obstruction.

Airway Obstruction by Endogenous Secretions

Prolonged anesthesia with dry gases results in inspissated bronchial secretions, which may contribute to respiratory difficulties postoperatively. Use of antisialogogues in the premedication prior to surgery may decrease the quantity of sputum and saliva, but increases their viscosity. Endotracheal intubation and inhalation anesthetics may provoke bronchorrhea and decrease mucociliary clearance. A weak cough and shallow breathing therefore may result in postoperative bronchial plugging with absorption atelectasis. This is most notably seen in smokers, in quadriplegics whose ability to clear secretions is severely diminished, and in patients with chronic obstructive pulmonary disease (COPD). Treatment consists of humidification of inspired oxygen, adequate analgesia to prevent thoracic or diaphragmatic splinting, encouragement to cough and to breathe deeply, and early active chest physiotherapy.

Aspiration

Due to the weakness of laryngeal protective reflexes and depression of the swallowing reflex, postoperative airway obstruction may be caused by a variety of substances that commonly accumulate in the oropharynx. Aspiration of blood, blood clot, dislodged teeth, vomitus, or pus can produce laryngospasm, bronchospasm, or obstruction at any level of the tracheobronchial tree. This is especially true after oral surgery, and it is prudent to provide care for such patients in the lateral position, slightly head down in order to encourage drainage of the pharynx through the mouth. Management of airway difficulties in these patients may be complicated by the presence of nasal packs or wired or banded jaws, but vigilance, adequate oral suction, and (when indicated) early intervention are usually sufficient to prevent problems. Nevertheless, the likelihood of aspiration after vomiting is higher when wires or bands are present, even if they are released quickly. Patients with a full stomach following emergency surgery, patients recovering following caesarean section, and those with symptomatic gastroesophageal reflux preoperatively must also be considered at high risk of postoperative regurgitation and aspiration. It is therefore advisable to extubate such patients in the left lateral position.

If vomiting occurs in any sedated patient,

he or she should be turned to the left lateral position with Trendelenburg tilt, allowing material to drain out of the mouth rather than into the larynx. The airway can then be thoroughly cleared with suction.

When aspiration is suspected, immediate intervention to limit its extent is essential. All PACU beds should therefore be equipped with suction devices at their head-end, and should be easy to quickly tilt into a head-down position. Measuring the pH of the vomitus may be prognostically valuable because very acidic vomitus (pH less than 2) presents a grave threat of chemical pneumonitis, often requiring prolonged respiratory support. The clinical course following aspiration of gastric contents with a pH greater than 2.5 is said to be less severe, but evidence to the contrary exists.[19] The lungs must be auscultated frequently for possible development of wheezes, rhonchi, and rales. Baseline data are collected, including a portable chest roentgenogram, along with an arterial blood sample for measurement of $PaCO_2$, pH, and PaO_2 breathing room air unless the patient is already hypoxemic. The most valuable therapeutic maneuvers are the early institution of chest physiotherapy, blind endotracheal suction to remove the aspirated material, and provision of supplemental humidified oxygen.

If aspiration of particulate matter is witnessed or confirmed by radiographic evidence of pulmonary collapse distal to the obstruction, early bronchoscopy is indicated. In cases of fluid aspiration, vigorous chest physiotherapy alone usually achieves re-expansion and clearance of the airway, but occasionally a patient develops acute respiratory failure that requires intubation, ventilation with positive end-expiratory pressure, and all supportive means pertinent to the care of the critically ill patient. Steroids are not indicated in acid aspiration,[20] nor is saline lavage useful, but bronchodilator therapy may minimize reactive bronchospasm. Sputum samples should be sent for Gram stain and culture. Acid aspiration is usually "sterile" in its early phase, whereas an anhydric stomach may contain fluid with significant bacterial colonization. It is generally preferable to withhold antibiotics until sputum culture results are available, unless the patient is immunocompromised or at particular risk from transient bacteremias (eg, prosthetic valve recipients).

Bronchospasm

Bronchospasm is more likely to occur in asthmatic patients and in smokers with a history of chronic bronchitis, but it may have multiple causes in the postoperative period. It may be provoked by aspiration of secretions (especially if acidic), by the presence of an endotracheal tube (especially if near the carina), or as part of an allergic response to drugs administered perioperatively. Anxiety and tachypnea may cause or exacerbate bronchospasm, or bronchospasm may be an early sign of pulmonary edema, preceding the more classic signs such as inspiratory rhonchi and pink, frothy sputum.

Bronchospasm should be treated promptly, because the excessive work required to overcome the increased airway resistance is difficult for the patient who is emerging from anesthesia. Hypercarbia is a likely consequence, as is hypoxia, which can occur in the most severe cases, even if 100% oxygen is administered.

Treatment of bronchospasm consists of supplemental oxygen by mask, removal of airway irritants (including the endotracheal tube if possible), and administration of bronchodilating aerosols such as salbutamol or terbutaline (β_2 mimetics), ipratropium bromide, atropine sulfate, or glycopyrrolate (anticholinergics), or beclomethasone (corticosteroid). Administration of nebulizers to intubated patients is inefficient due to "rain-out" of droplets in the endotracheal tube. Occasionally, intravenous therapy is necessary with β_2 mimetics and aminophylline infusion. Corticosteroids may be administered intravenously, but take several hours to become effective. In extreme situations (eg, anaphylactoid or anaphylactic reactions), administration of intravenous epinephrine (0.5 to 1 mg intravenously, or 0.5 to 2 μg/min by infusion) is appropriate. Re-intubation and ventilation, perhaps with a volatile anesthetic, should be reserved for those patients refractory to the above therapy.

PACU Management of Intubated Patients

Patients may be transferred to the PACU postoperatively with the endotracheal tube still in place, either for maintenance of a patent airway or to allow a prolonged period of positive-pressure ventilation. On arrival in the PACU, the endotracheal tube position must be checked because displacement (to endobronchial, pharyngeal, or esophageal sites) may occur during transport from the operating room. Subsequent management is dictated by assessing the adequacy of spontaneous ventilation, the character and quantity of sputum, the type and duration of surgery, the level of consciousness, and the anticipation of probable airway problems. Those patients likely to develop laryngeal edema should remain intubated until an air leak can be demonstrated around the endotracheal tube when the cuff is deflated and 15 cm H_2O or less positive-airway pressure applied. Patients with wired jaws or those unable to be cared for in the lateral or prone position should be free from nausea and awake enough to follow commands prior to extubation. In the mentally impaired or patients with acute cerebral or brain stem injuries, the medical and ethical issues pertaining to extubation in the face of compromised protective reflexes are complex and must be individualized according to general prognosis, degree of laryngeal competence, risk of gastroesophageal reflux, and the wishes of the patient, the family, and the primary physician.

Rare Complications of Intubation

Laryngeal injury following short-term endotracheal intubation is usually mild, with few problems other than transient sore throat and hoarseness. However, arytenoid dislocation, laryngeal laceration, pseudomembrane formation, and vocal cord paralysis have all been reported following elective endotracheal intubation for anesthesia.[21] The symptoms in such cases may be erroneously attributed to laryngeal edema; therefore, diagnosis of these injuries is often delayed. A high index of suspicion must therefore be maintained for all patients with significant symptoms who are being considered for discharge from the PACU.

References

1. Lunn JN, Mushin WW. Mortality Associated with Anaesthesia. London: Nuffield Provincial Hospitals Trust, 1982.
2. Cooper JB, Cullen DJ, Nemeskal R, Hoaglin DC, Gevirtz CC, Csete M, Venable C. Effects of information feedback and pulse oximetry on the incidence of anesthesia complications. Anesthesiology 67:686–694, 1987.
3. Opie JC, Chaye H, Steward DJ. Intravenous atropine rapidly reduces lower esophageal sphincter pressure in infants and children. Anesthesiology 67:989–990, 1987.
4. Forbes AR, Gamsu G. Lung mucociliary clearance after anesthesia with spontaneous and controlled ventilation. Am Rev Respir Dis 120:857–862, 1979.
5. Tomlin PJ, Howarth FH, Robinson JS. Postoperative atelectasis and laryngeal incompetence. Lancet 1:1402–1405, 1968.
6. Elpern EH, Jacobs ER, Bone RC. Incidence of aspiration in tracheally intubated adults. Heart Lung 16:527–531, 1987.
7. Burgess GE, Cooper JR, Marino RJ, Peuler MJ, Warriner RA. Laryngeal competence after tracheal extubation. Anesthesiology 51:73–77, 1979.
8. Pontoppidan H, Beecher HK. Progressive loss of protective reflexes in the airway with the advance of age. JAMA 174:2209–2213, 1960.
9. Morikawa S, Safar P, DeCarlo J. Influence of the head-jaw position upon upper airway patency. Anesthesiology 22:265–270, 1961.
10. Downes JJ, Godinez RI. Acute upper airway obstruction in the child. ASA Refresher Courses 8:29–48, 1980.
11. Koka BV, Jeon IS, Andre JM, MacKey I, Smith RM. Postintubation croup in children. Anesth Analg 56:501–505, 1977.
12. O'Sullivan JC, Wells DG, Wells GR. Difficult airway management with neck swelling after carotid endarterectomy. Anaesth Intensive Care 14:460–464, 1986.
13. Case history number 79. Steroid therapy for postintubation respiratory obstruction. Anesth Analg 53:588–591, 1974.
14. Goddard JE Jr, Phillips OC, Marcy JH. Betamethasone for prophylaxis of postintubation inflammation: A double-blind study. Anesth Analg 46:348–353, 1967.
15. Biller HF, Bone RC, Harvey, JE, Ogura JH. Laryngeal edema: An experimental study. Ann Otol Rhinol Laryngol 79:1084–1087, 1970.
16. Stinson TW III. A simple connector for transtracheal ventilation. Anesthesiology 47:232, 1977.
17. Hare RM. Respiratory obstruction after thyroidectomy. Anaesthesia 37:1136, 1982.
18. Rex MAE. A review of the structural and functional basis of laryngospasm and a discussion of the nerve pathways involved in the reflex and its clinical significance in man and animals. Br J Anaesth 42:891–899, 1970.
19. Schwartz DJ, Wynne JW, Gibbs CP, Hood CI, Kuck EJ. The pulmonary consequences of aspiration of gastric contents at pH values greater than 2.5. Am Rev Respir Dis 121:119–126, 1980.
20. Wynne JW, Modell JH. Respiratory aspiration of stomach contents. Ann Intern Med 87:466–474, 1977.
21. Komorn RM, Smith CP, Erwin JR. Acute laryngeal injury with short-term endotracheal anesthesia. Laryngoscope 83:683–690, 1973.

CHAPTER 42

Modern Airway Appliances and Their Long-Term Complications

Donna J. Wilson, R.N., M.S.N., R.R.T., and
Kenneth E. Shepherd, M.D.

Treatment of respiratory failure frequently requires use of artificial airways, including endotracheal or tracheostomy tubes. Although there have been advances in tube design and airway management, a number of complications may still occur. The incidence of such complications in today's practice is unknown; the high incidence usually quoted is based on old data. However, a knowledge of the potential hazards of modern airway appliances is important to patient care. Thus, in this chapter we review the pathogenesis, diagnosis, and management of these long-term airway problems. (Issues related to acute complications are covered in other chapters of this book and are not discussed in great detail here.) We also include an in-depth review of available airway appliances.

TRANSLARYNGEAL ENDOTRACHEAL INTUBATION

The complications associated with translaryngeal endotracheal intubation (TLEI) may occur during one or more of the following periods: (a) during insertion of the airway, (b) while the endotracheal tube is in the airway, (c) during extubation, and (d) after extubation.[1] The following text briefly reviews the incidence and pathogenesis of complications that arise while the endotracheal tube is in place and after extubation.

Major Complications of TLEI: General

Few studies are available that allow one to determine the exact incidence of complications. Prospective studies[2, 3] indicate that complications may occur in up to 62%[2] of all endotracheal intubations. Most of these lesions are minor and resolve spontaneously, but upper airway obstruction from prolonged TLEI can occur in less than 1%.[4] In this section, only complications common to both oro- and nasotracheal tubes that occur in the larynx and trachea are reviewed. In the following section, specific complications related to the route of intubation are discussed.

The cause and extent of laryngotracheal complications due to TLEI, regardless of route of intubation, result from a combination of factors that include (a) the small size and delicate anatomy of the larynx and trachea; (b) movement of the endotracheal tube with abrasion of the mucosa; (c) size, shape, and biologic properties of the tube; (d) cuff pressure; (e) duration of TLEI; and (f) aggravating factors such as hypotension, laryngotracheitis, and corticosteroid therapy.[1-3, 5, 6]

The larynx is the site of most of the serious complications of TLEI.[6] Laryngeal damage is invariably found after TLEI due, at least in part, to the small anatomic size of the glottis. Because endotracheal tubes fit tightly in this area, the thin epithelial lining is easily disrupted.[6]

Laryngeal injury is usually located over the medial aspects of the vocal cords and bodies of the arytenoid and inner posterolateral aspects of the cricoid cartilage.[5] The amount of injury (erythema, inflammation, and mucosal ulceration) is influenced also by the size of the endotracheal tube and by the duration of TLEI.[3, 6] Such an injury rarely may occur following brief periods of TLEI (24 hours or less) due to such factors as rough instrumentation, tubes that are too large, or accelerated inflammation due to tissue reactions to a substance found in the tubes.[7] The majority of patients who develop significant complications, however, have been intubated for longer intervals. Fortunately, most laryngeal lesions heal spontaneously.[1, 3, 4, 6] Long-term complications can be serious in the minority of patients who have required prolonged TLEI. These include laryngeal granuloma, vocal cord adhesions, and stricture.[1, 3, 6, 8]

In addition to laryngeal injury, tracheal injury may occur either at the cuff site or, less commonly, at the level of the tip of the endotracheal tube. Tracheal injury at the cuff site is thought to result from ischemia of the tracheal mucosa. This occurs when the cuff-to-tracheal wall pressure exceeds muscosal capillary perfusion pressure.[9] This is discussed in more detail in the tracheostomy section. Cuff-site injury is usually located between the third and seventh tracheal rings.[5] The movement between the endotracheal tube and tracheal mucosa can also lead to mucosal changes, usually located on the anterior tracheal wall below the level of cuff trauma.[5]

In addition to laryngotracheal injuries, other complications of TLEI include acquiring a nosocomial infection, risk of tube displacement with possible aspiration or hypoxemia, patient discomfort from the tube, as well as difficulty in communication.

Thus, complications of TLEI are common, but seldom are clinically severe.[6] As outlined above, the cause and extent of laryngotracheal complications, regardless of the route of intubation, result from a combination of factors that include the small size of the larynx and trachea, movement of the endotracheal tube, and excessive cuff pressure.

The complications of TLEI, including the development of tracheal stenosis that becomes clinically significant, are similar to those caused by tracheostomy, and their diagnosis is discussed later in this chapter.

Major Complications of TLEI: Oro- and Nasotracheal

As discussed in the previous section, the relative safety of TLEI is well established. A review of the long-term complications of prolonged oral and nasal intubation and the literature to support the superiority of one technique over the other is discussed. This literature is, in general, confusing, with many authors' conclusions in conflict with other conclusions. However, the major points influencing the choice between nasal and oral intubation are largely dependent on the considerations summarized in Table 42–1 and briefly discussed below.

There is literature to support the use of the oral route. It is generally accepted that oral TLEI is safer in patients with bleeding or clotting disorders, nasal trauma, or obstruction and paranasal sinus disease.[10] Additionally, oral TLEI can usually be placed more rapidly in emergent situations.[11] These tubes generally have larger bores and shorter lengths, as compared with nasal tubes. As a result, such tubes have a lesser chance of kinking, facilitate suctioning, and allow better access for bronchoscopy.[8, 10, 11] These tubes, however, may be poorly tolerated by patients and have several other disadvantages compared to other airway tubes (Table 42–1).[11] For example, there are reports that the nasal route is associated with less tracheolaryngeal injury,[14] is safer in patients with unstable cervical spines,[10] and is more comfortable than oral TLEI.[10, 13]

Review of the available literature shows conflicting opinions concerning nasal tubes and incidence of airway injury. Although some

Table 42–1. ADVANTAGES AND DISADVANTAGES OF VARIOUS AIRWAY APPLIANCES

Type	Advantages	Disadvantages
Oral endotracheal tube	Easy to insert Large bore; work of breathing less. Shorter length: easier to suction. Less acute angle; less likely to kink	Requires laryngoscopy Easily dislodged Poorly tolerated by some patients Patients require more sedation Occluded by patient biting tube Oral hygiene difficult Patient has difficulty swallowing Unable to communicate Lip laceration Difficult to stabilize Inadvertent extubation common
Nasal endotracheal tube	Easily secured Tolerated better by patient Insert blindly when neck motion or visualization is limited Allow for oral hygiene Able to swallow Requires less sedation Communication; mouthing of words	Skilled personnel for placement Nasal passageway limits size of tube Tube kinking due to curvature Inability to drain sinuses; sinusitis Obstruction of eustachian tube; otitis media Nasal soft tissue injury Laryngeal pathology
Tracheostomy tube	Most comfortable Easiest to suction Communication; mouthing words, talking or fenestrated trach tubes Able to swallow Resinsertion of trach tube relatively easy with mature stoma No laryngeal injury	Surgical procedure Complications postsurgery Bleeding Pneumothorax Subcutaneous emphysema Infection Posterior tracheal wall rupture during insertion False passage in subcutaneous tissue Stenosis, stoma; cuff Granulation tissue formation Innominate artery erosion

suggest that laryngotracheal injury does not correlate with the route of TLEI,[2, 10, 12] one small study did suggest that long-term oral intubation caused laryngeal damage more often than did nasal intubation[14]; this may be due to factors that include smaller tube size and less tube movement. In patients with cervical spine injuries, it has been shown in cadaver studies that the cervical spine moves during both orotracheal and nasotracheal TLEI.[10, 15] Although neither route seems to be as safe as cricothyroidotomy,[10] nasal intubation, when performed fiberoptically or blindly with minimal neck manipulation, has generally been found to provide rapid and safe access to the airway. Additionally, nasotracheal intubation allows nursing access to the oral cavity, and this route is often better tolerated by the patient than oral TLEI.[13] However, the study by Fletcher and associates[16] did not find any significant difference in patient comfort between the two routes.

Of the disadvantages of nasal TLEI, the one of greatest concern is infection. Various infections appear to be related to nasal TLEI.

These include sinusitis,[17–19] parotitis,[20] and otitis media[10] with the potential spread of infection to other sites.[10, 17, 18] All of the local infectious complications are due to obstruction of drainage from the sinuses,[17, 18] parotid glands,[20] and the middle ear. These local infections can be an occult source of fever and hypermetabolism. More importantly, delay in diagnosis can result in the seeding of bacteria to other sites, leading to meningitis[18] or systemic sepsis.[10, 17, 19]

In conclusion, although both routes of TLEI present unique associated problems, as outlined above, they both generally provide well-tolerated, safe, long-term airways. The available, often conflicting, studies do not clearly identify one procedure as clearly superior to the other.[10] The decision to use one route over the other requires an individualized clinical decision. Because of the potential seriousness of nasal intubation–associated infections,[10, 17, 18, 20] however, it may be prudent to limit the number of days a nasal tube remains in place.

The diagnosis and treatment of tracheal stenosis caused by TLEI is outlined in subsequent sections. The diagnosis of paranasal sinusitis requires a high index of suspicion when the intubated patient develops an unexplained hypermetabolic state and fever.[17] The finding of mucopurulent nasal discharge should heighten this suspicion. Standard, four-view sinus radiographs with the addition of Waters' view yield a diagnostic accuracy of 90%.[17] Involvement of the sphenoid or ethmoid sinuses is best diagnosed with computed tomography (CT) or sinus tomography.[17, 19, 21] Puncture of the involved sinuses gives the definitive diagnosis and guides therapy.[17]

Diagnosis of parotitis is suggested when swelling and erythema occur over the parotid gland. Gram's stain and culture of the exudate from Stensen's duct guide antibiotic therapy. All of these local complications are treated by changing from the nasal route of TLEI to facilitate drainage and antibiotics directed at the infecting pathogens. Decongestants may or may not be of added value in sinusitis after the nasal tube is removed.[17] Surgical drainage may be necessary in some cases.[21]

Optimal Timing for Changing from TLEI to Tracheostomy

Tracheostomy is seldom performed acutely for control of the airway. Endotracheal intubation or cricothyroidotomy is usually performed instead because of the markedly increased risk of complications of emergency tracheostomy.[22] Tracheostomy is, however, frequently used as a secondary procedure for prolonged mechanical ventilation.[6] Optimal timing for conversion from TLEI to tracheostomy in most patients is a difficult decision. In the following discussion, we present the data available to guide the clinician in making this decision.

Tracheostomy and TLEI both carry risks of airway damage. The decision to continue TLEI or convert to a tracheostomy is usually based on weighing the relative risks and benefits of each procedure in an individual patient (see Table 42–1).

If it appears that the patient may soon extubate, tracheostomy is generally deferred. Tracheostomy carries a small but definite risk of preoperative morbidity and mortality.[1, 6, 11, 22] Some of the data on the potential for complications favor prolonged TLEI over tracheostomy. Some authors have found no significant relationship between the duration of TLEI or tracheostomy and the overall rate of laryngotracheal injury,[2] whereas others have found more frequent and severe airway lesions associated with early tracheostomy.[23] El-Naggar and colleagues[23] found an eight-fold greater incidence of contamination of the airway by new organisms with tracheostomy. Because a duration of TLEI beyond which there occurs an unacceptable high incidence of serious complication has not been defined,[6] some now leave in endotracheal tubes for 4 to 6 weeks if the patient requires it.[24]

Other data in the literature suggest that the length of time a patient has TLEI should be shorter in duration. Prolonged TLEI is not without risks and has the potential for causing laryngotracheal damage.[1–3, 5, 6, 25] As TLEI times lengthen, the incidence of acute and chronic airway injuries increases.[3] A prospective study showed that the nature and severity of the laryngotracheal injury change dramatically after more than 7 days of TLEI.[3] The posterior glottis becomes damaged, and surgical repair of this injury is difficult.[3, 22] Long-term TLEI may also increase the risk of laryngotracheal injury from a subsequent tracheostomy.[3, 6, 22, 26]

Despite a large number of studies, the conclusion must be that although prolonged intubation with either TLEI or tracheostomy is reasonably safe,[27] both present inherent hazards for prolonged airway management.[22] Based on the available data, no generalized principle can be established with certainty concerning the proper timing (if any) of tracheostomy, and the clinician must make an individualized decision based on factors such as likelihood that the patient will soon tolerate extubation, possible better patient tolerance of tracheostomy,[11, 22] and surgical risk.[22]

It has been our experience that the widespread practice of very prolonged intubation (greater than 3 weeks) has led to increased referrals of patients with cuff stenosis of the trachea with associated laryngeal injuries.[27, 28] Although surgical results for uncomplicated cuff stenosis are excellent,[28] laryngeal repair is more difficult.[27, 29] In light of our experience, therefore, we have tended to take a cautious view in the debate concerning the length of time that TLEI is relatively safe.[27] This policy is in keeping with the recent recommendations of some,[3, 26] but not all, authors.[6, 24]

TRACHEOSTOMY

Tracheostomy is a well tolerated surgical procedure with a low associated mortality

($<5\%$).[1, 6, 26] However, complications may occur in up to 66% of patients[2] and may occur early or late in the postoperative period. In this section, early complications are mentioned briefly, and the pathogenesis, diagnosis, and management of late complications are discussed in detail.

Early Complications of Tracheostomy

These complications recently reviewed in detail,[1, 26] are outlined in Table 42–2 and are dealt with only briefly here.

The most common acute operative complications of tracheostomy are pneumothorax (1% to 5%),[26] mediastinal or subcutaneous emphysema (13%),[1, 2] and major postoperative bleeding (5%).[30] Complications that occur less frequently include injury to the esophagus, the recurrent laryngeal nerve, thyroid gland, or content of the carotid sheath, and cardiac arrest due to hypoxemia.[1, 2, 30]

The major early complication of tracheostomy is inadvertent tube dislodgement during the first few postoperative days, before the tracheostomy site has had time to develop a secure tract.[26, 31, 32] Efforts to reinsert a tracheostomy tube may generate a false passage, compress the trachea, and lead to respiratory arrest.[26] If it is not immediately apparent that tube placement can succeed on the first attempt, the airway should be intubated from above (TLEI) or, if time allows, a pediatric laryngoscope can be used to allow guided replacement of the tube.[26]

Late Complications of Tracheostomy

The major late complications are listed in Table 42–2 and are discussed below.

Table 42–2. MAJOR COMPLICATIONS OF STANDARD TRACHEOSTOMY PROCEDURES

Early	Late
Pneumothorax	Pneumonia
Pneumomediastinum	Tracheal stenosis
Subcutaneous emphysema	Tracheoinnominate fistula
Incisional hemorrhage	Tracheoesophageal fistula
Aspiration	
Tube displacement	Swallowing dysfunction
	Stomal infection

Adapted from Heffner JE, Miller KS, Sahn SA. Tracheostomy in the intensive care unit. II: Complications. Chest 90:430–436, 1986; with permission.

Pulmonary Infections

The majority of patients (up to 100%) with a tracheostomy have their lower airways colonized by bacteria.[26, 33, 34] This leads to nosocomial pneumonia in up to 66% of patients who require long-term tracheostomy.[35]

Several factors predispose these patients to airway colonization and subsequent pneumonia, including increased binding of bacteria to tracheal mucosa, decreased tracheal mucociliary clearance, and tracheal wound infections.[26, 36]

Avoidance of nosocomial pneumonia requires meticulous tracheostomy care.[26, 37] Good pulmonary toilet, proper humidification of inspired gases, tracheal wound care, and nutritional support can decrease the number of nosocomial pneumonias. Although establishing a precise bacteriologic diagnosis of nosocomial pneumonia is very difficult in this setting,[38] timely antimicrobial therapy may lead to improved outcomes.

Tracheal Stenosis

Tracheal stenosis develops in three main regions of the airway: subglottic area, cuff site, and stoma site. Subglottic stenosis is rare, but can develop if the tracheostomy is performed too high, resulting in damage to the cricoid cartilage.[26] Alternatively, subglottic stenosis may be attributed to laryngeal damage from the use of "oversized" endotracheal tubes[29] or from prolonged endotracheal intubation[6] preceding tracheostomy.

Tracheal damage leading to stenosis at the cuff site still occurs despite changes in cuff design and materials and transition to high volume–low pressure cuffs.[26, 39–42] The development of this stenosis is related to pressure necrosis.[9] Briefly, the mucosa becomes inflamed, ulcerated, and necrotic, resulting in exposure and fragmentation of cartilaginous rings when the cuff-to-tracheal wall pressure exceeds mucosal capillary perfusion pressure (usually 20 to 30 mm Hg).[9, 26] With persistent inflammation, tracheal architecture is destroyed to such a degree that attempts at healing produce only cicatricial scar.[9]

The advent of high volume–low pressure cuffs has markedly reduced the rate of tracheal stenosis at the cuff site (from 2.7% to 5.8%,[43, 44] to 0.3%[43]). Despite improvements in design, these cuffs still have the potential to cause significant damage to the trachea, especially if management of cuff inflation is not careful.[26, 45] The cuff pressure may exceed capillary perfusion pressure for many reasons. These include patient factors such as hypotension, or can be due to overinflation of the cuff,[26, 46, 47] changes in cuff pressure secondary to tracheal wall movement during mechanical ventilation,[48] or by use of improper-sized cuffs.[49] Whatever the mechanism, tracheal damage of various degrees may ensue.[5] The development of high volume–low pressure cuffs and careful management of cuff inflation has greatly decreased the incidence of cuff-related tracheal injury; now most tracheal stenoses occur at the tracheostomy stoma.[2, 26]

Tracheostomy can produce considerable tracheal damage at the stoma site that can subsequently lead to stenosis.[6, 26] Various factors including the initial dimensions of the tracheal incision,[6, 50, 51, 52] selection of "oversized" tracheal tubes,[6, 26, 52] excessive movement of the tracheal tube within the stoma,[6, 50, 51] and ongoing stomal infections, contribute to subsequent airway stricture at this site.[6, 26]

Prevention of tracheal stoma strictures begins at the time of surgery. The cartilage removed cannot regenerate once the tracheostomy tube is removed. Because cartilage healing must occur by fibrosis and wound contraction,[6] proper surgical technique is imperative to prevent significant inward collapse of the tracheal walls as a consequence of the healing process. Selection of a proper-sized tube[6, 26, 52] and avoidance of excessive traction on the tube[26] reduce irritation of the stomal site and prevent excessive scarring.[6] Chronic inflammation and infection of the stoma site, likely to lead to excessive granulation tissue formation,[6] should be prevented by local care including topical betadine application (if recalcitrant).[26]

Tracheomalacia

The incidence of tracheomalacia is difficult to establish with certainty. In one series of 100 patients with known or suspected upper airway obstruction, the authors found tracheomalacia in 35%.[53] This complication can be seen at the cuff or stomal site and the area between; it is thought to be due to thinning of the tracheal wall.

Tracheomalacia may be due to excessive removal of cartilage at the time of tracheostomy or may be due to incomplete erosion through the tracheal cartilage secondary to pressure necrosis or infection.[6, 54, 55] The increased compliance of the affected tracheal segment may become symptomatic. Diagnosis

can be made by bronchoscopy, fluoroscopy, or cinefluorography.[53] Resection of the malacic segment is the surgical procedure of choice for symptomatic upper airway obstruction.[53]

Tracheoinnominate Fistula

One of the most dramatic complications of tracheostomy is the development of a tracheoinnominate fistula (TIF). Bleeding that occurs 48 or more hours after surgery for tracheostomy is caused by TIF formation in 50% of instances.[26, 56] This life-threatening complication occurs in approximately 2% of patients and, even with appropriate and urgent management, only 25% of these patients survive.[26]

Many factors predispose to the development of a TIF. It can be due to inflammation, ulceration, necrosis, and dissolution of tracheal cartilage in the area of the tracheostomy tube cuff that involves the nearby innominate artery. This is often related to ischemic pressure necrosis from excessive cuff pressures,[56] as previously discussed. TIF formation may be related to the tracheal site selected for creation of the tracheotomy and to the length of the tube. If the tracheotomy site is created too low in the trachea, erosion directly into the artery can occur.[57] Alternatively, a tracheostomy tube whose tip lies too low can erode through the tracheal wall into the artery.[26]

Tracheoinnominate fistulas can be largely prevented by performing the tracheostomy above the third cartilaginous ring, using tubes of proper length, and minimizing cuff pressures.[26] If hemorrhage does develop, all such patients should be examined in the operating room.[56] The operation of choice is resection of the innominate artery in contact with the tracheal erosion and suture of the divided ends so that further contact of the artery with the trachea is prevented.[56, 57]

Hemorrhage may need to be controlled emergently, prior to transfer to the operating room. Weissman[57] devised a rapid method to control this type of hemorrhage that requires minimal equipment and skill when re-inflation of the tracheostomy tube cuff fails to temporarily control the bleeding.

By making a small incision in the suprasternal notch, a finger tunnel is made. Bleeding can then be controlled without interfering with the airway by compressing the innominate artery against the posterior surface of the sternum. The hand and finger of the person compressing the artery are prepped into the operative field and the surgical procedure is undertaken.[57]

Tracheoesophageal Fistula

Tracheoesophageal fistula (TEF) occurs in less than 1% of patients.[2, 23, 26, 54, 58, 59] When it occurs early after surgery, it is often due to poor surgical technique, with incision of the posterior tracheal wall.[26] Later occurrences are related to tracheal damage caused by poorly fitting tracheostomy tubes or excessive cuff pressures.[26, 58] Poor nutritional status and a nasogastric tube that impinges against the tracheostomy cuff also have been identified as risk factors for development of a TEF.[26, 58]

Copious secretions, violent coughing following swallowing, air leak with an intact cuff, and abdominal distension suggest the diagnosis.[26, 58] Direct visualization of the trachea usually establishes the diagnosis. If direct tracheal visualization fails, esophagoscopy or CT are alternative methods with the potential to diagnose this complication.[60] Operative repair of the fistula when the patient's overall condition permits is indicated.[58, 61, 62]

Other Complications

There are, in addition, many other late complications associated with prolonged intubation. These include aspiration,[63] recurrent pneumonias,[26, 38] dysphagia and swallowing dysfunction,[1, 22, 26] persistent open stoma[6] and cosmetically unacceptable scars at the stoma site.[6]

TRACHEAL STENOSIS

Diagnosis

Clinically, most patients are symptom free for a variable period following removal of the endotracheal or tracheostomy tube. They then present with complaints of coughing, wheezing, inability to clear secretions, dyspnea on exertion[26] and, in extreme cases, respiratory arrest.[64] These are nonspecific symptoms and may initially be attributed to other diagnoses, such as chronic bronchitis.[65] One must have a high clinical suspicion of tracheal stenosis in any patient who develops such respiratory symptoms after tracheostomy.

The physical examination may be nondiagnostic, and stridor may not be heard if only listened for during quiet breathing. Chest radiography may also be unrevealing if narrowing of the tracheal air column is not noted. Pulmonary function testing with close examination of the shape of the flow–volume loop and the finding that the peak expiratory flow rate is reduced out of proportion to the forced expiratory volume in 1 second (FEV_1) generally suggests the diagnosis of tracheal stenosis[66–69] and excludes alternate diagnoses such as emphysema, chronic bronchitis, or asthma. Flow–volume loops are relatively insensitive indicators of mild to moderate tracheal stenosis[26, 66, 68] and may fail to demonstrate the characteristic flow-limiting plateaus in patients with severe tracheal stenosis complicated by coexisting severe obstructive lung disease.[70, 71]

Of available diagnostic modalities, inspiratory and expiratory lateral soft-tissue radiographic views of the neck complemented with fluoroscopy are usually adequate to diagnose tracheal stenosis.[26, 65, 72] Although some authors have reported contrast laryngotracheography to be useful,[53] it is not routinely performed because it can acutely worsen symptomatic strictures. CT is not a primary technique for evaluating the trachea, because it is insensitive for detecting short stenoses.[26] Magnetic resonance imaging (MRI) seems to have potential for the evaluation of upper airway obstruction, but does not yet have an established role in the diagnosis of tracheal stenosis in adults.[73] A newer noninvasive technique—acoustic reflection—does, however, show some promise in confirming tracheal stenosis in patients with normal flow–volume loops.[74] More clinical experience with this technique is needed before its usefulness can be fully defined.

Treatment

There are two main approaches for dealing with symptomatic tracheal stenosis: laser and surgical. The newest approach involves laser therapy. Although some studies have reported favorable results,[26, 70, 75] adverse outcomes have been documented[76, 77] and the overall experience is still limited. It appears, however, that laser therapy may be appropriate for limited lesions or in rare instances of web-like stenoses and granulomas.[78]

Silicon T tubes can be placed surgically in selected cases to provide patients with an essentially normal airway and voice.[78] The tubes may be used for long-term or permanent maintenance of an extensively damaged upper airway which, for local or systemic reasons, is not suitable for a primary reconstruction.[11, 78]

Resection of the stenotic segment with a primary end-to-end anastomosis, however, still appears to be definitive treatment of choice for the majority of cases of symptomatic tracheal stenosis.[26, 64] Overall, surgical results for tracheal stenosis are excellent[28]; laryngeal repair is more difficult, but good results are obtainable.[29] Surgical approach to the trachea varies widely according to the level, nature, and extent of the lesion and whether the lesion can be approached electively or requires emergent surgery.[28, 29, 78, 79] In addition to exposure of the trachea itself, the surgical plan must provide exposure for anatomic mobilization of the lung, the hilus of the lung, or the carina, so that primary reconstruction can follow tracheal resection.[28, 79] Details of the surgical management of tracheal stenosis are beyond the scope of this chapter and are the focus of Chapter 29.

SUMMARY

In this section of the chapter we have briefly discussed some of the issues surrounding TLEI and tracheostomy. Many complications can result from TLEI, by both the oral and nasal routes. These include trauma to the airway with resultant laryngotracheal injury. The extent to which the duration of TLEI affects the severity of such injury remains controversial. The appropriate duration of TLEI cannot be defined, and there are no absolute guidelines concerning the correct timing of converting to tracheostomy.

Tracheostomy, like TLEI, is a reasonably safe adjunct in the management of patients requiring prolonged respiratory support. The potential benefits of tracheostomy over TLEI, such as sparing further direct laryngeal injury and permiting speech that may provide psychologic benefit, must be weighed against potential disadvantages of tracheostomy. These include early complications (eg, pneumothorax, inadvertent tube displacement) and late complications (eg, stomal site stenosis).

Over the years, many changes have occurred in airway management. In the following text, the focus is on the specific modern airway appliances that are available.

MODERN AIRWAY APPLIANCES

There are a wide variety of physical characteristics of tracheostomy tubes from the different manufacturers. Tubes differ in single or double cannula, neck flange, rigidity, cuff design, size, and length.

Tracheostomy tubes can be either double or single cannula. The single-cannula tracheostomy tube includes the outer cannula and the obturator. The double cannulae include outer and inner cannula and the obturator. The obturator is used to guide the outer cannula through the stoma into the trachea. The obturator has a smooth and tapered tip that extends approximately 1 cm from the end of the outer cannula. If a tracheostomy tube has a Magill tip, then an obturator is not provided.

The outer cannula maintains the patency of the tracheostomy stoma and is where the cuff is attached. The outer cannula on most tubes has a 15-mm adapter for direct connection to the manual resuscitator or ventilator circuit. Other tubes have the 15-mm male adapter attached to the inner cannula.

The outer cannula is attached to the neck flange. The neck flange can be stationary, adjustable, or swivel. The stationary type should lie flush with the neck, to prevent excessive movement of the tube. The adjustable flange allows the length of the tube to vary. One manufacturer makes a swivel flange; this allows the tube to conform to patient anatomic variations.

The rigidity of a tube is determined by its composition. Today, most tubes are made of polyvinyl chloride (PVC) and range from hard to soft. All the PVC tubes are disposable. These tubes are available in either single or double cannulae, with or without a cuff. The metal tubes are made of stainless steel or sterling silver and are reusable tubes. These tubes do not have a cuff, but a latex cuff can be placed. This is not advisable because of the potential problem of cuff slippage. There are silicone and silastic tubes; these tubes are very soft, flexible, and the least irritating to the tracheal mucosa.

The angle at which the cannula is attached to the neck flange is critical. If this angle is too much in either direction, the tip of the cannula can create pressure on the posterior or anterior wall of the trachea. Most tracheostomy tubes have an angle of 90 to 120 degrees. The outer cannula of the plastic tracheostomy tubes is radiopaque or metal, so that placement of the tube can be visualized for proper location in the trachea.

Today, most tracheostomy tubes have high volume–low pressure cuffs. The shape of these cuffs varies from cylindrical or sausage-shaped to tapered or pear-shaped. These cuffs are soft, thin-walled, compliant, conform to tracheal contours, and provide an adequate seal to protect the lower airway from aspiration. The major advantage of this large-volume cuff is that the intracuff pressure is evenly distributed onto the tracheal mucosa, thus minimizing the complications of tracheal lesions.

To ensure an adequate cuff seal at a low intracuff pressure, the diameter of the cuff should be larger than the tracheal diameter. Mackenzie and associates[4] report the average adult tracheal diameter is 24.3 mm in males and 20.5 mm in females. For example, a Portex #8.0-mm internal diameter (ID) tracheostomy tube with 8 mL in the cuff has a cuff diameter of 30 mm. Cuff-related trauma is due to cuff movement with head flexion and extension. If the tube moves within a large diameter cuff with head motion, this may minimize cuff movement and tracheal trauma. However, the design of the large-volume cuff does not ensure low pressure if the cuff is overinflated. A rule to remember is to maintain the cuff seal at the lowest volume and pressure required. The two methods of cuff inflation are minimal occlusive volume (MOV) or minimal leak volume (MLV).[80] If a patient is known to aspirate, the cuff should be inflated using MOV method; but in the majority of patients, MLV is used. A cuff should be completely deflated before slowly inflating the cuff in 1 mL increments. Using MLV, the cuff is inflated to the point where there is a slight leak heard at the end of the inspiratory phase of a positive-pressure breath. MLV technique may avoid the possibility of overinflation.[81] In general, the cuff on an artificial airway should not be routinely deflated. The cuff should only be deflated whenever it is necessary to (1) remove secretions pooled above the cuff, (2) evaluate the cuff volume with an audible cuff leak, and (3) give the patient the ability to speak. Upon reinflation of the cuff, pressure within the cuff must be maintained at levels less than the tracheal arterial pressure of approximately 30 mm Hg; otherwise, tracheal circulation will be compromised. The cuff pressure can be checked using a manometer (cm H_2O or mm Hg) connected to the one-way valve of the inflation line. This pressure is measured on a routine basis, with each tracheostomy tube change and after each cuff deflation–inflation procedure. The cuff pressure should be maintained less than 20 mm Hg to ensure that blood flow is adequate in the tracheal mucosa.

A different type of low-pressure, large-volume cuff is the Fome Cuf tracheostomy tube (Bivona Inc., Gary, IN). This is a large, foam-filled cuff with a silicone covering. The cuff is self inflating; when exposed to atmospheric pressure, it spontaneously expands. For insertion, the cuff must be completely deflated (approximately 35 mL). Even in the deflated state, the diameter of the tube at the cuff site is larger than other plastic tubes; therefore, passage into the stoma may be more difficult. This tube is used in the setting of tracheomalacia, when the cuff pressure and volume of a standard tube are excessive. The problem of cuff leak is common when a patient is on mechanical ventilation and the peak inspiratory pressures are greater than 45 cm H_2O. A seal can be created by adding air into the cuff in 1-mL increments and then clamping the inflation line. The Bivona Fome Cuff provides a side port airway connector. This connector attaches to the 15-mm adapter of the artificial airway and the ventilator connection. The tracheostomy tube cuff inflation port is attached to the sideport of the connector. Therefore, during the inspiratory phase of a positive-pressure breath, air will inflate the cuff to create an adequate seal. This connector has eliminated a cuff leak in patients who require high peak airway pressures for ventilation.

The ID of tracheostomy tubes is how the size of tubes are classified. Various tracheostomy tube sizes are listed in Table 42–3. The size of the tube is printed on the tracheostomy tube neck flange. There is approximately 3 mm difference between the internal and outer diameter in most tubes. The Jackson metal tube (Pillings, Fort Washington, PA) and the double-cannula tube by Shiley (Irvine, CA) are sized by the Jackson equivalent number, ie, a #6 tube is equal to a #7.0 mm ID. Thus, one should always select a tube by the ID.

Tracheostomy tubes have a size and length relationship. The smaller the internal diameter, the shorter the tube; this is illustrated in Table 42–4. If a small ID tube is needed in a

Table 42–3. COMPARABLE SIZES OF TRACHEOSTOMY TUBES (Portex / Bivona / NCC / Shiley)

Internal Diameter (mm)	Outer Diameter (mm)
5.0	7.0
6.0	8.3–8.5
7.0	9.6–10.0
8.0	11.0–11.3
9.0	12.0–12.7
9.5	13.3
10.0	13.3–14.0
11.0	15.3

Table 42–4. TRACHEOSTOMY TUBE SIZE CHART

	Portex		Length (mm) Shiley		Jackson*
Size	Standard	Extra	Single Cannula	Double Cannula	Stainless Steel
6.0 mm ID	67	—	67	—	69
7.0 mm ID	73	84	80	78	69
8.0 mm ID	78	95	89	—	69
8.5 mm ID (#8)	—	—	—	84	69
9.0 mm ID	84	106	99	—	69
10.0 mm ID (#10)	84	—	105	84	69

*Jackson #7 extra long: 85 mm.
ID, internal diameter.

longer length, a custom tube can be made from an endotracheal tube with an adjustable flange. Also, various manufacturers make extra-long tubes in sizes 7.0 mm ID to 10 mm ID. In patients with a short bullneck or in obese patients, the Portex (Wilmington, MA) extra-length tube is suggested. This tube has an increased distance from the neck flange to the bend, then drops vertically. Shiley makes a long, single-lumen cannula tube. This tube has a shorter distance from flange to its circular, less vertical bend and is used when problems exist in sealing a standard tube because of anatomic variation.

Talking Tracheostomy Tubes

All patients with a cuffed tracheostomy tube who have the ability to mouth words are candidates for a talking tracheostomy tube. The ability to phonate often relieves anxiety and frustration for the patient, family, and health care professional, because most of us cannot read lips well. The talking tracheostomy tube is a standard tube with a cuff to provide airway protection and positive-pressure ventilation.[82] This tube allows the patient to speak while the cuff is inflated. There is a cuff inflation port and a speaking port. The speaking port is a small tube that is set into the curvature of the tube; one end stops just above the cuff, and the other end is external on the patient. The external end has a two-way connector; one end is attached to a gas source (compressed gas or oxygen), and when the other end is occluded, the patient can speak. The gas attached to the speaking port exits from the opening above the cuff and is forced through the vocal cords, allowing the patient to speak (Fig. 42–1). The amount of gas flow attached to the speaking port ranges from 4 to 8 L/min. There are

patients who have a clear voice at 4 L/min, and others who require more. The patient should be told that his or her voice will not be normal, but lower pitched. Before using the speaking port, the patient's upper airway requires suctioning and the tube should be checked for proper alignment. The patient is instructed to speak in short sentences, because constant flow through the vocal cords will cause the voice to fade away.

There are several manufacturers that make talking tracheostomy tubes. Portex (Wilmington, MA) makes the "Talk" tube and Bivona (Gary, IN) has a talking tube with an air-filled or "foam" cuff; these are single-lumen cannula cuffed tube. Implant Technologies, Inc. (Minneapolis, MN) makes the COMMUNItrach I; this is a double-lumen cannula cuffed tube. The design of this tube is different. The gas source is connected to the speaking port and the gas moves into the air channels between the inner and outer cannulae, exiting through air vents in the outer cannula and directing upward toward the vocal cords, allowing vocalization. Talking tracheostomy tubes come in sizes 7.0 mm ID to 10.0 mm ID, and do not come extra long.

Poor voice quality can be a problem with a talking tube due to tube position or occlusion of the talking port with mucus. When the flow of gas is connected to the talking port for speaking and the gas extrudes through the stoma, this is due to a very large stoma or tube position. The flow of gas for talking that exits above the cuff may be positioned parallel to the stoma or in the pretracheal tissue; therefore, in most cases the tube is not long enough. In this situation, a larger size tube is required for a longer length. Then the exit of gas for talking will be positioned centrally in the trachea, below the stoma, and the flow will exit the upper airway, allowing vocalization. Secretions often occlude the talking port, caus-

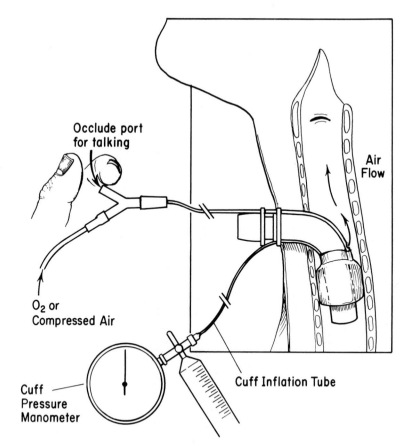

Figure 42–1. Talking tracheostomy tube.

ing poor voice quality. The talking port tubing can be cleaned with the instillation of acetylcysteine (Mucomyst), then by the application of suction to the port to remove secretions.[83] This can be done daily or whenever necessary.

Another aspect of this tube allows one to evaluate swallowing function. This is done with the cuff in the inflated position to maintain an adequate seal for airway protection. The patient is given a measured amount (30 mL of water with a vegetable dye, methylene blue) to drink; after swallowing is completed, connect a sputum trap with suction to the talking port and suction. This will remove any fluid that is pooling on top of the cuff. Evaluate the returns for amount and color in the sputum trap. This technique gives an estimate of potential aspiration.

Fenestrated Tracheostomy Tubes

Fenestrated tracheostomy tubes are used to allow a patient to breathe, cough, and speak using normal glottic function. The fenestration is a window cut into the outer cannula of a cuffed or cuffless tracheostomy tube, allowing increased flow to the upper airway[84] (Fig. 42–2). The precut fenestrated cuffed or cuffless tubes are made by two manufacturers, Portex and Shiley, and are available in sizes of 5.0 mm to 9.0 mm ID.

A cuffed fenestrated tube is a standard cuffed tube with a precut fenestration, inner cannula, and plug. When the fenestration is open by removal of the inner cannula, the cuff deflated, and the outer cannula plugged, the patient may breathe and talk via the upper airway. Mechanical ventilation and airway protection are provided when the fenestration is occluded with the inner cannula, the plug removed, and the cuff inflated.

Candidates for a cuffed fenestrated tube should have the ability to protect their airway and breathe spontaneously for 2 hours or more without the need of mechanical ventilation. Airway protection can be evaluated with a methylene blue test. The adequacy of the protective airway reflexes should be tested with the tracheostomy tube cuff deflated. Evaluation of the swallowing mechanism should include assessment of oral motor function, swal-

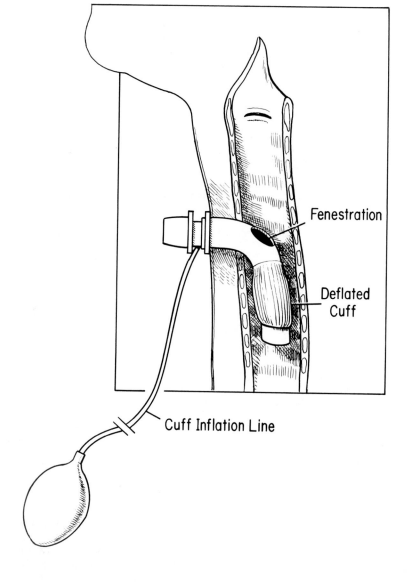

Fenestration

Deflated
Cuff

Cuff Inflation Line

Figure 42–2. Bedside technique for measuring fenestration.

lowing reflex, and cough. With the patient in a high Fowler's or sitting position, the lower and upper airways are suctioned and the cuff is deflated. Water or gelatin (20 to 30 mL) with a few drops of methylene blue dye is given to the patient to swallow. When this is finished, the cuff is inflated, the patient is deep tracheal suctioned, and the color of the secretions is evaluated. The test is considered negative if no dye appears in the aspirate; if any dye appears in the aspirate, the test is considered positive. This test should be negative before placement of a fenestrated tube. Another test to evaluate swallowing function is a modified barium swallow. This test is usually performed by the speech pathology department.

Before placement of the fenestrated tube, the upper airway should be evaluated. Once the artificial airway is removed, cover the stoma with gauze and evaluate the patient's breathing pattern. If inspiratory stridor or retractions are present, the fenestrated tube will not be placed and a cuffed tracheostomy tube will be inserted. The patient will require a bronchoscopy for airway evaluation.

Placement of the fenestration in the airway is most important for proper functioning and to prevent complications. The fenestration should not touch the tracheal wall, but lie within the lumen of the trachea. This position can be determined by bedside measurement or with a lateral neck radiograph. The bedside measurement is done with sterile pipe cleaners

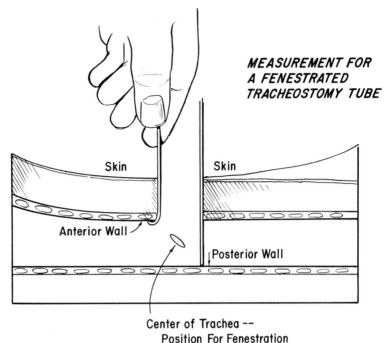

Figure 42–3. Proper positioning of a cuffed, fenestrated tracheostomy tube in the trachea. The cuff is deflated, the inner cannula is removed to open the fenestrations, and the tube is plugged to allow the patient to breathe and speak normally.

MEASUREMENT FOR A FENESTRATED TRACHEOSTOMY TUBE

Skin   Skin

Anterior Wall

Posterior Wall

Center of Trachea --
Position For Fenestration

to determine the distance of the anterior and posterior tracheal wall-to-skin measurement (Fig. 42–3). These distances are placed next to the precut fenestrated tube to ensure that the fenestration will be located in the lumen of the trachea. In the neck radiograph, the distance between the tracheal air column and skin is measured. If the fenestration is not in the proper position, granulation tissue can form in the fenestration, causing bleeding and airway obstruction. Frequently, the fenestration is occluded by the anterior or posterior tracheal wall. If the precut fenestrated tubes are not adequate, then one can customize one's own tube. Using your bedside measurements, place them next to a tracheostomy tube, mark the tube, then cut the fenestration out with a scalpel. Be sure all edges are smooth and that the fenestration is not larger than the lumen of the tube; otherwise, the tube may be structurally weak and kink.

Once the tube is placed, the fenestrations can be examined by direct vision with a flashlight on a routine basis and, if placement is in question, a flexible bronchoscope or a flexible laryngoscope can be used.

Patients with vocal cord paralysis, mild stenosis, tracheomalacia, laryngeal tumors, neuromuscular disease, COPD, those who are quadriplegic, or patients who emotionally are unable to tolerate plugging may have difficulty

breathing with their cuffless or cuffed fenestrated tube plugged. A possible solution is the Passy-Muir tracheostomy speaking valve (Passy & Passy, Inc., Irvine, CA)[85] (Fig. 42–4). This is a one-way valve that will fit on any tube with a 15-mm adapter. The valve opens on inspiration, bypassing upper airway pathology and thus making it easier to inspire; then on expiration, the valve closes and air is directed via the upper airway, allowing vocalization (Fig. 42–5). This valve should not be used in the unconscious patient or with patients with severe upper airway pathology.

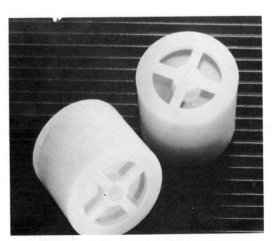

Figure 42–4. Passy-Muir speaking valve.

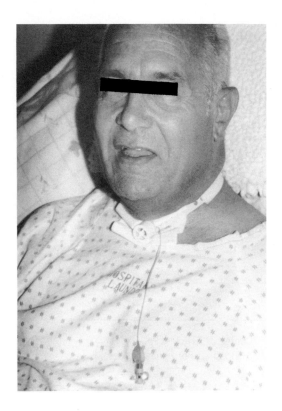

Figure 42–5. This patient has muscular dystrophy. He has difficulty speaking in full sentences due to muscle weakness; therefore, placement of a Passy-Muir speaking valve creates easier and clearer speech. This valve is placed on a cuffed, fenestrated tube with the cuff deflated and the inner cannula removed.

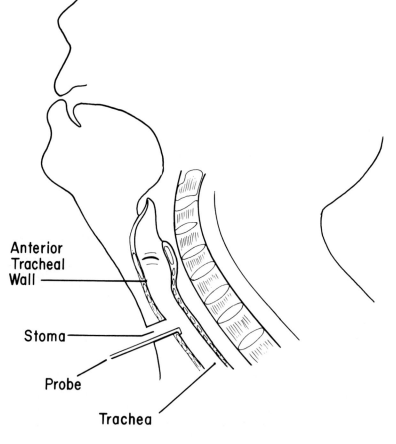

Figure 42–6. Measurement for trach button. Place probe through stoma and hook onto anterior tracheal wall, then mark at skin to determine the length of stoma track.

Anterior
Tracheal
Wall

Stoma

Probe

Trachea

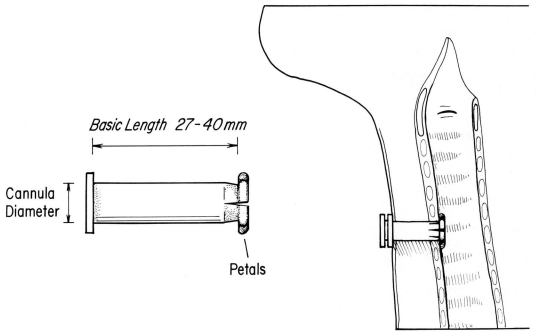

Figure 42–7. Olympic trach button. Cannula length is available in two sizes, to be adapted to fit most patients. The button maintains stoma patency and allows access for suctioning and normal respiration.

Buttons

The purpose of the Olympic Trach button, Kistner tracheostomy tube, and the Montgomery silicone tracheal cannula is to maintain the stoma patency when there is some doubt as to the patient's ability to maintain his or her airway without a tracheostomy tube in place. There are other reasons for placement of these tubes, such as easy access for suctioning the lower airway, sleep apnea (leaving the plug open during sleep), vocal cord paralysis, and in neurologic disorders such as myasthenia gravis. Before each appliance is placed, a sterile pipe cleaner or probe is placed in the stoma, then pulled back so that the length from the anterior tracheal wall to skin can be measured and marked (Figs. 42–6 and 42–7). The individual cannula length can be made smaller and therefore can be adapted to fit almost any patient. Each of these appliances is available in longer cannula lengths as well. These tubes extend only to the inner surface of the anterior tracheal wall and therefore do not cause any obstruction in the tracheal lumen. It is most important that the measurement is correct. If placement is in question, a flexible laryngoscope or bronchoscope can be used.

T Tube

The T tube is used to maintain an adequate tracheal airway. It serves as both a stent and tracheostomy tube. The T tube is supplied with a plug that allows for normal respiration and vocalization. The T tube does not protect against aspiration, nor can it be used routinely as a conduit for positive-pressure ventilation (Fig. 42–8).

The T tube is made of silicone. The characteristics of silicone are (1) it initiates little or no tissue reaction, (2) it does not harden with prolonged exposure to body temperature and secretions, and (3) mucus does not readily adhere to the very smooth surface. In addition, the ends of the tube are tapered to prevent injury to the mucosa.

Indications for a T tube are a palliative measure for patients with unresectable cancer of the trachea, inadequate trachea for repair due to previous tracheal surgery, medical contraindications to tracheal surgery, or in patients with temporary tracheal inflammation. This tube is placed and removed in the operating room.

SUMMARY

This chapter has reviewed the many aspects of artificial airways and their complications. Unfortunately, the lack of sufficient contemporary data makes it impossible to resolve many of the long-standing questions related to

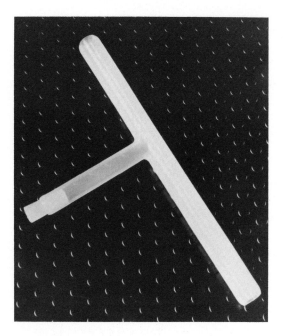

Figure 42–8. T tube (Hood Laboratories; Pembroke, MA) serves as a tracheal stent.

artificial airways (eg, optimal design of tubes, incidence of complications, and duration of TLEI). However, this chapter serves as a useful reference for those involved in the care of patients who require (or have required) artificial airways until large multicenter cooperative investigations are performed.

References

1. Stauffer JL, Silvestri RC. Complications of endotracheal intubation, tracheostomy, and artificial airways. Repir Care 27:417–434, 1982.
2. Stauffer JL, Olson DE, Petty TL. Complications and consequences of endotracheal intubation and tracheostomy. Am J Med 70:65–76, 1981.
3. Whited RE. A prospective study of laryngotracheal sequalae in long-term intubation. Laryngoscope 94:367–377, 1984.
4. Mackenzie CF, Shin B, McAslan TC, Blanchard CL, Cowley RA. Severe stridor after prolonged endotracheal intubation using high-volume cuffs. Anesthesiology 50:235–239, 1979.
5. Burns HP, Dayal VS, Scott A, van Nostrand AWP, Bryce DP. Laryngotracheal trauma: Observations on its pathogenesis and its prevention following prolonged orotracheal intubation in the adult. Laryngoscope 89:1316–1325, 1979.
6. Colice GL. Prolonged intubation versus tracheostomy in the adult. J Intensive Care Med 2:85–107, 1987.
7. Guess WL, Stetson JB. Tissue reactions to organotin-stabilized polyvinyl chloride (PVC) catheters. JAMA 204:118–122, 1968.
8. Mackenzie CF. Compromises in the choice of orotracheal or nasotracheal intubation and tracheostomy. Heart Lung 12:485–492, 1983.
9. Grillo HC, Cooper JD, Geffin B, Pontoppidan H. A low-pressure cuff for tracheostomy tubes to minimize tracheal injury: A comparative clinical trial. J Thorac Cardiovasc Surg 62:898–907, 1971.
10. Heffner JE. Tracheal intubation in mechanically ventilated patients. Clin Chest Med 9:23–35, 1988.
11. Wilson DJ. Airway appliances and management. Current Respiratory Care 80–89, 1988.
12. Rashkin MC, Davis T. Acute complications of endotracheal intubation: Relationship to reintubation, route, urgency and duration. Chest 89:165–167, 1986.
13. Lake KB, van Dyke JJ. Prolonged nasotracheal intubation. Heart Lung 9:93–97, 1980.
14. Dubick MN, Wright BD. Comparison of laryngeal pathology following long-term oral and nasal endotracheal intubations. Anesth Analg 57:663–668, 1978.
15. Aprahamian C, Thompson BM, Finger WA, Darin JC. Experimental cervical spine injury model: Evaluation of airway management and splinting techniques. Ann Emerg Med 13:584–587, 1984.
16. Fletcher R, Olsson K, Helbo-Hanson S, Nihlson C, Henderstrom P. Oral or nasal intubation after cardiac surgery? A comparison of effects on heart rate, blood pressure and sedation requirements. Anaesthesia 39:376–378, 1984.
17. Deutschman CS, Wilton P, Sinow J, Dibbell D, Konstantinides FN, Cerra FB. Paranasal sinusitis associated with nasotracheal intubation: A frequently unrecognized and treatable source of sepsis. Crit Care Med 14:111–114, 1986.
18. Grindlinger GA, Niehoff J, Hughes SL, Humphrey MA, Simpson G. Acute paranasal sinusitis related to nasotracheal intubation of head-injured patients. Crit Care Med 15:214–217, 1987.
19. Knodel AR, Beekman JF. Unexplained fevers in patients with nasotracheal intubation. JAMA 248:868–870, 1982.
20. Pruett TL, Simmons RL. Nosocomial gram-negative bacillary parotitis. JAMA 251:252–253, 1984.
21. O'Reilly MJ, Reddick EJ, Black W, Carter PL, Erhardt J, Fill W, Maughn D. Sado A, Klatt GR. Sepsis from sinusitis in nasotracheally intubated patients: A diagnostic dilemma. Am J Surg 147:601–604, 1984.
22. Heffner JE, Miller KS, Sahn SA. Tracheostomy in

the intensive care unit. I: Indications, techniques, management. Chest 90:269–274, 1986.

23. El-Naggar M, Sadagopan S, Levine H, Kantor H, Collins VJ. Factors influencing choice between tracheostomy and prolonged translaryngeal intubation in acute respiratory failure: A prospective study. Anesth Analg 55:195–201, 1976.

24. Lewis F. Discussion of Brooks et al. Management of acute and chronic disorders of the trachea and subglottis. Am J Surg 150:24–31, 1985.

25. Colice GL, Munster AM, Haponik EF. Tracheal stenosis complicating cutaneous burns: An underestimated problem. Am Rev Respir Dis 134:1315–1318, 1986.

26. Heffner JE, Miller KS, Sahn SA. Tracheostomy in the intensive care unit. II: Complications. Chest 90:430–436, 1986.

27. Rie M, Wilson RS. Acute respiratory failure. In Tinker J, Rapin M (eds). Care of the Critically Ill Patient. New York: Springer-Verlag, 1983; pp. 311–340.

28. Grillo HC. Surgical treatment of postintubation tracheal injuries. J Thorac Cardiovasc Surg 78:860–875, 1979.

29. Grillo HC. Primary reconstruction of airway after resection of subglottic laryngeal and upper tracheal stenosis. Ann Thorac Surg 33:3–18, 1982.

30. Orringer MB. Endotracheal intubation and tracheostomy. Surg Clin North Am 60:1447–1464, 1980.

31. Price DG. Techniques of tracheostomy for intensive care unit patients. Anaesthesia 38:902–904, 1983.

32. Wright MM, Shearer AJ. Tracheostomy tube insertion and replacement. Anaesthesia 39:717, 1984.

33. Bryant LR, Trinkle JK, Mobin-Uddin K, Baker J, Griffin WO. Bacterial colonization profile with tracheal intubation and mechanical ventilation. Arch Surg 104:647–651, 1972.

34. Niederman MS, Ferranti RD, Zeigler A, Merrill WM, Reynolds HY. Respiratory infection complicating long-term tracheostomy: The implication of persistent gram-negative tracheobronchial colonization. Chest 85:39–44, 1984.

35. Cross AS, Roup B. Role of respiratory assistance devices in endemic nosocomial pneumonia. Am J Med 70:681–685, 1981.

36. Neiderman MS, Merrill WW, Ferranti RD, Pagano KM, Palmer LB, Reynolds HY. Nutritional status and bacterial binding in the lower respiratory tract in patients with chronic tracheostomy. Ann Intern Med 100:795–800, 1984.

37. Selecky PA. Tracheostomy: A review of present day indications, complications and care. Heart Lung 3:272–283, 1974.

38. Tobin MJ, Grenvik A. Nosocomial lung infection and its diagnosis. Crit Care Med 12:191–199, 1984.

39. Loeser EA, Hodges M, Gliedman J, Stanley TH, Johansen RK, Yonetani D. Tracheal pathology following short-term intubation with low- and high-pressure endotracheal tube cuffs. Anesth Analg 57:577–579, 1978.

40. McGinnis GE, Shively JG, Patterson RL, Magovern GJ. An engineering analysis of intratracheal tube cuffs. Anesth Analg 50:557–564, 1971.

41. Steen JA, Lindholm CE, Brdlik GC, Foster CA. Tracheal tube forces on the posterior larynx: Index of laryngeal loading. Crit Care Med 10:186–189, 1982.

42. Dobrin P, Canfield T. Cuffed endotracheal tubes: Mucosal pressures and tracheal wall blood flow. Am J Surg 133:562–568, 1977.

43. Lewis FR, Schlobohm RM, Thomas AN. Prevention of complications from prolonged tracheal intubation. Am J Surg 135:452–457, 1978.

44. Andrews MJ, Pearson FG. Incidence and pathogenesis of tracheal injury following cuffed tracheostomy with assisted ventilation: Analysis of a two-year prospective study. Ann Surg 173:249–263, 1971.

45. Ching NP, Ayers SM, Paegle RP, Linden JM, Nealon TF Jr. The contribution of cuff volume and pressure in tracheostomy tube damage. J Thorac Cardiovasc Surg 62:402–410, 1971.

46. Magovern GJ, Shively JG, Fecht D, Thevoz F. The clinical and experimental evaluation of a controlled-pressure intratracheal cuff. J Thorac Cardiovasc Surg 64:747–756, 1972.

47. Brooks R, Bartlett RH, Gazzaniga AB. Management of acute and chronic disorders of the trachea and subglottis. Am J Surg 150:24–31, 1985.

48. Badenhorst CH. Changes in tracheal cuff pressures during respiratory support. Crit Care Med 15:300–302, 1987.

49. Bernard WN, Yost L, Jones D, Cothalis S, Turndorf H. Intracuff pressures in endotracheal and tracheostomy tubes: Related cuff physical characteristics. Chest 720–725, 1985.

50. Pearson FG, Goldberg M, da Silva AJ. Tracheal stenosis complicating tracheostomy with cuffed tubes: Clinical experience and observations from a prospective study. Arch Surg 97:380–394, 1968.

51. Geffin B, Grillo HC, Cooper JD, Pontoppidan H. Stenosis following tracheostomy for respiratory care. JAMA 216:1984–1988, 1971.

52. Goldberg M, Pearson FG. Pathogenesis of tracheal stenosis following tracheostomy with a cuffed tube: An experimental study in dogs. Thorax 27:678–691, 1972.

53. Stitik FP, Bartelt D, James AE Jr, Proctor DF. Tantalum tracheography in upper airway obstruction: 100 experiences in adults. AJR 130:35–41, 1978.

54. Dane TEB, King EG. A prospective study of complications after tracheostomy for assisted ventilation. Chest 67:398–404, 1975.

55. Harley HRS. Laryngotracheal obstruction complicating tracheostomy or endotracheal intubation with assisted respiration. Thorax 26:493–533, 1971.

56. Jones JW, Reynolds M, Hewitt RL, Drapanas T. Tracheo-innominate artery erosion: Successful surgical management of a devastating complication. Ann Surg 184:194–204, 1977.

57. Weissman BW. Tracho-innominate artery fistula. Laryngoscope 84:205–209, 1974.

58. Thomas AN. The diagnosis and treatment of tracheoesophageal fistula caused by cuffed tracheostomy tubes. J Thorac Cardiovasc Surg 65:612–619, 1973.

59. Arola MK, Puhakka H, Makela P. Healing of lesions caused by cuffed tracheostomy tubes and their late sequelae: A follow-up study. Acta Anaesth Scand 24:169–177, 1980.

60. Leeds WM, Morley TF, Zappasodi SJ, Giudice JC. Computed tomography for diagnosis of tracheoesophageal fistula. Crit Care Med 14:591–592, 1986.

61. Grillo HC, Moncure AC, McEnany MT. Repair of inflammatory tracheoesophageal fistula. Ann Thorac Surg 22:112–119, 1976.

62. Hilgenberg AD, Grillo HC. Acquired nonmalignant tracheoesophageal fistula. J Thoracic Cardiovasc Surg 85:492–498, 1983.

63. Cameron JL, Reynolds J, Zuidema GD. Aspiration in patients with tracheostomies. Surg Gynecol Obstet 136:68–70, 1973.

64. Attar S, Hankins J, Turney S, Mason GR, Ramirez

R, McLaughlin J. Tracheal obstruction. Ann Thorac Surg 16:555–567, 1973.

65. Weber AL, Grillo HC. Tracheal stenosis: An analysis of 151 cases. Radiol Clin North Am 16:291–308, 1978.

66. Miller RD, Hyatt RE. Obstructing lesions of the larynx and trachea: Clinical and physiologic characteristics. Mayo Clin Proc 44:145–161, 1969.

67. Hyatt RE, Black LF. The flow–volume curve: A current perspective. Am Rev Respir Dis 107:191–197, 1973.

68. Miller RD, Hyatt RE. Evaluation of obstructive lesions of the trachea and larynx by flow–volume loops. Am Rev Respir Dis 108:475–481, 1973.

69. Shim C, Corro P, Park SS, Williams MH Jr. Pulmonary function studies in patients with upper airway obstruction. Am Rev Respir Dis 106:233–238, 1972.

70. Gelb AF, Tashkin DP, Epstein JD, Zamel A. Nd-YAG laser surgery for severe tracheal stenosis physiologically and clinically masked by severe diffuse obstructive pulmonary disease. Chest 91:166–169, 1987.

71. Jett JR: The flow–volume loop and main-stem bronchial obstruction. Am Rev Respir Dis 138:1379–1380, 1988.

72. James AE Jr, MacMillan AS Jr, Eaton SB, Grillo HC. Roentgenology of tracheal stenosis resulting from cuffed tracheostomy tubes. AJR 109:455–466, 1970.

73. Fisher MR. Magnetic resonance of the chest. Chest 95:166–173, 1989.

74. Hoffstein V, Zamel N. Tracheal stenosis measured by the acoustic reflection technique. Am Rev Respir Dis 130:472–475, 1984.

75. Gelb AF, Epstein JD. Nd-YAG laser treatment of tracheal stenosis. West J Med 141:472–475, 1984.

76. Simpson GT, Strong MS, Shapshay SM, Healy GB, Vaughn CW. Predictive factors of success or failure in the endoscopic management of laryngeal and tracheal stenosis. Ann Otol Rhinol Laryngol 91:384–388, 1982.

77. Goodman RL, Hulbert WC, King EG: Canine tracheal injury by neodymium-YAG laser irradiation. Chest 91:745–748, 1987.

78. Grillo HC. Role of surgical therapy in upper airway disease. Pulmonary Perspectives 5:1–3, 1988.

79. Grillo HC. Surgical approaches to the trachea. Surg Gynecol Obstet 129:347–352, 1969.

80. Crabtree-Goodnough SK. Reducing tracheal injury and aspiration. Dimensions of Critical Care Nursing 7:324–331, 1988.

81. Off D, Braun SR, Tompkins B, Bush G. Efficacy of the minimal leak technique of cuff inflation in maintaining proper intracuff pressures for patient's with cuffed artificial airways. Respiratory Care 28:1115–1119, 1983.

82. Safar P, Grenvick A. Speaking cuffed tracheostomy tube. Crit Care Med 3:23–26, 1975.

83. Shinnick JP, Freedman AP. Acetylcysteine and speaking tracheostomy tube [letter]. JAMA 246:1771, 1981.

84. Trout C, Shapiro BA. A standard pre-cut fenestrated tracheostomy tube. Respiratory Care 17:173–176, 1972.

85. Passy V. Passy-Muir tracheostomy speaking valve. Otolaryngology 95:247–250, 1986.

Index

Note: Page numbers in *italics* refer to illustrations; page numbers followed by t refer to tables.